Nursing Now

Nursing Now

Today's Issues, Tomorrow's Trends

SECOND EDITION

Joseph T. Catalano, RN, PhD, CCRN
Professor of Nursing
East Central University
Ada, Oklahoma

 F. A. DAVIS COMPANY • Philadelphia

F. A. Davis Company
1915 Arch Street
Philadelphia, PA 19103

Printed in the United States of America

Last digit indicates print number: 10 9 8 7 6 5 4 3 2 1

Acquisitions Editor: Melanie J. Freely
Developmental Editor: Mari Fraser
Production Editor: Elena Coler
Designer: Christine Cantera
Cover Designer: Louis J. Forgione

As new scientific information becomes available through basic and clinical research, recommended treatments and drug therapies undergo changes. The author(s) and publisher have done everything possible to make this book accurate, up to date, and in accord with accepted standards at the time of publication. The authors, editors, and publisher are not responsible for errors or omissions or for consequences from application of the book, and make no warranty, expressed or implied, in regard to the contents of the book. Any practice described in this book should be applied by the reader in accordance with professional standards of care used in regard to the unique circumstances that may apply in each situation. The reader is advised always to check product information (package inserts) for changes and new information regarding dose and contraindications before administering any drug. Caution is especially urged when using new or infrequently ordered drugs.

Library of Congress Cataloging in Publication Data

Catalano, Joseph T.
  Nursing now: today's issues, tomorrow's trends/Joseph T. Catalano.–2nd ed.
    p. cm.
  Rev. ed. of: Contemporary professional nursing. c1996.
  Includes bibliographical references and index.
  ISBN 0-8036-0496-3 (alk. paper)
  1. Nursing–Vocational guidance–United States. 2. Nursing–Practice–United States. 3. Nursing–Social aspects–United States. 4. Nursing–Philosophy. I. Catalano, Joseph T. Contemporary professional nursing. II. Title.
  [DNLM: 1. Nursing. WY 16 C357n 1999]
RT82.C33 1999
610.73–dc21
DNLM/DLC
for Library of Congress
                                                                99-40516
                                                                CIP

Preface

It is difficult to believe how much has changed in health care and nursing since the first edition of *Contemporary Professional Nursing* was published. And it is with a great deal of excitement that we bring you the second edition, now renamed *Nursing Now: Today's Issues, Tomorrow's Trends*.

As you probably have already noticed, we have made many substantial revisions in this text. The text is divided into five major units. The format is now more interactive, and five new chapters have been included. We have added questions entitled "What Do You Think?" throughout the book to encourage reflection and discussion. The "journal format" makes the book more appealing visually.

We have been listening to what our readers have been telling us about nursing and what they wanted added. From these recommendations, we have added five new chapters written by experts in their respective fields: Chapter 12, Understanding and Dealing with Difficult People; Chapter 13, Cultural Diversity; Chapter 14, Spirituality and Health Care; Chapter 15, Nursing Informatics; and Chapter 17, Forensic Nursing: An Emerging Specialty. Actually, Chapter 17 started out as an add-on section to another chapter; however, after reviewing the nursing literature and trends in current nursing practice, we decided to include a separate chapter on forensic nursing.

Also, Chapter 16, The Politically Active Nurse, and Chapter 18, The Health-Care Delivery System, were completely rewritten by contributing authors to reflect current developments and trends in health care.

Other revisions in this edition include an updated glossary; extensive use of boxes to amplify the text; an expansion of the chapters on critical thinking, ethics, and legal issues; the addition of many new case studies; and an updated chapter on the NCLEX-CAT RN to reflect recent changes by the National Council of State Boards of Nursing. You will also find the addition of a list of Internet resources (Site Seeing) for each chapter.

We will continue to have the *Contemporary Professional Nursing Update* during the years when the book is not being revised. As with the last update, it will be on-line at the F.A. Davis Website: http://www.fadavis.com. Use of the Website has the advantage of allowing both students and professors to access the update. If you have any suggestions or recommendations for the next update, please e-mail your ideas to F.A. Davis. Please note also that an additional chapter, Historical Perspectives, is also available at the F. A. Davis Website.

As with the first edition, the material presented in the second edition is appropriate for issues and trends courses at various points throughout the typical curriculum of a nursing program. Several professors have told us that they use part of the text for their Introduction to Nursing courses for the freshman/sophomore years, and they use other sections in their senior-level seminars or issues and trends courses.

As we enter the new millennium, it is important to keep in mind this old adage: "Nothing is certain except change." The revisions and additions to this book represent the changes that have occurred in a mere 3-year period. It is a certainty that the new century will bring about changes and progress in health care and nursing that we can only dream about. Genetic research is poised to find not only cures but also preventions for cancer, heart disease, contagious diseases, and genetic disorders. Technology is on the verge of eliminating seizure disorders and Parkinson's disease with implantable electronic devices. Procurement of organs for transplantation may not be an issue in the near future if scientists are able to "grow" new organs from a few cells in the laboratory, as they are already doing with human skin.

All these changes will affect nurses and nursing. New ethical and legal issues will arise; career opportunities will change; and the knowledge that a nurse must have to practice safely will increase. It sometimes seems overwhelming. However, nurses as a group and nursing as a profession have always been and will continue to be highly adaptable to changes in the health-care system while maintaining their primary focus—the health and well-being of the client. The only way that nurses will be able to effectively practice their profession in the health-care system of the future is to remain firmly rooted in those values and beliefs that have always served as their source of strength. Membership in professional organizations will become increasingly important as nursing moves into the twenty-first century so that the profession's message will be heard loud and clear.

We hope that this book will help our future nurses become familiar with the important current issues concerning health care and nursing and the trends that will affect the profession far into the future. The nursing profession needs highly skilled nurses who can teach, do research, and obtain advanced degrees so that nursing can take its rightful place on the health-care team. Students who have a clear understanding of what it means to be a professional and are willing to invest the effort to attain their goals will be leaders well into the next century.

JOSEPH T. CATALANO, RN, PHD, CCRN

Contributors

Tonia Aiken, RN, BSN, JD
President and CEO
Aiken Development Group
New Orleans, Louisiana

Anne W. Davis, RNC, PhD
Associate Professor
East Central University
Ada, Oklahoma

Mary Evans, RN, JD
316 N. Tejon
Colorado Springs, Colorado

Deborah Finfgeld, RN, PhD
Assistant Professor
University of Missouri
Columbia, Missouri

Anita G. Hufft, RN, PhD
Dean of Nursing
Indiana University
New Albany, Indiana

Lynne M. Patzek Miller, RN, MSN,
  CNS, CNA
Director of Care Management
Bucks County Physician Hospital Alliance
Doylestown, Pennsylvania

Donna Gentile O'Donnell, RN, MSN
Deputy Health Commissioner (Formerly)
Health Commissioner's Office, Policy
  and Planning
Philadelphia, Pennsylvania

Cindy Peternelj-Taylor, RN, MSC
Associate Professor
University of Saskatchewan
Saskatoon, Saskatchewan
Canada

Nancy C. Sharts-Hopko, RN, PhD, FAAN
Professor
Villanova University
Villanova, Pennsylvania

Kathleen Mary Young, RN,C, MA
Instructor
Western Michigan University
Kalamazoo, Michigan

Consultants

Faith M. Addiss, RN, BSN
Instructor
Bryant & Statton
Buffalo, New York

Judith Allender, RN,C, MSN, EdD
Professor
California State University
Fresno, California

Julia W. Aucoin, RN,C, DNS
Assistant Professor
North Carolina Central University
Durham, North Carolina

Sister Rosita Brennan, CSSF, DNSc
Chair, Department of Associate Nursing
Felician College
Lodi, New Jersey

Esther Levine Brill, RN, PhD
Professor
Long Island University
Long Island, New York

Deborah Castellucci, CRNP, PhD
Chairperson, Nursing Department
Alvernia College
Reading, Pennsylvania

Patricia Cullen, RN, EdD
Associate Professor
Gwynedd-Mercy College
Gwynedd Valley, Pennsylvania

Nancy Dillard, RN, DNSc
Associate Director, Baccalaureate Nursing
Ball State University
Muncie, Indiana

Jane Elliott, PhD
Associate Director
Southside Regional Medical Center
Petersburg, Virginia

Branwynne Evans, RN, PhD
Nursing Department Head
Yakima Valley Community College
Yakima, Washington

Susan S. Gerberich, RN, PhD, CNS
Assistant Professor
University of Akron
Akron, Ohio

Lou Ella Humphrey, MSN, EdD, RNCS
Professor
Texarkana College
Texarkana, Texas

Louise Jasinski, MSN, CS
Interim Dean of Nursing
Oakland Community College
Waterford, Michigan

Ella Kick, RN, DNSc
Nursing Department Chair
Ashland University
Ashland, Ohio

Sally Knox, PhD, MSN
Professor
University of Florida
Gainesville, Florida

Deirdre Krause, PhD, ARNP, CS
Associate Professor
Lynn University
Boca Raton, Florida

Hope Moon, RN, MSN
Assistant Professor
Lorain County Community College
Elyria, Ohio

Debbie Fischer Peterson, RN, MS
Adjunct Assistant Professor
Montana State University
Billings, Montana

Larry Purnell, PhD
Acting Chair, Nursing Department
University of Delaware
Newark, Delaware

Mary L. Richards, RN, PhD
Professor Emeritus
Arizona State University
Tempe, Arizona

Patricia Lawless Ryan, MA, MSN
Assistant Professor
Gwynedd-Mercy College
Gwynedd Valley, Pennsylvania

Rosanne Schwartz, APRN-C, PhD
Associate Professor
Brigham Young University
Provo, Utah

Rachel Spector, RN, PhD,
  CTN, FAAN
Associate Professor
Boston College
Chestnut Hill, Massachusetts

Mary Thibault, MSN, MEd
Professor
Owen Community College
Toledo, Ohio

Carole E. Torok, RN,C, PhD
Associate Professor
SUNY Institute of Technology at
  Utica/Rome
Utica, New York

Contents

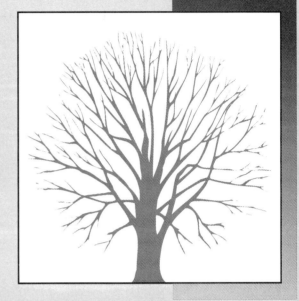

The Growth of Nursing as a Profession

1

The Development of Nursing as a Profession

> ➢ *Joseph T. Catalano*

Learning Objectives

After completing this chapter, the reader will be able to:

1. Define the terms *position, job, occupation,* and *profession.*

2. Compare the three approaches to defining a profession.

3. Analyze those traits defining a profession that nursing has attained.

4. Evaluate why nursing has failed to attain some of the traits that define a profession.

5. Correlate the concept of power with its important characteristics.

Since the time of Florence Nightingale, each generation of nurses, in its own way, has fostered the movement to professionalize the image of nurses and nursing. The struggle to change the status of nurses from that of female domestic servants to one of high-level health-care providers who base their protocols on scientific principles has been a primary goal of nursing's leaders for many years. Yet some people, both inside and outside of the profession of nursing, question whether the search for and attainment of professional status is worth the effort and price that must ultimately be paid.

At some levels in nursing, the question of **professionalism** takes on immense significance. However, to the busy **staff nurse**—who is trying to allocate patient assignments for a shift, distribute the medications at 9 A.M. to 24 clients, and supervise two aides, a licensed practical nurse (LPN) or licensed vocational

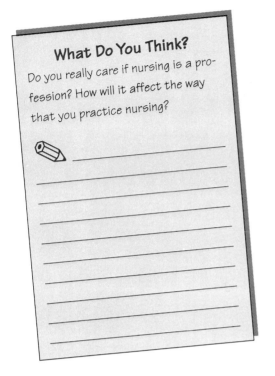

What Do You Think?

Do you really care if nursing is a profession? How will it affect the way that you practice nursing?

nurse (LVN), and a nursing student—the issue may not seem very significant at all.

Indeed, when nurses were first developing their identity separate from that of physicians, there was no thought about their being part of a **profession.** Over the years, however, as the scope of practice has expanded and the responsibilities have increased, nurses have increasingly begun to consider what they do as professional activities.

This chapter presents some of the current thought concerning professions and where nursing stands in relationship to these viewpoints.

APPROACHES TO DEFINING A PROFESSION

Terminology and the definition of terms, as with most complex and controversial issues,

play an important part in any discussion of nursing as a profession. In common usage, terms such as *position, job, occupation, profession, professional,* and *professionalism* are often used interchangeably and incorrectly. The following definitions will clarify what is meant by these terms within this text.

Position: A group of tasks assigned to one individual.

Job: A group of positions that are similar in nature and level of skill that can be carried out by one or more individuals.

Occupation: A group of jobs that are similar in type of work and that are usually found throughout an industry or work environment.

Profession: A type of occupation that meets certain criteria (discussed later in this chapter) that raise it to a level above that of an occupation.

Professional: A person who belongs to and practices a profession. (The term *professional* is probably the most misused of all these terms when describing people who are clearly involved in jobs or occupations, such as a "professional truck driver," "professional football player," or even a "professional thief").

Professionalism: The demonstration of high-level personal, ethical, and skill characteristics of a member of a profession.[1]

Experts in social science have been attempting to develop a "foolproof" approach to determine what constitutes a profession for almost 100 years but with only minimal success. Three common models are the process approach, the power approach, and the most widely accepted trait approach.

Process Approach

The process approach views all occupations as points of development into a **profession** along a continuum ranging from position to profession.

Continuum of Professional Development:

Position ⟷ Profession

Using this approach, the question becomes not whether nursing and truck driving are professions, but where they are located along the continuum. Occupations, such as medicine, law, and the ministry, are widely accepted by the public as being closest to the professional end of the continuum.[2] Other occupations may be less clearly defined.

The major difficulty with this approach is that it lacks criteria on which to base judgments. Final determination of the status of an occupation or profession depends almost completely on public perception of the activities of that occupation. Nursing has always had a rather poor public image when it comes to being viewed as a profession.

Power Approach

The power approach uses two criteria to define a profession: (1) how much independence of practice does this occupation have; and (2) how much power does this occupation control? The concept of power is discussed later in this chapter, but in this context it refers to political power. Political power goes hand in hand with income levels and monetary resources. Therefore, an important contributing characteristic to determine whether an occupation qualifies as a profession according to this approach is the amount of money that the person in that occupation earns.[3]

Using this determinant, occupations such as medicine, law, and **politics** would clearly be considered professions. The members of these occupations earn high incomes, practice their skills with a great deal of independence, and exercise significant power over individuals, the public, and the political community, both individually and in organized groups. The ministry is generally perceived as having power and influence. However, most persons in this group, except for a few individuals

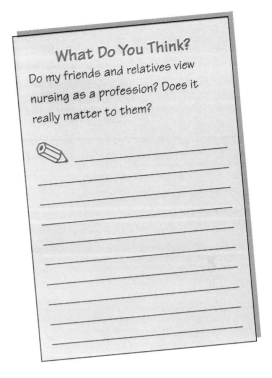

What Do You Think?

Do my friends and relatives view nursing as a profession? Does it really matter to them?

such as television evangelists, have relatively low income levels. Nursing, of course, with its relatively poor salaries, low membership in organizations, and perceived lack of political power, would clearly not meet the power criteria for a profession.

The question that comes to mind is whether power, independence of practice, and high incomes are the only elements that determine professional status. Although those three factors confer status in our culture, other elements can be considered as significant in how a profession is viewed. For example, for many, members of the clergy have a great deal of power when they act as counselors, speakers of the truth, and community leaders.

Trait Approach

Of the many researchers and theorists who have attempted to identify the traits that

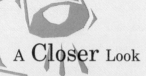

A Closer Look

CHALLENGES OF AN AGING NATION

The complexity of issues in today's health-care system challenges the professional nurse to look beyond the narrow confines of the individual client to a more comprehensive perspective of each situation. The following case study demonstrates some of the elements that need to be evaluated in the care of an elderly client.

Case Study

Clara, who is 108 years old, is admitted through the hospital emergency room (ER) for nonspecific complaints of chest pain and dizziness. This is the third time that she has come to the hospital with this complaint in the last month. Although previous examinations and tests have shown no acute disease process, the ER physician thought that because of her age and long history of coronary artery disease, Clara should be monitored and evaluated more closely. Clara has no private insurance, but she is covered under Medicare, Parts A and B, with supplemental coverage from a small insurance company in her state.

Despite her age, Clara is mentally alert and competent. She lives by herself in a small apartment and manages basic daily care, including shopping and cleaning, with only minimal assistance from friends. She has no living family members, except for a few aging cousins in a distant state. She is taking several medications at home. These medications include diltiazem (Cardizem) for her heart problems, ranitidine (Zantac) for a hiatal hernia, and papaverine (Pavabid) to increase her general circulation.

After a complete physical examination, including several laboratory tests and an electrocardiogram (ECG), she is scheduled for a cardiac catheterization. A significant block is seen in one of the major coronary arteries, and the physicians decide to perform an angioplasty on the artery. She is admitted to the intensive care unit (ICU) after the procedure, where she also receives 2 units of blood because she is anemic. She recovers without incident and is discharged 5 days after her admission. The total cost for her hospitalization, including tests and angioplasty, is more than $15,000.

Clara is not a typical client for her age group. Many medical experts would categorize the treatment given her as overtreatment because of the current emphasis on quality of life, death with dignity, and the futility of treating the hopelessly ill. Yet, as people in the United States continue to age, it is more likely that Clara will become the norm rather than the exception. Many issues—ethical, financial, and others—surround this case.

In an era of cost containment and reform, financial concerns are always near the top. Almost everyone admits that the Medicare reimbursement system is, at best, arbitrary and inconsistent, and at worst, disorganized and wasteful. Because of the concern about paying for expensive complicated procedures (e.g., angioplasty) that may not necessarily improve the quality of life and for which less expensive alternatives may exist, the system seems to force physicians to select modes of care that the elderly often consider substandard. In general, if a physician were to perform an angioplasty on a 108-year-old person, this treatment would be classified as excessive; yet, given this client's mental state and quick return to a normal life, it would appear to have been the correct course of action.

Related to the cost issue is the ethical issue of distributive justice. The terms currently used to define this problem are the rationing of health care and limiting access to health care. The elderly, through the various entitlement programs, consume a large proportion of the national budget. This cost is borne mainly by young and middle-aged workers through their taxes. Is it fair that the young be required to carry the burden for the care of the old?

The problems posed by an ever-aging population will only worsen in the twenty-first century. Decisions will have to be made about where best to spend the limited resources for health care. Basic questions, such as whether it is better to spend 65 cents to immunize a 4-year-old child or to spend $10,000 to perform an angioplasty on a 108-year-old woman, will challenge health-care providers of the future. It seems that blanket policies, such as are used now, will be inadequate to deal with these complex issues. Development of geriatric consultation teams at all facilities will make it possible to evaluate on an individual basis the case of each client 65 years or older who is admitted to the facility. Decisions could then be made about which type of care would be most appropriate, including the client's input, as well as what can be done to improve the quality of that individual's life. This will allow clients like Clara to live their lives to the fullest and to end their days with dignity and respect.

From Curtin, LH: How much is enough? Nurs Man 25:30–31, 1994.

define a profession, Flexner,[4] Bixler,[5] and Pavalko[6] are most widely accepted as the leaders in the field. These three social scientists have determined that the following common characteristics are important:

- High intellectual level
- High level of individual responsibility and **accountability**
- Specialized body of knowledge
- Knowledge that can be learned in institutions of higher education
- Public service and altruistic activities
- Public service valued over financial gain
- Relatively high degree of **autonomy** and independence of practice
- Need for a well-organized and strong organization representing the members of the profession and controlling the quality of practice
- A **code of ethics** that will guide the members of the profession in their practice
- Strong professional identity and commitment to the development of the profession
- Demonstration of professional competency and possession of a legally recognized license

NURSING AS A PROFESSION

How does nursing compare with other professions when measured against these widely accepted professional traits? The profession of nursing meets most of the criteria but falls short in a few areas.

When Nursing Meets the Criteria of a Profession

High Intellectual Level of Functioning

In the very early stages of the development of the practice of nursing, this criterion did not apply. Florence Nightingale raised the bar for education, and graduates of her school were considered to be highly educated compared with other women of that time. However, most of the tasks performed by these early nurses are generally considered, by today's standards to be menial and routine. On the other hand, as health care has advanced and made great strides in technology, pharmacology, and all branches of the physical sciences, a high level of intellectual functioning is required for even relatively simple nursing tasks, such as taking a client's temperature or blood pressure using automated equipment. Nurses use **assessment** skills and knowledge, have the ability to reason, and make routine judgments based on clients' conditions daily. Without a doubt, professional nurses must and do function at a high intellectual level.

High Level of Individual Responsibility and Accountability

Not too long ago, a nurse was rarely, if ever, named as a **defendant** in a malpractice suit. The public, in general, did not view nurses as having enough knowledge to be held accountable for errors that were made in client care. This is not the case in the health-care system today. Nurses are often the primary, and frequently the only, defendants named when errors are made that result in injury to the client. Nurses must be accountable and demonstrate a high level of individual responsibility for the care and services that they provide.

The concept of accountability has legal, ethical, and professional implications that include accepting responsibility for actions taken to provide **client** care as well as accepting responsibility for the consequences of actions that are not performed. A nurse can no longer state that "the physician told me to do it" as a method of avoiding responsibility for his or her actions.

A Specialized Body of Knowledge

Nursing has been and always will be eclectic in the sense that it draws a large portion of its knowledge from many areas of science. In the early history of nursing, most of the skills practiced by those who claimed to be nurses were based either on traditional ways of doing things or on the intuitive knowledge of the individual nurse. As nursing has developed into an identifiable, separate discipline, a specialized body of knowledge called "nursing science" was compiled through the research efforts of nurses who hold advanced educational degrees. Although this body of specialized nursing knowledge is relatively small, it forms a theoretical basis for the practice of nursing today. As more nurses obtain advanced degrees, conduct research, and develop philosophies and theories about nursing, this body of knowledge will increase in scope.

Public Service and Altruistic Activities

Almost all major nursing theorists, when defining nursing, include a statement that refers to a goal of helping clients to adapt to illness and to achieve their highest level of functioning. The public (variously referred to as consumers, patients, clients, individuals, or humans) is the focal point of all nurs-

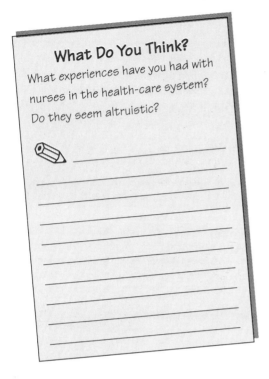

become disappointed. Although the pay scale has increased tremendously during the 1990s, nursing is, at best, a middle-income occupation. Surveys among students entering nursing programs continue to indicate that the primary reason for wishing to become a nurse is to "help others" or "make a difference" in someone's life and to have "job security." Rarely do these beginning students include "to make a lot of money" as their motivation.[7]

The Well-Organized and Strong Professional Organization

This type of organization represents the members of the profession and controls the quality of professional practice. Nursing has never been at a loss for nursing organizations. The National League for Nursing (NLN) and the American Nurses Association (ANA) are the two major national organizations that represent nursing in today's health-care system. The NLN is primarily responsible for regulating the quality of the educational programs that prepare nurses for the practice of nursing, whereas the ANA is more concerned with the quality of nursing practice in the daily health-care setting. These and other organizations are discussed in more detail in Chapter 2.

Both of these organizations are well organized, but neither can be considered powerful when compared with other professional organizations, such as the American Medical Association (AMA) or the American Bar Association (ABA). One reason for their lack of strength is that fewer than 15% of all nurses in the United States are members of any professional organization at the national level.[3] Many nurses do belong to specialty organizations that represent a specific area of practice, but these lack sufficient political power to produce changes in health-care laws and policies at the national level.

ing models and nursing practice. The public service function of nursing has always been recognized and acknowledged by society. This acknowledgment has been manifested by society's willingness to continue to educate nurses in public, tax-supported institutions as well as in private schools. In addition, nursing has been viewed universally as being an altruistic profession. From its earliest days, when dedicated nurses provided care for victims of deadly plagues with little regard for their own welfare, to today, when nurses are found in remote and often hostile areas, providing care for the sick and dying, or working 12-hour shifts, being "on call," or working rotating shifts, the perception is that nurses are selfless individuals who place the lives and well-being of their clients above their personal physical safety.

Few individuals enter nursing in order to become rich and famous. It is likely that those who do so for these reasons quickly

Professional Role of the Community Health Nurse

The Fayez family came to the United States from Cairo, Egypt, in 1976. After spending 6 months with distant relatives in Daly City, California, Anwar and his wife Fatma moved into an apartment of their own, and Anwar continued the job that his uncle Hussain had helped him get in the construction business. Fatma has never worked outside the home. In 1979, Mr. and Mrs. Fayez had their first child, a daughter named Randa. Two years ago, Fatma miscarried in her fourth month of pregnancy and lost a male child. At this point in their lives, Fatma is 6 months pregnant and Anwar owns and operates his own small construction and roofing company in the Richmond area of San Francisco. Sherief is a healthy looking boy who does well in school, and Randa is in the first grade.

The public health nurse, who is a family nurse practitioner assigned to the Fayez family for their child and prenatal care, has made two visits to the family's home. On both occasions the nurse noticed that Mrs. Fayez looked very fatigued and short of breath. Both Sherief and Randa were very quiet during the visits. Anwar often boasted of his son's achievements in school and said little about Randa. Fatma was showing some slight edema in both feet, and the nurse noticed during these visits (both in the evening) that Fatma was frequently getting up to serve the family tea and food. Mr. Fayez described how Sherief's teachers complained about his "aggressive behavior in school." Mrs. Fayez was concerned about her daughter's "finicky" eating habits. During both visits the nurse noticed an older, conservatively dressed woman who sat quietly during the early part of the visit and communicated to the family members in Arabic. She always left the room soon after the nurse arrived, and the nurse sensed that the family acknowledged her with a great deal of respect.

Traditionally, men of Egyptian origin have low expectations of nurses based on their experiences with the relatively poorly educated nurses in their home country. However, they do place a high value on good health and health-care practices.

In this community setting, what might the nurse do to demonstrate her competency to this family? Are there any health-care practices that she might introduce to this family?

From Purnell, LD, and Paulanka, BJ: *Transcultural Health Care,* with permission.
FA Davis, Philadelphia, 1998.

The Nurses' Code of Ethics

Nursing has several codes of ethics that are used to guide nursing practice. The ANA Code for Nurses, the most widely used in the United States, was first published in 1971 and last updated in 1985. The ANA Code of Ethics is currently being revised to make it more relevant to current nursing practice. This code of ethics is recognized by other professions as a standard with which others are compared. The nurses' code of ethics and its implications are discussed in greater detail in Chapter 6.

Competency and Professional License

Members of the nursing profession have demonstrated competency in practice and have a legally recognized **license** to practice the profession. Nurses must pass a national licensure examination to demon-

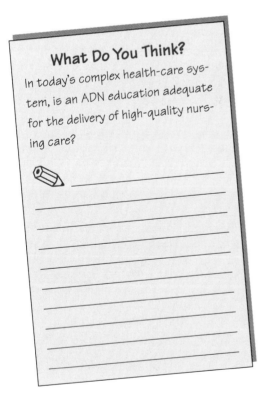

What Do You Think?

In today's complex health-care system, is an ADN education adequate for the delivery of high-quality nursing care?

strate that they are qualified to practice nursing. Only after passing this examination are nurses allowed to practice. Interim permits granted, which were used several years before the advent of the computerized examination, are used today in only a few locations. The granting of a nursing license is a legal activity conducted by the individual state under the **regulations** contained in that state's nurse practice act.

When Nursing Falls Short of Meeting the Criteria of a Profession

Activities are learned in institutions of higher education. Before Florence Nightingale practiced nursing, people considered it to be unnecessary, if not outright dangerous, to educate nurses through independent nursing programs in publicly supported educational institutions. As nursing has developed, particularly in the United States, the recognition of the intellectual nature of the practice, as well as the vast amount of knowledge required for the job, has led to a belief by some nursing leaders that college education for nurses is now a necessity. Since 1950, however, many attempts to require all nurses to be educated in institutions of higher education have been resisted and ultimately rejected by the more numerous diploma and **associate degree nursing programs.**

Nursing is the only major discipline that does not require its members to hold at least a baccalaureate degree in order to obtain licensure. Although the number of diploma programs in nursing has decreased tremendously since 1990, associate degree programs continue to maintain high enrollment and graduate large numbers of individuals. At issue is whether a **baccalaureate degree nursing program** should be the minimum requirement for entry-level nurses.

Autonomy and Independence of Practice

Historically, the handmaiden or servant relationship of the nurse to the physician was widely accepted. It was based on several factors, including social norms. For example, women became nurses, whereas men became physicians; and women were subservient to men, the nature of the work being such that nurses cleaned and physicians cured. In terms of the relative levels of education of the two groups, the average nursing program lasted for 1 year, whereas physician education lasted for 6 to 8 years. Unfortunately, despite efforts to expand nursing practice into more independent areas through updated nurse practice legislation, nursing retains its subservient image. In reality, nursing is both an independent and interdependent discipline. Nurses in all health-care settings must work closely with physicians, hospital administrators, pharmacists, and other groups in the provision of care. In some cases, nurses in **advanced practice** roles, such as **nurse practitioners,** can and do establish their own independent practices. Actually, most state **nurse practice acts** allow nurses more independence in their practice than they realize. To be considered a true profession, nursing will need to be recognized by other disciplines as having practitioners who practice nursing independently.

Professional Identity and Development

The issue of job versus career is in question here. A job is a group of positions that are similar in nature and level of skill that can be carried out by one or more individuals. There is relatively little commitment to a job, and many individuals move from one job to another with little regard to the long-term outcomes. A career, in contrast, is usually viewed as a person's major lifework, which progresses and develops as the person grows older. Careers and professions have many of the same characteristics, including a formal education, full-time employment, requirement for lifelong learning, and a dedication to what is being achieved. Although an increasing number of nurses view nursing as their life's work, many still treat nursing more as a job.

The problem becomes circular. The reason why nurses lack a strong professional identity and do not consider nursing a lifelong career is because nursing does not have full status as a profession. Until nurses are fully committed to the profession of nursing, identify with it as a profession, and are dedicated to its future development, nursing will probably not achieve professional status.

EMPOWERMENT IN NURSING

One of the concerns that has plagued nurses and nursing almost from its devel-

What Do You Think?

From your point of view, you have experienced the following samples of "power" demonstrated by nurses:

_____

_____

_____

_____

You feel that nurses should/should not use power because:

_____

_____

_____

_____

opment as a separate health-care specialty is the relatively large amount of personal responsibility shouldered by nurses combined with a relatively small amount of control over their practice. Even in the more enlightened atmosphere of today's society with its concerns about equal opportunity, equal pay, and collegial relationships, many nurses still seem uncomfortable with the concepts of power and control in their practice. Their discomfort may arise from the belief that nursing is a helping and caring profession whose goals are separate from issues of power. Historically, nurses have never had much power, and previous attempts at gaining power and control over their practice have been met with much resistance from groups who benefit from keeping nurses powerless. Nevertheless, all nurses use power in their daily practice, even if they do not realize it. Until nurses understand the sources of their power, how to increase it, and how to use it in providing client care, they will be relegated to a subservient position in the health-care system.

The Nature of Power

The term *power* has many meanings. From the standpoint of nursing, power is probably best defined as the ability or capacity to exert influence over another person or group of persons. In other words, power is the ability to get other people to do things even when they do not want to do them. Although power in itself is neither good nor bad, it can be used to produce either good or bad results.

Power is always a two-way street. By its very definition, when power is exerted by one person, another person is affected, that is, the use of power by one person requires that another person give up some of his or her power. Individuals are always in a state of change, either increasing their power or

losing some, the balance of power rarely remains static. **Empowerment** refers to the increased amount of power that an individual, or group, is either given or gains.

The Origins of Power

If power is such an important part of nursing and the practice of nurses, where does it come from? Although there are many sources, some of them would be inappropriate or unacceptable for those in a helping and caring profession. The following list includes some of the more accessible and acceptable sources of power that nurses should consider using in their practice.[3,8,9] These sources are:

- Referent
- Expert
- Reward
- Coercive
- Legitimate
- Collective

Referent Power

The referent source of power depends on establishing and maintaining a close personal relationship with someone. In any close personal relationship, one individual often will do something he or she would really rather not do because of the relationship. This ability to be able to change the actions of another is an exercise of power. Nurses often obtain power from this source when they establish and maintain good therapeutic relationships with their clients. Clients take medications, tolerate uncomfortable treatments, and participate in demanding activities that they would clearly prefer to avoid because the nurse has a good relationship with them. Likewise, nurses who have good collegial relationships with other nurses, departments, and physicians are often able to obtain what they want from these individuals or groups in providing care to clients.

Expert Power

The expert source of power derives from the amount of knowledge, skill, or expertise that an individual or group has. This power source is exercised by the individual or group when knowledge, skills, or expertise is either used or withheld in order to influence the behavior of others. Nurses should have at least a minimal amount of this type of power because of their education and experience. It follows logically that increasing the level of nurses' education will, or should, increase this expert power. As nurses attain and remain in positions of power longer, the increased experience will also aid with the use of expert power. Nurses in advanced practice roles are good examples of those who have expert power. Their additional education and experience provide these nurses with the ability to practice skills at a higher level, compared with nurses prepared at the basic education level.

Nurses access this expert source of power when they use their knowledge to teach, counsel, or motivate clients to follow a plan of care.

> 66 99 *Nurses access this expert source of power when they use their knowledge to teach, counsel, or motivate clients to follow a plan of care.*

Nurses can also use this source of power when dealing with physicians. By demonstrating their knowledge of the client's condition, recent laboratory tests, and other elements that are vital in the client's recovery nurses demonstrate their expert power. This knowledge may increase the amount of respect that they are given by physicians.

The Power of Rewards

The reward source of power depends on the ability of one person to grant another some type of reward for specific behaviors or changes in behavior. The rewards themselves can take on many different forms, including personal favors, promotions, money, expanded privileges, and eradication of punishments. Nurses, in their daily provision of care, can use this source of power to influence client behavior. For example, a nurse can give a client extra praise for completing the prescribed range-of-motion exercises. There are many aspects of the daily care of clients over which nurses have a substantial amount of reward power. This reward source of power is also the underlying principle in the process of behavior modification.

Coercive Power

The coercive source of power is the flip side of the reward source. The ability to punish, withhold rewards, and threaten punishment is the key element underlying the coercive source of power. Although nurses do have access to this source of power, it is probably one that they use minimally, if at all. Not only does the use of the coercive source of power destroy therapeutic and personal relationships, but it can also be considered unethical and even illegal in certain situations. Threatening clients that they will get an injection if they do not take their oral medications may motivate them to take those medications, but it is generally not considered to be a good example of therapeutic communication technique.

Legitimate Power

The legitimate source of power depends on a legislative or legal act that gives the individual or organization a right to make decisions that they might not otherwise have the authority to make. Most obviously, political figures and **legislators** have this source of power. But this power can also be disseminated and delegated to others through legislative acts. In nursing, the state board of nursing has access to the legitimate source of power because of its establishment under the nurse practice act of that state. Similarly, nurses have access to the legitimate source of power when they are licensed by the state under the provisions in the nurse practice act or when they are appointed to positions within a health-care agency. Nursing decisions made about client care can come only from individuals who have a legitimate source of power to make those decisions, that is, licensed nurses.

Collective Power

The collective source of power is often used in a broader context than individual client care and is the underlying source for many other sources of power. When a large group of individuals who have similar beliefs, desires, or needs becomes organized, a collective source of power exists. For individuals who belong to professions, the professional organization is the focal point for this source of power. The main goal of any organization is to influence those policies that affect the members of the organization. This influence is usually in the form of political activities carried out by politicians and **lobbyists.**

Professional organizations that can deliver large numbers of votes have a powerful means of influencing politicians. The use of the collective source of power contains elements of reward, coercive, expert, and even referent sources. Each source may come into play at one time or another.

How to Increase Power in Nursing

Despite some feelings of powerlessness, nurses really do have access to some important, and rather substantial, sources of power. What can nurses, either as individuals or as a group, do in order to increase their power?

Professional Unity

Probably the first, and certainly the most important, way in which nurses can gain power in all areas is through professional unity. The most powerful groups are those that are best organized and most united. The power that a professional organization has is directly related to the size of its membership. According to the ANA, there are approximately 3,000,000 nurses in the United States. It is not difficult to imagine the power that the ANA could have to influence legislators and legislation if all of those nurses were members of the organization rather than the 250,000 who actually do belong. This point—that nurses need to belong to their nursing national organization—cannot be emphasized too much.

Political Activities

A second way in which nurses can gain power is by becoming involved in **political action.** Although this produces discomfort in many, nurses must realize that they are affected by politics and political decisions in every phase of their daily nursing activities.

The simple truth is that if nurses do not become involved in politics and participate in important legislation that influences their practice, someone other than nurses will be making those decisions for them. Nurses need to become involved in political activities from local to national levels. The average legislator knows little about issues such as clients' rights, national health insurance, quality of nursing care, third-party reimbursement for nurses, and expanded practice roles for nurses. Yet, they make decisions about these issues almost daily. It would seem logical that more informed and better decisions could be made if nurses took an active part in the legislative process.

Accountability and Professionalism

A third method of increasing power is by demonstrating the characteristics of accountability and professionalism. Nursing has made great strides in these two areas in recent years. Nurses, through professional organizations, have been working hard to establish standards for quality client care. More important, nurses are now concerned with demonstrating competence and delivering high-quality client care through processes such as peer review and evaluation. By accepting responsibility for the care that they provide and by setting the standards to guide that care, nurses are taking the power

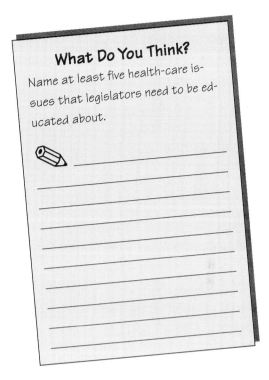

What Do You Think?

Name at least five health-care issues that legislators need to be educated about.

to govern nursing away from non-nursing groups.

Networking

Finally, nurses can gain power through establishing a nurse support network. It is common knowledge that the "old boy" system remains alive and well in many segments of our seemingly enlightened twentieth century society. The "old boy" system, which is found in most large organizations ranging from universities to businesses and governmental agencies, provides individuals, usually men, with the encouragement, support, and nurturing that allows them to move up quickly through the ranks in the organization to achieve high administrative positions. Nursing and nursing organizations have never had this type of system for the advancement of nurses. Part of this system of doing business involves never criticizing another "old boy" in public, even though there may be major differences of opinion in private. Presentation of a united front is extremely important in maintaining power within this system.

Part of the difficulty in establishing a nurse support network arises from the fact that nurses really have not been in high-level positions for very long. The framework for a support system for nurses is now in place; and with some commitment to the concept and activity, it can grow into a well-developed network to allow the brightest, best, and most ambitious people in the profession to achieve high-level positions.

FUTURE TRENDS IN THE NURSING PROFESSION

Clearly, it would be difficult to make an airtight case for nursing as a profession. Yet nursing does meet many of the criteria proposed for a profession. Although it would probably be most accurate to call nursing a developing or aspiring profession, for the purposes of this book nursing will be referred to as a profession. Only when nurses begin to think of nursing as a profession, work toward raising the educational standards for entry level, and begin practicing independently as professionals, will the profession become a reality for nursing. The movement of any discipline from the status of occupation to one of profession is a dynamic and ongoing process with many considerations.

The experts predict another period of shortage for professional nurses extending well into the twenty-first century. In the past, the way that nursing shortages were handled was to use a "quick-fix" method of producing more nurses in a shorter period of time by reducing the educational requirements. The current nursing education system is producing approximately 40,000 graduates from diploma and associate degree programs every year.[10] Although this number may help alleviate the nursing shortage, the more critical question to ask is whether this level of education is going to prepare nurses to meet the challenges of a rapidly changing and demanding health-care system into the twenty-first century.

As the national employment picture continues to evolve for registered nurses from bedside caregivers to coordinators of care, and financial resources become stressed, perhaps more nurses will begin to look on what they do as a lifelong commitment. Professional commitment is a complicated issue, but little doubt exists that nurses will not have increased independence of practice until they begin to demonstrate that they are professionals committed to the field of nursing.

Conclusion

Ongoing changes in the health-care system will have a major impact on how, where, and even who practices nursing. Unless nurses become involved in decisions about the direction in which health care is going, band together as a profession, and exert some of the tremendous potential power that they have, politicians, physicians, hospital administrators, and insurance companies will ultimately be shaping their future.

Nursing has taken great strides forward in achieving professional status in the health-care system. Currently, many nurses accept the premise that nursing is a profession and therefore are not very concerned about furthering the process. Even as nursing has matured and evolved into a field of study with an identifiable body of knowledge, the questions and problems that have plagued this profession persist. In addition, advances in **technology,** management, and society have raised new questions about the nature and role of nursing in the health-care system. Only by understanding and exploring the issues of professionalism will nurses be prepared to practice effectively in the present and meet the complex challenges of the future.

References

1. Holl, RM: Characteristics of the registered nurse and professional beliefs and decision making. Crit Care Nurse Q 17(3):60–66, 1994.
2. Moloney, MM: Professionalization of Nursing. JB Lippincott, Philadelphia, 1986.
3. Smith, GR: Power and health care reform. J Nurs Educ 33:194–197, 1994.
4. Flexner, A: Medical Education in the United States and Canada, Carngie Foundation: New York.
5. Bixler, GK: The professional status of nursing. AJN, 59(8): 1142-1147.
6. Pavalko, J: The Professions. Clarendon Press, Oxford, 1971.
7. McCloskey, M, and Grace, HK: Current issues in nursing, ed 4. CV Mosby, St. Louis, 1994.
8. Fitzpatrick, ML: Prologue to Professionalism. Robert J. Brady, Bowie, MD, 1983.
9. Kalisch, BJ, and Kalisch, PA: The Politics of Nursing. JB Lippincott, Philadelphia, 1996.
10. American Nurses Association, Nursing Social Policy Statement. Washington D.C.,1996

BIBLIOGRAPHY

American Nurses Association: Nursing's Agenda for Health Care Reform. American Nurses Association, Kansas City, 1992.

Brink, PJ: The difference between a job and a career. West J Nurs Res 10:5–6, 1988.

Bunting, S, and Campbell, J: Feminism and nursing: Historical perspectives. Adv Nurs Sci 12:11–24, 1990.

Carroll, V, and Morin, K: Workplace violence affects one-third of nurses. Am Nurse 30(5):15, 1998.

Curtin, LH: How much is enough? Nurs Mon 25:30–31, 1994.

De Tornyay, R: Reconsidering nursing education: The report of the Pew Health Professions Commission. J Nurs Educ 13:296–301, 1992.

Hoffman, S: Nurses must unify to bring change for patients and profession. Am Nurse 29(6):5–7, 1998.

Hunt, R: Community-based nursing: Philosophy or setting? Am J Nurs 98(10):44–49, 1998.

Loscalzo, F: The essence of nursing is touching another soul. AACN News 15(10):3, 1998.

McCloskey, M: Many issues influence profession. Am Nurse 22:7, 1992.

McKinley, M: The power of our practice: Look to our roots. AACN News 15(9):2, 1998.

Munro, N: Public policy: A new paradigm grows from grass roots. Crit care Nurse 18(5):76–85, 1998.

Nicoll, LH: Nurses' Guide to the Internet, ed 2. JB Lippincott, Philadelphia, 1998.

Purnell, LD, and Paulanka, BJ: Transcultural Health Care. FA Davis, Philadelphia, 1998.

Sandhaus, S: Migrant health: A harvest of poverty. Am J Nurs 98(9):52–65, 1998.

Siebber, JR, et al: Missing in action: Nurses in the media. Am J Nurs 98(12):55–56, 1998.

Wilson, J: Healing and curing. Oklahoma Nurse 43(1):4–5, 1998.

Critical Thinking Exercises

✔ Distinguish between an occupation and a profession.

✔ Is nursing a profession? Defend your position.

✔ Discuss four ways in which nursing can improve its professional status.

✔ Name the three sources of power to which nurses have the most access. Discuss how nurses can best use these sources of power to improve nursing, nursing care, and the health-care system.

2

The Evolution of Licensure, Certification, and Nursing Organizations

➤*Joseph T. Catalano*

Learning Objectives

After completing this chapter, the reader will be able to:

1. Identify the purposes and needs for nurse licensure.
2. Distinguish between permissive and mandatory licensure.
3. Explain why institutional licensure is unacceptable in today's health-care system.
4. Evaluate the importance of nurse practice acts.
5. Analyze the significance of professional certification.
6. Evaluate the importance of nursing organizations in the nursing profession.

Almost from the inception of nursing, societal needs and expectations have been the driving forces behind the establishment of the standards that guide the profession. In the early days of nursing when health care was relatively primitive and society's expectations of nurses were low, there was little demand for regulations or controls over and within the profession. However, as technology and health care have advanced and become more complex, there has been a corresponding increase in societal expectations for nurses. All nurses now accept licensure and **certification** examinations as given in today's health-care system. But where did these examinations come from? And what do they mean to the profession? This chapter explores the answers to these questions.

Rather than looking on the advent of sophisticated telecommunications, growing information technologies, redesigned health-care organizations, and increasing **health-care consumer** demands with fear and trepidation, nurses should consider this as an exciting time of growth and opportunity. In today's health-care system, nurses have an almost unlimited number of ways to provide new and creative nursing care for clients in all settings. As society's needs and expectations change, so will the regulations and standards that help define nursing practice. Through their professional nursing organizations, nurses can help shape health-care regulations that establish the most freedom to provide effective care while maintaining the goal of protection of the public. It is likely that in the future state boards of nursing will look much different, just as the profession of nursing will differ from that of its past.

2.1 Reasons the State Boards of Nursing May Revoke a Nursing License

- Conviction for a serious crime
- Demonstration of gross negligence or unethical conduct in the practice of nursing
- Failure to renew a nursing license while still continuing to practice nursing
- Use of illegal drugs or alcohol during the provision of care for clients, or the use carries over and affects client's care
- Willful violation of the state's nurse practice act

THE DEVELOPMENT OF NURSE PRACTICE ACTS

A nurse practice act is state legislation that regulates the practice of nurses to protect the public and make nurses accountable for their actions. Nurse practice acts establish state boards of nursing (SBN) and define specific SBN powers regarding the practice of nursing within the state. Rules and regulations written by the SBsN become **statutory laws** under the powers delegated by the state **legislature.**

Although nurse practice acts differ from one state to another, the SBsN have many powers in common. All SBsN have the power to grant licenses, to accredit nursing programs, to establish standards for nursing schools, and to write specific regulations for nurses and nursing in general in that state. Of particular importance is the SBsN's power to deny or revoke nurse licenses (Box 2–1).

Other functions of nurse practice acts include defining nursing and the scope of practice, ruling on who can use the titles regis-

tered nurse (RN) and licensed practical nurse/licensed vocational nurse (LPN/LVN), setting up an application procedure for licensure in the state, determining fees for licensure, establishing requirements for renewal of licensure, and determining responsibility for any regulations governing expanded practice for nurses in that particular state.

THE NEED FOR LICENSURE

Imagine what the quality of health care would be if anyone could walk into a hospital, claim to know how to care for clients, and be given a job as a nurse. This situation might sound impossible in today's health-care system, but not too long ago it was the norm rather than the exception.

Throughout the last half of the nineteenth century, and the first half of the twentieth century, rapid growth in health-care technology led to the increasing use of hospitals as the primary source of health care. Individuals who were qualified to provide this care, however, were in short supply. There

2.2 Key Points in the New York State Licensure Bill (1904)

- Established minimum educational standards
- Established the minimum length of basic nursing programs at 2 years
- Required all nursing schools to be registered with the state board of regents (who oversee all higher education)
- Established a state board of nursing (SBN) with five nurses as members
- Formulated rules for the examination of nurses
- Formulated regulations for nurses who, if violated, could lead to the revocation of licensure

Hirsh, IL: Statement on nursing's scope describes how two levels of nurses practice. Amer Nurse 20:13, 1988.

were wide variations both in the abilities of those who claimed to be nurses and in the quality of the care that they provided. Paradoxically, nursing leaders who had always advocated some type of **credentialing** for nurses to ensure competency found that their attempts to initiate registration or licensure met with strong opposition from physician groups, hospital administrators, and practicing nurses themselves.[1]

EARLY ATTEMPTS AT LICENSURE

Although the idea of registering nurses had been in existence for some time, Florence Nightingale was the first to establish a formal register for graduates of her nursing school. In the United States and Canada, there was widespread recognition of the need for some type of credentialing of nurses as far back as the middle 1800s. The first organized attempt to establish a credentialing system was initiated in 1896 by the Nurses Associated Alumnae of the United States and Canada (later to become the American Nurses Association). As with other early attempts at licensure, it was met with resistance and eventually failed.[2]

Several nursing leaders, including Lillian Wald, Annie Goodrich, and Isabel Stewart, recognized the inconsistent quality of nursing care and the need for licensure to protect the public. In 1901, after an extensive and lengthy campaign to educate the public, physicians, hospital administrators, and nurses themselves about the need for licensure, the International Council of Nurses passed a resolution that required each state to establish a licensure and examination procedure for nurses. It took 3 years before the state of New York, through

What Do You Think?

Think of five infractions that you think, if committed by nurses, should lead to revocation of a nurse's licensure.

the New York Nurses Association, developed a licensure bill that passed the legislature (Box 2–2).

Other states that followed New York's lead were North Carolina, New Jersey, and Virginia. Although these states had bills that were weaker than New York's nurse practice act, passage of such legislation was considered a major accomplishment for several reasons. Women did not even have the right to vote in general elections at the time these bills were passed. In addition, few requirements and regulations for licensure existed during this period in the history of the United States, even for the medical profession.

THE IMPORTANCE OF LICENSURE EXAMINATIONS

The thought of having to take an examination that can determine whether or not one can practice nursing can make even the best student anxious. Adding to the tension is the fact that the examination is given outside of the academic setting, by computer, and is created by individuals other than the students' teachers. (See Chapter 9 for a detailed discussion of NCLEX- CAT, RN.)

Some type of objective method, however, to prove that the individual is qualified to practice nursing safety is necessary to protect the public from unqualified practitioners. Early attempts at creating licensure examinations for nurses were met with resistance. Although all states had some form of licensure examination by 1923, the format and length of the examinations varied widely. Some states required both written and practical examinations to demonstrate safety of practice, whereas others added an oral examination.

Although licensure was and is a state-controlled activity, the major nursing organizations in the United States eventually realized that in order to have some consistency of quality across the country, a single examination that all nurses needed to pass should be devised. The American Nurses Association (ANA) Council of State Boards of Nursing was organized in 1945 to oversee development of a uniform examination for nurses that could be used by all state boards of nursing. The National League of Nursing Testing Division developed such a test, which was implemented in 1950. Originally the test was simply called the State Board Examination, but it was renamed the National Council Licensure Examination (NCLEX) in 1987. In 1994, the computerized version of the examination was implemented—the National Council Licensure Examination–Computerized Adaptive Testing, for Registered Nurses (NCLEX-CAT, RN).

Licensure for nurses has undergone a major change. States are currently in the process of implementing the Mutual Recognition Model for Nursing Licensure, which will allow nurses licensed in one state to practice nursing in other states that belong

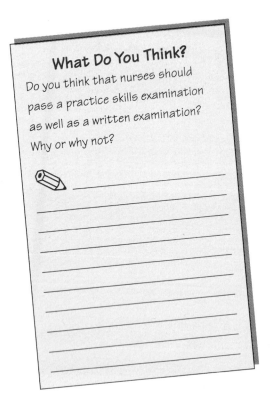

What Do You Think?

Do you think that nurses should pass a practice skills examination as well as a written examination? Why or why not?

Mutual Recognition Model of Nursing Licensure

The Delegate Assembly of the National Council of State Boards of Nursing has begun the process of developing a mutual recognition model of nursing licensure that would allow nurses licensed in one state to practice in other states without the necessity of seeking additional licensure. Although all the particular policies have not been formulated at this time, the proposed system would likely be similar to what is currently being used by nurses in the military, who can practice anywhere in the United States as long as they have a valid license from one state.

The movement toward a national licensure has been encouraged by several trends and developing issues in health care. These include the trend of nurses to increase their practice across state lines, the use of new technologies in numerous settings often located in different states, and the need by employers for quick approval for practice. Major issues that influence the movement include the demand by health-care consumers for qualified practitioners without regard to state boundaries, efficient and cost-effective use of limited registration and management resources for licensure, and questionable compliance with state requirements for licensure.

Many difficult issues remain to be resolved by the boards of nursing as they work toward the goal of national licensure. These issues include determining who would be responsible for disciplining nurses who violate the state practice act or code of ethics, requirements for demonstration of currentness of education and practice skills, setting a uniform licensure fee scale, and development of a national nursing database to monitor nurses across state lines.

However, this movement is seen by many as an historic turning point in nursing that will affect every nurse in the United States. Mutual recognition will usher in a new and innovative method of regulation of nursing licensure and nursing practice, again demonstrating the nursing profession's creative leadership in health care.

Modified from News: National Council of State Boards of Nursing, Inc., Publication No. 132. NANDA, Philadelphia, August 25, 1997, with permission.

to their regional agreement. The eventual goal is to have a "universal" nursing license that will allow nurses to practice in all states without having to become relicensed each time they cross a state border.

REGISTRATION VERSUS LICENSURE

The terms *registration* and *licensure* are often used interchangeably, although they are not synonymous. They serve a similar purpose, but some technical differences exist.

Registration

Registration is the listing, or registering, of names of individuals on an official roster who have met certain pre-established criteria. Before universal licensure by the states, any health-care institution that wanted to know whether a person applying for a position had met the standards for that position by graduating from a school of nursing or by passing an examination could call the school and see whether the applicant's name appeared on the official roster or register, hence the origin of the term *registered nurse*. With the advent of state board examinations, an institution merely has to call the SBN to find out whether the individual is registered or licensed.

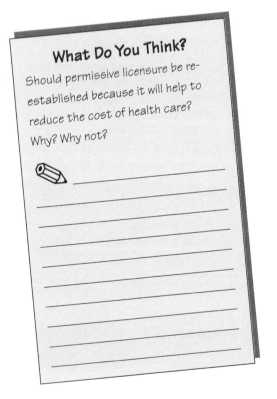

What Do You Think?

Should permissive licensure be re-established because it will help to reduce the cost of health care? Why? Why not?

Licensure

Licensure is an activity conducted by the state through the enforcement powers of its regulatory boards to protect the public's health, safety, and welfare by establishing professional standards. Licensure for nurses, as for other professionals who deal with the public, is necessary to ensure that everyone who claims to be a nurse can function at a minimal level of competency and safety. There are several different types of licensure.

Permissive Licensure

Permissive licensure allows individuals to practice nursing as long as they do not use the letters "RN" after their names. Basically, permissive licensure protects the "registered nurse" designation but not the practice of nursing itself. Under a permissive licensure law, anyone could carry out the functions of an RN, regardless of their level of education, without having to pass an examination indicating competency. Health-care administrators seem to support the concept of permissive licensure because it allows them to employ less-educated and lower-paid employees rather than the more highly paid RNs. However, they also recognize that the quality of care decreases when the education level of health-care providers is lower. Although most early licensure laws were permissive, all states now have **mandatory licensure.**

Mandatory Licensure

Mandatory licensure requires anyone who wishes to practice nursing to pass a **licensure examination** and become registered by the SBN. Because different levels of nursing practice exist, different levels of licensure are necessary. At the technical level, the individual must take and pass the licensed practical nurse (LPN)/licensed vocational nurse (LVN) examination; at the professional level, the individual must take and pass the RN examination.

Mandatory licensure forced SBNs to distinguish between the activities that nurses at different levels could legally perform. The scope of practice defines the boundaries for each of the levels: advanced practice nurse (APN), RN, and LPN/LVN. As more levels of nursing education (e.g., the associate degree in nursing [ADN]) have been added, however, lines dividing the different scopes of practice have become blurred. In the current health-care system, it is not unusual to find LPNs/LVNs performing activities that are generally considered professional.

A particularly confusing element in today's health-care system is the use of unlicensed individuals to provide health care. The advent of certified nurses assistants (CNAs) and unlicensed assistive personnel (UAP) has led to widespread use of such individuals in all health-care settings. Although they must be supervised by an RN or LPN/LVN, these individuals are sometimes illegally assigned nursing tasks much more advanced than their levels of training. (See Chapter 8 for a more detailed discussion of delegation.) Despite the fact that permissive licensure is no longer legal, CNAs and UAP appear to fall under an unofficial type of permissive licensure.

Institutional Licensure

Although universally rejected by every major nursing organization, **institutional licensure** has become a reality for many other types of health-care workers, such as respiratory therapists and physical therapists. In some state legislatures, bills have been introduced to allow **foreign graduate nurses** and nurses who are licensed in foreign countries to work in specific institutions without taking the American licensure examination. Up to this point, these bills have been stopped by the state nursing or-

ganizations before they could become law. Institutional licensure has been proposed periodically over the years as an alternative to governmental licensure.

The idea behind institutional licensure is that the individual health-care institution will be permitted to determine which individuals are qualified to practice nursing within general guidelines established by an outside board. Although this type of licensure appeals to hospitals and nursing homes because it would allow them to hire individuals with less education at a reduced cost, it has some serious difficulties associated with it.

Probably the most critical problem is the lack of any external control to determine a minimal level of competency. The designations of RN and LPN/LVN would be virtually meaningless under institutional licensure. These nurses would not be under the control of a state **licensing board** and thus

What Do You Think?

Why would health-care institutions be in favor of institutional licensure? How would it affect health care either positively or negatively?

would not be held to the same **standards of practice** as other nurses who were licensed by the states. A second problem is that nurses who wished to move to a new place of employment would have to undergo whatever licensure procedure the new institution had established before being allowed to work there. Currently nurses who move from one state to another can obtain **licensure by endorsement** by having the state recognize their nursing license from the original state of licensure. This process is generally referred to as **reciprocity.**

CERTIFICATION

At first glance, not much difference may be seen between certification and licensure. Strictly defined, licensure can actually be considered a type of legal certification. In the more widely accepted use of the term, however, certification is a granting of credentials to indicate that an individual has achieved a level of ability higher than the minimal level of competency indicated by licensure.[3] As technology increases and the health-care environment becomes more complex and demanding, nurses are finding a need to increase their knowledge and skill levels beyond the essentials taught in their basic nursing courses. Certification acknowledges the attainment of increased knowledge and skills and provides nurses with a means to validate their own self-worth and competence.

Some certification also carries with it a legal status, like licensure; but in many cases certification merely indicates a specific professional status. The public, employers, and even nurses themselves have difficulty understanding what certification means. Another element that adds confu-

> " " *certification is a granting of credentials to indicate that an individual has achieved a level of ability higher than the minimal level of competency indicated by licensure*

sion to the understanding of the process of certification is that a large number of groups can offer certification. These are usually professional specialty groups like the National Association of Pediatric Nurse Associates and Practitioners (NAPNAP) and the American Association of Critical Care Nurses (AACN), but they can also be national organizations like the National League for Nursing (NLN) of the ANA.

Individual Certification

The most common type of certification is called individual certification. When a nurse has demonstrated that he or she has attained a certain level of ability above and beyond the basic level required for licensure in a defined area of practice, that nurse can become certified. Usually some type of written and practical examination is required to demonstrate this advanced level of skill. The American Nurses Credentialing Center (ANCC) offers certifications in more than 40 areas that are widely recognized. Almost all nurses with individual certification are required to maintain their skills and competencies through continuing education and a specified number of continuing education units (CEUs). Recertification may be achieved through CEUs or retaking of the certification examination.

Organizational Certification

Organizational certification is the certification of a group or health-care institution by some external agency. It is usually referred to as accreditation and indicates that the institution has met standards established by either the government or by a non-governmental agency. Often the ability of the institution to collect money from insurance companies or the federal government depends on whether or not the institution is certified by a recognized agency. Most hospitals are accredited by the Joint Commission on Accreditation of Healthcare Organizations (JCAHO) as a minimum level of accreditation.

Advanced Practice

Some state governments may either award or recognize certification granted to nurses in areas of advanced practice. In these cases, the certification becomes a legal requirement for practice at the APN level. Depending on the individual state's nurse practice act, nurses thus certified fall under regulations in the state's practice act that control the type of activities nurses may legally carry out when they perform advanced roles. For example, many states recognize the position of nurse **midwife** as an advanced practice role for nurses. In these states, a nurse midwife is allowed to practice those skills allowed under the nurse practice act of that state after obtaining certification. Generally nurse midwives are allowed to conduct prenatal examinations, do prenatal teaching, and deliver babies vaginally in uncomplicated pregnancies. They are not usually allowed to perform cesarean sections.

An independent certification center was proposed in 1978 to establish uniform criteria and standards and to oversee all certification activities. Although it would eliminate much of the current confusion about certification and would help with the legal recognition of advanced practice nurses, this proposal has not yet been acted upon because of opposition from physician and health-care administration groups.

Unfortunately, there is no uniformity among states in the recognition of certification of advanced practice nurses. Some states recognize almost all certifications and have provisions in their nurse practice acts to help guide these practices. Other states have very little legal recognition of certification levels and thus few guidelines for practice. This confusion may result from so many different organizations offering certification in different areas. In some advanced practice areas, like nurse practitioners, two or more organizations may offer certification for the same title. The certification standards vary from organization to organization, and the method of determining certification may also be different.

It is expected that advanced practice nurses will play a larger role in the rapidly evolving health-care system of the future. What that role will be depends on how well governmental organizations and the public understand the contributions practitioners can make as **primary care** providers. Without a uniform definition of this spe-

What Do You Think?

Think of some creative ways that advanced practice nurses can practice in the health-care system of the future.

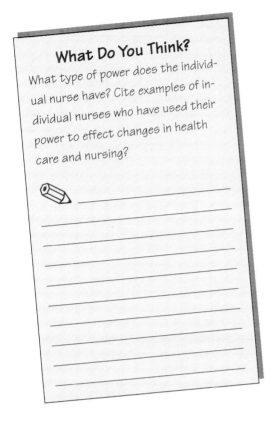

What Do You Think?

What type of power does the individual nurse have? Cite examples of individual nurses who have used their power to effect changes in health care and nursing?

cialty, such nurses will not be utilized to their full potential.

Licensure and certification are both methods of granting credentials to demonstrate that an individual is qualified to provide safe care to the public. Without proof of competency, the profession of nursing would become chaotic, disorganized, and even dangerous. It is important for nurses to keep a watchful eye on pending legislation and practices that health-care institutions are initiating. Many of these proposals and practices are covert ways of reintroducing permissive and institutional licensure.

NURSING ORGANIZATIONS AND THEIR IMPORTANCE

The establishment of a professional organization is one of the most important defining characteristics of a profession. Many professions have a single major professional organization to which most of its members belong and several specialized suborganizations that members may also join. Professions with just one major organization generally have a great deal of political power.

Nurses need and use power in every aspect of their professional lives, ranging from supervising nonlicensed personnel to negotiating with the administration for increased independence of practice. Clearly an individual nurse probably does not have much power, but for nurses as a group, the potential is increased exponentially by the organization. The dedication to high-quality nursing standards and improved methods of practice by the major nursing organizations have led to improved care and increased benefits to the public as a whole.

National nursing organizations need the participation and membership of all nurses in order to claim that they are truly representative of the profession. A large membership allows the organization to speak with one voice when making its values about health-care issues known to politicians, physicians groups, and the public in general.

The National League for Nursing

Purposes

The primary purpose of the National League for Nursing (NLN) is to maintain and improve the standards of nursing education. The NLN is also a strong force in community health nursing, occupational health nursing, and nursing service activities. Its bylaws state that its purpose is to foster the development and improvement of hospital, industrial, public health, and other organized nursing services and of nursing education through the coordinated action of nurses, allied professional groups, citizens, agencies, and schools so that the nursing needs of the people will be met.

Membership

Although membership is open to individual nurses, the primary membership in the NLN comes in the form of agency membership, usually through schools of nursing. One of the major functions of this organization, through the National League for Nursing Accrediting Commission (NLNAC), is to accredit schools of nursing through a self-study process. The schools are given a set of criteria or **essentials for accreditation** and are then required to evaluate their programs against these criteria. After the evaluation report is written and sent to the NLNAC, site representatives visit the school to verify the information in the report and see whether the school has met the criteria. If the school meets the evaluation criteria, it is accredited for up to 8 years. NLNAC accreditation of a school of nursing indicates that the school meets national standards. In some work settings, it is a requirement that a nurse be a graduate of an NLNAC-accredited school of nursing before the nurse can be hired or accepted into many master's level nursing programs.

Other Services

Other services and activities that the NLN carries out include testing, evaluating new graduate nurses, supplying career information and continuing education workshops and conferences for all levels of nursing, publishing a wide range of literature and videotapes covering current issues in health care, and compiling statistics about nursing, nurses, and nursing education.

American Association of Colleges of Nursing

Purposes

The American Association of Colleges of Nursing (AACN) was established to help col-

Site Seeing

Agency for Health Care Policy and Research (AHCPR)
http://www.ahcpr.gov/ info@ahcpr.gov

American Association of Colleges of Nursing
http://www.aacn.nche.edu/
Contact: mail to:webmaster@aacn.nche.edu

American Nurses Association
http://www.ana.org/
http://www.nursingworld.org/
Contact: mail to:webfeedback@ana.org

Canadian Nurses Association
http://www.cna-nurses.ca/
Contact: mail to:cna@cna-nurses.ca

National League for Nursing
http://www.nln.org/
Contact: mail to:nlnweb@nln.org

NURSE WWW Information Server
http://medsrv2.bham.ac.uk/nursing/
Contact: Denis Anthony
mail to:cudma@csv.warwick.ac.uk

Nursing NCLEX
http://www.kaplan.com:80/nclex/

Nursing Student WWW Page
http://www2.csn.net/~tbracket/htm.htm
Contact: Tim Brackett
mail to:Tim.Brackett@uchsc.edu

Student Nurse Information Center
http://glass.toledolink.com/~ornrsg/
Contact: mail to:ornrsg@toledolink.com

Sigma Theta Tau International Nursing Honor Society
http://stti-web.iupui.edu/
Contact: Waiping Kam
mail to:waiping@stti-sun.iupui.edu

leges with schools of nursing to work together to improve the standards for higher education for professional nursing. The AACN, through the Commission on Collegiate Nursing Education (CCNE), has developed standards for the accreditation of baccalaureate schools of nursing and is poised to become a major accreditation agency, competing with the NLNAC. The AACN has developed and published a set of guidelines for the education of professional nursing students that is widely used as the theoretical basis for baccalaureate curricula.

Membership

Only deans and directors of programs that offer baccalaureate or higher degrees in nursing with an upper-division nursing major are permitted membership.

American Nurses Association

Purposes

The American Nurses Association (ANA) grew out of a concern with the quality of nursing practice and the care that nurses were providing. The major purposes for the existence of the ANA, as stated in its by-laws, include improvement of the standards of health and the access to health-care ser-vices for everyone, improvement and maintenance of high standards for nursing practice, and promotion of the professional growth and development of all nurses, including economic issues, working conditions, and independence of practice.[4]

Membership

Membership in the ANA is limited to 52 constituents—50 state organizations and Washington, DC, and Puerto Rico. An individual joins a state organization and through the state organization indirectly is a member of ANA. Certain discounts in membership are offered for new members and new graduate nurses. Various levels of membership are available for nurses who work part-time or those who are retired. The ANA makes every effort to encourage individual nurses to join the organization. Unfortunately, most nurses do not belong to this potentially powerful, politically active, and very influential organization.

Each state has the opportunity to determine what is needed from each member to run the state association; the amount of the dues that is sent to ANA is predetermined. Although dues are not inexpensive (they change a little from year to year but are less than $200 per year), the ANA offers various plans for payment, such as three equal payments over the course of a year or monthly payroll deductions. Because of the efforts of the ANA, nurses' salaries have risen to a point where this sum is affordable.

Other Services

When nurses pursue advanced education and levels of practice, as many are doing today, the ANA ANCC is essential for testing and certification of many of these practice levels. Although other organizations offer advanced practice certification, without the ANCC, there would be even less standardization for and less recognition of these

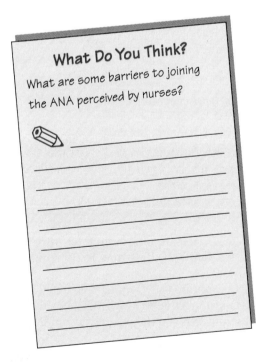

What Do You Think?

What are some barriers to joining the ANA perceived by nurses?

practitioners by the public, physicians, or lawmakers.

Another important issue that the ANA has been involved in is the entry-level education requirement for professional nurses. The ANA has supported the baccalaureate degree as the minimum educational requirement for nurses for the last 25 years. The ANA will be in the forefront of the debate over **entry into practice,** which will continue into the twenty-first century.

Additional functions carried out by the ANA include the establishment and continual updating of standards of nursing practice. These standards are the yardstick against which nurses are measured and held accountable by courts of **law.** The ANA also established the official code of ethics that guides professional practice.

Many of the political and economic activities of the ANA are carried out in the halls of legislatures and offices of legislators. The ANA Political Action Committee (PAC) is one of the most powerful in Washington, DC. (See Chapter 16 for more detailed discussion.) Such activities have a profound effect on the role that nurses play and will continue to play in health care well into the twenty-first century. Successful PAC activities require money and the power of a large, unified membership. The ANA-PAC seeks to influence legislation about nurses, nursing, and health care in general. It has been and will be a strong voice in the formulation of current national health-care reform.

Another important function of the ANA is economic. In many states, the ANA is the official **bargaining agent** for nurses in the negotiation of **contracts** with hospitals, nursing homes, and other health-care agencies that employ nurses. However, collective bargaining is done on a state-to-state basis—some states are **collective bargaining units** and others are not. (See Chapter 11 for more detailed discussion.) Professional organizations represent professional groups better than a labor union that has little knowledge of professional activities or needs.

The National Student Nurses' Association

Purposes

The National Student Nurses' Association (NSNA) is an independent legal corporation established in 1953 to represent the needs of nursing students. Working closely with the ANA, which offers services, an official publication, and close communication, the NSNA consists of state chapters that represent student nurses in those particular states.

The main purpose of the NSNA is to help maintain high standards of education in schools of nursing, with the ultimate goal of educating high-quality nurses who will provide excellent health care. Students' ideas, concerns, and needs are extremely important to nursing educators. Most nursing programs have committees in which students are asked to participate, including curriculum development and evaluation techniques. It is important that students belong to these committees and actively participate in the committees' activities.

Membership

Membership consists of all nursing students in registered nurse programs. Students can join at the local, state, or national level, or at all levels if desired. Dues are low, with a discount for the first year's membership.

Other Services

Additionally, the NSNA is concerned with developing and providing workshops, seminars, and conferences that deal with current issues in nursing and health care, with a wide range of subjects, from ethical and

What Do You Think?

What professional organizations do you belong to? Make two lists. The first list should contain advantages to belonging to the NSNA. The second list should cover disadvantages of belonging to the SNA. Which list is longer? Why?

1. Advantages

_____

_____

_____

_____

_____

_____

_____

2. Disadvantages

_____

_____

_____

_____

_____

_____

Many benefits exist for student nurses who belong to the NSNA. A number of scholarships are available through this organization to members of the NSNA. Members receive the official publication of the organization, *Imprint,* and the NSNA News, keeping the student nurse current on recent developments in health care and nursing. The student member also has political representation on issues that may affect the student now or in the future. Some of the issues include educational standards for practice, standards of professional practice, and health insurance. The NSNA is also concerned with the difficulty that many nursing students from minority groups experience in the educational process. The Breakthrough project is an attempt by the NSNA to help such students enter the profession of nursing.

Student nurses who join the NSNA experience firsthand the operation, activities, and benefits of a professional organization. In schools with active memberships, the NSNA can be a very exciting and useful organization for students. Many NSNA chapters are involved in community activities that provide services at a local level and allow the student to practice "real" nursing. These services include providing community health screening programs for hypertension, lead poisoning, vision, hearing, and birth defects; setting up information and education programs; giving immunizations; and working with groups concerned with drug abuse, child abuse, drunk driving, and teen pregnancy. All nursing students should be encouraged to belong to this organization.

The International Council of Nurses

Membership in the International Council of Nurses (ICN) consists of national nursing organizations, and it serves as the international organization for professional nursing. The ANA is one member among 104 nursing associations around the world. Each mem-

legal concerns to recent developments in pharmacology, test-taking skills, and professional growth. Student nurses who belong to the NSNA and who take an active part in its functions are much more likely to join the ANA after they graduate. Professional identity and professional behavior are learned. By beginning the process during the formal school years, student nurses develop professional attitudes and behaviors that they will continue for the rest of their lives.

ber nation sends delegates and participates in the international convention held every 4 years. The quadrennial conventions or congresses are open to all nurses and delegates from all nations.

The goal of the ICN is to improve health and nursing care throughout the world. The ICN coordinates its efforts with the United Nations and other international organizations when appropriate in the pursuit of its goal.

Some issues that have been the focus of concern by the ICN are social and economic welfare of nurses, the changing role of nurses in the present health-care environment, the challenges being faced by the various national nursing organizations, and how government and politics affect the nursing profession and health care. Overseeing the ICN is the Council of National Representatives. This body meets every 2 years and serves as the governing organization. ICN headquarters is located in Geneva, Switzerland.

Sigma Theta Tau

Sigma Theta Tau is an honorary organization that was established in colleges and universities to recognize those individuals who have demonstrated leadership or made important contributions to professional nursing. It is international in scope, and candidates are selected from among senior nursing students or graduate or practicing nurses.

The organization has its headquarters in Indianapolis, where it has a large library open to members to use for scholarly activities and research. It also boasts the first "on-line" nursing journal, which can be accessed by any nurse with a computer anywhere in the world. Local chapters of Sigma Theta Tau collect and distribute funds to nurses who are conducting **nursing research.** The organization also holds educational conferences and recognizes those who have made contributions to nursing.

Grassroots Organizations

A growing trend in contemporary nursing has been the formation of grassroots nursing organizations. In reality, all nursing organizations start as the grassroots efforts of local nursing groups who are trying to solve a particular problem. Over time, these small grassroots organizations become more structured, larger, and eventually become national or international when they spread to other areas across the country or world. Unfortunately, the large organizations tend to lose sight of the fundamental issues they were originally formed to solve, or they are unable to deal effectively with local problems.

Grassroots organizations usually have relatively small memberships; are localized to a town, city, or sometimes a state; and attempt to solve a problem or deal with an issue that the members feel is not being adequately handled by a large national organization. They may be created as a completely new and separate organization, or they may break away from a larger, established group. Because all the members of the grassroots organizations are passionately concerned about only one or two issues at a time that affect them directly, they tend to work hard to effect change and can bring a great deal of concentrated power to bear upon those, such as legislators, who make the decisions about the issues.

A number of techniques that are often frowned upon by the more established organizations are used by grassroots groups to attain their goals. In addition to the traditional techniques of writing letters, sending e-mail, and calling legislators, grassroots groups actively seek media attention, march on capitol buildings and state houses, introduce resolutions, and testify before committee hearings. Their success varies from issue to issue and location to location.

Two examples of successful grassroots efforts are found in California and Pennsylva-

BOX

2.3 Case Study

Juanita R., an RN at a large, inner-city hospital, has been working on her off-hours as a volunteer in a storefront clinic to treat the indigent and underserved population of that part of the city. The clinic clientele is primarily Mexican-American, as are the majority of the 20 nurses working at the clinic. Because all the nurses, including a family nurse practitioner, volunteer their time and receive no pay, the small private grant that Juanita had managed to secure was adequate to cover the cost for rental of the building, basic supplies for the clinic, and a few medications. However, the grant is about to run out and is nonrenewable.

Juanita first tried to obtain money from the hospital to keep the clinic going, but she was told that the hospital was having its own financial problems because of managed care demands and could not spare any money. At a staff meeting of the nurses from the clinic, the nurses decided to band together and form a grassroots organization called the Store-Front Clinic Nurses in order to focus their efforts on obtaining funds to keep the clinic open. They printed and passed out flyers, called local and city politicians, encouraged the patrons of the clinic to talk to people they knew, and even called the local television station for an interview about their plight.

Although most of the nurses' effort went unrewarded, a large pharmaceutical company became aware of their plight and wanted to provide a sizable financial stipend to the clinic, in addition to supplying free medications, for a period of at least 5 years. In addition to their philanthropic interests, the pharmaceutical company also wanted to gather long-term data about a newly developed antihypertensive medication. The company would provide the medication free to the clients at the clinic, the majority of whom had some degree of hypertension, and all the nurses would have to do is take and record the clients' blood pressure readings and complete "reported side effects" forms on each client. Client identifier codes, rather than

What Do You Think?

1. What are the main issues in this case study?

2. What ethical principles are being violated? What is the ethical dilemma that Juanita is facing?

3. Are there any other solutions to this problem?

names, would be used to maintain confidentiality. Juanita, as the group's coordinator, would be responsible for coordinating and preserving the data.

Although Juanita saw it as an answer to her prayers, she was concerned about the medication project. The pharmaceutical company said that no research consent forms were needed because the medica-

tion had already been through clinical trials and had received approval by the Food and Drug Administration. Juanita called another meeting of her nurses to discuss the issue. Without the grant, the clinic would close, but if they accepted the grant, they would have to participate in a medication research project that made Juanita feel uncomfortable.

---

nia. The California Nurses Association decided to break away from the American Nurses Association because it was not addressing some key state issues such as length of hospital stays, reduction in professional nursing staffs, and the preoccupation with profit of **managed care.** The grassroots group in Pennsylvania formed a completely new organization, the Nurses of Pennsylvania (NPA), and focused their energies on the trend to replace licensed registered nurses with unlicensed technicians, sometimes called "downskilling."

Special-Interest Organizations

The historical origins of special-interest organizations in nursing are even older than those of the main national organizations. For example, the Red Cross, established in 1864, is one of the oldest special-interest organizations that nurses have been involved with. Like the Red Cross, most specialty organizations in nursing were founded when a group of nurses with similar concerns sought professional and individual support. These organizations usually start out small and informal, then increase in size, structure, and membership over a number of years. There were relatively few of these organizations until 1965, when an explosion in specialty organizations in nursing took

place. During the next 20 years, almost 100 new organizations were formed, with the associated effect of diminishing membership levels in the ANA.

Specialty organizations are usually organized according to clinical practice area. Organizations exist for almost every clinical specialty and subspecialty known in nursing, such as obstetrics/gynecology, critical care, operating room, emergency room, and occupational health, to less known areas such as flight nurses, urology, and cosmetic surgery. Another focal area for these organizations is education and ethics (Box 2–3). Organizations such as American Association of Colleges of Nursing and the Western Interstate Commission for Higher Education fall into this category. Often organizations focus on the common **ethnic group,** cultural, or religious backgrounds of nurses. The National Association of Hispanic Nurses and the National Black Nurses Association represent this type of specialty organization.

Although many of these organizations promote the personal and professional growth of their membership, they also carry out many other activities. Particularly important among these activities is establishing the standards of practice for the particular specialty area. Much as the ANA establishes overall standards of practice for nursing in general, the specialty organizations establish standards for their particular clinical areas. Providing educational services for their members is another important activity of specialty organizations. Conferences, workshops, and seminars in the clinical area represented are important venues for nurses to keep current on new developments and to maintain high standards of practice.

How many of these specialty nursing organizations are there? No one really knows. Many such organizations are informal and run by volunteers. Organizations are continually being formed, while others are being disbanded. Should nurses belong to these organizations? The answer is yes, but only after they belong to the ANA. Many of the larger specialty organizations have recognized this fact and have established close ties with the ANA. The ANA, in its turn, is well aware of the membership bleed-off from the specialty organizations and has initiated efforts to become more involved in the specialty nursing areas.

Before nurses join a specialty organization, they should determine whether its purposes are at odds with those of the ANA. Many of the large specialty organizations have their own lobbyists in both state and national legislatures. Because the legislators really do not know the differences between the various nursing organizations, they can become easily confused over health-care issues if they are receiving pressure from two nursing groups representing opposing sides of the same issue. At this point, legislators may simply surmise that nurses really do not know what they want and vote on an important issue without regard to nurses and nursing.

Conclusion

Nursing, in its journey toward professionalism, has been propelled and shaped by its nursing organizations, which were the main vehicles for the development of educational and practice standards, initiation of licensure, promotion of advanced practice, and general improvement in the level of care nurses provided. From their beginnings, nursing organizations have served as channels of communication between nurses, consumers of health care, and other health-care professionals. In many cases, the nursing organizations have served as a focus of power for the profession to influence those important **health policies** that affect the whole nation. That continued unity is essential for the survival of nursing.

The tendency toward specialization has led to an ever-increasing number of nursing organizations, however, each focusing on a particular practice field within the profession. This trend has diluted the unity and ultimately lessened the power that nursing as a profession can exert in health-care issues. Although it is important to recognize the complexity of today's health-care system and the pluralism inherent in nursing, unity of opinion on major issues is essential if nursing is to have any influence on the future of the profession. The challenge for nurses in the future is to use the diversity in the profession as a positive force and to unite as a group on important issues. Awareness of earlier development of nursing organizations provides a perspective for the current situation and can act as a framework for planning the future.

Critical Thinking Exercises

✔ Develop a strategy for increasing the membership in the ANA.

✔ A labor union is attempting to organize the nurses at your hospital. Is it better for the professional nursing organization to represent the nurses? Why?

✔ A new graduate nurse is working in the intensive care unit (ICU) of a large hospital. She wants to join a nursing organization but only has a limited amount of money to spend. Her coworkers in the ICU want her to join the AACN, but she would also like to join the ANA. Basing her decision on economic and professional issues, which organization should she join?

✔ Compare and contrast certification and licensure. Should certification be legally recognized? Justify your answer.

References

1. Donahue, MP: Nursing: The Finest Art. CV Mosby, St. Louis, 1996.
2. McKinley, M: The power of our practice: Look to our roots. AACN News 15(9):2, 1998.
3. American Nurses Association: Nursing's social policy statement. ANA, Washington, DC, 1995.
4. American Academy of Nursing: The Evolution of Nursing Professional Organizations: Alternatives for the Future. ANA, Kansas City, 1987.

BIBLIOGRAPHY

American Nurses Association: Federation of Specialty Nursing Organizations and ANA—A History. ANA, Kansas City, 1980.

Bower, K: Case Management by Nurses. ANA, Washington, DC, 1992.

Christman, L: Opinion: Knowledge is power. Reflections 17:40, 1992.

Cristy, T: First fifty years. Am J Nurs 9:1778–1784, 1971.

De Tornyay, R: Reconsidering nursing education: The report of the Pew Health Professions Commission. J Nurs Educ 31:296–301, 1992.

Edmunds, MW: Council's pursuit of national standardization for advanced practice meets resistance. Nurse Pract 17:81–83, 1992.

Hoffman, S: Nurses must unify to bring change for patients and profession. American Nurse 29(6):5–7, 1997.

Joel, LA: Hungry for the truth. Am J Nurs 96(3): 23-28, 1996.

Maffeo, R: Divorcing the UAP: Heresy or solution? American Nurse 30(1):5, 1998.

Mohr, WK: Values, ideologies and dilemmas: Professional and occupational contradictions. J Psychosoc Nurs 33(1):29–34, 1995.

Moloney, M: Professionalization of Nursing: Current Issues and Trends. JB Lippincott, Philadelphia, 1992.

Munro, N: Public policy: A new paradigm grows from grass roots. Critical Care Nurse 18(5):76–85, 1998.

News. *National Council of State Boards of Nursing, Inc.,* Publication No. 132, August 25, 1997.

Nicoll, LH: Nurses' Guide to the Internet, ed 2. JB Lippincott, Philadelphia, 1998.

Stewart, M: Health care community faces the year 2000. American Nurse 29(6):24, 1997.

Sullivan, TJ: Collaboration: A Health Care Imperative. McGraw-Hill, New York, 1998.

Tanner, CA: Accreditation under siege. J Nurs Educ 35(6):243–244, 1996.

Trossman, S: Stepping onto the stage: RNs take on the role of political player. American Nurse 29(6):1–18, 1997.

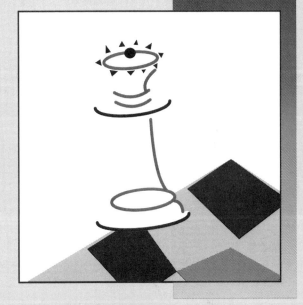

Theory and Education

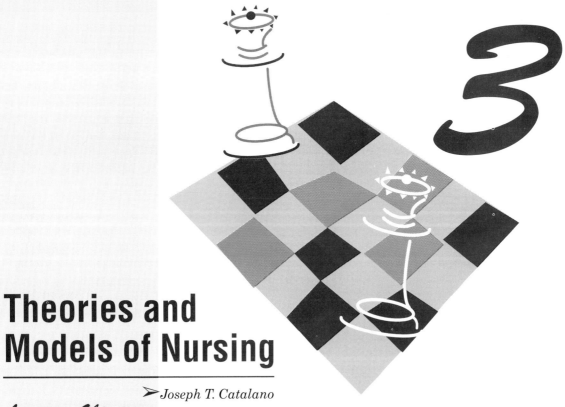

Theories and Models of Nursing

➤ *Joseph T. Catalano*

Learning Objectives

After completing this chapter, the reader will be able to:

1. Explain why theories and models are important to the profession of nursing.
2. Analyze the four key concepts found in nursing theories and models.
3. Interrelate systems theory as an important element in understanding nursing theories or models.
4. Evaluate how the four parts of all systems interact.
5. Synthesize three nursing theories, identifying how the different nursing theorists define the key concepts in their theories.

For many nurses, and for most nursing students, the terms *theory* and *model* evoke images of textbooks filled with abstract, obscure words and convoluted sentences. The visceral response is often "Why is this important, I want to take care of real people!" The simple answer is: Understanding and using nursing theories or models will help you to be a better nurse and provide better care to real people.

DIFFERENCES BETWEEN THEORY AND MODEL

Although the terms *theory* and *model* are not synonymous, in nursing practice they are often used interchangeably. Strictly speaking, a theory refers to a speculative statement involving some element of reality that has not been proved. For example, the theory of rela-

43

tivity has never been proved, although the results have often been observed. The nursing profession tends to use the term *theory* when attempting to explain apparent relationships between observed behaviors and their effects on a client's health. In this nursing context, the goal of a theory is to describe and explain a particular nursing action in order to make a **hypothesis** or predict its effect on a client's outcome, such as improved health or recovery from illness. For example, the action of turning an unresponsive client from side to side every 2 hours should help prevent skin breakdown and improve respiratory function.

A model, on the other hand, is a hypothetical representation of something that exists in reality. The purpose of a model is to attempt to explain a complex reality in a systematic and organized manner. For example, a hospital organizational chart is a model that attempts to demonstrate the interrelationships of the various levels of the hospital's administration.

Although a model tends to be more concrete than a theory, they both help explain and direct nursing actions. This ability, using a systematic and structured approach, is one of the key elements that raises nursing from a task-oriented job to the level of a real profession. With the use of a **conceptual model,** nurses can provide intelligent and thoughtful answers to the question "What do nurses do?" Consider this scenario:

Mr. X had surgery for intestinal cancer 4 days ago. He has a colostomy and needs to learn how to take care of it at home because he is going to be discharged from the hospital in 2 days. When the nurses attempt to teach him colostomy care, he looks away, makes sarcastic personal comments about the nurses, and generally displays a belligerent and hostile attitude.

Without an understanding of the underlying dynamics involved, the nurse's reactions to this client's behavior might be to become sarcastic and scold the client about his behavior or simply to minimize the amount of contact with him.[1] This type of response will not improve Mr. X's health status (Box 3–1). If the nurses knew, however, and understood the dynamics of the grief theory, they would realize that Mr. X was probably in the anger stage of the grief process. This understanding would direct the nurse to allow, or even to encourage, Mr. X to express his anger and **aggressiveness** without condemnation, and to help him deal with his feelings in a constructive manner. Once Mr. X gets past the anger stage, he can move on to taking a more active part in his care and thus improve his health status. The **client goals** would then be achieved.

If a researcher were to stop 10 people at random on the street and ask the question, "What do nurses do?", he or she would likely get 10 different answers. But the confusion about nurses' activities extends far beyond the public at large. What if the researcher asked 10 hospital administrators, 10 physicians, or even 10 nurses the same question? It could be anticipated that the answers would vary almost as much as the answers from lay people. In an attempt to identify what exactly it is that nurses do, McCloskey and Bulechek, two nurse researchers at the University of Iowa, have been conducting a research project since 1990 to develop a **taxonomy** of the **interventions** that nurses use in their practice. This research has been called Nursing Interventions Classification (NIC), the Iowa Interventions Project, or simply the Iowa Project.[2–5]

The first results, published in 1994, categorized and ranked 336 interventions that nurses use when they provide care to clients. A follow-up study was conducted about 2 years after the original and published in 1996. This study categorized and ranked 433 interventions used by nurses. A partial list

3.1 What Do Nurses Really Do?

At first glance, it would seem that everybody knows that nurses take care of clients. But what constitutes care? A study conducted by the faculty of the University of Iowa, called the Nursing Interventions Classification (NIC) or simply the Iowa Project, has identified 336 tasks or interventions that nurses are responsible for in their care of patients. Not all nurses carry out all 336 of these tasks all the time, but during an average career, a nurse would likely be involved in the majority of these tasks (see Closer Look Tables 3–1 and 3–2).

This project is an excellent example of how a nursing theory led to a research pro-ject that developed information that can be used by nurses in their daily practice. Based on the belief that nursing inter ventions are specific actions that a nurse can perform to bring about the resolution of a potential or actual health-care problem, the NIC attempted to identify and classify nursing interventions. It also attempted to rank those interventions according to the number of times a nurse was likely to perform one during a working day. The goal of the project was to develop a nursing information system that could be incorporated into the current information systems of all clinical facilities. By using the NIC system, hospital administrators,

A Closer Look Table 3.1	**Interventions Frequently Used by Individual Nurses**		
INTERVENTION	% WHO USE	INTERVENTION	% WHO USE
Several times a day		Teaching: procedure	26
Active listening	80	Presence	26
Medication administration	65	Mutual goal setting	25
Emotional support	64		
Infection control	62	**Weekly**	
Medication administration: parenteral	60	Diarrhea management	27
Medication administration: oral	59	Urinary catheterization	27
Touch	57	Referral	26
Positioning	57	Blood products administration	26
Analgesic administration	55	Fever treatment	25
Intravenous (IV) therapy	53		
Skin surveillance	53	**Monthly**	
Presence	53	Postmortem care	34
Pressure management	51	Dying care	33
		Culture brokerage	33
Daily		Seizure management	30
Hope instillation	32	Guilt work facilitation	30
Family involvement	31	Ostomy care	28
Decision-making support	30	Urinary retention care	26
Sleep enhancement	28	Spiritual support	25
Family mobilization	27	Seizure precautions	25
Teaching: disease process	27	Amputation care	25
Foot care	27	Wound irrigation	25
Family support	26		

3.1 What Do Nurses Really Do? *(continued)*

physicians, nurses, and even the public should be better able to recognize and evaluate the multiple interventions that nurses are responsible for in their daily work.

It is a generally acknowledged fact that nurses, as the largest single group of health-care providers, are essential to the welfare and care of most clients. Yet, in an age of health-care reform, nurses are finding it increasingly difficult to delineate the specific contributions they make to health care. And if nurses themselves are unable

A Closer Look
Table 3.2 — Interventions with Highest Use Rates

INTERVENTION	% WHO USE	INTERVENTION	% WHO USE
Survey of Organizations (n = 28)		Medication management	90
Active listening*	100	Teaching: procedure/treatment*	90
Referral	100	Anxiety reduction	90
Limit setting	97	Calming technique	90
Communication enhancement	97	Simple relaxation therapy	90
Emotional support*	97	Infection protection	90
Support system enhancement	97	Vital signs monitoring*	90
Discharge planning	97	Intravenous (IV) insertion	90
Health system guidance	97	IV therapy	90
Patient rights protection	97		
Teaching: disease process*	97	Survey of Individuals (n = 277)	
Health screening	97	Emotional support	98
Risk identification	97	Presence	98
Coping enhancement	93	Active listening	97
Counseling*	93	Decision-making support	94
Decision-making support	93	Hope instillation	92
Hope instillation	93	Family involvement	92
Touch	93	Coping enhancement	91
Family involvement	93	Teaching: disease process	91
Medication administration: parenteral	93	Anxiety reduction	91
Teaching: prescribed medication	93	Communication enhancement	91
Teaching: individual*	93	Teaching: prescribed medication	90
Environmental management	93	Touch	90
Environmental management: safety	93	Infection control	90
Infection control*	93	Counseling	88
Specimen management	93	Environmental management: safety	87
Self-responsibility facilitation	90	Teaching: individual	87
Humor	90	Vital signs monitoring	87
Values clarification	90	Humor	86
Caregiver support*	90	Infection protection	86
Admission care	90	Environmental management: comfort	85
Analgesic administration*	90	Pain management	85
Medication administration	90	Security enhancement	85
Medication administration: oral	90	Discharge planning	85
Medication administration: topical	90		

*These interventions, along with pain management, airway management, and nutrition management, were reported most often among all reporting organizations. Taken together, they represent core interventions across nursing specialties.

to define the care they provide, how are the reformers, politicians, and even the public going to be able to identify the unique contribution made by nursing?

Unfortunately, many of the contributions that nurses make to health care are currently invisible because there is no method of classification for them in computerized database systems now in use. Commonly used nursing interventions such as active listening, emotional support, touch, skin surveillance, or even family support cannot be measured and quantified by most current information systems.

The large number of different interventions used daily by nurses demonstrates the complex and demanding nature of the profession. The breadth and depth of knowledge and skills demanded of nurses on a daily basis is much greater than is found in many other health-care professions.

One study found that nurses working in general medical/surgical units during a 6-month period were likely to care for 500 clients with more than 600 individual diagnoses (many clients have multiple diagnoses). These researchers also found that the physical demands of the work were actually less difficult and tiring than dealing with the emotional and technical demands of handling the huge amounts of information generated by the care given.

From McCloskey, JC, and Grace, CK: Current issues in nursing, ed 5. Mosby–Year Book, St. Louis, 1997; and Bulechek, GM, et al: Nursing interventions used in nursing practice. Am J Nurs 94(10):59–61, 1994.

is found in Closer Look Table 3–1. McCloskey and Bulechek[6] also investigated what nursing interventions were commonly used by nurses in specialty settings. Forty specialty areas responded, and the researchers were able to develop a table that lists what core skills are used by each organization. This type of research helps identify the important contributions made by nursing to the health and well-being of clients. It also demonstrates the complex and demanding nature of the nursing profession.

KEY CONCEPTS COMMON TO NURSING MODELS

Although nursing models vary in terminology and approach to health care, there are four **concepts** that are common to almost all of them: client or patient (individual or collective), health, environment, and nursing. Each nursing model has its own specific definition of these terms, but the underlying definitions of the concepts are similar.

Client

The concept of client (or patient) is central to all nursing models, because it is the client who is the primary recipient of nursing care. Although the term *client* is usually used to refer to a single individual, it can also refer to small groups or to a large collective of individuals (for community health nurses, the community is the client).

The concept of client has changed over the years as the knowledge and understanding of human nature developed and increased. A client constitutes more than a person who simply needs **restorative care** and comes to a health-care facility with a

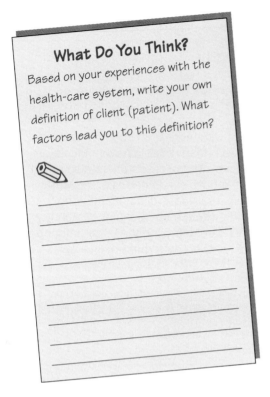

What Do You Think?

Based on your experiences with the health-care system, write your own definition of client (patient). What factors lead you to this definition?

disease to be cured. Clients are now seen as complex entities affected by various interrelating factors, such as the mind and body, the individual and the environment, and the person and the person's family. When nurses talk about clients, the term *biopsychosocial* is often used to express the complex relationship between the body, mind, and **environment.**

A client, in many of the nursing models, does not have to have an illness in order to be the central element of the model (this explains the current preference of using the term *client* over the term *patient*). This is also one of the clearest distinctions between medical models and nursing models. Medical models tend to be restrictive and are almost exclusively devoted to curing diseases and to restoring health. Nursing models tend to be **holistic;** they are concerned with curing disease and restoring a client's health, but they also focus on prevention of disease and maintenance of health. A healthy person is just as important to many nursing models as the person with a disease.

Health

Like the concept of client, the concept of health has undergone much development and change over the years as knowledge has increased. Originally thought of as an absence of disease, a more current realistic view is that of health as a continuum, ranging from a completely healthy state where there is no disease to a completely unhealthy state, which results in death. At any given time in their lives, everyone is located somewhere along the health continuum and may move closer to one side or the other depending on circumstances and health status.[7]

Health is difficult to define because it varies so much from one individual to another. For example, a 22-year-old bodybuilder who has no chronic diseases perceives health differently than an 85-year-old who has diabetes, congestive heart failure, and vision problems. The perception of health also varies from one culture to another and at different historical periods within the same culture. In some past cultures, a sign of health was pure white skin, whereas in the modern American culture, a dark bronze suntan has been more desirable as a sign of health, although there is an increasing recognition of the harmful effects of ultraviolet light on the skin.

Environment

The concept of environment is another element in most current nursing models. Nursing models often broaden the concept of environment from the simple physical environment to include elements such as living conditions, public sanitation, and air and water quality. Factors such as interpersonal relationships and social interactions are also included.

Some internal environmental factors that affect health include the personal psychological processes, religious beliefs, sexual orientation, personality, and emotional responses. It has long been known that individuals who are highly self-motivated and internally goal directed (i.e., type A personality) tend to develop ulcers and have myocardial infarctions at a higher rate than the general population.[1] Medical models, which are primarily illness oriented, although acknowledging this factor, may not consider it to be treatable. Nursing models that consider personality as one of the environmental factors that affect health are more likely to attempt to modify the individual's behavior (internal environment) to decrease the risk of disease.

Like the other key concepts found in nursing models, the concept of environment is used so that it is consistent within a particular model's overall context. Nursing models try to show how various aspects of environment interrelate and how they affect the client's health status. In addition, nursing models treat environment as an active element in the overall health-care system and assert that positive alterations in the environment will improve the client's health status.

Nursing

The culminating concept in all the various nursing models is nursing itself. After consideration of what it means to be a client, what it means to be healthy, and how the environment influences the client's health status either positively or negatively, the concept of nursing delineates the function and role nurses have in their relationship with clients. Historically, the profession of nursing has been interested in providing

What Do You Think?

Do you consider yourself to be healthy? What factors make you healthy? What factors are indicators of illness?

basic physical care (i.e., hygiene, activity, nourishment), psychological support, and relief of discomfort for clients. But modern nursing, although still including these basic elements of client care, has expanded into areas of health care that were only imagined a generation ago.

In the modern nurse-client relationship, the client is no longer the passive recipient of nursing care. The relationship has been expanded to include clients as key partners in curing and in the health maintenance process. In conjunction with the nurse, clients set goals for care and recovery, take

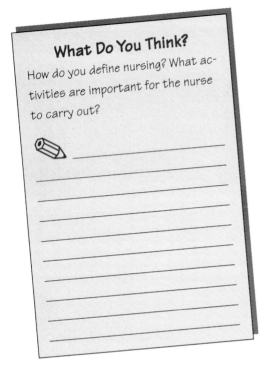

What Do You Think?

How do you define nursing? What activities are important for the nurse to carry out?

an active part in achieving those goals, and help in evaluating whether or not those actions have achieved the goals.[8]

Because of the broadened understanding of environment, several nursing models include manipulation of environmental elements that affect health as an important part of the nurse's role. The environment may be directly altered by the nurse with little or no input from the client, or the client may be taught by the nurse to alter the environment in ways that will contribute to curing disease, increasing comfort, or improving the client's health status.[9]

To analyze and understand any nursing model, it is important to look for these four key concepts: client, health, environment, and nursing. These concepts should be clearly defined, closely interrelated, and mutually supportive. Depending on the particular nursing model, one element may be emphasized more than another. The resultant role and function of the nurse depend on which element is given greater emphasis.

GENERAL SYSTEMS THEORY

A widely accepted method for conceptualizing and understanding the world and what is in it is derived from a systems viewpoint. Generally understood as an organized unit with a set of components that interact and affect each other, a system acts as a whole because of the interdependence of its parts.[10] As a result, when part of the system malfunctions or fails, it interrupts the function of the whole system rather than affecting merely one part. Humans, plants, cars, governments, the health-care system, the profession of nursing, and almost anything that exists can be viewed as a system. The terminology and principles of systems theory pervade American society.

Although general systems theory in its pure form is rarely, if ever, used as a nursing model, its process and much of its terminology underlie many nursing models. Elements of general systems theory in one form or another have found their way into many textbooks and much of the professional literature. General systems theory often acts as the unacknowledged **conceptual framework** for many educational programs. An understanding of the mechanisms and terminology of general systems theory is helpful in providing an orientation to understanding nursing models.

General systems theory, sometimes referred to simply as **systems theory,** is an outgrowth of an innate intellectual process. The human mind has difficulty comprehending large, complex entities as a single unit. As a result, the mind automatically divides that entity into smaller, more manageable fragments and then examines each fragment separately. This is similar to the process of deductive reasoning, in which a single complex thought or theory is broken down into smaller, interrelated pieces. All scientific disciplines, from physics to biology and social sciences (e.g., sociology and psychology), use this method of analysis.

Systems theory, however, takes the process a step further. After analyzing or breaking down the entity, systems theory attempts to put it back together by showing how the parts work individually and together within the system. This interrelationship of the parts makes the system function as a unit. And often, particularly where the system involves biologic or sociologic entities, the system that results is greater than the sum of its parts. For example, a human can be considered to be a complex, biosocial system. Humans are made up of a large number of smaller systems such as the endocrine system, neurologic system, gastrointestinal system, urinary system, and so forth. Although each of these systems is important, in and of themselves they do not make a human. Many animals have the same systems, yet the human is more than the animal and more than the sum of the systems.

Although the early roots of general systems theory can be traced as far back as the 1930s, von Bertalanffy is usually credited with the formal development and publication of general systems theory around 1950.[11] His major achievement was to standardize the definitions of the terms used in systems theory and make the concept useful to a wide range of disciplines. Systems theory is so widely applicable because it reflects the reality that underlies the basic human thought processes.

Very simply, a system is defined as a set of interacting parts. The parts that compose a system may be similar or they may vary a great deal from each other, but they all have the common function of making the system work well to achieve its overall purpose. A school is a good example of how the dynamics and interrelatedness of a system work. A school as a system consists of a large number of units including buildings, administrators, teachers, students, and various other individuals (e.g., counselors, financial aid personnel, bookkeepers, and maintenance persons). Each of these individuals has a unique job but also contributes to the overall goal of the school, which is to provide an education for the students and also to further the development of knowledge through research.

All systems consist of four key parts: the system itself (i.e., whether an **open system** or a **closed system**); **input** and **output; throughput;** and a **feedback** loop.

Open and Closed Systems

A system is categorized as either being open or closed. In reality, very few systems are completely open or completely closed. Rather, they are usually a combination of both open and closed systems.

Open systems are those in which relatively free movement of information, matter, and **energy** into and out of the system exists. In a completely open system there would be no restrictions on what moves in and out of the system, thus making its boundaries difficult to identify. Most systems have some control on the movement of information, energy, and matter around them. This control is maintained through the semipermeable nature of their boundaries, which allows some things in and keeps some things out as well as allowing some out while keeping others in. This control on input and output leads to the dynamic equilibrium found in most well-functioning systems.

Theoretically, a closed system prevents any movement into and out of the system. In this case, the system would be totally static and unchanging. Probably no absolutely closed systems exist in the real world, although there are systems that may tend to be closed to outside elements. A stone, for example, considered as a system, seems to be very nearly a perfectly closed system. It does not take anything in or put anything out. It does not change very much over long periods. In reality, though, it is affected by a number of elements in nature. It absorbs moisture when it is damp, freezes when cold, and becomes hot in the summer. Over long periods, these factors may cause the stone to crack, break down, and eventually become topsoil.

Systems that nurses deal with frequently are relatively open. Primarily, the client can be categorized as a highly open system that requires certain input elements and has output elements also. Other systems that nurses commonly work with (e.g., hospital administrators and physicians) are generally considered to be open systems, although their degree of openness may vary widely.

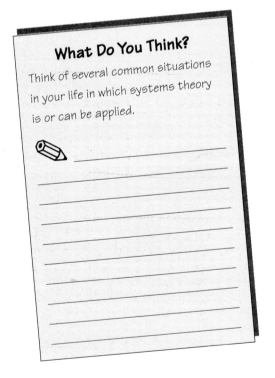

What Do You Think?

Think of several common situations in your life in which systems theory is or can be applied.

Input and Output

The processes by which a system interacts with elements in its environment are called input and output. Input is defined as any type of information, energy, or material that enters the system from the environment through its boundaries. Conversely, output is defined as any information, energy, or material that leaves the system and enters the environment through the system's boundaries. The **end product** of a system is a type of output that is not reusable as input. Open systems require relatively large amounts of input and output.

Throughput

A third term, sometimes used in relationship to the system's dynamic exchange with the environment, is throughput. Throughput is a process that allows the input to be changed so that it is useful to the system. For example, most automobiles operate on some form of liquid fossil fuel (input) such as gasoline or diesel. However, going to the gas station and pouring liquid fuel on the roof of the car will not produce the effects desired when most people buy fuel for their cars. But if the fuel is put into the gas tank, it can be transformed by the carburetor or fuel injection system into a fine mist, which when mixed with air and ignited by a spark plug burns rapidly to produce the force necessary to propel the car. Without this internal process (throughput) found in the car, liquid fuel is not a useful form of energy.

Feedback Loop

The fourth key element of a system is the feedback loop. The feedback loop allows the system to monitor its internal functioning so that it can either restrict or increase its input and its output and maintain the highest level of functioning.

Two basic types of feedback exist. Positive feedback leads to change within the system, with the goal of improving the system. Students in the classroom, for example, receive feedback from the teacher in several ways; it may be in the form of direct verbal statements such as "good work on this assignment" or feedback by examination and homework grades.

Feedback is considered positive if it produces a change in student's behavior, such as motivating him or her to study more, spending more time on assignments, or preparing more thoroughly for class. Negative feedback maintains stability; that is, it does not produce change. Negative feedback is not necessarily bad for a system. Rather, when a system has reached its peak level of functioning, negative feedback helps it maintain that level. For example, an athlete who has reached his or her peak level of performance through long hours of practice knows what type of practice is required to stay at that level of ability. Negative feedback, in the form of optimal times in the case of runners or number of pounds lifted in the case of weightlifters, indicates that no changes in practice patterns are required.

> **" "** *Positive feedback leads to change within the system, with the goal of improving the system.*

The feedback loop is an important element in systems theory. It makes the process circular and links the various elements of the system together. Without a feedback loop, it is virtually impossible for the system to have any meaningful control over its input and output.

Feedback loops are used at all levels in a hospital. Nurses get feedback about the care that they provide both from clients and from their supervisors. The hospital administration gets feedback from clients and accrediting agencies. Physicians get feedback from clients, nurses, and the hospital administration. Systems theory is present, if sometimes unseen, in almost all health-care settings. Professional nurses need to be able to understand and identify the components of systems theory when they are encountered to improve their nursing practice and quality of care.

MAJOR NURSING THEORIES AND MODELS

At least 15 published nursing models (or theories) have been used to direct nursing education and nursing care.[12] The six nursing models discussed here (Table 3–1) have been selected because they are the most widely accepted and are good examples of how the concepts of client, health, environment, and nursing are used to explain and guide nursing actions. Discussion of these theories is not intended to be exhaustive, but rather to provide an overview of the main concepts of the **nurse theorist.** It is important to understand the terms used in the theories as defined by their authors and to see the interrelationship between the elements in each theory as well as the similarities and differences among the various different models.

The Roy Adaptation Model

As developed by Sister Callista Roy, the Roy Adaptation Model of nursing is very closely related to systems theory.[13] The main **goal** of this model is to allow the client to reach his or her highest level of functioning through **adaptation.**

Client

The central element in the Roy Adaptation Model is man (a generic term referring to

ISSUES IN PRACTICE

Looking to the Future—The Pew Report

As the profession of nursing enters the new millennium, the employment sooth-sayers are unable to agree on projections of how many nurses will be required to keep the health-care system running smoothly nor where in the health-care system nurses will be needed. Consider the following data collected by the U.S. Bureau of the Census Current Population Survey, Division of Nursing, the Pew Commission, and the Buerhaus and Staiger data collection agency:

- RN employment growth has been flat for the past 5 years. (1993–1998)
- LPN employment has decreased during the same period. (1993–1998)
- RN wage growth has decreased during the past 5 years.
- LPN wage growth has increased during the same period.
- RN unemployment rate is less than 2%.
- LPN unemployment rate is less than 3%.
- The majority of RNs (60%) are employed in hospitals, but is less than 5 years ago. (1993)
- States with well-developed managed care systems have fewer RNs employed in the hospital setting, more employed in home health care.
- UAP employment has increased markedly during the past 3 years in all states and in all employment areas. (1995–1998)
- Nursing school enrollments have decreased during the past 2 years. (1995–1998)
- There are more than 2.5 million RNs in the United States; 83% are actively employed in nursing.
- RN average age is 44.3 years.
- 10% of RNs are from minority groups.
- 42.1% of RNs have a BS or higher degree (32% BSN; 9.5% MSN; 0.6% PhD)
- Projected graduates from nursing schools through the year 2020 will remain approximately the same, with the majority graduating from associate degree programs.

What conclusions can be drawn from these data as a predictor for the nursing profession into the twenty-first century? The answer seems to depend on whether the prophet is a true believer in supply side or demand side economics.

The supply side prophets project that there will be a severe nursing shortage during the next 10 to 20 years and a need for as many as 300,000 more RNs. They base this projection on the declining nursing school enrollment numbers and the increasing age of the current pool of registered nurses.

Demand side prophets take a much different view of the employment situation for nurses in the twenty-first century. Based on projected market needs, population characteristics, technology, income, and the movement toward managed care, they have taken the position that the health-care market will not be willing to pay for more RNs and therefore will replace them with LPNs and UAPs. Overall, by the year 2020, demand siders predict an excess of RNs and declining salaries.

Regardless of the approach used to project the future for professional nursing, there are many critical questions regarding both nursing and health care that need to be answered.

- How will the profession deal with the projected nursing shortage or surplus?
- How will the profession increase the number of graduates with BSN degrees?
- How can nursing be reconfigured in a market-driven health-care environment?
- Will nursing graduates be prepared to practice in evolving health-care settings and systems?

From Rice, B: CIC work in year 2: Data gathering, analysis, and work force modeling. Colleagues in Caring Newsletter, October 1997, p. 3–9 Buerhaus, P: Is another RN shortage looming? Nurs Outlook 46(3):103–108, 1998; and de Tornyay, R: Reconsidering nursing education: The report of the Pew Health Professions Commission. J Nurs Educ 13:296–301, 1992.

humans in general, or the client in particular, collectively or individually). Man is viewed as a dynamic entity with both input and output. As derived from the context of the four modes in the Roy Adaptation Model, the client is defined as a biopsychosocial being who is affected by various stimuli and displays behaviors to help adapt to the stimuli. Because the client is constantly being affected by stimuli, adaptation is a continual process.[13]

Input are called stimuli and include internal stimuli that arise from within the client's environment as well as stimuli coming from external environmental factors such as physical surroundings, family, and society. The output in the Roy Adaptation Model is the behavior that the client demonstrates as a result of stimuli that are affecting him or her.

Output, or behavior, is a very important element in the Roy Adaptation Model, because it provides the **baseline data** about the client that the nurse obtains through assessment techniques. In this model, the output (behavior) is always modified by the client's internal attempts to adapt to the input, or stimuli. Roy has identified four internal adaptational activities that clients use and has called them the four adaptation modes: (1) the physiologic mode (using internal physiologic process), (2) the self-concept mode (developed throughout life by experience), (3) the role function mode (dependent on the client's relative place in society), and (4) the interdependence mode (indicating how the client relates to others).

Health

In the Roy Adaptation Model, the concept of health is defined as the location of the client along a continuum between perfect health and complete illness. Health, in this

Table 3.3 Comparison of Selected Nursing Models

NURSING THEORY	CLIENT	HEALTH	ENVIRONMENT	NURSING
Roy Adaptation Model	Man—as a dynamic system with input and output	A continuum—the ability to adapt successfully to illness	Both internal and external stimuli that affect behaviors	Multistep process that helps the client adapt and reach the highest level of functioning
Orem Self-Care Model	Humans—biologic, psychologic social beings with the ability for self-care	Ability to live life to the fullest through self-care	The medium through which the client moves	Helping the client achieve health through assistance in self-care activities
King Model of Goal Attainment	Person—exchanges energy and information with the environment to meet needs	Dynamic process to achieve the highest level of functioning	Personal, interpersonal, and social systems and the external physical world	Dynamic process to identify and meet the health care needs of the person
Watson Model of Human Caring	Individual—has needs, grows, and develops to reach a state of inner harmony	Dynamic state of growth and development leading to full potential as a human being	Those factors the client must overcome to achieve health	Science of caring that helps clients reach their greatest potential
Johnson Behavioral System Model	Person—a behavioral system that is an organized and integrated whole composed of seven subsystems	A balanced and steady state within the behavioral system of the client	All those internal and external elements that affect client behavior	Activities that manipulate the environment and help clients achieve the balanced state of health
Newman Health Care Systems Model	An open system that constantly interacts with internal and external environment	Relatively stable internal functioning of the individual in a high state of wellness (stability)	Internal and external stressors that produce change in the client	Identifies boundary disruption and helps clients in activities to restore stability

model, is rarely an absolute. Rather, "a person's ability to adapt to stimuli, such as injury, disease, or even psychological stress, determines the level of that person's health status." For example, a client who was in an automobile accident, had a broken neck, and was paralyzed but who eventually went back to college, obtained a law degree, and became a practicing lawyer would, in the Roy Adaptation Model, be considered to have a high degree of health because of the ability to adapt to the stimuli imposed.

Environment

The Roy Adaptation Model's definition of environment is synonymous with the concept of stimuli. The environment consists of all those factors that influence the client's behavior, either internally or externally. This model categorizes these environmental elements, or stimuli, into three groups: (1) focal, (2) contextual, and (3) residual.

Focal stimuli are environmental factors that most directly affect the client's behavior and require most of his or her attention. Contextual stimuli form the general physical, social, and psychological environment from which the client emerges. Residual stimuli are factors in the client's past, such as personality characteristics, past experiences, religious beliefs, and social norms that have an indirect effect on the client's health status. Residual stimuli are often very difficult to identify because they may remain hidden in the person's past memory or may be an integral part of the client's personality.

Nursing

In the Roy Adaptation Model, nursing becomes a multistep process, similar to the **nursing process,** to aid and support the client in the attempt to adapt to stimuli in one or more of the four adaptive modes. To determine what type of help is required to promote adaptation, the nurse must first assess the client. The primary **nursing assessments** are of the client's behavior (output). Basically, the nurse should try to determine whether the client's behavior is adaptive or maladaptive in each of the four adaptational modes previously defined. Some first-level assessments of the pneumonia client might include a temperature of 104°F, a cough productive of thick green sputum, chest pain on inspiration, and signs of weakness or physical debility, such as the inability to bring in wood for the fireplace or to visit friends.

A second-level assessment should also be made to determine what type of stimuli (input) are affecting the client's health care status. In the case of the client with pneumonia, this might include a culture and sensitivity of the sputum to identify the invasive bacteria, assessment of the client's clothes to determine whether they were adequate for the weather outside, and an investigation to find out whether any neighbors could help the client when he or she is discharged from the hospital.

After performing the assessment, the nurse analyzes the data and arranges them in such a way so as to be able to make a statement about the client's adaptive or maladaptive behaviors, that is, identifies the problem. In current terminology, this identification of the problem is called a **nursing diagnosis.**

After the problem has been identified, goals for optimal adaptation are established. Ideally, these goals should be a collaborative effort between the nurse and the client. A determination of the actions that need to be taken to achieve the goals is the next step in the process. The focus should be on manipulation of the stimuli to promote optimal adaptation. Finally, an evaluation is made of the whole process to evaluate whether the goals have been met. If the goals have not been met, the nurse must then determine why, not how, the activities should be modified to achieve the goals.[11]

The Orem Self-Care Model

Dorothea E. Orem's model of nursing is based on the belief that health care is each individual's own responsibility. The model is aimed at helping clients direct and carry out activities that either help maintain or improve their health.[14]

Client

As with most other nursing models, the central element of the Orem model is the client who is a biologic, psychological, and social being with the capacity for self-care. Self-care is defined as the practice of activities that individuals initiate and perform on their own behalf to maintain life, health, and well-being. Self-care is a requirement both for maintenance of life and for optimal functioning.

Health

In the Orem Self-Care Model, health is defined as the person's ability to live fully within a particular physical, biologic, and social environment, achieving a higher level of functioning that distinguishes the person from lower life forms. Quality of life is an extremely important element in this model of nursing. A person who is healthy is living life to the fullest and has the capacity to maintain that life through self-care. An unhealthy person is an individual who has a self-care deficit. This deficit is indicated by the inability to carry out one or more of the key health-care activities. These activities have been categorized into six groups: (1) air, water, and food; (2) excretion of waste; (3) activity and rest; (4) solitude and social interactions; (5) hazards to life and well-being; and (6) being normal mentally under universal self-care. This group of unhealthy individuals also includes adults with diseases and injuries, young and dependent children, the elderly, and the disabled.

Universal Self-Care

In the Orem model, self-care is a two-part concept. The first type of self-care is called universal self-care and includes those elements commonly found in everyday life that support and encourage normal human growth, development, and functioning. Persons who are healthy, according to the Orem Model, carry out the activities listed in order to maintain a state of health. To some degree, all these elements are necessary activities in maintaining health through self-care.[15]

The second type of self-care comes into play when the individual is unable to conduct one or more of the six self-care activities. This second type of self-care is called health deviation self-care. Health deviation self-care includes those activities carried out by individuals who have diseases, injuries, physiologic or psychological stress, or other health-care concerns. Activities such as seeking health care at an emergency room or clinic, entering a drug **rehabilitation** unit, joining a health club or weight control program, or going to a physician's office fall into this category.

Environment

Environment, in the self-care model, is the medium through which clients move as they conduct their daily activities. Although less emphasized in this model, the environment is generally viewed as a negative factor on a person's health status because many environmental factors detract from the ability to provide self-care. Environment includes social interactions with others, situations that

Nursing

The primary goal of nursing in the Orem model is to help the client conduct self-care activities in such a way as to reach the highest level of human functioning. Because there is a range of levels of self-care ability, three distinct levels, or systems, of nursing care are delineated, based on the individual's ability to undertake self-care activities. As clients become less able to care for themselves, their nursing care needs increase.

A person who is able to carry out few or no self-care activities falls into the wholly compensated nursing care category in which the nurse must provide for most or all of the client's self-care needs. Examples of clients who require this level of care include comatose and ventilator-dependent clients in an intensive care unit, clients in surgery and the immediate recovery period, women in the labor and delivery phases of child birth, and clients with emotional and psychological problems so severe as to render them unable to conduct normal activities of daily living.

Clients in the partially compensatory category of nursing care can meet some to most of their own self-care needs, but still have certain self-care deficits that require nursing intervention. The nurse's role becomes one of identifying these needs and carrying out activities to meet them until the client reaches a state of health and is able to meet the needs personally. Examples of this level of nursing care include the postoperative client who can feed himself and do basic activities of daily living (ADLs) but is unable to care for his or her catheter and dressings, or a client with newly diagnosed diabetes who has not yet learned the technique of self-administered insulin injections.

Clients who are able to meet all of their basic self-care needs require very little or no nursing interventions. These clients are recipients of the supportive developmental category of nursing care, in which the nurse's main functions are to teach the client how to maintain or improve health and to offer guidance in self-care activities and provide emotional support and encouragement. Also, the nurse may adjust the environment to support the client's growth and development toward self-care or may identify community resources to help in the self-care process. Conducting prenatal classes, arranging for discharge planning, providing child screening programs through a community health agency, and organizing aerobic exercise classes for postcoronary clients all are nursing actions that belong in the supportive developmental category of care.

Nursing care is carried out through a three-step process in the Orem model. Step 1 determines whether nursing care is needed. This step includes a basic assessment of the client and identification of self-care problems and needs. Step 2 determines the appropriate nursing care system category and plans nursing care according to that category. Step 3 provides the indicated nursing care or actions to meet the client's self-care needs.

Five Methods

In the Orem model, step 3, the provision of nursing care (**implementation** phase), is carried out by helping the client through one or a combination of five nursing meth-

> " " *The primary goal of nursing in the Orem model is to help the client conduct self-care activities in such a way as to reach the highest level of human functioning.*

ods:[12] (1) acting for or doing for another person; (2) guiding another person; (3) supporting another person (physically or psychologically); (4) providing an environment that promotes personal development; and (5) teaching another person.

The King Model of Goal Attainment

The current widely accepted practice of establishing health-care goals for clients, and directing client care to meet these goals, has its origins in the King Model of Goal Attainment developed by Imogene M. King. It is also called the King Intervention Model.[16]

The King model also noted that nursing must function in all three system levels found in the environment: personal, interactional, and social. The primary function of nursing is at the personal systems level, whereby care of the individual is the main focus. However, nurses can effectively provide care at the interactional systems level, at which they deal with small- to moderate-sized groups in activities such as group therapy and in health promotion classes. Finally, nurses can provide care at the social systems level through activities such as programs in community health. In addition, the role of nursing at the social systems level can be expanded to include involvement in policy decisions that have an effect on the health-care system as a whole.

Client

As in other nursing models, the focal point of care in the King model is the person or client. The client is viewed as an open system that exchanges energy and information with the environment, a personal system with physical, emotional, and intellectual needs that change and grow during the course of life. Because these needs cannot be met completely by the client alone, interpersonal systems are developed through interactions with others depending on the client's perceptions of reality, communications with others, and transactions to reduce stress and tension in the environment.

Environment

Environment is an important concept in the King model and encompasses a number of interrelated elements. The personal and interpersonal systems or groups are central to King's conception of environment. They are formed at various levels according to internal goals established by the client.

Personal Systems. At the most basic level are the personal systems, where an interchange takes place between two individuals who share similar goals. An example of such a personal system is a client-nurse relationship.

Interpersonal Systems. At the intermediate level are the interpersonal systems that involve relatively small groups of individuals who share like goals, for example, a formal weight-loss program in which the members have the common goal of losing weight. Human interactions, communications, role delineation, and stress reduction are essential factors at this level.

Social Systems. At the highest level are social systems that include the large, relatively homogeneous elements of society. The health-care system, government, and society in general are some important social systems. These social systems have as their common goals organization, authority, power, status, and decision. Although the client may not be in direct interaction with the social systems, these systems are important because the personal and interpersonal systems necessarily function within larger social systems. Evoking the principle of nonsummativity, whenever one part of an open system is changed, all the other parts of the system feel the effect. For example, a decision made at the governmental level to reduce **Medicare** or **Medicaid** payments may affect when and how often a client can use health-care services such as doctor's office visits, group therapy, or emergency room care.

The King model also includes the external physical environment that affects a person's health and well-being. As the person moves through the world, the physical setting interacts with the personal system to either improve or degrade the client's health-care status.

Health

Viewed as a dynamic process that involves a range of human life experiences, health exists in people when they can achieve their highest level of functioning. Health is the primary goal of the client in the King model. It is achieved by continually adjusting to environmental **stressors,** maximizing the use of available resources, and setting and achieving goals for one's role in life. Anything that disrupts or interferes with people's ability to function normally in their chosen roles is considered to be a state of illness.

Nursing

The King model considers nursing to be a dynamic process and a type of personal system based on interactions between the nurse and the client. During these interactions, the nurse and the client jointly evaluate and identify the health-care needs, set goals for fulfillment of the needs, and consider actions to take in achieving those goals. Nursing is a multifaceted process that includes a range of activities such as the promotion and maintenance of health through education, the restoration of health through care of the sick and injured, and preparation for death through care of the dying.[11]

The process of nursing in the King model includes five key elements considered central to all human interactions: (1) action; (2) reaction; (3) interaction; (4) transaction; and (5) feedback.

The Watson Model of Human Caring

Although the concept of caring has always been an important, if somewhat obscure, element in the practice of nursing, the Watson

Model of Human Caring defines caring in a detailed and systematic manner. In the development of her model, Jean Watson used a philosophical approach rather than the systems theory approach seen in many other nursing models. Her main concern in the development of this model is to balance the impersonal aspects of nursing care that are found in the technologic and scientific aspects of practice with the personal and interpersonal elements of care that grow from a humanistic belief in life. Watson is also one of the very few theorists who openly recognizes the client's and family's spirituality and spiritual beliefs as an essential element of health.[17]

Client

The concept of client or person in the Watson model is not well developed as separate from the concept of nursing. The individuality of the client is a key concern. The Watson model views the client as someone who has needs, who grows and develops throughout life, and who eventually reaches a state of internal harmony. The client is also seen as a gestalt, or whole, who has value because of inherent goodness and capacity to develop. This gestalt, or holistic, view of the human being is a recurring theme in the Watson model; it emphasizes that the total person is more important to nursing care than the individual injury or disease process that produced the need for care.

> " " *Watson makes a clear distinction between the science of nursing and the practice of curing (medicine).*

Environment

Environment in the Watson model is a concept that is also closely intertwined with the concept of nursing. Viewed primarily as a negative element in the health-care process, the environment consists of those factors that the client must overcome to achieve a state of health. The environment can be both external physical and social elements and internal psychological reactions that affect health.

Health

To be healthy according to the Watson model, the individual must be in a dynamic state of growth and development that leads to reaching full potential as a human. As with other nursing models, health is viewed as a continuum along which a person at any point may tend more toward health or more toward illness. Illness, in the Watson model, is the client's inability to integrate life experiences and the failure to achieve full potential or inner harmony. In this model, the state of illness is not necessarily synonymous with the disease process. If the person reacts to the disease process in such a way as to find meaning, then that response is considered to be healthy. A failure to find meaning in the disease experience leads to a state of illness.

Nursing

Watson makes a clear distinction between the science of nursing and the practice of curing (medicine).[12] She defined nursing as the science of caring in which the primary goal is to assist the client reach the greatest level of personal potential. The practice of curing involves the conduct of activities that have the goal of treatment and elimination of disease.

The process of nursing in the Watson model is based on the systematic use of the scientific problem-solving method for decision making. In order to best understand nursing as a science of caring, the nurse should hold certain beliefs and be able to initiate certain caring activities.

Values. Basic to the beliefs necessary for the successful practice of nursing in the Watson model is the formation of a humanistic altruistic system of values based on the tenet that all people are inherently valuable because they are human. In addition, the nurse should have a strong sense of faith and hope in people and their condition because of the human potential for development.

Caring. A number of activities are important when practicing nursing according to Watson's caring way. These activities include establishing a relationship of help and trust between the nurse and the client; encouraging the client to express both positive and negative feelings with acceptance; manipulating the environment to make it more supportive, protective, or corrective for the client with any type of disease process; and assisting in whatever way deemed appropriate to meet the basic human needs of the client.

The Johnson Behavioral System Model

By integrating systems theory with behavioral theory, Dorothy E. Johnson has developed a model of nursing that considers client behavior to be the key to preventing illness, and also to restoring health when illness occurs. Johnson holds that human behavior is really a type of system in itself that is influenced by input factors from the environment and has output that in its turn affects the environment.[12]

Client

Drawing directly on the terminology of systems theory, the Johnson model describes the person, or client, as a behavioral system that is an organized and integrated whole.

The whole is greater than the sum of its parts because of the integration and functioning of its **subsystems.** In the Johnson model, the client as a behavioral system is composed of seven distinct behavioral subsystems. In turn, each of these seven behavioral subsystems contains four structural elements that guide and shape the subsystem.

Security. The first behavioral subsystem is the attachment or affiliate subsystem, which has security as its driving force. The type of activity that this subsystem undertakes is, for the most part, inclusion in social functions, and the behavior that is observed from this subsystem is social interactions.

Dependency. The second behavior subsystem is the dependency subsystem and has as its initiating force the goal of assisting or helping others. The primary type of activity involved is nurturing and promoting self-image. The observable behaviors that are a result of this activity include approval, attention, and physical assistance of the person.

Taking In. The third behavioral subsystem is called the ingestive subsystem and has as its driving force the meeting of the body's basic physiologic needs of food and nutrient intake. Correspondingly, its primary activity is seeking and eating food, which manifests itself in the behavior of eating.

Eliminative Behavior. The fourth behavioral subsystem is the eliminative; its goal is removal of waste products from the system. Its primary activity is means of elimination, which is observed as the behavior of expelling waste products.

Sexual Behavior. The fifth behavioral subsystem is sexual behavior and is found in the Johnson model's description of the person. The sexual subsystem has gratification and procreation of the species as its goals. It involves the complex activities of identifying gender roles, sexual development, and actual biologic sexual activity. It manifests itself in courting and mating behaviors.

Self-Protection. The sixth behavioral subsystem is called the aggressive subsystem, and its driving force is the goal of self-preservation. All the actions that individuals undertake to protect themselves from harm, either internal or external, derive from this subsystem and are shown in actions toward others and the environment in general.

Achievement. The seventh, and final, behavioral subsystem is identified as achievement. Achievement has as its driving force the broad goal of exploration and manipulation of the environment. Gaining mastery and control over the environment is the primary activity of this subsystem; it can be demonstrated externally when the individual shows that learning has occurred and higher-level accomplishments are being produced.[18]

As with all open systems, the behavioral system that makes up the person seeks to maintain a dynamic balance by regulating input and output. This regulation process takes the form of adapting to the environment and responding to others. However, the Johnson model sees human behavior as being goal directed, which leads the person to constant growth and development beyond the maintenance of a mere steady state.

Health

A state of health exists, according to the Johnson model, when balance and steady state exist within the behavioral systems of the client. Under normal circumstances, the human system has enough inherent flexibility to maintain this balance without external intervention. At times, however, the system's balance may be disturbed to such a degree by physical disease, injury, or emotional crisis as to require external assistance. This out-of-balance state is the state of illness.

Environment

In the Johnson model, the environment is defined as all of those internal and external elements that have an affect on the behavioral system. These environmental elements include obvious external factors, such as air temperature and relative humidity; sociologic factors, such as family, neighborhood, and society in general; and the internal environment, such as bodily processes, psychological states, religious beliefs, and political orientation. All seven behavioral subsystems of the client are involved with his or her relationship to the environment through the regulation of input and output. The client is continually interacting with the environment in the attempt to remain healthy by maintaining an internal dynamic balance.

Nursing

In the Johnson model, nursing is an activity that helps the individual achieve and maintain an optimal level of behavior (state of health) through the manipulation and regulation of the environment.[11] Nursing has functions in both health and illness. Nursing interventions to either maintain or regain health involve four activities in the regulation of the environment: (1) restricting harmful environmental factors, (2) de-

> " " *The Johnson model sees human behavior as being goal directed, which leads the person to constant growth and development beyond the maintenance of a mere steady state.*

fending the client from negative environmental influences, (3) inhibiting adverse elements from occurring, and (4) facilitating positive internal environmental factors in the recovery process.

As a professional, the nurse in the Johnson model provides direct services to the client. By interacting with, and sometimes intervening in, the multiple subsystems that are found in the client's environment, the nurse acts as an external regulatory force. The goal of nursing is to promote the highest level of functioning and development in the client at all times. Nursing actions include helping the client act in a socially acceptable manner, monitoring and aiding with biologic processes necessary for maintenance of a dynamic balance, demonstrating support for medical care and treatment during illness, and taking actions to prevent illness from recurring. In this model, nursing makes its own unique contribution to the health and well-being of individuals and provides a service that is complementary to that provided by other health-care professionals.

The Neuman Health-Care Systems Model

As envisioned by Betty Neuman, the Health-Care Systems Model focuses on the individual and his or her environment and is applicable to a variety of health-care disciplines apart from nursing. Drawing from systems theory, the Neuman model also includes elements from stress theory with an overall holistic view of humanity and health care.[19]

Client

In this model, the client is viewed as an open system that interacts constantly with internal and external environments through the system's boundaries. The client-system's boundaries are called lines of defense and resistance in the Neuman model and may be represented graphically as a series of concentric circles that surround the basic core of the individual. The goal of these boundaries is to keep the basic core system stable by controlling system input and output.

Neuman classifies these defensive boundaries according to their various functions. The internal lines of resistance are the boundaries that are closest to the basic core and thus protect the basic internal structure of the system. The normal lines of defense are outside the internal lines of resistance; they protect the system from common, everyday environmental stressors. The flexible line of defense surrounds the normal line of defense and protects it from extreme environmental stressors. The general goal of all of these protective boundaries is to maintain the internal stability of the client.

Health

Health, then, in the Neuman model is defined as the relatively stable internal functioning of the client. Optimal health exists when the client is maintained in a high state of wellness or stability. As in other nursing models, health is not considered an absolute state, but rather a continuum that reflects the client's internal stability while moving from wellness to illness and back. It takes a considerable amount of physical and psychological energy to maintain the stability of the person who is in good health.

The opposite of a healthy state, illness exists when the client's core structure becomes unstable through the effects of environmental factors that overwhelm and defeat the lines of defense and resistance. These environmental factors, whether internal or external, are called stressors in this model.

Environment

The environment is composed of internal or external forces or stressors that produce change or response in the client. Stressors may be helpful or harmful, strong or weak.

Stressors are also classified according to their relationship to the basic core of the client-system. Stressors that are completely outside the basic core are termed extrapersonal stressors and are either physical in nature, such as atmospheric temperature, or sociologic, such as living in either a rural or urban setting. Interpersonal stressors arise from interactions with other human beings. Marital relationships, career expectations, or friendships are included in this group of interpersonal stressors. Those stressors that occur within the client are called intrapersonal and include involuntary physiologic responses, psychological reactions, and internal thought processes.

Nursing

The nurse's role in the Neuman model is to identify at what level or in which boundary a disruption in the client's internal stability has taken place, and then to aid the client in activities that strengthen or restore the integrity of that particular boundary. The Neuman model expands the concept of client from the individual to include families, small groups, the community, or even society in general.

Nursing's main concern in this model is either to identify stressors that will disrupt a defensive boundary in the future (prevention) or to identify a stressor that has already disrupted a defensive boundary, thereby producing present instability (illness).[19] The Neuman model is based on the nursing process, and identifies three levels of intervention: primary, secondary, and tertiary.

A **primary intervention** has as its main goal the prevention of possible symptoms that could be caused by environmental stressors. Teaching clients about stress management, giving immunizations, or encouraging aerobic exercises to prevent heart disease are examples of primary interventions. A **secondary intervention** is aimed at treating symptoms that have already been produced by stressors. Many of the actions that nurses perform in the hospital or clinic (e.g., giving pain medications or teaching a client with cardiac disease about the benefits of a low-sodium diet) fall into this secondary intervention category. **Tertiary care** actions seek to restore the client's system to an optimal state of balance by adapting to negative environmental stressors. Teaching a client how to care for a colostomy at home after discharge from the hospital is an example of nursing activities at the tertiary level.

TRENDS FOR THE FUTURE IN NURSING THEORY

Although the search for the perfect nursing model continues, the emphasis in recent years has shifted from developing new theories to the application of existing theories to nursing practice. Also, the new theorists seem to be more interested in expanding existing nursing theories by including such concepts as cultural diversity, spirituality, family, and social change rather than starting all over again from the beginning. A good example of this trend is the cultural meaning centered theory that was published by Mendyka and Bloom.[20] This theory expands the King model by adding a cultural perspective (Box 3–2).

One of the more recent of the established nursing theories is the Man-Living-Health Model proposed by Parse. Although her original work started in 1981, a more developed form of her theory was published in 1987.[21] Parse's theory stresses the elements of experience, personal **values,** and lifestyle choices in the maintenance of health.

In this theory, the client can be any person or family who is concerned with the quality of their life situation. The client is viewed as an open, whole being who is influenced by past and present life experiences. The ability to make free choices is essential in this theory.

The client, through choices that are made, interacts with the environment to influence health either positively or negatively.

Health, for Parse, is an ongoing process. By making free choices, the client's health status is continually unfolding. In addition, health is determined by lived experiences, synthesis of values, and the way the client lives.

Therefore, the main role of nursing in the Parse model is to guide the client in finding and understanding the meaning of their lives. Once the client chooses a healthy life situation, then the nurse can further increase the quality of the client's life and improve his or her health status. The ability to change the client's health related values is an important skill for nurses to master in this model.

Parse never really defines the concept of environment in relationship to her theory. Specifically, it seems to be any health-related setting, but it can also be expanded to include past and present experiences.

As with any developing science, nursing will continue to change and respond to the

---

3.2 Remember Graduation Day? What Happened to the Dream?

Graduation day is a big event in most individuals' lives. Graduation day from a school of nursing often leaves an indelible imprint on the graduating nurse's brain. The keynote speaker congratulates the new nurses on their achievements in nursing school and for their choice of such a noble profession.

By 1 year after graduation, many of these same new graduates would have difficulty visualizing themselves in a noble profession. Because of the hours, the stress, and the seeming lack of rewards, nurses quickly fall into the view that nursing is a job rather than a profession. It becomes essential to reexamine periodically why they chose this profession in the first place.

There is no greater calling than to help those in need. Care of the patients and their families should always be foremost in the nurse's mind and heart. If the nurse does not do it, who else will care, clean a draining wound, and speak softly to a grieving family? Who else will convert the unspoken movements and gestures of a patient into a nursing diagnosis and care plan? Who else will look past the myriad of tubes, wires, and machines to acknowledge a frightened, helpless patient?

Only nurses have the education, the strength, and the ability to deliver high-quality care to every patient who seeks help. If the patient is viewed as the hub in the wheel of health care, and the members of the health-care team as spokes focused on the care of the patient, then the importance of the profession of nursing becomes evident. All members of the health-care team, as the spokes of the wheel, touch, support, and guide the patient along his or her path to recovery.

Many of the things that nurses do as part of their daily tasks take on a great deal of significance to the patients under their care. Simple tasks such as introducing themselves as the primary care provider, calling the patient by name, touching the patient with a reassuring hand, and explaining what will happen to the patient and what can be expected next are small, but vital elements in patient care. Through these types of actions, nurses lessen the fear and hasten the recovery of those under their care.

From Lasscar, DA: What ever happened to nursing? American Nurse 27(1):4, 1995.

dynamic trends of society. Older nursing models will either be replaced by new ones or modified to include developing concepts. Indeed, one of the hallmarks of a sound nursing theory or model is its flexibility and ability to adapt to new discoveries. The increasing number of **independent nurse practitioners** and other advanced practice nurses are testing nursing theories as they have never been tested before. The theories that are flexible, realistic, and usable in actual practice will survive and remain as the pillars of professional nursing. Others that are too theoretical or rigid will fall by the wayside and become mere footnotes in nursing texts.

Conclusion

As nursing takes its rightful place among the other helping professions, nursing theory will take on additional importance. Nursing theory and models are the systematic conceptualizations of nursing practice and how it fits into the health-care system. Nursing theories help describe, explain, predict, and control nursing activities to achieve the goals of client care. By understanding and using nursing theory, nurses will be better able to incorporate theoretical information into their practice to provide new ways of approaching nursing care and improving nursing practice.

The development of nursing theory and models indicates a maturing of the profession. As the knowledge associated with the profession increases, becomes unique, more complex, and better organized, the general body of nursing science knowledge also increases. Only when nursing has a well-developed body of specialized knowledge will it be fully recognized as a separate scientific discipline and a true profession.

Critical Thinking Exercises

Mrs. McCann, an 88-year-old woman, has been a resident of St. Martin's Village, a lifetime care community, since her husband died 8 years ago. Her health status is fair. She has adult-onset diabetes controlled by oral medication and a scar from a tumor behind her left ear that was removed surgically. The wound from this tumor removal has never healed completely, and it has continuously oozed a serous fluid requiring a dressing.

At St. Martin's Village, Mrs. McCann has her own apartment, which she maintains with minimal assistance, receives one hot meal each day in a common dining room, and has access to a full range of services such as a beauty shop, recreational facilities, and a chapel. She is generally happy in this setting. She has no immediate family nearby, and the cost of the facility was covered by a large, one-time gift from her now deceased husband.

Recently, she has become much weaker and has had difficulty walking, attending activities including meals, and changing the dressing on her ear. The nurse at St. Martin's Village is sent to evaluate this client.

✔ Select two nursing models and apply the principles of the model to this case study. Make sure that you include the concepts of client, health, environment, and nursing.

References

1. Aguilera, DC: Crisis Intervention: Theory and Methodology. CV Mosby, St. Louis, 1990.
2. Bulechek, GM, et al: Nursing interventions used in nursing practice. Am J Nurs 94(10): 61, 1994.
3. Rice, B: CIC work in year 2: Data gathering, analysis, and work force modeling. Colleagues in Caring Newsletter, October 1997 p. 3–4.
4. Titler, MG, et al: Use of the nursing interventions classification by critical care nurses. Critical Care Nurse 16(4):38–54, 1996.
5. Tripp-Reimer, T, et al: The dimensional structure of nursing interventions. Nurs Res 45(1):7–10, 1996.
6. McCloskey, JC, et al: Nursing interventions core to specialty practice. Nurs Outlook 46(3):67–76, 1998.
7. Mitchell, PR, and Grippando, GM: Nursing Perspectives and Issues. Delmar, Albany, NY, 1993.
8. McCann-Flynn, JB, and Heffron, PB: Nursing: From Concept to Practice. Robert J. Brady, Bowie, MD, 1984.
9. Riehl-Sisca, JP: Conceptual Models for Nursing Practice. Appleton-Lange, E. Norwalk, CT, 1989.
10. Putt, A: General Systems Theory Applied to Nursing. Little, Brown, Boston, 1978.
11. Stevens, BJ: Nursing Theory: Analysis, Application, Evaluation. Little, Brown, Boston, 1984.
12. Fawcett, J: Analysis and Evaluation of Conceptual Models of Nursing. FA Davis, Philadelphia, 1989.
13. Roy, C, and Andrews, HA: The Roy Adaptation Model: The Definitive Statement. Appleton-Lange, E. Norwalk, CT, 1991.
14. Orem, DE: Nursing: Concepts of Practice. Mosby–Year Book, St. Louis, 1991.
15. Leininger, MM (ed): Cultural Care Diversity and Universality: A Theory of Nursing. National League for Nursing, New York, 1992.
16. King, IM: King's theory of goal attainment. Nursing Science Quarterly 5:19–25, 1992.
17. Watson, J: Nursing: Human Science and Human Care: A Theory of Nursing. Appleton Century Crofts, E. Norwalk, CT, 1985.
18. Schaefer, KM, and Pond, JB: Levine's Conservation Model: A Framework for Nursing Practice. FA Davis, Philadelphia, 1991.
19. Neuman, B: The Neuman Systems Model. Appleton & Lange, E. Norwalk, CT, 1989.
20. Mendyka, BE, and Bloom, FR: Reaffirming the relevance of culture for nursing. Scholarly Inquiry for Nursing Practice 11(3):179–197, 1997.
21. Parse, RR: Man-Living-Health: Theory of Nursing. Wiley, Philadelphia, 1987.

BIBLIOGRAPHY

Belgin, MA, and Tripp-Reimer, T: Implications of nursing taxonomies for middle-range theory development. Advanced Nursing Science 19(3):37–49, 1997.

Buerhaus, P: Is another RN shortage looming:? Nurs Outlook 46(3):103–108, 1998.

Donahue, MP: Nursing the Finest Art: An Illustrated History, ed 2. CV Mosby, St. Louis, 1996.

Lasscar, DA: Whatever happened to nursing? American Nurse 27(1):4, 1995.

McCloskey, JC, and Bulechek, GM. Nursing Interventions Classification (NIC). Mosby–Year Book, St. Louis, 1996.

McCloskey, JC, and Grace, CK: Current Issues in Nursing, ed 5. Mosby–Year Book, St. Louis, 1997.

Nicoll, LH: Nurses' Guide to the Internet, ed 2. JB Lippincott, Philadelphia, 1998.

Nightingale, F: Notes on Nursing: What It Is and What It Is Not. Harrison, London, 1859 (Reprinted by JB Lippincott, Philadelphia, 1966).

Sullivan, TJ: Collaboration: A Health Care Imperative. McGraw-Hill, New York, 1998.

von Bertalanffy, L: General Systems Theory: Foundation, Development, and Applications. George Braziller, New York, 1968.

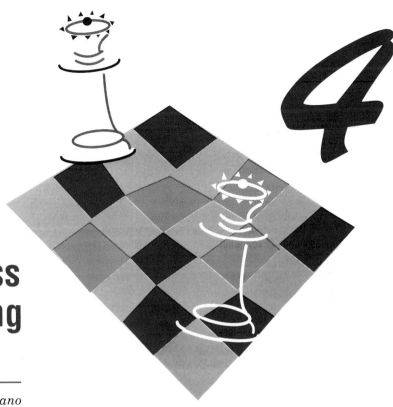

The Process of Educating Nurses

> *Joseph T. Catalano*

Learning Objectives

After completing this chapter, the reader will be able to:

1. Compare the major differences between the diploma, associate degree nursing, and bachelor of science in nursing educational programs.

2. Discuss at least three types of advanced nursing degrees.

3. Distinguish between the different types of doctoral degrees available to nurses.

4. Explain the concept of advanced practice for nurses.

Unlike many other professions, nursing has several related, but unique, educational pathways that lead to licensure and professional status. Indeed, the current system of nursing education creates a great deal of confusion about nursing, not only among the public, but even among nurses themselves. Perhaps the belief that "a nurse is a nurse is a nurse is a nurse" developed from the fact that even though registered nurses may be prepared in educational programs that vary in length, orientation, and content, the graduates all take the same licensing examination, and, superficially, all seem to be able to provide the same level of care. The licensure examination measures knowledge at the minimal level of safe practice. The workplace has not provided pay differences to distinguish levels of education despite studies showing performance differences.

PARADIGM SHIFTING IN NURSING EDUCATION

Current changes in health care are being driven by a number of powerful societal forces that are producing a gradual but inevitable reshaping of health-care delivery. Although insulated to some degree from these forces, nursing education is beginning to recognize that their graduates need to be prepared with knowledge and skills that are different from those that have been traditionally needed by a hospital-based, physician-directed health-care system. The most powerful of these forces of change are the movement towards a market-driven health-care economy, the wider use of capitated managed care for financing coverage, the increasing age and diversity of the American population, and the rapid leaps forward in health care and information technology.

According to the Department of Health and Human Services, Division of Nursing, in a report based on a survey conducted in 1996, only 60% of registered nurses remained employed in hospitals, down from 66% in 1992.[1] The remainder were employed in a wide variety of settings, including private practice, public health agencies, home health care, primary nursing-school–operated nursing centers, **ambulatory care centers,** insurance and managed care companies, education, and health-care research. There is also an ever-growing group of **emerging health occupations** that have not yet been officially recognized by professional organizations.

The Pew Health Professions Commission Report, sometimes referred to as the Pew Report, was a major study of health care and nursing education that also reinforces the belief that there is a need for reform in nursing education.[2,3] Its recommendations for all schools preparing health-care professionals are comprehensive and include issues such as expanding the scientific basis of the programs, promoting interdisciplinary education, developing cultural sensitivity, establishing new alliances with managed care companies and government, and increasing the use of computer technology and interactive software. The Pew Report also recommended a differentiated practice structure to simplify and consolidate the titles that it uses for the various levels of practitioners so that there is just one title for each level.

As more and more health care shifts to ambulatory and community-based settings, nursing educators need to re-evaluate whether the graduates of their programs are adequately prepared to meet the demands posed by these areas of care. Nursing educators also need to evaluate their own educational and skill preparation in light of these changing needs.

THE NURSE OF THE FUTURE

The nurse of the future will need to practice with self-reliance, independence, and flexibility. They will be required to have well-developed decision-making skills based on critical-thinking ability, a working knowledge of community resources, and computer and technical competencies, as well as the ability to deliver high-quality client education. Nurses in the future will also be required to deliver high-quality care while working within the constraints of a managed care system and tight cost control measures.

Will nursing education ever be able to prepare a graduate who fulfills all the qualities for *the nurse of the future?* Certainly not without alterations so that the graduate will obtain the essential tools to build on as they advance in their careers.

It is important to remember that hospital-based acute care nursing practice will always have an important place in any health-care system. Hospitals will always exist. Highly skilled, acute care nurses will always find a place to practice. It is a generally accepted fact that the older population requires more health care of all types— acute, chronic, and community based. Although the current health-care system is experiencing a gradual decrease in the utilization of acute care beds, this trend is likely to reverse as the "baby boomers" become the senior citizens.

Paradigm shifting in nursing education does not need to be an either/or proposition. It is sometimes felt that nursing education is *either* acute care focused *or* it is community focused. Nursing education in the future will need to combine the two so that the graduate can practice with competence in either or both settings. The skills are similar; however, the emphasis may be different. Although many hospital skills can and are being done by nonnurses at a cheaper cost—for example, the use of emergency medical technicians (EMTs) in the emergency room—nursing education must still impart important skills to its graduates, such as critical thinking, therapeutic relationship, **primary care** and **case management,** and comfort with a consumer-driven health-care system.

Critical thinking has been a buzzword in nursing education for the past several years. Although critical thinking has many different definitions, it is generally recognized as the ability to use basic core knowledge and decision-making skills in deciding and resolving situations where there is a relatively small amount of data and a high degree of risk and ambiguity. Although not always called critical thinking, nursing has long been concerned with the ability to make good judgments and decisions about client care. (See Chapter 5 for a fuller discussion of critical thinking.) At a fundamental level, the nursing process is a type of critical thinking. Unfortunately, in the health-care system of the future, a nurse's critical thinking skills must go far beyond those of the basic nursing process. Nursing education will need to prepare students for more advanced critical thinking by exposing them to real-life situations that require the use of creativity, intuition, analysis, and deductive and inductive reasoning. These situations are introduced in the classroom as case studies and are reinforced in the clinical setting through guided experiences and mentoring.

Therapeutic relationship skills have been long stressed by mental health nursing faculty as a key element in the treatment of psychiatric problems. In reality these therapeutic relationship skills are essential for all nurses to fulfill their roles as health-care providers and healers. Although these skills are currently being taught in a limited and focused way in most schools of nursing, they need to be expanded to involve directed services and relationship-centered care nursing.

Relationship-centered nursing care is client focused and revolves around the client's trust in, value of, and understanding of the nurse's skills and role in the healing process. The client must be able to feel comfortable with the nurse and share his or her understanding of both illness and health. Currently, in many licensed practical nurse/licensed vocational nurse (LPN/ LVN) programs and schools offering the associate degree in nursing, clinical experiences consist of one-time, 8-hour provision of care for an acute or chronically ill client. Little time is spent in follow-up care. However, some bachelor of nursing science (BSN) programs have expanded clinical experiences to include **discharge planning** and follow-up home health-care experiences. To meet the demands of the future health-care system, all nursing education programs must be able to develop learning experiences for students that involve care for selected individuals or families over extended periods of time, perhaps ranging from several weeks to several semesters.

Care management is a general term that refers to a method of coordinating care

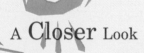

CRITICAL THINKING: A STRATEGY FOR SOLVING PROBLEMS

Nurses have always been required to make clinical decisions that are based on a strong body of knowledge. Nurses have constantly been challenged to use their reasoning ability to recognize and choose appropriate courses of action for clients in changing situations. These are exercises in critical thinking. Why then is all the renewed current emphasis being placed on critical thinking?

The critical thinking skills that nurses have long used informally in client care are even more crucial in a rapidly changing consumer-oriented health-care system. The ability to use logical and analytic skills in conjunction with intuitive and creative problem-solving abilities is required to survive the vagaries of the current health-care system. For example, nurses frequently deal with controversial ethical issues such as the right to die. By using a critical thinking approach to this type of issue, nurses can identify the essential elements and work toward a satisfactory resolution of the dilemma. In addition, nurses who can integrate logical elements with the more intuitive thinking have a much better chance to provide care in a flexible individualized way.

Nurses have been traditionally educated in a system that stressed logical and systematic approaches to solving client problems. Emphasis was placed on didactic knowledge and manual skill perfection as the measures of a nurse's success in the health-care system. This approach worked well in a system in which clients viewed themselves as merely recipients of care. In today's society, more clients insist on taking an active part in their care, participating at all levels ranging from the actual physical care to the final decision-making process. Nurses who were professionally prepared under the old system are finding it difficult to adjust to the new consumer-focused health-care system.

Although critical thinking has a number of different definitions, the key elements common to many of the definitions include the ability to solve problems creatively both by processing technical information logically and by using intuition to guide the application of that information. The ability to use intuition in conjunction with a logical approach to problems allows nurses to make fast and accurate decisions about care, while helping the client deal with his or her emotions and physical needs. This type of thinking is much more difficult to teach than simple logical problem solving such as the nursing process.

An important first step in learning real critical thinking is the identification and recognition of the nurse's style of processing information. Many nurses rely on a logical and analytic approach to do this. Once a nurse's personal style is identified, allowing or even requiring that nurse to use a different approach expands her or his ability to adapt to different situations.

Critical thinking in the current health-care system is an extremely important skill. Nurses who can use creative methods to solve problems at the bedside are essential for the survival of the profession. Sharing with other nurses experiences in which critical thinking was used to solve problems increases the insight of both participants into the process. Nursing can only be strengthened when nurses understand that creative problem solving is the key to meeting the needs of future health-care consumers.

From Brookfield, S: On impostorship, cultural suicide, and other dangers: How nurses learn critical thinking. J Cont Educ Nurs 24:197–205, 1993; Snyder, M: Critical thinking: A foundation for consumer-focused care. J Cont Educ Nurs 24:206–210, 1993.

either with an individual client or on a system-wide basis. **Case management,** a new entity in a health-care system driven by the urge for cost-effective care, usually is associated with coordinating care for an individual client as he or she moves from one level to another through the health-care system. Case management is now a certified specialty. Almost all of the proposals for revisions in the health-care system include the **case manager** as an important element in the overall management of care. Currently, case managers do not have to be registered nurses. Many individuals with degrees in social work and human resources as well as registered nurses are serving in the capacity of case managers. Perhaps the ideal situation would be to function as a **health-care team,** with both a registered nurse and a social worker coordinating all aspects of the client's care.

As case managers, nurses will be responsible for developing **clinical pathways** and also for directing and guiding the overall health care of a specific group of clients. Case management includes not only overseeing the clients' care while they are in the hospital but also following clients through their rehabilitation at home, long-term follow-up, health-care practices, and developmental stages.

The knowledge and thinking required by an effective case manager go far beyond what is currently required of new graduates. Nurses must be able to understand not only the immediate disease process but also the long-term outcomes and factors that influence the disease. Case managers must also practice health-focused nursing and primary levels of intervention. Decisions will need to be made about care from a broad **database** as well as an understanding of the client's abilities, knowledge level, and even financial status.

Nursing education will be severely challenged to provide experiences to prepare students for this role. Students must be allowed to experience the authority, accountability, and responsibility of guiding a client's health care over an extended period. It might be beneficial to combine the learning experiences mentioned earlier in establishing the therapeutic relationship with the managed care experience.

A consumer-driven health-care system is at one and the same time the nurse's dream

Delegation: An Essential Element in the RN's Role

With the trend in health care toward increasing the use of unlicensed assistive personnel (UAP), the ability to make decisions about what responsibilities can be delegated and to whom has become a major responsibility of RNs. Delegation involves the transfer of authority to a competent individual to do a selected nursing task in a specific situation. When the nurse delegates a task or series of tasks to a UAP, the UAP is responsible for performing the task; however, the RN retains the ultimate responsibility and accountability for the total nursing care of the client. Although delegation of tasks is not a new role for RNs, its sudden increase has made many RNs uncomfortable, particularly if their education program has not prepared them for assuming this responsibility.

Guidelines for delegation were established by the National Council of State Boards of Nursing in 1990. According to these guidelines, the decision to delegate should be based on:

- Determination of the task, procedure, or function that is to be delegated
- Staff available
- Assessment of client needs
- Consideration of the potential delegatee's abilities
- Consideration of the level of supervision available and a determination of the level and method of supervision required to ensure safe practice

Schools of nursing should include classes on delegation as the requirements for nurses to develop the skill of delegation increases in importance. Making a decision about whether or not to delegate a nursing task based on UAP job description, client circumstances, difficulty of the task, and staffing patterns involves a high level of decision-making skills. In making this sort of decision, the RN often places her or his license, career, and future on the line.

From National Council of State Boards of Nursing, Inc., newsletter, June 22, 1995.

and nightmare. Many widely used nursing models or theories claim to be client-centered, which translates into being consumer driven. Yet, when these models are put into practice, the care given is more provider driven than anything else. A client/consumer-driven health-care system means that the care given is defined by the consumer and the outcomes are also determined by the

consumer. The nurse must be able to accept the authority of the group or community as a determinant of health care. The nurse's role becomes one of a partner in guiding, implementing, and overseeing ways to deliver requested health care for a given community.

Many nursings programs, particularly baccalaureate programs, include a course in community health and home-health-care nursing. A requirement of these courses is often to have the students do a community survey in which they determine the needs of the community as they perceive them. Currently, many of these courses have been modified so that the students learn from the community what the community perceives to be their own needs.

> 66 99 *Since 1965, the ANA has upheld the belief that baccalaureate education should be the basic level of preparation for professional nurses.*

Paradigm shifting is never easy. Major paradigm shifts in thinking and acting are even more difficult. Nursing education will face a huge paradigm shift in the very near future. How educators meet these challenges will, to a large extent, shape the future of professional nursing well into the next century. However, the process has already begun.

ANA POSITION PAPER ON EDUCATION FOR NURSES

After evaluating the changes that occurred in the health care system during the 1950s and studying the projected educational needs for nurses, the American Nurses Association (ANA) published a paper in 1965 that took a stand on an issue that was, and still is, highly controversial. Although written almost 40 years ago, this document is still relevant to many of the issues in nursing education today.

For full appreciation of the significance of this paper, it must be examined from a historical perspective. The overall purpose of the ANA has always been to ensure high-quality nursing care to the public by fostering high standards of nursing practice. In addition, the ANA was concerned with furthering the professional and educational advancement of nurses as well as protecting the occupational welfare of nurses. To achieve these goals, the ANA took responsibility for establishing the scope of practice for nurses and for guaranteeing the competence of those who claim the title of nurse.

After World War II, there was an explosion of scientific and technologic knowledge used in health care. The educational level of the population was also increasing, thus resulting in greater public demand for higher-quality health care. In re-evaluating the nature and scope of nursing practice, and the type and level of quality of education needed to meet these new demands, the ANA reached the conclusions that are presented in its position paper.

Since 1965, the ANA has upheld the belief that baccalaureate education should be the basic level of preparation for professional nurses. Specifically, the ANA concluded that:

> "The education for all those who are licensed to practice nursing should take place in institutions of higher education; minimum preparation for beginning professional nursing practice at the present time should be the baccalaureate degree education in nursing; minimum preparation for beginning technical nursing practice at the present time should be associate degree education; education for assistants in the health care service occupations should be short, intensive pre-service programs in vocational education institutions rather than on the job training."[4]

There were several assumptions on which the ANA based this position paper:

1. Nursing is a helping profession and, as such, provides services that contribute to the health and well-being of people.

2. Nursing is of vital significance to the individual receiving services; it meets needs that cannot be met by the person, the family, or other persons in the community.
3. The demand for the services of nurses will continue to increase.
4. The professional practitioner is responsible for the nature and quality of all nursing care that clients receive.
5. The services of professional practitioners of nursing will continue to be supplemented and complemented by the services of nurse practitioners who will be licensed.
6. Education for those in the health-care professions must increase in depth and breadth as scientific knowledge expands.
7. The health care of the public, in the amount and to the extent needed and demanded, requires the services of large numbers of health occupation workers, in addition to those licensed as nurses, to function as assistants to nurses. These workers are presently designated nurses' aides, orderlies, assistants, and attendants.
8. The professional association must concern itself with the nature of nursing practice, the methods for improving nursing practice, and standards for membership in the professional association.[4]

The rationale for taking such a strong stand on the future of nursing education derived from recognition by the profession of its heritage, its immediate problems, the emerging social issues and trends, the nature of nursing practice, and the extent to which nurses could realistically enact changes for continued professional progress. The ANA drew on Florence Nightingale's vision of nursing and nursing education, which emphasized the value of education for the development of the profession. It was important to Nightingale that schools of nursing be independent of hospitals and that they have a strong theoretical component on which to base clinical practice.

By recognizing the increasing complexity of society, the ANA realized that nursing was not only becoming more specialized but was also moving toward greater interdependence with other groups in society. One of these key groups was the U.S. federal government. As the government began increasing aid for nursing education, educational facilities expanded, providing greater opportunities for professional advancement. Larger numbers of students with more varied backgrounds were recruited into the profession, requiring greater flexibility in nursing education programs to accommodate their needs. Schools of nursing were, at the same time, also hard-pressed to meet the attendant demands of science and technology that were changing the traditional role of nurses. In addition to expanding roles for nurses, greater consumer awareness and expectations were placing new demands on the abilities of nurses.

Even in 1965, the ANA recognized that nurses were required to master a very large and extremely complex body of knowledge. In addition, nurses had to be able to make critical and independent decisions about client care.

Effects of the ANA Paper on Education

The implications of this paper were far-reaching and highly controversial. The ANA paper affected many different elements of society and the health-care industry.

Hospitals recognized that they would no longer retain their traditional role of preparing nurses for practice. Even though pressure to move nursing education from hospital-based diploma schools to institutions of higher education had been building for some time, in the mid-1960s, a full 75% of the graduating nurses were awarded diplomas.[5]

Colleges and universities were hard pressed to develop undergraduate and graduate programs quickly for nursing majors. The relatively few and small baccalaureate programs in existence at the time were called on to expand their programs rapidly. It also became evident that a clear distinction between technical and professional programs needed to be made.

To this day, the ANA remains firmly committed to its stand that all nursing education should be housed in institutions of higher learning. Even 40 years after this statement was made, the profession of nursing is still trying to reach a consensus on the issue of basic educational preparation for entry into practice.

A similar resolution was again proposed by the ANA in 1985, but it also met strong opposition and was never enacted. As recently as 1996, the American Association of Colleges of Nursing (AACN) presented its own position paper emphasizing the belief that the baccalaureate degree should be the minimal requirement for entry into the nursing profession. The most influential reason why these proposals have not been adopted has been economic, not conceptual.

Continuing discussion and efforts to bring about collaborative agreement on nursing education is a goal that the profession must work toward. Only after the issue of basic entry-level education for professional nursing is resolved, and when nurses, like all other professionals, obtain their knowledge from recognized schools of higher education, will nursing as a profession be able to resolve its other important problems. Advancement of clinical practice, preparation for advanced practice roles, and increased body of nursing knowledge all depend on baccalaureate entry-level education for professional nurses.

HOSPITAL-BASED DIPLOMA SCHOOLS

The Nightingale School of Nursing was a diploma school in the strict use of the term. When nurses graduated from this school they were given a diploma, not an academic degree. The first graduates from the

Nightingale School soon began to establish their own schools of nursing based on the Nightingale model and adhered to her philosophy of nursing education. These were also diploma schools. After an initial period of uncertainty and trepidation, both physicians and hospital administrators began to recognize that when the quality of nurses was improved so too was the overall quality of their hospitals. They also understood that these types of schools that were closely associated with hospitals could provide a source of free, or inexpensive, labor. Diploma schools sprang up throughout Europe so that, in time, each hospital had its own school of nursing. Many of Nightingale's principles and concerns about nursing education were abandoned during this period of growth.

> 66 99 *Both physicians and hospital administrators began to recognize that when the quality of nurses was improved so too was the overall quality of their hospitals.*

In the United States, developments in nursing education, as with health care in general, lagged behind those in Europe. It was not until the mid-1870s that the first school of nursing was established in the United States. This was a diploma school that was attached to the New England Hospital for Women.[6] As in Europe, the idea of diploma schools quickly caught on, and within 10 years almost every large hospital in the United States had its own diploma school of nursing. These schools had very little in common with the Nightingale School of Nursing. There was no uniformity in curriculum, length of program, or requirements. To guarantee adequate enrollment, candidates were again being recruited from the lowest levels of society.

The hospitals used the student nurses as the major source of free labor for their facilities. There was little or no classroom or theoretical study. The students learned exclusively by hands-on experience during their 12- to 14-hour work shifts. Most of the students consisted of young, single women recruited just after they graduated from high school. The students were confined to dormitories on the hospital property. The dormitories were monitored closely by a housemother who enforced the rigorous rules of behavior and dismissed students for even minor infractions of the rules. The early diploma schools of nursing were organized and administered on a model that was similar to the strictest of the religious orders.

The nurses who graduated from these schools were proficient in basic nursing skills and could assume positions in the hospital where they were trained on in home nursing where they worked on a case-by-case basis without any additional orientation or education. Only head nurses (often also the instructor) worked in the hospital after graduation. Because of the 24-hour-a-day, 7-day-a-week socialization process administered by these schools, diploma graduate nurses tended to be very submissive to authority and willing to carry out any duty to please the physician, administrator, or head nurse. Before the advent of licensure examinations and standardization of practice, nurses from diploma schools were often limited to employment in their own training institutions or in the home-health-care setting.

Diploma schools of nursing remained relatively unchanged in the United States until 1949 when the National Nursing Accrediting Service, working under the guidance of the National League for Nursing Education, became the licensing body for all schools of nursing who voluntarily sought accreditation. The first formal accreditation of nursing schools occurred in the early 1950s. In 1952, the National League for Nursing (NLN) assumed accrediting responsibilities for all schools of nursing.[7] Accreditation by the National League for Nursing Accrediting Commission (NLNAC) has always been and remains a voluntary undertaking.

In order to be accredited by the NLN, schools of nursing had to meet specific **outcome criteria** and teach specific content in their curricula. Many of the diploma schools of nursing could not or would not comply with these criteria and eventually closed. Some of the requirements for the schools that did choose to comply with the NLN included a 3-year course of study meeting the criteria established by the state board of nursing, using only faculty with baccalaureate or higher degrees in nursing, developing a unique philosophy for their school, and demonstrating how that philosophy was implemented through learning objectives, course objectives, and outcome criteria, and by showing an adequate pass rate on the State Board or National Council Licensure Examination (NCLEX).

One of the key factors that all state boards of nursing were concerned about was that the school should be able to demonstrate that the students were not being used as unpaid hospital personnel while they were in their education and training programs. When students could no longer be used as free labor, diploma nursing schools went from being virtually free to the hospital to being very expensive. Not only did they still have to pay for the room and board of the students, but they also now had to hire and pay additional staff because the students could no longer be included in the overall staff numbers. Even more diploma schools closed because of the financial burdens to the hospitals. The schools that stayed open began increasing their tuition rates to the point where they were as expensive as programs granting academic degrees.

The 1960s and 1970s brought an increased awareness that nurses should be educated in institutions of higher education and receive academic degrees and not just diplomas for nursing to be considered a full profession.

Many diploma schools during this period became associated with universities and converted their curricula into degree-granting programs. According to the 1997–1998 statistics published by the NLN, there are only 121 accredited diploma programs still functioning. They are of universal high quality and meet all the standards necessary for NLN accreditation. The main emphasis remains on preparing nurses who are highly competent in the technical nursing skills through extensive hands-on practice in the clinical setting, but elements of leadership, humanities, and general sciences are also included in the classroom setting.[8]

ASSOCIATE DEGREE NURSING

The associate degree nursing (ADN) program was developed by Mildred Montague as a short-term solution to the nursing shortage experienced after World War II.[9] Originally designed to prepare students for technical nursing practice, the 2-year ADN programs were offered through community colleges with an emphasis on developing the skills necessary to provide high-quality bedside care in less time than BSN programs. A successful pilot program for ADNs was conducted by Montague at Teachers' College in Columbia University in New York City in 1952 to prepare technical nurses who could assist professional nurses. It demonstrated that community college–based programs could attract large numbers of students, prove cost effective, and produce skillful technical nurses in half the time required for BSN programs.[10]

Early on, there was some heated debate concerning licensure and titling for this group of nurses. The technical orientation of the curriculum was, and is, very similar to that the LPNs, but the location of the programs in the community college setting and the increased theoretic orientation seemed to elevate these programs to a higher educational plane. It was finally decided that the

ADN graduates should take the registered nurse (RN) licensure examination rather than the LPN/LVN examination.

The emphasis on technical skills of the ADN programs met a need in the health-care system of the 1960s and 1970s. By the early 1980s, there were more than 800 ADN programs across the United States; as of 1997, the number was 892, with more than 64,000 students attending.[11] Graduates from these programs soon exceeded the number of graduates from all the BSN and LPN/LVN programs combined.

Although it is possible to complete the requirements for an ADN in 2 academic years, most programs actually take at least 3 years to complete for a new student who has no prior college credit.[11] ADN graduates have a proven track record for providing safe bedside care for clients from the first day they are hired. They function well as team members, and after a period of orientation can assume responsibility for the care of clients who are more acutely ill.

BACCALAUREATE EDUCATION IN NURSING

The development of schools of nursing in the university and college setting was a gradual process that extended over several decades. Only a few collegiate nursing programs were established during the years when the diploma programs were expanding. Some of these early collegiate programs were a hybrid mixture of college-level classes and diploma school clinical experiences that still granted only a diploma rather than an academic degree. Early attempts at college-level nursing programs sometimes took the form of "pre-nursing" courses over a 1- or 2-year period that prepared students to enter upper division schools of nursing. Generally acclaimed as the first university program to be completely conducted in the higher education setting, the University of Minnesota School of Nursing was opened in 1909. In 1923, the Yale School of Nursing began accepting students; it is considered the first autonomous college of nursing in the United States.

The number of university-based nursing programs gradually increased over the years, and by the beginning of World War II there were 76 programs granting baccalaureate degrees in nursing. These programs tended to specialize in preparing nurses for public health nursing, teaching, administration, and supervisory positions in hospitals. Although all these programs included a clinical component, the emphasis was more on theoretical knowledge, development of decision-making skills, and leadership. Universities in general enjoyed rapid growth immediately after World War II, and higher education nursing programs expanded along with the universities. Many military nurses prepared by the Cadet Nurse Corps during World War II went back to school under the G.I. Bill to complete their baccalaureate degrees.

During this rapid growth period, these baccalaureate degree programs were plagued with problems similar to those found in the diploma programs during their own rapid expansion period. Primarily, the lack of uniformity in content, curriculum, and even length of programs was problematic. It was difficult to find qualified faculty because most of the nurses up to this time had received their education in diploma programs. No doctorate degrees existed in nursing; few nurses had master's degrees; and only a smattering of nurses had baccalaureate degrees. During the late 1940s and early 1950s, awareness began to develop that there was a need to stratify nursing education programs into technical levels and professional levels. It became apparent that all health-care professionals should have, at minimum, a baccalaureate degree.[12]

The NLN began to develop strict criteria for the accreditation of baccalaureate nursing programs. These criteria included courses in general education, general sciences, humanities, and language as well as specific nursing courses. They required a certain number of hours to be spent in the clinical setting practicing nursing skills, a faculty prepared at the master's degree level, and the availability of laboratory and library facilities for the students. Faculty-to-student ratios were limited, particularly in the clinical setting, and outcome criteria were required for the students.[13]

Although all university level baccalaureate degrees in nursing have the same number of required credit hours and educational requirements for baccalaureate degrees, there are three avenues for attaining this degree. The BSN degree fulfills the criteria to be known as a professional degree. It meets the overall requirements for a college baccalaureate degree (124 credit hours, 65 hours of nursing major, and most of the general education requirements), but does not meet all the general education requirements for an academic bachelor of science (BS) degree. Although this degree is usually obtained in a traditional college setting, it can also be obtained through an **external degree** program where the student has to meet the criteria for the BSN.

The second approach is found in programs that offer a bachelor of science degree with a major in nursing (BS Nursing). This degree is the full academic college degree and guarantees that the person holding it has met all of the general education, science, and major subject requirements. According to statistics published by the NLN for academic year 1997–1998, there are 529 accredited programs offering baccalaureate degrees in nursing.

A third avenue that may be pursued is sometimes called the **career ladder** program (see section on Ladder Programs).

> **" "** *It became apparent that all health-care professionals should have, at minimum, a baccalaureate degree.*

PRACTICAL/VOCATIONAL NURSING

The practical/vocational nurse, in one form or another, has been a part of the health-care system in the United States for more than 100 years. Although the earliest formal schools of practical/vocational nursing were started around 1890, informal training programs for this level of nursing probably existed well before this time—for example, in the Young Women's Christian Association (YWCA), particularly in New York City. These programs took uneducated girls who had migrated from rural areas and farms to the cities in search of employment and taught them a useful trade with which they could support themselves. With no regulation or accreditation for the early practical/vocational nurse programs, there were wide variations in the quality, length, and focus of what was being taught. Generally, the students were taught to provide home care, similar to that given by private duty nurses, for clients ranging from newborns to the elderly and invalid.

The number of practical/vocational nursing programs gradually increased over the next 50 years. Graduates of these 3-month programs were beginning to find employment in hospitals and nursing homes as well as in areas of private duty. During the nurse shortage after World War I, many hospitals found that these relatively undereducated nurses, after receiving on-the-job training in the hospital, could function at a fairly high level of skill, and at a much reduced cost. The word got around, and soon the number of these unlicensed nurses grew.

By the late 1930s, the ANA saw the need to regulate the quality of the practical/vocational nursing programs in order to protect public safety. It was not until 1938 that the state of New York took seriously the ANA's recommendation for compulsory licensure for practical/vocational nurses and enacted the first law requiring such licensure. In 1960, all practical/vocational nurses were required to pass a licensure examination before they could practice. These nurses are now referred to as licensed practical nurses (LPNs). In Texas and California, these nurses are called licensed vocational nurses (LVNs).

Although education for LPNs or LVNs varies slightly from one state to another, there are some common characteristics. Most of the programs are from 9 months to 12 months and are measured in clock hours rather than academic hours. They are often offered in hospitals, high schools, vocational schools, or trade schools, although some programs are conducted in community colleges or even in universities. Orientation of the curricula in these programs is highly technical and emphasizes the learning of skills in the setting of a hospital or nursing home with less emphasis on theoretical knowledge. As a **technician,** it is much more important for practical/vocational nurses to learn how to do something than why it is being done.

The stated scope of practice for the practical/vocational nurse involves providing care for clients in hospitals, nursing homes, or the home setting for those who have stable conditions. LPNs/LVNs are to be under the supervision of an RN or a licensed physician. However, in the real world, LPNs/LVNs are often required to provide care well outside of their scope of practice, often functioning in leadership roles or providing care in acute settings with highly unstable clients. LPNs/LVNs are often hired when there are shortages of registered nurses to fill the gaps in client care. Many associate degree RN programs have developed a ladder curriculum whereby an LPN/LVN can go back to school for a shorter period, often receiving credit for years of experience, complete the pro-

> 66 99 *However, in the real world, LPNs/LVNs are often required to provide care well outside of their scope of practice, often functioning in leadership roles or providing care in acute settings with highly unstable clients.*

gram in 1 year, and then take the RN licensure examination.

LADDER PROGRAMS

Career ladder, educational ladder, **articulation,** or educational mobility programs have become increasingly popular as a result of an interest in **upward mobility,** educational articulation, and **career mobility.** A ladder program allows nurses to upgrade their education and move from one educational level to another with relative ease and without loss of credits from previous education. Each ladder program is developed according to the philosophy of the particular nursing school, may use any one of a number of curricular patterns, uses one of several means of **advanced placement,** or granting credit for previous education, and must meet NLNAC accreditation standards. Ladder programs take several different forms. Some ladder programs provide a **competency-based education** that allows the students to proceed at their own pace as long as they fulfill required educational outcomes.

The LPN/LVN–to–ADN ladder allows individuals who have been licensed as LPNs/LVNs to take a minimal number of courses in an associated degree program to obtain their ADN and then take the NCLEX-RN, CAT to become licensed as registered nurses. Programs vary widely as to how many credits they will accept from the LPN/LVN programs and how many courses the students take to complete the degree. Some of the requirements for number of hours are out of the control of the nursing programs, because they have been established as general education requirements of the college or are state regents requirements.

There are also LPN/LVN-to-BSN ladder programs that allow licensed LPNs/LVNs to either challenge out of a number of courses or grant them credit for nursing courses based on previous experience and demonstrated competency. Students who enter these types of ladder programs usually spend more time in school than the LPN/LVN-to-ADN programs. In addition to meeting the requirements of the BSN, they also have to meet the general education requirements for a baccalaureate degree and complete 124 hours of college-level courses.

Nursing education has seen a marked increase in the number of ADN-to-BSN, and diploma-to-BSN ladder programs, sometimes called **two plus two (2+2) programs.** These programs admit individuals who are already licensed as registered nurses but who have either a diploma or associate degree. These programs may take several different forms. Upper division baccalaureate programs work exclusively with ADN-RNs, have no generic students and are designed exclusively to meet the educational needs of students who are already RNs. Other programs accept ADN or diploma graduates as students, in addition to generic students. These schools often have separate programs for ADN or diploma RNs that allow them to take examinations to prove educational knowledge and nursing proficiency (**challenge examinations**) in specific classes, thus granting credit for their nursing experience. The RNs then take advanced-level nursing courses such as Community Health/Home Health Care, Leadership, and Critical Care, which are not commonly found in diploma or ADN programs. In either case, on completion of the degree requirements, these nurses are granted a baccalaureate degree. Some of these programs have an **open curriculum** that allows students to enter and leave the program freely. There are 418 such programs accredited by the NLNAC.[11]

A growing trend in educational ladder programs is the ADN-to-MSN programs. Schools that offer this type of ladder must have an MSN program in place. The ADN students that enter these programs are given credit for prior classes and work experience and take both undergraduate and graduate level courses, receiving a BSN along the way to obtaining the MSN. These programs vary a great deal from school to school and may require from 3 to 5 semesters of classes. Often they are offered on a part-time basis, with many evening and weekend classes to meet the needs of working students.

Another type of educational ladder program that is less common is the nurse practitioner (NP)-to-MSN program. These programs admit nurse practitioners who graduated from programs that allowed the student to become certified but did not include enough credit hours for a master's degree. Again, the students are granted credit for past classes and work experience and often are allowed to challenge a certain number of core courses. Then they take the remaining required courses and are granted an MSN at graduation.

MASTER'S AND DOCTORAL LEVEL EDUCATION

The baccalaureate degree is considered a generalist degree that exposes a student to a wide range of subjects during the 4 years spent in college. The master's degree, on the other hand, is a specialist's degree.[14] Students who pursue a master's degree concentrate their study in one particular subject area and become expert in that given area.

Master's degree nursing programs have been in existence almost from the time baccalaureate level nursing programs were started. These early master's degree in nursing programs were designed for students who had baccalaureate degrees in other majors, such as biology, who wanted to become nurses. After completion of an additional 36 to 42 credit hours in nursing courses only, these students were awarded the MSN, and could then take the licensure examination for registered nurses.

Today, most master's degree in nursing programs are restricted to registered nurses who have the baccalaureate degree. Many of these programs require at least 1 year of clinical practice after the BSN and require approximately 36 to 46 college credit hours. Most students who enter master's degree programs attend classes on a part-time basis while they are working and may take up to 5 years to complete the requirements. Many universities have recognized this trend and have tailored their programs to meet the needs of these part-time students; the universities now offer courses in the evening, on weekends, or 1-day-a week programs. There are 296 accredited master's degree programs across the United States.[11]

There are a number of available areas of study for those pursuing master's degrees in nursing. Some of the more popular areas include nursing administration, community health, psychiatric mental health, adult health, maternal-child health, gerontology, rehabilitation care, nursing education, and some more advanced areas of practice, such as anesthesiology, pediatric nurse practitioner (PNP), family nurse practitioner, geriatric nurse practitioner (GNP), and obstetric-gynecology nurse practitioner.[15] Most of these programs require the student to pass a comprehensive written or oral examination, and some courses require the student to write an extensive research thesis before graduation.

There are two basic types of master's degrees in nursing. The master's of science in nursing (MSN) is the professional degree, and the master's of science with a major in nursing degree (MS Nursing) is the formal academic degree.[16] In practice, however, little differentiation is made between the two. Almost all master's programs accredited by the NLNAC require the applicant to have at least a 3.0 grade point average (GPA) and to demonstrate academic proficiency by achieving a satisfactory score on the Graduate Record Examination (GRE) or the

Miller's Analogy Test before admission. The GRE is also used to recommend remedial coursework needed to correct deficiencies before the master's program is undertaken.

In the evolution of the various levels of education, the baccalaureate degree is a generalist's degree, the master's degree is a specialist's degree, and the doctoral degree is a generalist's degree, although at a much higher academic level than that of the baccalaureate degree. Actually, the major purpose of early doctoral degrees was to prepare the individual to conduct advanced research in a particular area of interest.

Currently there is a wide range of available doctoral degrees for nurses. The doctor of philosophy (PhD) degree is the most accepted academic degree and is designed to prepare individuals to conduct research. The doctor of education (EdD) degree is considered to be a professional degree, although in many programs there is little difference between the courses of study taken by the EdD and PhD candidates. In other programs, the PhD focuses primarily on research, whereas the EdD focuses more on administration in the educational setting. The classes and research credits differ somewhat between the two degrees.

Since the 1970s, other doctoral programs for nurses have been developed that stress the clinical rather than academic nature of nursing.[17] These include the doctor of nursing science (DNSc) and the doctor of science in nursing (DSN), which is a clinically oriented nursing degree. The doctor of nursing (DN or ND) degree is for the person with a BS or MS in a field other than nursing who wants to pursue nursing as a career. It is a generalist's degree at a basic level of education. In addition, for nurses who wish to pursue a career in higher education, the doctor of nursing education (DNEd) degree is available.

Despite the wide range of doctoral degrees in nursing, there are relatively few programs across the United States that offer these degrees. Many nurses who seek them may obtain them in fields such as higher education, psychology, college teaching, and adult education.

The requirements for doctoral education are similar, even though the specific degrees being sought are different. The student must have attained a master's degree and must have achieved a satisfactory score on the GRE. Often there is an admission interview and preprogram examination that must be passed before the candidate can be formally admitted to the program. Doctoral programs are at least 60 college credit hours in length, require many statistics and research courses, and often have a residency requirement. Before the doctoral degree can be granted, the student must successfully complete both oral and written comprehensive examinations, as well as write a doctoral dissertation explaining the conduct of a major research project.

Some individuals pursuing doctoral degrees do so on a part-time basis while they are working full-time, whereas others attend classes full-time while working full-time, often completing the program in 3 to 4 years. Many programs require that the individual complete all the requirements within a 10-year time period. Although this may seem a like a long time, it is not unusual for the dissertation process itself to take 2 to 3 years.

Nurses with master's or doctoral degrees are regarded as leaders in the profession of nursing. Many of the larger hospitals across the United States require their head nurses and supervisors to have master's degrees and their directors of nursing to have doctorates. Of course, in higher education, the minimal requirement for teaching is the master's degree, and the doctorate is preferred. Nurses with these advanced degrees provide direction and leadership for the profession through their publications, research, and theory development. As health-care delivery becomes more complicated, larger numbers of nurses with advanced degrees will be required.

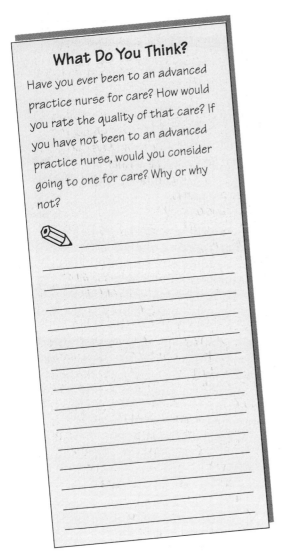

What Do You Think?

Have you ever been to an advanced practice nurse for care? How would you rate the quality of that care? If you have not been to an advanced practice nurse, would you consider going to one for care? Why or why not?

EDUCATION FOR ADVANCED PRACTICE

Advanced practice is one of those often misused terms in nursing that adds to the public's confusion about educational levels of those in the profession. Sometimes referred to as **expanded role** or practice, nurses who obtain certification are allowed to practice at a higher and more independent level depending on the nurse practice act of their individual state. Advanced practitioners diagnose illnesses, prescribe medications, conduct physical examinations, and refer clients to specialists for more intensive follow-up care. These nurses practice nursing under their own licenses as **independent practitioners** but often work closely with a physician so that they can quickly refer clients' medical problems that lie outside their scope of practice.

The nurse practitioner levels of nursing are most widely accepted as advanced practice areas for nursing. These include the pediatric nurse practitioner (PNP), the neonatal nurse practitioner (NNP), the geriatric nurse practitioner (GNP), the obstetrics-gynecology nurse practitioner, the family nurse practitioner (FNP), the rehabilitation nurse practitioner (RNP), the psychiatric nurse practitioner, and the nurse midwife. The certified registered nurse anesthetist (CRNA) and nurse midwife are the oldest of the advanced practice certificates for nurses and are already well accepted in the medical community. Other advanced practice nurses experience varying levels of acceptance from physicians (Boxes 4–1 and 4–2), although the public in general likes the care they receive from advanced practice nurses. All states now have granted some type of **prescriptive authority** to nurse practitioners.

In the past, nurses with baccalaureate degrees, or even associate degrees in California as late as the 1990s, could attend highly concentrated courses of study for 1 to 2 years and become increasingly proficient in a particular specialty area without, however, obtaining an MSN. They could then take the certification examination and become certified as nurse practitioners. Currently, most nurse practitioner programs are offered in major universities, requiring students to complete the master's degree before allowing them to take the certification examination.

One level of nursing that falls under the umbrella of advanced practice is the **nurse**

4.1 Wanted: Nurse Practitioners—Good Pay and Great Working Conditions

Although slow to evolve, physicians' attitudes toward nurse practitioners have made a 180-degree turnaround in the past few years. As managed care stresses and seeks more economical methods of delivering cost-effective primary care, nurse practitioners have experienced an increase in demand for their services. The shift of care from hospital-based to community-based services has many physicians looking at nurse practitioners from a new perspective.

Physicians are beginning to recognize that modern health care is a team process involving physicians, nurses, dietitians, social workers, and nurse practitioners. Not only do nurse practitioners expand the physicians' practice by allowing for increased numbers of clients to be treated, they also offer a unique aspect to the care. The additional time that nurse practitioners spend with clients, coupled with their traditional nurse orientation toward caring, produces an atmosphere in clinics, physicians' offices, and health-care facilities where clients perceive that they are important and the focus of the care.

The National Advisory Council on Nurse Education and Practice estimates that the United States had only 20,000 certified nurse practitioners of all types in 1993. The Council projects that by the year 2020, the United States will require almost 100,000 nurse practitioners to meet the primary health-care needs of a predominantly managed care system.

Schools of nursing are responding to this trend by increasing the number of master's level nurse practitioner programers. All nurse practitioner programs are reporting full classes. Many nurses who have been practicing for several years view the move to nurse practitioner as a method to advance in nursing without moving to an administrative or desk job far away from direct client care. Also, many nurses who were classified as clinical specialists recognized the uncertainty of this position and began entering nurse practitioner programs.

Managed health-care institutions are beginning to recognize that nurse practitioners excel at health promotion and management of clients with chronic and disabling diseases. When nurse practitioners keep clients healthier and out of the hospital, the managed systems can keep their costs lower. Relatively simple practices routinely performed by nurse practitioners, like calling clients to see whether they are taking their blood pressure medications, drawing blood samples to monitor clients' conditions, or simply listening attentively to client complaints, add a humanistic touch to the cold world of medical treatment. Clients tend to be more willing to follow health-care teaching if they feel the health-care provider is really interested in them as a person.

Across the nation, more and more physicians are beginning to use or considering using nurse practitioners in their practice. They recognize that the key to success in a managed health-care world is to keep clients as healthy as possible. Nurse practitioners are particularly well suited to provide wellness and health maintenance care because of both their education and their orientation toward caring.

From Job security, better pay spur nurses to better training. St. Louis Post Dispatch, August 25, 1997, 10BP–13BP.

4.2 Misplaced Loyalty

Tisha S., a senior nursing student, was acting as the team leader during her final clinical experience. Jamie D., a close friend of Tisha's, was one of three junior nursing students in Tisha's team that day. Because of some personal problems, Jamie had been late and unprepared for several clinical experiences. She was informed by her instructor that she might fail unless she showed marked improvement during clinical training.

Claire, B., a 64-year-old woman with diabetes and possible renal failure, was one of Jamie's clients. Mrs. B. was having a 24-hour urine test to help determine her renal function. After the test was completed later that afternoon, she was to be discharged and treated through the renal clinic. Jamie understood the principles of the 24-hour urine test and realized that all the urine for the full 24 hours needed to be saved. But she became busy caring for another client and accidentally threw away the last specimen before the test ended. She took the specimen container to the laboratory anyway.

At the end of the shift, when Jamie was giving her report to Tisha, she confided that she had thrown away the last urine specimen but begged Tisha not to tell the instructor. This mistake would mean that the test would have to be started over again, and Mrs. B. would have to spend an extra day in the hospital. Out of friendship, Tisha agreed not to tell the instructor, rationalizing that they had got almost all the urine and she was going to be treated for renal failure anyway. When the instructor asked Tisha for her final report for the day, she specifically asked if there had been any problems with the 24-hour urine test. What would be the consequences of telling the truth and of not telling the truth?

specialist, or **clinical nurse specialist (CNS).** Although there are a few schools that offer specific clinical nurse specialists curricula, more often these nurses are self-classified as clinical nurse specialists after completing a master's degree, or some additional education, in a particular clinical area. However, in a few states, such as Ohio, the clinical nurse specialist designation requires a master's degree and a special licensing examination. CNSs are usually hired by hospitals and often function as in-service educators for the hospital.

In 1988, an amendment to the New York Nurse Practice Act established a separate scope of practice and title protection for nurse practitioners (NPs). Subsequent to the NP amendment, there has been some confusion regarding which of the advanced nurs-ing practice categories are included within the scope of practice particularly by clinical nurse specialists, nurse midwives, and certified nurse anesthetists. This confusion, especially in psychiatric mental health nursing and nurse anesthesia, is related to the legal interpretations of the NP amendment. The resultant debate about this issue has led to a clearer definition and understanding of the term advanced practice nurse.

The career opportunities for advanced practice nurses are numerous.[18] Many nurse practitioners work for county health departments, rural clinics, and on Native American reservations; others work in hospitals, with physicians in private practice, and in rehabilitation centers. They have even established their own independent clinics. They provide primary health-care services in areas where there is a lack of primary care physicians. Although many of these areas are traditionally rural, today inner-city areas also often have need for this type of health care.

In addition, a common element of several proposed national health-care plans is the requirement that a client seeking entry into the health-care system be evaluated by a primary health-care practitioner before referral to any specialized health-care practitioner. Although the family practice physician, or general practitioner, would be the most common primary health-care provider to evaluate the client, the nurse practitioner could also function in this role. If any of these proposed health-care plans are adopted on a national level, the demand for nurse practitioners will increase tremendously.

Conclusion

In today's rapidly changing health-care environment, there is an ever-increasing need for health-care professionals who are educated to practice at the highest levels.[1] It is imperative that the schools that will be educating future nurses be responsive to the changes, challenges, and demands of an ever more sophisticated and technologically advanced health-care system. Nursing education is an important part of a much larger network of health-care systems, including the service and practice sector, government and regulatory agencies, and licensing and credentialing institutions. All of these interact with each other and together form what is called the health-care system.

The nursing profession has, over the years, developed a number of different types of education programs in an attempt to meet the demands of a growing health-care system. Some of the programs that were developed for specific needs that no longer exist should be examined for their usefulness and viability in today's advanced health-care atmosphere. Perhaps their resources could be rechanneled to programs that are more in tune with current needs. Students should carefully evaluate programs that they might enter and decide which one best meets their care goals. Meanwhile nursing education continues to develop innovative approaches to help nurses meet the demands for more education, more technical skills, and more leadership ability. The ladder programs are a good example. By recognizing the dynamic state of nursing education, and implementing changes that respond to or even anticipate changes in the health-care system, the nursing profession will continue as one of the pillars of the health-care system.

Educators in nursing have begun to recognize that it is impossible to teach nursing students everything they need to know in the short time allowed for formal education. The demands of the changing health-care system will make that goal even more difficult. However, it may not be necessary to teach nursing students everything. It is more important to teach these students the thinking, decision-making, and management skills that will allow them to adjust to an ever-changing and developing health-care system.

Name _____

Course _____

Instructor _____

Date _____

Critical Thinking Exercises

✔ Discuss why the current educational system for nurses leads to confusion over the role and scope of practice for nurses.

✔ The literature reports that there will be a nursing shortage well into the twenty-first century. What aspects of health-care reform are likely to produce changes in nursing education? Identify possible changes that may occur in nursing education because of the projected nursing shortage. Will these changes be beneficial or harmful to the profession of nursing?

✔ What historical factors had an important influence on the development of nursing education as it is currently conducted in the United States?

✔ What should the minimum level of education be for the professional nurse— ADN, BSN, or MSN? Defend your position.

References

1. Buerhaus, P: Is another RN shortage looming? Nurs Outlook 46(3):103–108, 1998.
2. de Tornyay, R: Reconsidering nursing education: The report of the Pew Health Professions Commission. J Nurs Educ 13:296–301, 1992.
3. de Tornyay, R: Critical challenges for nurse educators. J Nurs Educ 35(4):146–147, 1996.
4. American Nurses Association: Position Paper on Education. American Nurses Association, Kansas City, MO, 1965.
5. Fitzpatrick, ML: Prologue to Professionalism. Brady, Bowie, MD, 1983.
6. Jamieson, EM, et al: Trends in Nursing History. WB Saunders, Philadelphia, 1968.
7. Hegner, BR, and Caldwell, E: Nursing Assistant: A Nursing Process Approach, ed 6. Delmar Publishers, Albany, NY, 1995.
8. National League for Nursing, Trends in Baccalaurate Education, June, 1998.
9. Ketefian, S: Moving beyond traditional boundaries. J Prof Nurs 9:25–31, 1993.
10. Calhoun, J: The Nightingale pledge: A commitment that survives the passage of time. Nursing & Health Care 14:130–136, 1993.
11. National League for Nursing, 1992.
12. O'Neal, EH, and Hare, DM: Prospectives on Health Care Professions. Duke University Press, Durham, NC, 1990.
13. National League for Nursing: Characteristics of Baccalaureate Education in Nursing. Council of Baccalaureate and Higher Degrees, National League for Nursing, New York, 1987.
14. Forni, PR: Nursing's diverse master's programs: The state of the art. Nursing & Health Care 8:770–775, 1987.
15. Lipman, TH, and Deatrick, JA: Enhancing specialist preparation for the next century. J Nurs Educ 33:53–58, 1994.
16. Kalisch, PA, and Kalisch, BJ: The Advance of American Nursing, ed 3. JB Lippincott, Philadelphia, 1995.
17. American Association of Colleges of Nursing: Indicators of quality in doctoral programs in nursing. J Prof Nurs 3:72–74, 1987.
18. Houston, CJ, and Fox, S: The changing health care market: Implications for nursing education. Nurs Outlook 46(3):109–114, 1998.

BIBLIOGRAPHY

American Association of Colleges of Nursing: The baccalaureate degree in nursing as minimal preparation for professional practice. AACN, Washington DC, 1996.

American Association of Colleges of Nursing: Non-hospital clinical sites increase. News Release, October, 1995.

Canavan, K: Faculty refocus educational mission. American Nurse 28(26):1, 1996.

Canavan, K: Nursing education on the cusp of shift in focus. American Nurse 28(26):1, 1996.

Clarke, PN, and Cody, WK: Nursing theory-based practice in the home and community. Advances in Nursing Science 17:41–53, 1994.

Department of Health and Human Services, Division of Nursing: National Sample Survey of Registered Nurses, March, 1996.

Diamond, K: Primary nurse directs interdisciplinary care for cardiac patient. AACN News 14(11):14–15, 1998.

Diploma programs in nursing accredited by the NLNAC, 1996–1997. Nursing & Health Care: Perspectives on Community 17(5):268–269, 1996.

Evans, ML, et al: Nursing care and patient satisfaction. Am J Nurs 98(12):57–62, 1998.

Hunt, R: Community-based nursing: Philosophy or setting? Am J Nurs 98(10):44–49, 1998.

Keepnews, D: The national sample survey of RNs: What does it tell us. American Nurse 30(3):11, 1998.

Lindeman, C: Curriculum changes needed in nursing education. Am Nurse 28(26):6, 1996.

Loscalzo, F: The essence of nursing is touching another soul. AACN News 15(10):3, 1998.

Malone, B: The power of nursing education. Am Nurse 28:4, 1996.

Marks, D: Nurse-managed health centers gain recognition for innovation. American Nurse 29(4):10, 1997.

National League for Nursing: Characteristics of Associate Degree Education in Nursing. Council of Associate Degree Programs, National League for Nursing, New York, 1992.

National League for Nursing: Criteria and Guidelines for Accreditation of Associate Degree Programs, ed 7. Council of Associate Degree Programs, National League for Nursing, New York, 1991.

National League for Nursing: Education Outcomes of Associate Degree Programs Roles and Competencies. Council of Associate Degree Programs, National League for Nursing, New York, 1990.

Nicoll, LH: Nurses' Guide to the Internet, ed 2. JB Lippincott, Philadelphia, 1998.

Nicoteri, JA: Critical thinking skills. Am J Nurs 98(10): 62–68, 1998.

Oesterle, M, and O'Callaghan, D: The changing health care environment: Impact on curriculum and faculty. Nursing & Health Care: Perspectives on Community 2(17):78–81, 1996.

Rode, D, et al: The therapeutic use of technology. Am J Nurs 98(12):32–35, 1998.

Seymer, LR: Selected Writings of Florence Nightingale. Macmillan, New York, 1954.

Stewart, M: Health care community faces the year 2000. American Nurse 29(6):24, 1997.

Strategies advance family-centered care philosophy. AACN News 15(10):5, 1998.

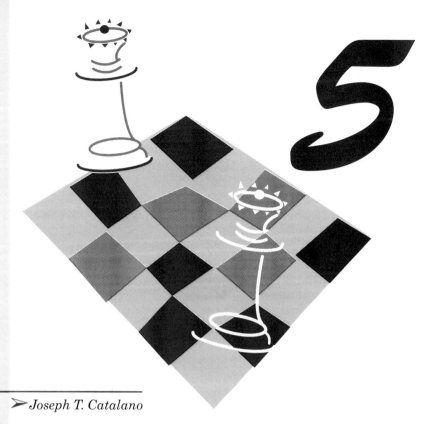

Critical Thinking

➤ *Joseph T. Catalano*

Learning Objectives

After completing this chapter, the reader will be able to:

1. Demonstrate logical, rational, and creative critical thinking.
2. Describe the steps of the critical thinking process in resolving a client care issue.
3. Apply critical thinking to client care.
4. List five characteristics of critical thinking.

One of the most important responsibilities that nurses have is to make correct and safe decisions in a variety of client care situations. The decisions made by nurses affect the health status, recovery time, and even the life or death of a client. For example, the critical care nurse must decide when to give certain medications based on changes in the client's condition. The emergency room nurse must decide which client is treated first based on the extent of his or her injuries. The hospital staff nurse must decide what PRN medication to give for which set of symptoms. The home health nurse must decide when to call the physician about a change in a client's condition.

The process by which these decisions are made involves the use of critical thinking. Critical thinking is based on reason and reflection, knowledge and instinct derived from experience. It has also been defined as "the art of thinking about thinking." It is both an attitude about and an approach to solving problems. Critical thinking helps nurses make decisions about problems for which there are no simple solutions. Often nurses have to make these decisions with less than complete information.

Although critical thinking has always been used by nurses to some degree and recognized as important in the provision of care, its status increased greatly when the National League for Nursing Accrediting Commission (NLNAC) designated critical thinking as one of its mandatory outcome objectives in 1992. Since then, schools of nursing have been challenged to demonstrate where and how they teach and measure critical thinking in the curriculum. It is fairly easy to claim: "Yes, we teach our students how to think critically," but much more difficult to accurately define what critical thinking actually is and then demonstrate that the graduates of the program have attained and can use the skill.

A definition is a short statement that identifies and distinguishes something from all other things so that it can be recognized. Generally, things that are easy to define have one or a few definitions. Things that are more difficult to define tend to have many definitions that may or may not overlap. It would seem that critical thinking falls into the latter category. There are at least 10 different definitions for critical thinking that have been developed over the years by the various experts in the subject. Perhaps a better approach to recognizing and developing critical thinking is to look at the characteristics that seem to be common in most of the definitions.

CHARACTERISTICS OF CRITICAL THINKING

Critical Thinking Is Creative

Nurses who think creatively explore new ideas and alternative ways of solving client care problems. Creative thinkers are able to bring together bits of knowledge or information that may initially seem unrelated and formulate them into a plan that leads to effective decision making and solves the problem by finding connections between the thoughts and concepts. This process is similar to the linear approach used in the nursing process. All the situational variables must be considered, and decision making becomes more complex as the number of variables increase.

Example of Creative Thinking

In a small hospital, a policy was instituted that required all post–cesarean delivery clients to be monitored in the recovery room just like all other postoperative clients. Because the operating room (OR) nurses were on call for the recovery room, they thought

What Do You Think?

Identify two situations that you have been involved with that required critical thinking. How did you resolve these situations? What elements of critical thinking did you use?

✎ _____

_____

_____

_____

_____

_____

_____

_____

_____

_____

that they were being required to do more work with no additional staff. The circulating and scrub obstetric (OB) nurses could go home after the delivery. The OR nurses became very resentful of the extra call for the postdelivery clients and often called in sick the day after they were required to attend a postcesarean client. This practice left the OR short staffed during the day and led to increased tension and frequent unfriendly confrontations between the OR and the OB nurses.

The nurse managers of the OB and OR units resolved the problem by instituting a policy of "cross-training" with the OR and OB nurses. OB nurses were taught how to monitor the recovery of postoperative clients and were rotated through recovery for 1 week every 2 months to keep these skills current. The OR nurses were taught how to assist at cesarean deliveries and were rotated through the OB unit for 1 week every 2 months. This system kept the staffing levels constant, and allowed the OB nurses to assist with the post–cesarean delivery clients. Although not everyone was happy with the practice, it did reduce the resentment levels between the two units and gave the nurses a better appreciation of the other nurses' responsibilities.

Critical Thinking is Logical, Rational, and Reflective

Although the critical thinking process is often expanded beyond fundamental logical thinking, it must always be based on rationales and facts rather than emotions or egocentric impulses. Intuition can play a part in critical thinking when it is recognized as a rational thought process that brings together and processes a number of factors at the subconscious level rather than a simple

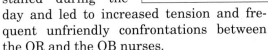 *Jumping to conclusions often produces poor decisions and negative results.*

"gut feeling." If at all possible, critical thinkers must take the time to collect as much data as they can, and examine it under the light of reason before making a decision or taking an action. Sometimes, decisions must at times be made on a limited amount of information in situations where there is a high degree of risk and ambiguity. In these situations, the nurse's past experiences resolving similar situations as well as intuition can help. However, in most cases merely jumping to conclusions often produces poor decisions and negative results. Logical reasoning is often divided into deductive and inductive reasoning.

Deductive logic or reasoning is a process whereby the individual proceeds from the general to the particular. The conclusions reached by deductive reasoning based on a valid argument are certain and true.

Example of Deductive Reasoning

Either John Smith or George Jones is to be given a dose of IV penicillin before surgery.

There was no order for IV penicillin for John Smith before surgery.

Therefore, George Jones is to be given IV penicillin before surgery.

The conclusion is valid. The rationale is that all of the information in the conclusion is found in the premises; therefore, the conclusion must logically follow if the premises are true.

Inductive logic or reasoning involves proceeding from the particular to the general. The conclusions reached by inductive reasoning are probable or contingent. Inductive reasoning is more frequently used in health-care situations than deductive reasoning because of the wide range of variables involved in client care.

Example of Inductive Reasoning

Mr. Jones has a bacterial lobar pneumonia.
   Antibiotics are usually used to treat this disease.
   Therefore, Mr. Jones should be given an antibiotic.

The conclusion is valid. The rationale is that the conclusion is uncertain because the use of the word "usually" in the premise leaves room for alternative conclusions.

Keep in mind that all critical thinking, including both inductive and deductive reasoning, is open to fallacies. A fallacy is generally defined as an error in reasoning that leads to a conclusion that does not follow from its premises.[1] Some arguments are valid, sound, or cogent, whereas others are false, illogical, and invalid. The most common type of fallacy seen in nursing is the *non sequitur,* a fallacy in which the conclusion does not follow from the arguments or premise. For example, a 72-year-old male client who had a colon resection and colostomy 12 days ago and who is being prepared for discharge expresses fear about returning to his one-room apartment in the inner city. He also has a heart murmur. On these two factors alone, a nursing diagnosis of "severe dependency needs" is formulated. Another common example of this fallacy is often seen when there are staffing shortages. It is not unusual for nursing supervisors to say to a staff nurse, "We need you to work this extra shift because everyone else called in. I know you take classes in the evening, but the clients always come first. Therefore, if you don't work, you might as well start looking for employment elsewhere." This situation also adds the element of irrelevant appeal to force.

People commit fallacies for various reasons. In some cases, individuals have such a strong ideological commitment to a religious, economic, or political belief that they refuse to listen to any ideas or opinions that contradict what they believe. Basically, their minds are closed to any alternative conclusions, thus they stick to their own conclusions regardless of the reasoning process. Some individuals have difficulty acknowledging that they have made a mistake and will refuse to see the lack of logic in their reasoning and conclusions. Still others must "win" at all cost and will subvert the critical thinking process and logic by abuse, twisting the other person's words, and using personal attacks. Being able to recognize conclusions that are valid or invalid is an important part of critical thinking.

For practice, analyze each of the following arguments, decide whether they are inductive or deductive, note whether they are valid or invalid, and give a rationale for the decision.

1. The largest city in a country is usually the capital of the country.

   New York City is the largest city in the United States.

   Therefore, New York City is the capital of the United States.

   Type of reasoning _inductive_
   Conclusion valid? ☐ Yes ☑ No
   Rationale: Because of the word "usually" there is room for alternative conclusions

2. All nurses are women.

   Pat is a nurse.

   Therefore, Pat is a woman.

   Type of reasoning _deductive_
   Conclusion valid? ☑ Yes ☐ No
   Rationale: conclusion called be drawn from both premises

3. Nora is a premature infant who weighs 1 pound.

   Nora has two congenital abnormalities—myelomeningocele and ventricular septal defect.

Premature infants with congenital abnormalities usually die within 2 weeks of birth.

Therefore, Nora will die within the next 2 weeks.

Type of reasoning __inductive__
Conclusion valid? ❏ Yes ☑ No
Rationale: _____

_____

4. In prison, criminals perform hard labor.

Tom is a prisoner performing hard labor.

Therefore, Tom is a criminal.

Type of reasoning __deductive__
Conclusion valid? ☑ Yes ❏ No
Rationale: _____

_____

5. 96% of nurses are women.

Terry is a nurse.

Therefore, Terry is probably a woman.

Type of reasoning __inductive__
Conclusion valid? ❏ Yes ☑ No
Rationale: _____

_____

6. Mary is staggering around the room.

Mary was just at a cocktail party.

Therefore, Mary drank too much alcohol.

Type of reasoning __inductive__
Conclusion valid? ❏ Yes ☑ No
Rationale: _____

_____

7. Almost every identified carcinogen causes cancer in animals.

Humans are animals.

Therefore, almost every identified carcinogen causes cancer in humans.

Type of reasoning __inductive__
Conclusion valid? ❏ Yes ☑ No
Rationale: _____

_____

8. O.J. owns a pair of Bruno Magli shoes.

Footprints from Bruno Magli shoes were found at the crime scene.

Therefore, O.J. committed the crime.

Type of reasoning __inductive__
Conclusion valid? ❏ Yes ☑ No
Rationale: __This conclusion is probable but not absolute__

9. Ada, Betty, and Clara are the staff nurse, the head nurse, and the supervisor (but not necessarily in that order).

Ada was beaten by the head nurse in a bridge game.

Betty is the supervisor's neighbor.

Betty is unbeatable at bridge when playing the other two nurses.

Clara wants to become a head nurse or supervisor.

a. Who is the head nurse? __Betty__
b. Who is the supervisor? __Ada__
c. Who is the staff nurse? __Clara__

Type of reasoning __deductive__

Rationale: _____

_____

_____

_____

_____

10. Smith, Jones, and Brown are a surgeon, a scrub nurse, and an OR tech (but not necessarily in that order).

The OR tech, who is an only child, earns the least amount of money.

Brown, who married Smith's sister, earns more than the scrub nurse.

Who is the surgeon? *Brown*

Who is the scrub nurse? *Smith*

Who is the scrub tech? *Jones*

Type of reasoning _*deductive*_

Rationale: _____

_____

_____

_____

_____

_____

Keep in mind that these exercises are simplified examples of inductive and deductive reasoning and are presented as an introduction to logical reasoning. However, using simple reasoning processes alone in client care decisions can lead to serious fallacies and error in judgment. All the other characteristics of critical thinking discussed here must be included for sound clinical decision making.

Critical Thinking is Independent

Nurses who think critically are not easily influenced by others with strong opinions. They demonstrate their autonomy by thinking for themselves and not passively succumbing to peer pressure or the belief system of the majority.

Example of Independent Thinking

An 82-year-old woman was brought into the emergency room (ER) by her family with complaints of "difficulty urinating." During the initial assessment, the RN noted that the client had +2 edema of her ankles and feet, congested lung sounds, and shortness of breath. The ER physician ordered a Foley catheter, urinalysis, and a consultation with a urologist for the urinary complaint. The RN pointed out the client's history of congestive heart failure (CHF) and current symptoms and also the fact that only 10 mL of urine was obtained when the catheter was inserted. The ER physician insisted that the problem was urinary and refused to discuss the client's condition any more.

While waiting for the urinalysis results, the client became increasingly short of breath and restless. The RN called for a chest x-ray and measurement of arterial blood gases (ABGs). The chest x-ray showed that 75% of the client's lung fields were filled with fluid, and the ABGs showed respiratory acidosis with hypoxia. The nurse asked the physician to order furosemide (Lasix) for the client based on these findings. The physician became angry, accused the nurse of practicing medicine, and refused to write the order. The nurse then called the client's attending physician, who decided to admit the client to the hospital and begin treatment with IV furosemide for the obvious CHF.

Critical Thinking Challenges Rituals and Assumptions About Client Care

A healthy, constructive questioning of long-used health-care practices prevents the nurse from the mindless provision of rote care. Improvement and advance in health-care practices occur only when nurses understand the rationale behind the practices, then accept or reject them based on evidence that they either do or do not work as intended.

Example of Challenging Rituals and Assumptions

A newly hired nurse was beginning her first shift on the obstetric (OB) unit when a 28-year-old client in her sixth month of pregnancy was admitted with abdominal cramps and vaginal bleeding. A spontaneous abortion was suspected. Another nurse who had worked on the OB unit for 10 years knew the client and her family. She told the newly hired nurse to call the client's sister (her number was on the chart), even though the client had not requested it. The newly hired nurse felt uncomfortable making the call and refused on the grounds that it was a violation of client **confidentiality.** The experienced nurse became angry at the refusal and berated the new nurse with the statement "We've been notifying the families of our clients for years and you're not going to change that practice."

The next day, the newly hired nurse had a conference with the OB unit nurse manager and arranged for several inservice presentations on the right to privacy.

Critical Thinking is Free of Bias and Prejudice

Biases are unjustified personal opinions. When a bias, as well as **stereotype,** is taken as fact, it becomes a prejudice. A belief is not true just because it has been in existence for a long period of time or because many people believe it. In order to use effective critical thinking, biases and stereotypes must be identified and eliminated.

Analyzing and viewing a situation from all points of view before arriving at a conclusion prevents the nurse from making one-sided decisions. It also helps determine bias or prejudice on the part of physicians, nurses, and even clients and the backlash effect that it may produce on other decision makers.

Recognition of bias does not always eliminate it, but helps the decision maker compensate for it when making the final decision.

Example of Bias- and Prejudice-Free Thinking

A homosexual, HIV-positive client with full-blown symptoms of AIDS is admitted to a medical/surgical unit for care. The nurse assigned to care for the client has very strong religious beliefs about homosexuality. She believes that her obligation as a nurse requires her to care for this client despite his diagnosis and sexual preference, yet she also believes that caring for this client would tacitly condone his sexual preferences and lifestyle. She tries to place herself in the client's situation and recognizes that an ill client deserves quality care without consideration of his beliefs or background.

Critical Thinking is Action Oriented

The goal of critical thinking in health care should always be the resolution of a problem or a method to improve client care. Critical thinking is used at all levels of the health-care system and is essential to the formulation and evaluation of policies and procedures, use of effective communication, and resolution of management and personnel conflicts.

Example of Action-Oriented Critical Thinking

A physician with a reputation for striking fear in the hearts of the nurses in the medical/surgical unit was in a particularly bad mood one day. After making his rounds, the physician criticized the care that the nurses were giving to his clients loudly and publicly in the nurses' station and proceeded to announce numerous mistakes that the nurses had made over the past year. The unit manager took the physician aside and told him that if he was having problems with the nurses on the unit, he should follow correct channels to file complaints and not make a scene in the nurses' station where many of the clients could hear him.

The physician became even more irate and stormed out of the unit directly to the office of the Director of Nursing (DON). He told the DON that he was filing an official **complaint** against the unit manager for unprofessional behavior, disrespect for a physician, and failure to follow medical orders. The DON told him that she would investigate the complaint and take appropriate action.

After talking with all the nurses on the medical/surgical unit and nurses on other units, as well as a number of physicians, it was discovered that the physician who filed the complaint was well known for his **capricious** and obnoxious behavior toward nurses. He was referred to the hospital medical board, reprimanded for his behavior toward the nurses, and required to drop the complaint about the manager of the medical/surgical unit. In addition, a special meeting was called for all the physicians practicing in the hospital to discuss the problem and to better understand what was involved regarding professional behavior.

CRITICAL THINKING SKILLS

Although there are different approaches to developing critical thinking, certain concepts are common to the skill. Some individuals seem to have an innate ability to master these concepts, whereas others have difficulty with them. As with most skills, practice and repetition increase efficiency and the ability to make safe decisions in complex nursing situations where there are multiple variables that affect the client's health status.

Concept 1: Identify the Problem

The saying "It's hard to know when you have arrived if you don't know where you are going" applies particularly well to critical thinking. If the underlying problem has not been identified, then it is almost impossible to develop a plan to solve it. One way to identify the underlying problem is to try to restate the issue as a declarative statement. For example, a public health nurse may identify that "sexually transmitted dis-

eases (STDs) among teenagers in our society is increasing at a rapid rate."

Concept 2: Gather Pertinent Data

It sometimes happens that when trying to apply critical thinking to the resolution of a problem, there is only a small amount of information that relates to the situation. On the other hand, in our information-oriented society, there may be an overabundance of data. It becomes necessary for the nurse to sort through the data, use the data that relate to the problem, and reject the data that are extraneous and perhaps misleading. In the previous example of STD in teenagers, the Internet can provide copious data, including general population statistics, racial and ethnic breakdowns, STD incidents by region, the most common STDs, treatment regimens, and even projections for the future.

Rational analysis and consideration of the data may produce a re-examination and refocusing of the problem. For example, after examining the abundance of information about teenage STD, the community health nurses may decide to focus their emphasis on dealing with the problem in their community rather than the entire state.

Concept 3: Identify and Challenge Assumptions, Beliefs, Ideas, and Issues

Developing a contextual awareness requires primarily the use of deductive reasoning. Contextual awareness is a very broad concept that is not merely limited to values but also includes everything that may have an affect on the client, such as physical symptoms and environment. Everyone, including nurses, has feelings and beliefs about all issues. Some of these beliefs are personal; some are cultural; some are stated overtly, whereas others remain deeply rooted but hidden in the unconscious. In any case, these beliefs influence how situations are perceived and what decisions are made.

In order to make solid decisions based on critical thinking, nurses must examine their own philosophy, beliefs, and value systems. **Values clarification** is an important element in critical thinking. At some point in the nurse's career, preferably in the early stages, he or she should make a list of all the things they consider as valuable. It should also be recognized that values are not static and that values will be added or deleted or will change in priority with time.

In addition, nurses must examine their own philosophy of nursing and health care as it relates to that of the agency for which they are working. Then, they need to compare how societal values relate to their own personal philosophy and that of the agency. Do societal values reflect or contradict the philosophy? How do the standards of care, the nurse practice act of the state, facility **protocols,** and even the code of ethics affect the care being provided?

Challenging assumptions and rituals of care requires use of inductive reasoning. The nurse needs to ask whether there are any assumptions about the care provided;

What Do You Think?

What five values are most important to you? How do these influence the way you act? What happens when these values conflict?

A Closer Look

PERSONAL VALUES

Listed below are a number of values that almost everyone has. Circle the ones that you feel are important to you, adding additional values as necessary. Then rank the values according to priority.

family
education
career
honesty
good health
respect
leisure time
nonjudgmental attitude
cooperative work relationships
professional integrity
competency
empathy
flexibility
trust
teamwork
dependability
punctuality
accountability
self-determination
independence

veracity
justice
commitment

_____
_____
_____
_____

what they are; how they affect care; and whether any of these assumptions can be challenged.

In much the same way, rituals about care should also be identified and challenged. What are the rituals that are done rotely without much thought? Are they beneficial, or can they be changed or eliminated?

The community health nurse, for example, may have the philosophy that an STD among teenagers represents a dangerous and serious threat to the health of the community. On the other hand, the community may have an underlying philosophy that teenage STD is to be expected and is only one of the rites of passage that must be experienced. Where such a major difference in philosophy exists, it would be extremely difficult for the nurse to implement any action that would resolve the problem.

Some assumptions that could be challenged might revolve around the cause of the problem. An increase in STDs among teenagers may be caused by (1) a lack of sexual education in school, (2) a lack of morals in our society, or (3) an atmosphere of permissiveness and egocentrism that is projected in the media.

One health department philosophy about teenagers that may need to be challenged might be that all teenagers are rebellious, uncooperative, and promiscuous, when in reality, many teenagers work well with others, are highly productive, and have high moral standards.

> **" "** *As a way of looking at the world, critical thinking allows the nurse to consider new ideas and then evaluate those ideas in light of accepted information as well as client and personal value systems.*

Nurses also need to learn and evaluate the value systems of those with whom they are working. Even though they may not agree with those values, it is important to recognize them and work with them when attempting to affect health. For example, when teaching a group of high-school students about STDs, it would be essential to know what their attitudes toward sex and health were. In all likelihood, these attitudes would be different from those of the nurse. An education program organized around only the nurse's belief and value system would be doomed to failure. Presenting the information from a viewpoint of the students would help them better understand and perhaps be more willing to accept it.

Concept 4: Imagine and Explore Alternatives Creatively

Once the nurse has identified the problem and explored the assumptions and rituals, he or she needs to consider the possible alternatives to care delivery. However, the nurse does not need to do this alone.

The information can be obtained from a variety of sources, such as written reports, surveys, and published articles. Information may also be obtained from others informally, such as in discussions with individuals who work in the field or have dealt with a similar problem before, or via feedback from the clients who are receiving the care. No matter what the source of information, it needs to be evaluated critically for accuracy, consistency, cause and effect, and biases.

A nurse using critical thinking will often be able to identify more than one solution to a problem. For example, possible solutions to the teenage STD problem may include providing condoms for all high-school students, performing tubal ligations on sexually active girls, or establishing strict nighttime curfews.

Although all of these solutions may be effective, the nurse would have to evaluate the cause-and-effect relationship, value, and consequences of each of these courses of action. A nurse who is a critical thinker would consider each one of these before implementing a course of action.

CRITICAL THINKING IN DECISION MAKING

Although critical thinking is used in all aspects of decision making, it is particularly important in the nursing process. It is important to remember that although the nursing process and critical thinking are interrelated and interdependent, *they are not identical.*

As a way of looking at the world, critical thinking allows the nurse to consider new ideas and then evaluate those ideas in light of accepted information as well as client and personal value systems. Nurses are constantly making decisions in both their professional and personal lives. By viewing critical thinking as a purposeful mental activity in which ideas are evaluated and decisions reached, nurses will be able to make ethical, creative, rational, and independent decisions related to client care.

Critical thinking, when applied to the nursing process, makes it a powerful client problem-solving tool. Critical thinking expands the usual linear nursing process into a gestalt that allows the nurse to sort through the multiple variables that are often encountered in client care. Effective use of critical thinking within the nursing process is evident when the nurse successfully applies knowledge from other disciplines in the resolution of client problems, deals with stressful environments, and creatively resolves unique nursing care problems.

Conclusion

Nurses practicing in today's health-care system are required to master many skills. Critical thinking underlies many of these skills. By examining assumptions, beliefs, propositions and meanings, nurses are able to make sound and valid decisions about client care. Critical thinking both underlies and expands the nursing process in the practical provision of nursing care. When students and nurses master critical thinking concepts and skills, they open their perspectives on client care. An important transformation occurs when students are taught how to think rather than what to think.

The profession of nursing is in an active state of change, continually developing new theories, redefining its practice, and adapting to changing **public policy** and social mandates. Nurses who use critical thinking in making nursing judgments tend to consider the client's human rights and be effective client advocates. These nurses will also be able to adapt the rules of the nursing process to meet a wide range of client needs.

Critical Thinking Exercises

Use the steps in the nursing process to provide a plan of care, including at least two nursing diagnoses, for the following client situation:

Mr. Y is 49 years old and has been complaining of chest pain starting in the center of his chest and radiating to his left arm and hand for 2 hours. He is having trouble breathing, is very pale, and has cool and moist skin. His pulse is 134 bpm and irregular; his blood pressure is 92/50 mm Hg; and his respiratory rate is 24 bpm. He is very anxious and expresses concern about having to leave his job as an accountant because of these symptoms. He is diagnosed as having an acute anterior myocardial infarction and is admitted to the intensive care unit.

✔ What key assessment does the nurse need to identify as essential to this client's problem?

✔ What problems does this client have that a nurse can treat independently? Write nursing diagnoses for these problems.

✔ What can be accomplished in the nursing treatment of this client's problems (goals)?

✔ What type of activities can the nurse undertake to achieve the goals (intervention)?

✔ What does the nurse need to look for to see whether the interventions have worked (evaluation)?

References

1. Beeken, JE, et al: Teaching critical thinking skills in undergraduate nursing students. Nurse Educator 22(3):37–39, 1997.

BIBLIOGRAPHY

Alfaro-LeFevre, R: Applying Nursing Process: A Step by Step Guide, ed 4. JB Lippincott, Philadelphia, 1998.

Benner, P: From Novice to Expert. Addison-Wesley, Menlo Park, CA, 1984.

Doenges, ME, et al: Application of Nursing Process and Nursing Diagnosis: An Interactive Text for Diagnostic Reasoning. FA Davis, Philadelphia, 1995.

Farrell, M: Planning for critical outcomes. J Nurs Educ 35:278–281, 1996.

Hunt, R: Community-based nursing: Philosophy or setting? Am J Nurs 98(10): 44–49, 1998.

Maslow, AH: Motivation and Personality. Harper & Row, New York, 1971.

Nicoll, LH: Nurses' Guide to the Internet, ed 2. JB Lippincott, Philadelphia, 1998.

Nicoteri, JA: Critical thinking skills. Am J Nurs 98 (10): 62–68, 1998.

Stewart, M: Health care community faces the year 2000. American Nurse 29(6):24, 1997.

Sullivan, TJ: Collaboration: A health care imperative. McGraw-Hill, New York, 1998.

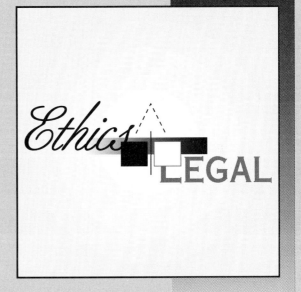

Professional Accountability

6

ETHICS IN NURSING

➤ *Joseph T. Catalano*

Learning Objectives

After completing this chapter, the reader will be able to:

1. Discuss and analyze the difference between law and ethics.

2. Define the key terms used in ethics.

3. Discuss the important ethical concepts.

4. Distinguish between the two most commonly used systems of ethical decision making.

5. Apply the steps in the ethical decision-making process.

Nurses who practice in today's health-care system soon realize that making ethical decisions is a common part of daily nursing care. However, experience shows that in the full curricula of many schools of nursing, the teaching of ethical principles and ethical decision making gets less attention than the topics of nursing skills, pathophysiology, and nursing care plans. As health-care technology continues to advance into the twenty-first century, it will become more and more difficult for nurses to make these ethical decisions. Many nurses thus feel the need to be better prepared to understand and deal with the complex ethical problems that keep evolving as they attempt to provide care for their clients.

Ethical decision making is a skill that can be learned. The ability to make sensible ethical decisions is based on an understanding of underlying ethical principles, ethical theories or systems, a decision-making model, and the profession's Code of Ethics. This skill, like others, involves mastery of the theoretical material and practice of the skill itself.

This chapter presents the basic information required to understand ethics, the code of ethics, and ethical decision making. It also highlights some of the important bioethical issues that confront nurses in the current health-care system.

IMPORTANT DEFINITIONS

In Western cultures, the study of ethics is a specialized area of philosophy, the origins of which can be traced to ancient Greece. In fact, certain ethical principles articulated by Hippocrates still serve as the basis of many of the current debates. Like most specialized areas of study, ethics has its own language and uses terminology in precise ways. The following are some key terms that are encountered in studies of health-care ethics.

Values

Values are ideals or concepts that give meaning to the individual's life. Values are derived most commonly from societal norms, religion, and family orientation and serve as the framework for making decisions and taking action in daily life. A person's values tend to change as his or her life situations change, as the person grows older, and as he or she encounters situations that cause value conflicts. For example, prior to the 1950s, pregnancy outside of marriage was unacceptable, and unmarried women who were pregnant were shunned and generally separated from society. Today, it is much more accepted, and it is not uncommon to see pregnant high-school students attending classes.

Values are usually not written down; however, at some time in their professional careers, it may be important for nurses to make a list of their values. This value clarification process requires that the nurse assess, evaluate, and then determine a set of personal values and prioritize them. This will help the nurse make decisions when confronted with situations in which the client's values differ from the nurse's own values. (See the values clarification exercise in Chapter 5, Box 5.2.)

Value conflicts that often occur in daily life can force an individual to select a higher priority value over a lower priority one. For example, a nurse who values both her career and her family may be forced to decide between going to work and staying home with a sick child.

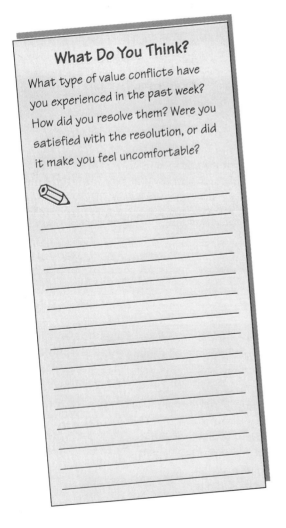

What Do You Think?

What type of value conflicts have you experienced in the past week? How did you resolve them? Were you satisfied with the resolution, or did it make you feel uncomfortable?

Morals

Morals are the fundamental standards of right and wrong that an individual learns and internalizes, usually in the early stages of childhood development. An individual's moral orientation is often based on religious beliefs, although societal influence plays an important part in this development. The word *moral* comes from the Latin word **mores,** which means customs or values. Moral behavior is often manifested as behavior in accordance with a group's norms, customs, or traditions. A moral person is generally someone who responds to another person in need by providing care and who maintains a level of responsibility in all relationships.[1] In many situations in which moral convictions differ, it is difficult to find a rational basis for proving one side right over the other. For example, animal rights' activists believe that killing animals for sport, their fur, or even food is morally wrong. Most hunters do not even think of the killing of animals as a moral issue at all.

Laws

Laws can generally be defined as rules of social conduct made by humans to protect society, and these laws are based on concerns about fairness and **justice.** The goals of laws are to preserve the species and promote peaceful and productive interactions between individuals or groups of individuals by preventing the actions of one citizen from infringing on the rights of another. Two important aspects of laws are that they are enforceable through some type of police force and that they should be applied equally to all persons.

Ethics

Ethics are declarations of what is right or wrong and of what ought to be. Ethics are usually presented as systems of value behaviors and beliefs; they serve the purpose of governing conduct to ensure the protection of an individual's rights. Ethics exist on several levels, ranging from the individual or a small group to the society as a whole. The concept of ethics is closely associated with the concept of morals in both their development and purposes. In one sense, ethics can be considered a system of morals for a particular group. There are usually no systems of enforcement for those who violate ethical principles.

A **code of ethics** is a written list of a profession's values and standards of conduct. The code of ethics provides a framework for decision making for the profession and should be oriented toward the daily decisions made by members of the profession.

An **ethical dilemma** is a situation that requires an individual to make a choice between two equally unfavorable alternatives. When ethical dilemmas are reduced to their

What Do You Think?

Identify a situation in which a law is or may be unethical. Which system has higher authority? How do you resolve the conflict?

Drug Experimentation and Informed Consent

Picture yourself in this situation. You are in the terminal stages of an incurable disease. Your physicians have used all the conventional and approved treatments that are normally used for this disease, but you are still getting progressively worse. Then, one morning, a new physician that you have never seen before enters your room and begins to tell you about an experimental drug that has been used on a few other clients who have the same disease as you do. This therapy has shown some promise for improvement or even a cure. He then offers to give you this drug, free of charge, if you are willing to participate in the experiment. You will have to sign a form that prevents you, or your family, from suing either the physician or the drug company if the experiment does not prove to be successful. What would you do?

If you are like most clients who find themselves in this situation, you would probably take the risk and try the new drug. But do you really understand what you are agreeing to? Have you really been informed about the consequences before you give consent?

Although this is a common method for testing new drugs, reports of drug trials that went wrong have brought the whole process under question. When 5 of 15 clients died after receiving an experimental drug for hepatitis B, attention began to focus on how well the participants were prepared for the risks incurred when receiving experimental drugs. The basic question is whether the consent given by any critically ill client can ever be considered informed.

Consent forms used for trial medications need to explain the nature of the experiment and the risks involved. It is difficult for the experimenters preparing these forms to determine how much information to provide and to phrase the form in such a way that the average client can understand it. Obviously, if the form is too detailed or complicated, some clients may refuse to undergo the treatment. On the other hand, if the form is too simple, the client may be agreeing to something for which full information has not been given. The consent form used for the new hepatitis B drug listed fatigue, nausea, skin rashes, bone marrow suppression, seizures, pain, and numbness in the arms and legs as the only major risk factors. A general disclaimer at the end of the form stated: "This is a new medication, and its side effects have not been completely described." It is interesting to speculate about how many patients would have taken this medication if "death" had been listed as one of the possible side effects.

Another factor that enters into the question of informed consent is coercion. Although the experimenters are not physically forcing these clients to take the trial medication, desperately ill clients tend to grasp at any glimmer of hope and may sign the consent form without understanding it, or even without reading it. And, of course, the physician who is explaining the new medication is going to try to put the medication and test in as positive a light as possible.

In new guidelines for experimental medication forms, it has been suggested that no mention of benefit or cure from the drug be made. It would be much more honest to let the client know that he or she is involved in research whose primary goal is to obtain new knowledge. If the medication should produce a benefit or cure, then it will have been successful and everyone is happy. But the client also needs to realize that the drug may produce worse symptoms, or even death, and those results are also beneficial to the experimenter.

From Altman, LK: Fatal drug trial raises questions about informed consent. New York Times, October 5, 1993, C-3.

elemental aspects, conflicts of one individual's rights with those of another, or one individual's obligations with the rights of another, or a combination of one group's obligations and rights conflicting with those of another group usually form the basis of the dilemma. By the very nature of an ethical dilemma, there can be no simple correct solution, and the final decision must often be defended against those who disagree with it. For example, a client went to surgery for a laparoscopic biopsy of an abdominal mass. After the laparoscope was inserted, the physician noted that the mass had metastasized to the liver, pancreas, and colon, and even before the results of the tissue biopsy returned from the laboratory, the physician diagnosed metastatic cancer with a poor prognosis. When the client was returned to his room, the physician told the nurses about the diagnosis but warned them that under no circumstances were they to tell the client about the cancer. When the client awoke, the first question that he asked the nurses was "Do I have cancer?" This posed an ethical dilemma for the nurses. If they were to tell the client the truth, they would violate the principle of fidelity to the physician. If they lied to the client, they would violate the principle of veracity.

KEY CONCEPTS IN ETHICS

In addition to the terminology used in the study and practice of ethics, several important principles often underlie ethical dilemmas. These principles include autonomy, justice, fidelity, beneficence, nonmaleficence, veracity, standard of best interest, and obligations.

Autonomy

Autonomy is the right of self-determination, independence, and freedom. Autonomy refers to the client's right to make health-care decisions for himself or herself, even if the health-care provider does not agree with those decisions.

Autonomy, as with most rights, is not absolute, and under certain conditions, limitations can be imposed on it. Generally these limitations occur when one individual's autonomy interferes with another individual's rights, health, or well-being. For example, a client generally can use his or her right to autonomy by refusing any or all treatments. In the case of contagious diseases (e.g., tuberculosis [TB]) that affect society, however, the individual can be forced by the health-care and legal systems to take medications

What Do You Think?

Must the nurse report the condition to the Department of Public Safety? Does the public's right to safety always supersede the client's right to self-determination and confidentiality? What if the nurse can convince June to take her medications and June has no more seizures?

to cure the disease. The individual can also be forced into isolation to prevent the disease from spreading. Consider the following situation:

June, who is the 28-year-old mother of two children, is brought into the emergency department after a tonic-clonic type seizure at a shopping mall. June is known to the emergency room (ER) nurses because she has been treated several times for seizures because she did not take her antiseizure medications. She states that the medications make her feel "dopey" and tired all the time and she hates the way that they make her feel.

Recently, June has started to drive one of her children and four other children to school in the neighborhood car pool 1 day a week. She also drives 62 miles one way on the interstate highway twice a week to visit her aging mother in a nursing home in a different city. The nurse who takes care of June this day in the ER knows that the state licensing laws require that an individual with uncontrolled seizures must report the fact to the Department of Motor Vehicles and is usually ineligible for a driver's license. When the nurse mentions that she is going to have to report the seizure, June begs her not to report it. She would have no means of taking her children to school or visiting her mother. She assures the nurse that she will take her medication no matter how it makes her feel.

Justice

Justice is the **obligation** to be fair to all people. The concept is often expanded to what is called **distributive justice,** which states that individuals have the right to be treated equally regardless of race, sex, marital status, medical diagnosis, social standing, economic level, or religious belief. The principle of justice underlies the first statement in the American Nurses Association (ANA) Code of Ethics for Nurses: "The nurse provides services with respect for human dignity and the uniqueness of the client unrestricted by considerations of social or economic status, personal attributes, or the nature of health problems."[2] Distributive justice sometimes includes ideas such as equal access to health care for all. As with other rights, limits can be placed on justice when it interferes with the rights of others. For example, a middle-aged home-

Issues

A Question of Distributive Justice

Jessica B. was diagnosed with acute lymphocytic leukemia at age 4. She is now 7 years old and has been treated with chemotherapy for the past 3 years with varying degrees of success. She is currently in a state of relapse, and a bone marrow transplant seems to be the only treatment that might improve her condition and save her life. Her father is a day laborer who has no health insurance, so Jessica's health care is being paid for mainly by the Medicaid system of her small state in the Southwest.

The current cost of a bone marrow transplant at the state's central teaching hospital is $1.5 million, representing about half of the state's entire annual Medicaid budget. Although bone marrow transplants are an accepted treatment for leukemia, this therapy offers only a slim chance for a total cure of the disease. The procedure is risky, and there is a chance that it may cause death. The procedure will involve several months of post-transplant treatment and recovery in an intensive care unit far away from the family's home and will require the child to take costly antirejection medications for many years.

The family understands the risks and benefits. They ask the nurse caring for Jessica what they should do. How should the nurse respond? Does the nurse have any obligations toward the Medicaid system as a whole?

less man who was diagnosed with type I, insulin-dependent diabetes mellitus demanded that Medicaid pay for a pancreas transplant. His health record showed that he refused to follow the prescribed diabetic regimen, drank large quantities of wine, and rarely took his insulin. The transplant would cost $48,000, which is the total cost of immunizing all the children in the state for 1 year.

Fidelity

Fidelity is the obligation of an individual to be faithful to commitments made to himself or herself and also to others. In health care, fidelity includes the professional's faithfulness or loyalty to agreements and responsibilities accepted as part of the practice of the profession. Fidelity is the main support for the concept of accountability, although conflicts in fidelity might arise from obligations owed to different individuals or groups.

For example, a nurse who was just finishing a very busy and tiring 12-hour shift may experience a conflict of fidelity when she is asked by a supervisor to work an additional shift because of the hospital's being short staffed. The nurse has to weigh her fidelity to herself against fidelity to the employing institution and against the fidelity to the profession and

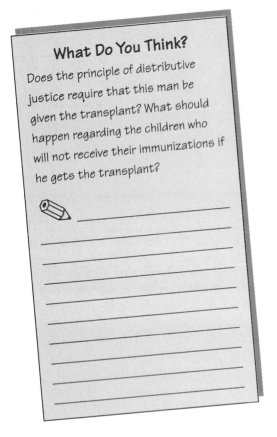

What Do You Think?

Does the principle of distributive justice require that this man be given the transplant? What should happen regarding the children who will not receive their immunizations if he gets the transplant?

clients to do the best job possible, particularly if she felt that her fatigue would interfere with the performance of those obligations.

Beneficence

Beneficence, one of the oldest requirements for health-care providers, views the primary goal of health care as doing good for clients under their care. In general, the term *good* includes more than providing technically competent care for clients. Good care requires that the health-care provider take a holistic approach to the client, including the client's beliefs, feelings, and wishes as well as those of the client's family and significant others. The difficulty in implementing the principle of beneficence is in determining what exactly is good for another and who can best make the decision about this good.

Consider the case of the man involved in an automobile accident who ran into a metal fence pole. The pole passed through his abdomen. Even after 6 hours of surgery, the surgeon was unable to repair all the damage. The man was not expected to live for more than 12 hours. When the man came back from surgery, he had a nasogastric tube inserted, thus the physician ordered that the client should have nothing by mouth (NPO) to prevent depletion of electrolytes. Although the man was somewhat confused when he awoke postoperatively, he begged the nurse for a drink of water. He had a fever of 105.7°F. The nurse believed the physician's orders to be absolute, thus she repeatedly refused the client water. He began to yell loudly that he needed a drink of water, but the nurse still refused his requests. At one point, the nurse caught the man attempting to drink water from the icepacks that were being used to lower his fever. This continued for the full 8-hour shift until the man died.

Nonmaleficence

Nonmaleficence is the requirement that health-care providers do no harm to their clients, either intentionally or unintentionally. In a sense, it is the opposite side of the concept of beneficence, and it is difficult to speak of one term without referring to the other. In current health-care practice, the principle of nonmaleficence is often violated in the short term to produce a greater good in the long-term treatment of the client. For example, a client may undergo painful and debilitating surgery to remove a cancerous growth in order to prolong his life.

By extension, the principle of nonmaleficence also requires that health-care providers protect those from harm who cannot protect themselves. This protection from harm is particularly evident in groups such as children, the mentally incompetent, the unconscious, and those who are too weak or debilitated to protect themselves. In fact, very strict regulations have developed around situations involving child abuse and the health-care provider's obligation to report suspected child abuse. (This issue is discussed in more detail in Chapter 7.)

Veracity

Veracity is the principle of truthfulness. It requires the health-care provider to tell the truth and not to deceive or mislead clients intentionally. As with other rights and obligations, limitations to this principle exist. The primary limitation is when telling the client the truth would seriously harm (principle of nonmaleficence) the client's ability to recover or would produce greater illness. Health-care providers often feel uncomfortable giving a client bad news, and they tend to avoid answering these questions truthfully. An uncomfortable feeling is not a good enough reason to avoid telling clients the truth about their diagnosis, treatments, or prognosis. Clients have a right to know this information. One common situation in which veracity is violated is in the use of placebo medications. At some point during their careers, most health-care providers will observe the placebo effect among some clients. Sometimes when a client is given a gel capsule filled with sugar powder and it seems to relieve the pain, this has the same effect as giving the person a narcotic, but without the side effects or potential for addiction. Of course, if the client was told that it was just a sugar pill (veracity), it would not have the same effect. How should nurses feel about this practice?

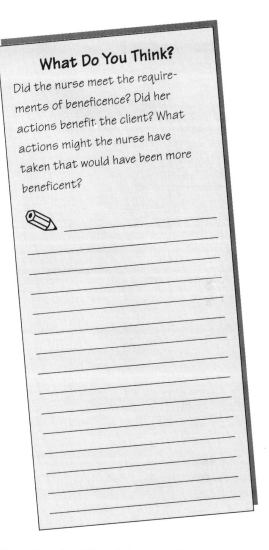

What Do You Think?

Did the nurse meet the requirements of beneficence? Did her actions benefit the client? What actions might the nurse have taken that would have been more beneficent?

Standard of Best Interest

Standard of best interest describes a type of decision made about a client's health care when the client is unable to make the informed decision regarding his or her own care. The standard of best interest is based on what health-care providers and the family decide is best for that individual. It is very important to consider the individual client's expressed wishes, either formally in a written declaration (e.g., a **living will**) or informally in conversation with family

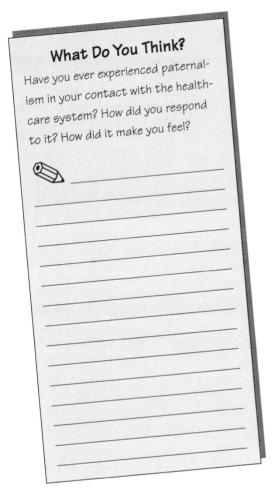

has been designated, the resolution of the dilemma can be a unilateral decision made by health-care providers. The making of a unilateral decision by health-care providers that disregards the client's wishes implies that the providers alone know what is best for the client; this is called paternalism.

Obligations

Obligations are demands made on an individual, a profession, a society, or a government to fulfill and honor the rights of others. Obligations are often divided into two categories.

Legal Obligations

Legal obligations are those that have become formal statements of law and are enforceable under the law. For instance, a nurse has a legal obligation to provide safe and adequate care for clients assigned to him or her.

Moral Obligations

Moral obligations are those based on moral or ethical principles but are not enforceable under the law. In most states, no legal obligation exists for a nurse on a vacation trip to stop and help an automobile accident victim.

Rights

Rights are generally defined as something owed to an individual according to just claims, legal guarantees, or moral and ethical principles. Although the term *right* is frequently used in both the legal and ethical systems, its meaning is often blurred in daily usage. Individuals sometimes mistakenly claim things as rights that are really privileges, concessions, or freedoms. Several classification systems exist in which differ-

members. Individuals can also legally designate a specific person to make health-care decisions for them in case they become unable to make decisions for themselves. The designated person then has what is called durable power of attorney for health care (DPOAHC). The Omnibus Budget Reconciliation Act (OBRA) of 1990 made it mandatory for all health-care facilities, such as hospitals, nursing homes, and home-health-care agencies, to provide information to clients about the living will and DPOAHC.

The standard of best interest should be based on the principle of beneficence. Unfortunately, when clients are unable to make decisions for themselves and no DPOAHC

Withdrawal of Informed Consent: A Case Study

Mrs. Hobbs was a 52-year-old unemployed teacher who received minor injuries when she fell down the steps at a neighbor's house. She was intoxicated at the time, and she had a long history of alcohol abuse. She was brought to the emergency department of a large city hospital and treated. She was also offered a chance for treatment in the alcohol dependency unit of the hospital at no charge if she agreed to participate in a study on the long-term effects of alcohol on the central nervous system. Dr. Wei, the chief investigator of the study, and Ms. Anderson, the nurse in charge of the unit, explained to Mrs. Hobbs that the study involved the administration of a medication that, over a period of time, might reduce the long-term effects of alcohol on the brain. The study required Mrs. Hobbs to be hospitalized and to be given an experimental medication intravenously for 45 days. She was also required to eat a well-balanced diet and take supplemental vitamins. After the risks and benefits of the study were discussed, Mrs. Hobbs signed the consent form and was admitted to the chemical dependency unit.

During the first 20 days of the study, Mrs. Hobbs was cooperative with the nursing staff, participated actively in the group therapy, and had a positive attitude about the program. Her physical condition, and her mental function continued to improve until the 25th day into the study. On that day, she awoke in the morning very agitated and slightly disoriented, and appeared somewhat depressed. She said she had "real bad cabin fever," and needed to "get out of this loony bin." She made the point that she was much better than when she was admitted and should be permitted to go home. When she was reminded that she had signed a consent form for the study and had agreed to participate for the full 45 days, she claimed that she did not remember signing it. Even after being shown the signed form, she denied it was her signature and stated that she was going home, like it or not.

On closer examination of the document, Ms. Anderson noted that the signature looked like a poorly scribbled "H." The chart also noted that although Mrs. Hobbs had been in rather severe alcohol withdrawal not long after she was admitted to the hospital until about 48 hours into her hospitalization. Mrs. Hobbs had not had any hallucinations and was generally oriented to person, place, and time.

Two questions arise from this case. First, because of Mrs. Hobbs' condition on admission, did she give a fully informed valid consent? Second, if an informed consent is valid, can the person who signed it ever withdraw the consent, and if so, when can this be done?

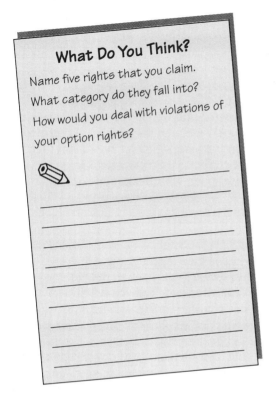

ent types of rights are delineated. The following three types of rights include the range of definitions.

Welfare Rights

Welfare rights (also called **legal rights**) are based on a legal entitlement to some good or benefit. These rights are guaranteed by laws (e.g., the **Bill of Rights** of the U.S. Constitution), and violation of such rights can be punished under the legal system. For example, citizens of the United States have a right to equal access to housing regardless of race, sexual preference, or religion.

Ethical Rights

Ethical rights (also called **moral rights**) are based on a moral or ethical principle. Ethical rights usually do not need to have the power of law in order to be enforced.

Ethical rights are, in reality, often privileges allotted to certain individuals or groups of individuals. Over time, popular acceptance of ethical rights can give them the force of a legal right. An example of an ethical right in the United States is the belief in universal access to health care. In the United States, it is really a long-standing privilege, whereas in many other industrialized countries, such as Canada, Germany, Japan, and England, universal health care is a legal right.

Option Rights

Option rights are rights that are based on a fundamental belief in the dignity and freedom of humans. These are **basic human rights** that are particularly evident in free and democratic countries such as the United States and much less evident in totalitarian and restrictive societies such as Iraq. Option rights give individuals freedom of choice and the right to live their lives as they choose, but within a given set of prescribed boundaries. For example, people may wear whatever clothes they choose, as long as they wear some type of clothing.

ETHICS COMMITTEES

Physicians, nurses, and other staff members often encounter ethical conflicts that they are unable to resolve on their own. In these cases, the interdisciplinary ethics committee can help the health-care provider to resolve the dilemma. An increasing number of health-care facilities, particularly hospitals, have instituted ethics committees that make their consultation services available to health-care providers.

The people who belong to the ethics committee vary somewhat from one institution to another, but almost all include a physician, a member of administration, an RN, a clergy person, a philosopher with a background in ethics, a lawyer, and a person from the community. Members of ethics committees should not have any personal agenda that they are promoting and should be able to make decisions without prejudice on the basis of the situation and ethical principles.

Depending on the institution, the scope of the ethics committee's duties can range widely, from very limited activity with infrequent meetings on an ad hoc basis to active promotion of ethical thinking and decision making through educational programs. Other common functions of ethics committees include making evaluations of institutional policies in the light of ethical considerations, making recommendations about complex ethical issues, and providing education programs for medical and nursing schools as well as the community. It is extremely important that nurses participate in these committees and that the ethical concerns of the nurses are recognized and addressed.

ETHICAL SYSTEMS

An ethical situation exists every time a nurse interacts with a client in a health-care setting. Nurses are continually making ethical decisions in their daily practice, whether or not they recognize it. These are called normative decisions. **Normative ethics** deal with questions and dilemmas that require a choice of actions when there is a conflict of rights or obligations between the nurse and the client, the nurse and the client's family, or the nurse and the physician. In resolving these ethical questions, these nurses often use just one ethical system, or they may use a combination of several ethical systems.

The two systems that are most directly concerned with ethical decision making in the health-care professions are **utilitarianism** and **deontology.** Both apply to

> 66 99 *An ethical situation exists every time a nurse interacts with a client in a health-care setting.*

bioethical issues, the ethics of life (or, in some cases, death). *Bioethics* and *bioethical issues* are terms that are in common use. These terms have become synonymous with health-care ethics and encompass not only questions concerning life and death but also questions of quality of life, life-sustaining and life-altering technologies, and biologic science in general. It is in the context of bioethics that the following discussion of these two systems of ethics is undertaken.

Utilitarianism

Ethical Precepts

Utilitarianism (also called **teleology,** consequentialism, or situation ethics) is referred to as the ethical system of utility. As a system of normative ethics, utilitarianism defines good as happiness or pleasure. It is associated with two underlying principles: "The greatest good for the greatest number," and "The end justifies the means." Because of these two principles, utilitarianism is sometimes subdivided into act utilitarianism and rule utilitarianism. According to rule utilitarianism, the individual draws on past experiences to formulate internal rules that are useful in determining the greatest good. With act utilitarianism, the particular situation in which a nurse finds himself or herself determines the rightness or wrongness of a particular act. In practice, the true follower of utilitarianism does not believe in the validity of any system of rules because the rules can change depending on the circumstances surrounding whatever decision needs to be made.

Situation ethics is probably the most publicized form of act utilitarianism. Joseph Fletcher, one of the best-known proponents of act utilitarianism, outlines a method of ethical thinking in which the situation itself determines whether the act is morally right or wrong. Fletcher views acts as good to the extent that they promote happiness and bad to the degree that they promote unhappiness. Happiness is defined as the happiness of the greatest number of people, yet the happiness of each person is to have equal weight. Abortion, for example, is considered ethical in this system in a situation where an unwed mother on welfare with four other children becomes pregnant with her fifth child. The greatest good and the greatest amount of happiness are produced by aborting this unwanted child.

Because utilitarianism is based on the concept that moral rules should not be arbitrary but should rather serve a purpose, ethical decisions derived from a utilitarian framework weigh the effect of alternative actions that influence the overall welfare of present and future populations. As such, this system is oriented toward the good of the population in general and also toward the individual in the sense that the individual participates in that population.

Advantages

The major advantage of the utilitarian system of ethical decision making is that many individuals find it easy to use in most situations. Utilitarianism is built around an individual's needs for happiness in which the individual has an immediate and vested interest. Another advantage is that utilitarianism fits well into a society that otherwise shuns rules and regulations. A follower of utilitarianism can justify many decisions based on the happiness principle. Also, its utility orientation fits well into Western society's belief in the work ethic and a behavioristic approach to education, philosophy, and life.

Truth telling is not an absolute requirement to the follower of utilitarianism.

The follower of utilitarianism will support a general prohibition against lying and deceiving because ultimately the results of telling the truth will lead to greater happiness than the results of lying. Yet truth telling is not an absolute requirement to the follower of utilitarianism. If telling the truth will produce widespread unhappiness for a great number of people and future generations, then it would be ethically better to tell a lie that will yield more happiness than to tell a truth that will lead to greater unhappiness. Although such behavior might appear to be unethical at first glance, the strict follower of act utilitarianism would have little difficulty in arriving at this decision as a logical conclusion of utilitarian ethical thinking.

Disadvantages

Some serious limitations to utilitarianism as a system of health care or bioethics exist. An immediate question is whether happiness refers to the average happiness of all or the total happiness of a few. Because individual happiness is also important, one must consider how to make decisions when the individual's happiness is in conflict with that of the larger group. More fundamental is the question of what constitutes happiness. Similarly, what constitutes the greatest good for the greatest number? Who determines what is good in the first place? Is it society in general, the government, governmental policy, or the individual? In health-care delivery and the formulation of health-care policy, the general guiding principle often seems to be the greatest good for the greatest number. Yet where do minority groups fit into this system?

Also, the tenet that the ends justify the means has been consistently rejected as a rationale for justifying actions. It is generally unacceptable to allow any type of action as long as the final goal or purpose is good. The Nazis in the 1930s and 1940s used this aphorism to justify many actions that may be viewed by others to be considerably less than good.

The other difficulty in determining what is good lies in the attempt to quantify such concepts as good, harm, benefits, and greatest. This problem becomes especially acute when dealing with health-care issues that involve individuals' lives. For example, an elderly family member has been sick for a long time, and that course of illness has placed great financial hardship on the family. It would be ethical under utilitarianism to allow this client to die or even to euthanize her to relieve the financial stress created by her illness.

> 66 99 *A follower of a pure form of the deontological system of ethical decision making believes in the ethical absoluteness of principles regardless of the consequences of the decision.*

Utilitarianism as an ethical system in the health-care decision-making process requires use of an additional principle of distributive justice as an ultimate guiding point. Unfortunately, whenever an unchanging principle is combined with this system, it negates the basic concept of pure utilitarianism. Pure utilitarianism, although easy to use as a decision-making system, does not work well as an ethical system for decision making in health care because of its arbitrary, self-centered nature. In the everyday delivery of health care, utilitarianism is often combined with other types of ethical decision making in the resolution of ethical dilemmas.

Deontology

Ethical Precepts

Deontology is a system of ethical decision making based on moral rules and unchanging principles. This system is also termed the formalistic system, the principle system of ethics, or duty-based ethics. A follower of a pure form of the deontological system of ethical decision making believes in the ethical absoluteness of principles regardless of the consequences of the decision. Strict adherence to an ethical theory, in which the moral rightness or wrongness of human actions is considered separately from the consequences, is based on a fundamental principle called the categorical imperative. It is not the results of the act that make it right or wrong, but the principles by reason of which the act is carried out. These fundamental principles are ultimately unchanging and absolute and derived from the universal values that underlie all major religions. Focusing on a concern for right and wrong in the moral sense is the basic premise of the system. Its goal is the survival of the species and social cooperation.

Rule deontology is based on the belief that standards exist for the ethical choices and judgments made by individuals. These standards are fixed and do not change when the situation changes. Although the number of standards or rules is potentially unlimited, in reality—and particularly in dealing with bioethical issues—many of these principles can be grouped together into a few general principles. These principles can also be arranged into a type of hierarchy of rules and include such maxims as the following: People should always be treated as ends and never as means; human life has value; one is always to tell the truth; above all in health care, do no harm; humans have a right to self-determination; and all people are of equal value. These principles echo such fundamental documents as the Bill of Rights and the Ameri-

6.1 **The American Hospital Association's Patient's Bill of Rights**

1. The patient has the right to considerate and respectful care.

2. The patient has the right to obtain from his doctor complete and current information about his diagnosis, treatment, and prognosis in terms the patient can be reasonably expected to understand. When it is not medically advisable to give such information to the patient, it should be made available to an appropriate person in his behalf. He has the right to know by name the doctor responsible for coordinating his care.

3. The patient has the right to receive from his doctor information necessary to give informed consent prior to the start of any procedure or treatment. Except in emergencies, such information for informed consent should include but not necessarily be limited to the specific procedure or treatment, the medically significant risks involved, and the probable duration of incapacitation. Where medically significant alternatives for care or treatment exist, or when the patient requests information concerning medical alternatives, the patient has the right to such information. The patient has the right to know the name of the person responsible for the procedure or treatment.

4. The patient has the right to refuse treatment to the extent permitted by law and to be informed of the medical consequences of his action.

5. The patient has the right to every consideration of his privacy concerning his own medical care program. Case discussion, consultation, examination, and the treatment are confidential and should be conducted discreetly. Those not directly involved in his care must have the permission of the patient to be present.

6. The patient has the right to expect that all communications and records pertaining to his care should be treated as confidential.

7. The patient has the right to expect that within its capacity a hospital must make reasonable response to the request of a patient for services. The hospital must provide evaluation, service, or referral as indicated by the urgency of the case. When medically permissible, a patient may be transferred to another facility only after he has received complete information and explanation concerning the needs for and alternatives to such a transfer. The institution to which the patient is to be transferred must first have accepted the patient for transfer.

8. The patient has the right to obtain information as to any relationship of his hospital to other health care and educational institutions insofar as his care is concerned. The patient has the right to obtain information as to the existence of any professional relationships among individuals by name who are treating him.

9. The patient has the right to be advised if the hospital proposes to engage in or perform human experimentation affecting his care or treatment. The patient has the right to refuse to participate in such research projects.

10. The patient has the right to expect reasonable continuity of care. He has the right to know in advance what appointment times and doctors are available and where. The patient has the right to expect that the hospital will provide a mechanism whereby he is informed by

his doctor or a delegate of the doctor of the patient's continuing health care requirements following discharge.

11. The patient has the right to examine and receive an explanation of his bill, regardless of the source of payment.

12. The patient has the right to know what hospital rules and regulations apply to his conduct as a patient.

From the American Hospital Association: A Patient's Bill of Rights. AHA Board of Trustees, 1973; revised 1992, with permission.

can Hospital Association's Patient's Bill of Rights (Box 6.1).

Advantages

The deontological system is useful in making ethical decisions in health care because it holds that an ethical judgment based on principles will be the same in a variety of given similar situations regardless of the time, location, or particular individuals involved. In addition, deontological terminology and concepts are similar to the terms and concepts used by the legal system. The legal system emphasizes rights, duties, principles, and rules. Significant differences, however, exist between the two. Legal rights and duties are enforceable under the law, whereas ethical rights and duties are usually not. In general, ethical systems are much wider and more inclusive than the system of laws that they underlie. It is difficult to have an ethical perspective on law without having it lead to an interest in making laws that govern health care and nursing practice.

Disadvantages

The deontological system of ethical decision making is not free from imperfection. Some of the more troubling questions include the following: What do you do when the basic guiding principles conflict with each other? What is the source of the principles? Is

there ever a situation where an exception to the rule will apply? Although various approaches have been proposed to circumvent these limitations, it may be difficult for nurses to resolve situations in which duties and obligations conflict, particularly when the consequences of following a rule end in harm or hurt being done to a client. In reality, there are probably few pure followers of deontology, because most people will con-

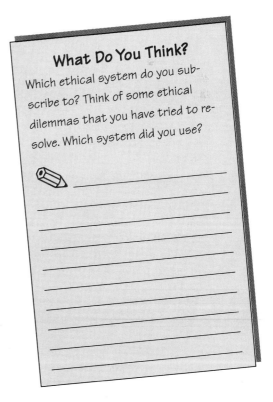

What Do You Think?

Which ethical system do you subscribe to? Think of some ethical dilemmas that you have tried to resolve. Which system did you use?

sider the consequences of their actions in the decision-making process.

APPLICATION OF ETHICAL THEORIES

Ethical theories do not provide recipes for resolution of ethical dilemmas. Instead, they provide a framework for decision making that the nurse can apply to a particular ethical situation.

At times, ethical theories may seem too abstract or general to be of much use to specific ethical situations. Without them, however, ethical decisions may often be made without reasoning or forethought and may be based on personal emotions. Most nurses in attempting to make ethical decisions combine the two theories presented here.

Nursing Code of Ethics

A code of ethics is generally defined as the ethical principles that govern a particular profession. Codes of ethics are presented as general statements and thus do not give specific answers to every possible ethical dilemma that might arise. These codes do, however, offer guidance to the individual practitioner in making decisions.

Ideally, codes of ethics should be reviewed periodically to reflect necessary changes in the profession and society as a whole. Although codes of ethics are not judicially enforceable as laws, consistent violations of the code of ethics by a professional in any field may indicate an unwillingness to act in a professional manner and will often result in disciplinary actions ranging from reprimands and fines to suspension of licensure.

Although similar, there are several different codes of ethics that nurses may adopt. In the United States, the American Nurses Association (ANA) Code of Ethics (Box 6.2) is the generally accepted code. There is also a Canadian Nurses Association Code of Ethics.

Site Seeing

Agency for Health Care Policy and Research (AHCPR)
http://www.ahcpr.gov/ info@ahcpr.gov

American Nurses Association
http://www.ana.org/
http://www.nursingworld.org/
Contact: mail to: webfeedback@ana.org

Bioethics Discussion Pages
http://www-hsc.usc.edu/~mbernste/
Contact: Maurice Bernstein, MD
DoktorMo@aol.com

Bioethics Online Service
http://www.mcw.edu/bioethics/index.html
Contact: Arthur R. Derse
aderse@its.mcw.edu

Boston College School of Nursing
http://www.bc.edu/bc-org/avp/son/default.html
Contact: Cathy Toran
toranca@bc.edu

Canadian Nurses Association
http://www.can-nurses.ca/
Contact: mail to:cna@can-nurses.ca

Global Health Network
http://www.pitt.edu/HOME/GHNet/GHNet.html
Contact: Amy Brenen
mail to:brenena@ghnet.org

Health Information Research Unit
http://hiru.mcmaster.ca/
Contact: haywarddr@fhs.mcmaster.ca

London Health Sciences Centre
http://spin.lhsc.on.ca/research/innovati/pathways/
Contact: wendy.schneidmiller@lhsc.on.ca

Nightingale
http://nightingale.con.utk.edu/index.htm
Contact: mail to:mackbo@utk.edu

The ANA Code of Ethics has been acknowledged by other health-care professions as one of the most complete. It is sometimes used as the benchmark against which other codes of ethics are measured. Yet, a careful

6.2 The American Nurses Association Code of Ethics*

1. The nurse provides services with respect for human dignity and the uniqueness of the client unrestricted by considerations of social or economic status, personal attributes or the nature of the health problems.
2. The nurse safeguards the client's right to privacy by judiciously protecting information of a confidential nature.
3. The nurse acts to safeguard the client and the public when health care and safety are affected by the incompetent, unethical, or illegal practice of any person.
4. The nurse assumes responsibility and accountability for individual nursing judgments and actions.
5. The nurse maintains competence in nursing.
6. The nurse exercises informed judgment and uses individual competence and qualification as criteria in seeking consultation, accepting responsibilities, and delegating nursing activities to others.
7. The nurse participates in activities that contribute to the ongoing development of the profession's body of knowledge.
8. The nurse participates in the profession's efforts to implement and improve standards of nursing.
9. The nurse participates in the profession's efforts to establish and maintain conditions of employment conducive to high-quality nursing care.
10. The nurse participates in the profession's efforts to protect the public from misinformation and misrepresentation and to maintain the integrity of nursing.
11. The nurse collaborates with members of the health professions and other citizens in promoting community and national efforts to meet the health needs of the public.

Reprinted with permission from *Code for Nurses with Interpretive Statements,* © 1985. American Nurses Publishing, American Nurses Foundation/American Nurses Association, 600 Maryland Avenue, SW. Suite 100W, Washington, DC 20024-2571, p1.

*Draft 7, proposed revisions

reading of this code of ethics reveals only a set of clearly stated principles that the nurse must apply to actual clinical situations. For example, the nurse involved in resuscitation will find no specific mention of **no code orders** in the ANA Code of Ethics. Rather, the nurse must be able to apply general statements such as "The nurse provides services with respect for human dignity" and "The nurse assumes responsibility and accountability for individual nursing judgments and actions" to the particular situation. At this time, the nursing code of ethics is undergoing revision to make it more relevant to current nursing practice.

DECISION-MAKING PROCESS IN ETHICS

Nurses, by definition, are problem solvers, and one of the important tools that nurses use is the nursing process. The nursing process is a systematic step-by-step approach to resolving problems that deal with a client's health and well-being.

Although nurses deal with problems related to the physical or psychological needs of clients, many feel inadequate when dealing with ethical problems associated with client care. Nurses in any health-care setting can, however, develop the decision-making skills necessary to make sound ethical decisions if they learn and practice using an ethical decision-making process.

An ethical decision-making process provides a method for the nurse to answer key questions about ethical dilemmas and to organize his or her thinking in a more logical and sequential manner. Although there are several ethical decision-making models, the problem-solving method presented here is based on the nursing process. It should be a relatively easy transition for the nurse to move from the nursing process used in the resolution of a client's physical problems to the ethical decision-making process for the resolution of problems with ethical ramifications.

The chief goal of the ethical decision-making process is to determine right and wrong in situations where clear demarcations are not readily apparent. This process presupposes that the nurse making the decision knows that a system of ethics exists, knows the content of that ethical system, and knows that the system applies to similar ethical decision-making problems despite multiple variables (see Box 6.2). In addition to identifying his or her own values, the nurse also needs an understanding of the possible ethical systems that may be used in making decisions about ethical dilemmas.

The following ethical decision-making process is presented as a tool for resolving ethical dilemmas (Fig. 6-1).

Step 1: Collect, Analyze, and Interpret the Data

Obtain as much information as possible concerning the particular ethical dilemma. Unfortunately, such information is sometimes very limited. Among the issues important to know are the client's wishes, the client's family's wishes, the extent of the physical or emotional problems causing the dilemma, the physician's beliefs about health care, and the nurse's own orientation to issues concerning life and death.

Many nurses, for example, face the question of whether or not to initiate resuscitation efforts when a terminally ill client is admitted to the hospital. Physicians often leave instructions for the nursing staff indicating that the nurses really should not resuscitate the client but should, instead, merely go through the motions to make the family feel better, which is sometimes referred to as a **slow-code order.** The nurse's dilemma is whether to make a serious attempt to revive the client or to let the client die quietly.

Important information that will help the nurse to make the decision might include:

- The mental competency of the client to make a no-resuscitation decision
- The client's desires
- The family's feelings
- Whether the physician previously sought input from the client and the family
- Whether there is a living will or DPOAHC

Many institutions have policies concerning no-resuscitation orders, and it is wise to consider these during data collection. After collecting information, the nurse needs to bring the pieces of information together in a manner that will give the clearest and sharpest focus to the dilemma.

Step 2: State the Dilemma

After collecting and analyzing as much information as is available, the nurse then needs to state the dilemma as clearly as possible. In this step, it is important to iden-

> ❝ ❞ *The chief goal of the ethical decision-making process is to determine right and wrong in situations where clear demarcations are not readily apparent.*

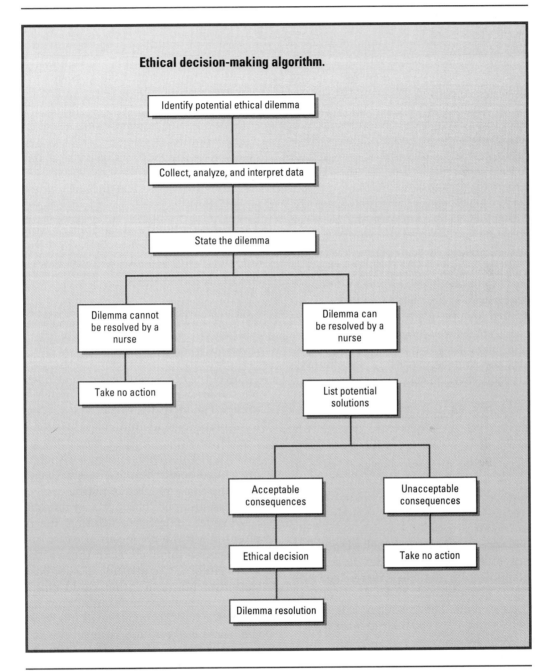

Ethical decision-making algorithm.

Identify potential ethical dilemma

Collect, analyze, and interpret data

State the dilemma

Dilemma cannot be resolved by a nurse

Dilemma can be resolved by a nurse

Take no action

List potential solutions

Acceptable consequences

Unacceptable consequences

Ethical decision

Take no action

Dilemma resolution

➤ Figure 6-1 Ethical decision-making algorithm.

(Adapted from Catalano, JT: Ethical decision making in the critical care patient. Critical Care Nursing Clinics of North America 9(1):45–52, 1997.)

tify whether the problem is one that directly involves the nurse or is one that can be resolved only by the client, the client's family, the physician, or the DPOAHC.

Recognizing the key aspects of the dilemma helps focus attention on the important ethical principles. Most of the time, the dilemma can be reduced to a few statements that encompass the key ethical issues. Such ethical issues often involve a question of conflicting rights, obligations, or basic ethical principles.

In the case of a no-resuscitation order, the statement of the dilemma might be: "The client's right to death with dignity versus the nurse's obligation to preserve life and do no harm." In general, the principle that the competent client's wishes must be followed is unequivocal. If the client has become unresponsive before expressing his or her wishes, then the family members' input must be given serious consideration. Additional questions can arise if the family's wishes conflict with those of the client.

Step 3: Consider the Choices of Action

After stating the dilemma as clearly as possible, the next step is to attempt to list, without consideration of their consequences, all possible courses of action that can be taken to resolve the dilemma. This brain-storming activity in which all possible courses of action are considered may require input from outside sources such as colleagues, supervisors, or even experts in the ethical field. The consequences of the different actions are considered later in this chapter.

Some possible courses of action for the nurse might include the following:

- Resuscitating the client to the nurse's fullest capabilities despite what the physician has requested
- Not resuscitating the client at all

- Only going through the motions without any real attempt to revive the client
- Seeking another assignment so as to avoid dealing with the situation
- Reporting the problem to a supervisor
- Attempting to clarify the question with the client
- Attempting to clarify the question with the family
- Confronting the physician about the question
- Consulting the institution's ethics committee

For nurses who are unsure about which issues can be referred to the ethics committee, the facility's policy and procedure manual can give direction.

Step 4: Analyze the Advantages and Disadvantages of Each Course of Action

Some of the courses of action developed during the previous step are more realistic than others. The identification of these actions becomes readily evident during this step in the decision-making process, when the advantages and the disadvantages of each action are considered in detail. Along with each option, the consequences of taking each course of action must be thoroughly evaluated.

Consider whether initiating discussion might anger the physician or cause distrust of the nurse involved. Both these responses may reinforce the attitude of submission to the physician, and either could make continuing to practice nursing at that institution difficult. The same result might occur if the nurse successfully resuscitates a client despite orders to the contrary. Failure to resuscitate the client has the potential to produce a lawsuit unless a clear order for no resuscitation has been given. Presenting the situation to a supervisor may, if the supervisor supports the physician, cause the nurse to be considered a troublemaker and thus have a negative effect on future evaluations. The same process could be applied to the other courses of action.

When considering the advantages and disadvantages, the nurse should be able to narrow the realistic choices of action. Other relevant issues need to be examined when weighing the choices of action. A major factor would be choosing the appropriate code of ethics. The ANA Code of Ethics should be part of many client-care decisions affected by ethical dilemmas.

Step 5: Make the Decision and Act on It

The most difficult part of the process is actually making the decision, following through with action, and then living with the consequences. Decisions are often made with no follow-through, because nurses are fearful of the consequences of their decisions. By their nature, ethical dilemmas produce differences of opinion and not everyone will be pleased with the decision.

In the attempt to solve any ethical dilemma, there will always be a question of the correct course of action. The client's wishes almost always supersede independent decisions on the part of health-care professionals. A collaborative decision made by the client, physician, nurses, and family about resuscitation is the ideal situation and tends to produce fewer complications in the long-term resolution of such questions.

Conclusion

Ethical dilemmas, by definition, are difficult to resolve. Rarely will a nurse find ethical dilemmas covered in policy, procedure, and protocol manuals, but nurses can develop the skills necessary to make appropriate ethical decisions. The key to developing these skills is the recognition and frequent use of an ethical decision-making model and application of the appropriate ethical theories to the dilemma. As an orderly approach in solving the often disorderly aspects of ethical questions encountered in nursing practice, the decision-making model presented in this chapter can be applied to almost every type of ethical dilemma. Although each situation is different, ethical decision making based on ethical theory can provide a potent tool for resolving dilemmas found in client-care situations.

Name _____

Course _____

Instructor _____

Date _____

Critical Thinking Exercises

1. Compare and contrast ethics with laws by delineating the purposes, scopes, and methods of enforcement of each.
2. Distinguish between the two types of obligations.
3. Compare the three categories of rights.
4. Analyze the following ethical dilemma case study using the ethical decision-making process:

✔ What are the important data in relation to this situation?

✔ State the ethical dilemma in a clear, simple statement.

✔ What are the choices of action and how do they relate to specific ethical principles?

✔ What are the consequences of these actions?

✔ What decision can be made?

Bill L., a veteran emergency room (ER) nurse, called the resident physician about a client just admitted to the ER after a fall from a ladder. The client, a 52-year-old man, had been fixing his roof when the accident occurred. He had suffered a minor head injury, a twisted ankle, and a badly bruised arm. He also had a long history of asthma and heavy smoking. Not long after his admission to the ER, the client became cyanotic, dyspneic, and semiconscious. By the time that the resident physician arrived, the nurse had prepared the client for endotracheal intubation and had already notified the personnel in the medical intensive care unit (MICU) that they would be receiving this client.

After a hasty evaluation of the client, the resident decided to perform an emergency tracheostomy before transporting the client to the MICU. While performing the tracheostomy, the physician severed a major blood vessel and the client hemorrhaged profusely. After several tense minutes, the endotracheal tube was inserted, and the client was quickly transported to the MICU. The client remained cyanotic and had great difficulty breathing. Shortly after leaving the ER, the nurse realized that the oxygen tank that the client had been connected to was empty. The client never regained consciousness and died 3 days after admission. His death was due to respiratory failure and not to the injuries sustained in the fall.

When the client's wife came to the unit to collect the deceased's belongings, the nurse was torn between telling her about the mistakes that were made in the treatment of her husband and remaining silent. What are the key ethical principles involved in this situation? Are there any statements in the ANA Code of Ethics that may help resolve this dilemma? What would be the consequences of informing the client's wife of the truth? What are the consequences of not informing her?

References

1. Gilligan, C, and Attanucci, J: Two moral orientations: Gender differences and similarities. Merrill-Palmer Quarterly 34(3):223–231, 1988.

2. American Nurses Association: Code for Nurses with Interpretive Statement. American Nurses Association, Kansas City, 1976.

BIBLIOGRAPHY

American College of Physicians: Ethics Manual, ed 4. Ann Intern Med 128:576–594, 1998.

American Nurses Association: Nursing's Social Policy Statement. American Nurses Association, Washington, DC, 1996.

Aiken, TD, and Catalano, JT: Legal, Ethical, and Political Issues in Nursing. FA Davis, Philadelphia, 1994.

Altman, LK: Fatal drug trial raises questions about informed consent. New York Times, October 5, 1993, C-3.

Bullough, UL: The Emergence of the Modern Nurse. Macmillan, New York, 1969.

Burkhardt, MA, and Nathaniel, AK: Ethics and issues in contemporary nursing. Delmar Publications, Albany, NY, 1998.

Campbell, G: Ethical principles must guide us. AACN News 15(1):1–12, 1998.

Catalano, JT: Critical care nurses and ethical dilemmas. Critical Care Nurse 11:16–21, 1991.

Catalano, JT: Ethical decision making in the critical care patient. Critical Care Nursing Clinics of North America 9(1):45–52, 1997.

Catalano, JT: Systems of ethics. Critical Care Nurse 12:91–96, 1992.

Crego, PJ, and Lipp, EJ: Nurse's knowledge of advanced directives. Am J Crit Care 7(3):218–223, 1998.

Curtin, LL: Ethics, discipline and discharge. Nursing Management 27(3):51–52, 1996.

Davis, AJ, et al: Ethical Dilemmas and Nursing Practice, ed 4. Appleton & Lange, E. Norwalk, CT, 1997.

Doheny, M, et al: The Discipline of Nursing. Appleton & Lange, E. Norwalk, CT, 1987.

Farquhar, M: Definitions of quality of life: A taxonomy. J Adv Nurs 22:502–508, 1995.

Fiesta, J: The Law and Liability: A Guide for Nurses. Wiley & Sons, New York, 1988.

Fiesta, J: Legal update, 1995. Nursing Management 25(5):22–24, 1996.

Fletcher, J: Situation Ethics. Westminster, Philadelphia, 1966.

Ford, RD (ed): Nurse's Legal Handbook. Springhouse, Springhouse, PA, 1985.

Frank, L: The ethical imperative to treat pain in infants: Are we doing the best we can. Critical Care Nurse 17(5):80–89, 1997.

French, PA: The Spectrum of Responsibility. St. Martin's Press, New York, 1991.

Guido, GW: Legal Issues in Nursing. Appleton & Lange, E. Norwalk, CT, 1997.

Jameton, A: Nursing Practice: The Ethical Issues. Prentice Hall, Englewood Cliffs, NJ, 1984.

Joel, LA: Hungry for the truth. Am J Nurs 96(3):7, 1996.

Howell, JH, and Sale, WF (eds): Life Choices: A Hastings Center Introduction to Bioethics. Georgetown University Press, Washington, DC, 1995.

Mappes, TA, and Zembaty, JS: Biomedical Ethics, ed 3. McGraw-Hill, New York, 1991.

Monarch, K: Insurance portability. Oklahoma Nurse 43(1): 11, 1998.

Munro, NL: Apply the rules of "people ethics." AACN News 15(11):2–15, 1998.

Nicoll, LH: Nurses' Guide to the Internet, ed 2. JB Lippincott, Philadelphia, 1998.

Quinn, CA, and Smith, MD: The Professional Commitment: Issues and Ethics in Nursing. WB Saunders, Philadelphia, 1987.

Sawyer, LM: Nursing code of ethics: An international comparison. Int Nurse Rev 36:145–148, 1989.

Stewart, M: Managed care law blocks quality care to indigent patients. American Nurse 29(6):12, 1997.

Thompson, JE, and Thompson, HO: Bioethical Decision Making for Nurses. Appleton-Century-Crofts, E. Norwalk, CT, 1985.

Thompson, JE, and Thompson, HO: Teaching ethics to nursing students. Nurs Outlook 37:84–88, 1989.

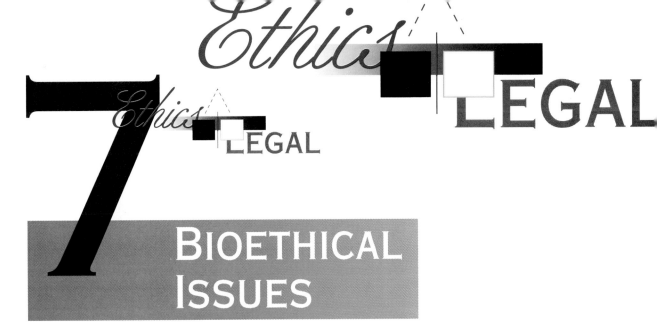

7

BIOETHICAL ISSUES

➤ *Joseph T. Catalano*

Learning Objectives

After completing this chapter, the reader will be able to:

1. Discuss the key ethical principles involved in:
   a. Abortion
   b. Genetic research
   c. Fetal tissue research
   d. Organ transplantation
   e. Use of scarce resources
   f. Assisted suicide
   g. Acquired immunodeficiency syndrome (AIDS)
   h. Children
2. Discuss the nurse's role in these ethical dilemmas.
3. Analyze and make a thoughtful ethical decision in a complex situation.

In the recent history of nursing, numerous biomedical and ethical dilemmas have arisen. Historically, nurses have been concerned with moral responsibility and ethical decision making. The nursing code of ethics and its frequent revisions demonstrate the profession's concern with providing ethical health care. The earliest codes of ethics made obedience to the physician the nurse's primary responsibility. The present code of ethics recognizes that the primary responsibility of the nurse is the client's well-being. This change in emphasis reflects the profession's increased self-awareness, independence, and growing accountability for its actions. Unfortunately, this new attitude has also heralded an era of increased tension, self-doubt, and ethical confusion. By examining the issues and identifying the key moral and ethical conflicts, nurses will be able to accept their moral responsibilities and make good ethical decisions.

In the course of their careers, nurses are likely to face ethical dilemmas. Although a complete analysis of every issue is beyond the scope of this book, some of the more common situations and their important ethical features are presented as examples of ways to analyze such dilemmas and to make informed decisions. The resolution of ethical dilemmas is never an easy task, and it is likely that someone may disagree with the decision.

ABORTION

Few issues evoke as strong an emotional reaction as abortion. Because of its religious, ethical, social, and legal implications, the abortion issue touches everyone in one way or another. There seems to be very little "middle ground." People are either strongly in favor of abortion or oppose it completely.

Elective abortion is the voluntary termination of a pregnancy before 24 weeks of gestation. An elective abortion may be either therapeutic or self-selected. Strictly speaking, a therapeutic abortion would be one performed in consultation with and on the recommendation of a physician or psychiatrist, based on the conclusion that the mother's health or psychological state would be damaged without the abortion. Self-selected abortions are those performed solely on the mother's own decision, without consultation with a physician or psychiatrist, usually for economic or convenience reasons. In the case of *Roe v. Wade* in 1973, the Supreme Court changed the legal status of elective abortion in the United States, but the ethical basis and moral status of this decision remain controversial.

A careful reading of the decision in *Roe v. Wade* reveals that the court made no decision about the ethics or morality of elective abortion. Rather, the court said that, according to the U.S. Constitution, all people have a right to determine what they can do with their bodies (i.e., the right to self-determination) and that such a right includes termination of a pregnancy.

The fundamental issues at the heart of the abortion debate center on the right of freedom of choice, which the court recognized, and the question of when life begins. Those who argue against abortion believe that life begins at the moment of conception and therefore hold that abortion is an act of killing. Proponents of abortion argue that the fetus is not really human until it reaches the point of development where it can live outside the mother's body (i.e., the age of viability). From a deontological standpoint, abortion represents a basic conflict of rights.

> " " *The fundamental issues at the heart of the abortion debate center on the right of freedom of choice, which the court recognized, and the question of when life begins.*

On one hand, a woman's rights to privacy, self-determination, and freedom of choice are at issue. In the United States, these rights are fiercely held and are considered to be issues of public policy and **constitutional law.** Indeed, these rights form the basis of the *Roe v. Wade* decision.

The conflicting right from the antiabortion side of the dilemma is the fetus's right to life. In most Western civilizations, particularly those that are based on Judeo-Christian beliefs, the casual and intentional taking of a human life is strongly prohibited. Life is the most basic good, because without it there can be no other rights. In general, the right to life is considered to be the most profound of the rights and is absolute in most situations.

When one is attempting to resolve the ethics and morality of abortion, these two conflicting rights need to be weighed against each other. Nurses are often placed in situations where they must help clients make decisions about abortion. Just as frequently, they are asked to participate in the procedure itself. In practice, ethical issues are always affected by the health-care provider's moral values. In the dilemma over abortion, nurses must analyze their own values and perceptions of their roles in order to make the best decisions. As a client **advocate,** should a nurse be for or against abortion? How can a nurse avoid influencing the woman's decision about abortion? Can a nurse ethically and legally refuse to assist at abortions? Ought the client's reason for wanting an abortion or her stage of pregnancy (first or second trimester, or later, requiring a partial-birth procedure) have any influence on the nurse's decision? These questions are not easily answered, but understanding the underlying principles involved in the issue may help to defuse some of the emotional impact that often surrounds this topic. As in all complicated ethical dilemmas, the nurse needs to remember that the client must receive competent, high-quality care regardless of the nurse's own personal values or moral beliefs.

GENETICS AND GENETIC RESEARCH

The ability to alter genetic material in such a way as to produce organisms that differ greatly from their original form is now a reality. Scientific and popular literature is filled with reports of new ways to identify and change the genetic material of all types of living creatures. Currently, genetically altered bacteria (e.g., *Escherichia coli*) are used to produce various medications, including a purer form of insulin. Genetically altered corn is now growing in very hot, dry places and is resistant to most insects. Abnormal genes that indicate individuals who are at risk for various types of cancer, Alzheimer's disease, and Down syndrome have been identified.

What Do You Think?

Do you support or reject elective abortion? On what ethical principles do you base your belief? What advice would you give to a pregnant teenager who wanted to have an abortion?

In the twentieth century, society has become so accustomed to the idea that science should be allowed to do whatever it is capable of doing that very few questions have been asked about the ethics of genetic engineering and research. As with most scientific research and techniques, the techniques of genetic engineering are ethically neutral. Procedures such as refining recombinant DNA, gene therapy, altering germ cells, and cloning other cells, in themselves, are neither good nor bad. The potential for misuse of these procedures is so great,

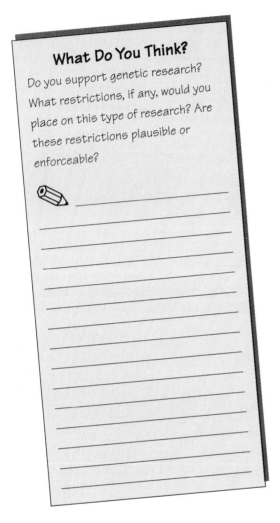

What Do You Think?

Do you support genetic research? What restrictions, if any, would you place on this type of research? Are these restrictions plausible or enforceable?

however, that it may permanently alter or even destroy the human race.

Several ethical issues need to be considered when genetic engineering and research are being conducted, including those involving the safety of genetic research, the legality and morality of genetic screening, and the proper use of genetic information. Recently proposed laws attempt to regulate genetic research to prevent the production of a supervirus or superbacteria that could exterminate the entire human population.[1]

With current technology, it is possible to detect genetic patterns in newborn infants that are linked to breast and colon cancer, heart disease, Huntington's disease, and Parkinson's disease. The advantage to insurance companies, which could screen individuals as early as infancy for costly and potentially lethal diseases later in life, is obvious: These individuals could be excluded from health and life insurance coverage, thus saving the insurance companies a great deal of money. Although this practice would most likely be unethical, the concept of mandatory genetic screening is not unrealistic. Because it requires just one blood sample from a person at some point during that person's life, it is possible that this type of screening could even be done without the individual's knowledge or consent.

Informed consent is discussed in Chapter 8. Confidentiality is at great risk of being violated by genetic screening. The confidentiality, trust, and fidelity that exist between the health-care provider and the client have been the basis of the therapeutic relationship. Information obtained through genetic screening can be used to benefit clients and to prepare them for future problems, or it can be released to insurance companies to give them grounds for refusal of coverage. In some cases, individuals may be denied employment based on the results of genetic testing. In this time of the information superhighway and vast computerized databases, very little of a client's health history remains confidential.[2]

An important ethical implication for nurses is the emotional impact that genetic information may have on the client. Knowledge of the possible long-term outcome of one's health, particularly if that knowledge is negative, may cause a client **anxiety,** or the person may become depressed or suicidal. Nurses must further hone their teaching and counseling skills to assist clients in dealing with implications of this type of information.

Obstetric nurses have been involved with genetic screening procedures for years.

Some of the most important information obtained from amniocentesis deals with the genetic composition of the fetus. It is important that the mother understand the procedure and the type of information it may yield and also that she gives informed consent for this procedure.

A strict ethical obligation exists for nurses to refuse to participate in mandatory, involuntary screening programs as well as a strict prohibition about revealing genetic test results to unauthorized individuals. Forcing clients who are strongly opposed to finding out information about their genetic status to be tested is clearly a breach of those clients' right to self-determination. However, much as the current practice of routine screening for diseases such as tuberculosis, hepatitis, and blood lead levels promotes the general health of the population, so does the screening for genetic diseases. Clients who are strongly opposed to such genetic screening must be allowed the option to refuse it to maintain their right to self-determination.

> 66 99 *Forcing clients who are strongly opposed to finding out information about their genetic status to be tested is clearly a breach of those clients' right to self-determination.*

THE USE OF FETAL TISSUE

Although it has just recently become news in the popular media, fetal tissue research has been conducted since at least the early 1990s. Traditional fetal tissue research has been generally limited to taking living cells from an aborted fetus and transplanting them into other people who have chronic or severe diseases. The procedure has been found to be helpful to a limited extent in the treatment of Alzheimer's disease and Parkinson's disease.

During 1997–2000, the Human Genome Project has added a new twist to this research. Rather than using tissue from aborted fetuses, scientists are now growing their own fetal tissue in the laboratory through **artificial insemination** and in vitro fertilization procedures. These test-tube fetuses are then dissected. Various fetal tissues are used for genetic and other types of research. The legal system has become aware of abuses of these procedures and has proposed legislation to control their use, including limiting the age of in vitro fetuses to 6 weeks. After 6 weeks, such fetuses will have to be destroyed.

Fetal tissue is highly desirable for research and transplantation because it lacks some of the genetic material that makes more mature tissues and organs more likely to cause rejection in the host. These fetal tissues are also in a rapid growth mode and naturally develop more quickly than do tissues from other sources. Scientists involved in this research see fetal tissue as one of the most important means of curing diseases.

Yet, even a superficial consideration of these procedures necessarily raises many important ethical issues. Basic to the ethics of this type of research is the source of the research material. In the past, most of the material came from elective abortions. Because of the immaturity and lack of differentiation of cells during the first trimester of pregnancy, however, the best fetal tissue comes from fetuses aborted during the second trimester. Most scientists agree that second-trimester fetuses have well-developed nervous, cardiovascular, gastrointestinal, and renal systems and are capable of feeling pain. Even though fetal tissue research has not led to an increase in abortions, the potential for abuse is tremendous.

It is also not definite whether the fetal tissue research scientists are paying others for these aborted fetuses. If payment is being made for aborted fetuses, it would seem to violate both the laws that prevent payment for organs used in transplantation and the moral respect for humanity. Questions also arise concerning who is giving permission for the use of fetuses in transplantation procedures. Does anyone really own them?

Another important ethical issue concerns the use of in vitro fertilization as a source for fetal tissue. Many religious groups question the morality of the procedure itself. Even if in vitro fertilization is considered ethical for procedures such as surrogate motherhood, is it ethical to create fetuses that are going to be used only for research and transplantation? From whom are the ova and sperm coming? Have the people from whom these have been obtained given permission for such use of their tissues? What about the rights of a fetus who was created in a test tube without ever having a hope of a normal life?

Despite a 1988 directive, which was extended indefinitely in 1990, to prevent the Department of Health and Human Services from using federal money for fetal tissue research, such research continues. Recent administrations have unofficially lifted the ban by allowing local biomedical ethical panels to make decisions about this type of research. Many of these panels, which consist mainly of research scientists, have ruled in favor of continuing research.

Nurses may have an important role to play in issues involving fetal tissue research. Although they will not likely be involved directly in research itself, nurses are often employed in facilities where elective abortions are performed. Nurses employed in such places must become aware of the issues involved in abortion. They also should know where the aborted fetuses are taken and how they are disposed of. Nurses should also remain informed about developing procedures and techniques regarding fetal tissue research; they should support legal and ethical efforts to control its abuses.

ORGAN TRANSPLANTATION

Despite widespread public and medical acceptance of organ transplantation as a highly beneficial procedure, ethical questions still remain. Whenever a human organ is transplanted, many people are involved, including the donor, the donor's family, medical and nursing personnel, and the recipient and his or her family. Society in general could also be added to this group, because of the high cost of organ transplantation, which is usually paid from tax money directly or indirectly in

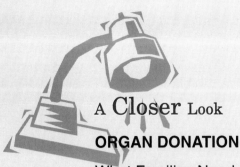

A Closer Look

ORGAN DONATION

What Families Need to Know

Seven Questions That Families Often Ask About Organ Donation and How You Should Answer Them

Many families refuse to donate a loved one's organs simply because they do not fully understand organ donation. By being prepared to address their concerns, you can help them make a decision they are comfortable with.

Here are the most common questions families ask about organ donation. Review them along with the answers so that you are prepared the next time that you need to counsel a family on this sensitive issue.

1. *Whose consent is needed to allow organ donation?*
   Consent must come from the patient's legal next of kin, even if the patient has a signed donor card or an organ donation sticker on his or her driver's license.

2. *How can you ask us to make this decision at such a tragic time?*
   "I know that this is a very stressful time for you, but I need to ask that you think about organ donation. Is it what your loved one would have wanted?
   I understand that you may not be able to say yes right now, and that's okay. However, if you decide to donate, we need to know as soon as possible so that any tissues or organs may be removed in time to help another person."

3. *What does brain death mean?*
   Brain death is an irreversible condition that occurs when blood no longer flows to the brain and the brain tissue dies. Although the brain is dead, other organs and tissues can function if supported by artificial means. A doctor will pronounce brain death only after everything possible has been done for your loved one and there is no chance of survival.

4. *Is the body disfigured when the organs are removed?*
   Surgeons use as few incisions as possible to recover the donated organs or tissues. Donation shouldn't interfere with an open casket funeral, if that's what you have planned.

5. *Will we be charged for donation costs?*
   No. All costs related to removal of the organs are covered by the donor program. However, you'll still be responsible for the funeral, burial arrangements, and related costs.

6. *How are recipients chosen?*
Recipients are chosen from the United Network of Organ Sharing, a national computer registry. They're selected according to degree of need, how long they've been on the waiting list, and certain medical criteria, such as blood type compatibility, tissue matching, and body size.
7. *We're not sure if our religion allows organ donation. What should we do?*
Many religions support organ donation, but if you're concerned, speak with your religious leader.

TERESA M. ODELL, RN
Coordinator, Nursing Staff Education
Cobb Hospital and Medical Center
Kennesaw, GA

From Odell, TM: Organ donation. What families need to know. Nursing 94 December 1994, p 321, with permission.

the form of increased insurance premiums. Each one of these persons or groups has rights that may conflict with the rights of others.

Currently, the two primary sources for organ and tissue donations are living related donors and **cadaver donors.** Most institutions that perform transplants or organizations that are involved in obtaining organs and tissues have developed elaborate procedures to help deal with the ethical and legal issues involved in transplantation. Despite these efforts, some ethical uncertainties remain whenever the issue of organ transplantation is raised. One particularly sensitive issue is exemplified when a child donates an organ, for example, a kidney transplant for a sibling, a procedure that poses some risk. Although parents are usually required to give consent for medical procedures for their children, by legal definition, a child younger than 18 years of age cannot give informed consent to such a procedure. It can be argued, however, that ethically the donor child, as a participant, should have input in making such a deci-

sion. At what age can a child have a say in the decision? Can a child be forced, for example, to donate a kidney even if he or she refuses? (See the discussion of children's ethics later in this chapter.)

One situation that illustrates this dilemma is that of a teenage girl who developed leukemia. The only way to save her life was to find a bone marrow donor who matched her genetic type. When no donor could be found, the parents decided to have another baby in the hope that the bone marrow of the second child would match that of the first child. After the baby was born, it was found that the bone marrow did indeed match, and when the child was old enough to donate safely, the bone marrow was taken and transplanted into the older child.

Despite the best efforts of the medical and legal community to establish criteria for death, some ethical questions still linger about what constitutes death. Because organs such as the heart, lungs, and liver need to come from a donor whose heart is still beating, some clinicians fear that there will be a tendency for physicians to declare that a person is dead before death actually occurs. The most widely accepted criterion for death is **brain death.** Some researchers, however, question whether the death of the brain actually means that a person ceases to exist as a human. Are there some other criteria that ought to be examined in conjunction with brain death?

One of the most difficult ethical issues involved in organ transplantation is the selection of recipients. Because fewer organs are available than the numerous people who need them, the potential ethical dilemmas are great. The **Uniform Anatomical Gift Act** was passed to increase the supply of organs for donation and attempt to reduce some of the confusion over organ donation. The national organ recipient list attempts to list and rank all people who need organs in a nondiscriminatory manner. Some important criteria for ranking include need, length of time on the list, potential for survival, prior organ transplantation, value to the community, and tissue compatibility.

Nurses can be, and often are, involved in some aspect of the organ donation process. Many states have passed laws that require the health-care workers to ask the family members of potential organ donors whether they have ever thought about their dead or dying loved one being used for organ donation. Many nurses, particularly nurses who work in critical care units, provide care for clients who may potentially become organ donors. Nurses in operating rooms may help in the actual surgical procedures that remove organs from a cadaver and transplant them into a recipient's body. Other nurses provide the postoperative care for clients who have received a transplanted organ. Home-health-care nurses give the follow-up care to such clients at home.

Nurses working with organ transplantation need to be sensitive to the potential for manipulation. Most people who are seeking organ transplantations are desperately ill or

What Do You Think?

How do you define death? Is brain death really death when the client's heart is still beating? How do you explain this idea to grieving families?

near death. They and their families can be very easily manipulated or can themselves become very manipulative. On the other side, the families of potential organ donors are usually distraught about the sudden and traumatic loss of a loved one. They too are vulnerable to psychological manipulation. Because of the emotionally fragile state present in the family of a trauma victim, they are vulnerable to guilt and grief. Health-care providers should avoid appealing to these emotions when obtaining permission to harvest organs for transplantation.

As a general rule, neither the donor nor his or her family should play any part in the selection of a recipient. Nurses need to avoid making statements or giving nonverbal indications of their approval or disapproval of potential recipients.

THE USE OF SCARCE RESOURCES IN PROLONGING LIFE

In these days of restructuring and downsizing, money for health care is in short supply. It is recognized that most public money allocated for health care is spent during the last year of life for many elderly clients. Expensive procedures, therapies, technologies, and care are provided to terminally ill individuals to extend their lives by a few days or even a few hours. It is not unusual to spend as much as $5000 a day on a client receiving care in an intensive care unit.

The traditional belief has been that life should be preserved at all cost and by any means available. Health-care providers feel uncomfortable when cost considerations are mentioned regarding treatments for terminally ill clients. Yet, in the context of current problems in society, such considerations are both economical and ethical realities. The necessity of conserving resources has forced society, through governmental action, to face this issue. All of the present proposed health-care plans take into consideration some type of cost-control measures related to restricting payment for client care. In addition, the **hospice care** movement and a growing number of physicians and other health-care professionals support **palliative** care for the terminally ill that provides pain relief and comfort measures but does not try to prolong the person's life (Box 7.1).

In reality, the current health-care system is already rationing care to some degree.

Many people who are not covered by health-care insurance do not seek health care. Groups such as the poor, who are covered by massive governmental programs, shy away from seeking health care because of the numerous restrictions placed on it. Individuals who are covered by insurance often have restrictions placed on them by the insurance companies.

The use of public funds for health care is an ethical issue that revolves around the principle of distributive justice. In this context, distributive justice requires that all citizens have equal access to all types of health care, regardless of their income levels, race, sex, religious beliefs, or diagnosis. Many complex issues are involved in this dilemma.

These issues go far beyond the questions of who gets what type of care and where and how the care takes place. Some type of **universal health-care coverage** is likely to be mandated for all Americans sometime in the future. Is it fair that some individuals (taxpayers) pay for the health care of others? Should individuals who contribute to their own poor state of health by smoking, drinking, taking illicit drugs, or overeating be provided with the same type of care as those who do not put themselves at risk? And who is going to make the decisions about who gets expensive treatment such as organ transplantations, experimental medications, placement in intensive care units, or life-extending technologies?

The use of criteria such as age, potential for a high-quality life, and availability of resources for determining who receives life-extending technologies is gaining wider acceptance. But is this a valid ethical position? Nurses are often involved in situations in which terminally ill clients are brought to the hospital for end-of-life care.

> 66 99 *In reality, the current health-care system is already rationing care to some degree.*

Many procedures and techniques commonly used to promote healing, cure, and recovery can also be used to maintain and prolong life. None is more controversial than tube feedings. It is a relatively simple procedure that is used in all areas of health care, from feeding premature infants in the neonatal intensive care unit to maintaining the elderly postoperative client at home under the supervision of home-health-care staff. Additionally, it is a way of maintaining nutrition and hydration, two of the most basic needs of life. Nurses who work with terminally ill clients often believe that once a feeding tube has been inserted, it cannot be removed for any reason because that would constitute active euthanasia, or mercy killing. But is that belief justified in all circumstances? Consider the following scenario:

Her large family, consisting of her husband of many years, three adult sons and two daughters, were very upset. Mrs. Ada Floral, 82 years old, had just suffered a massive stroke that rendered her unresponsive. Although she was breathing on her own, she had no voluntary movements and seemed to be completely paralyzed. Magnetic resonance imaging (MRI) showed a large area of bleeding around the midbrain and brainstem. Her pupils were constricted and unresponsive. The physician explained that the prognosis was extremely grave, and the likelihood of Mrs. Floral's survival was minimal.

However, the family members all agreed that "everything" should be done, so the physician reluctantly initiated aggressive medical therapy with IV glucocorticoids, osmotic diuretics, antihypertensives, and physical therapy. After a week, there was no change. The family wondered whether Mrs. Floral might be "starving to death" and asked the physician to have a feeding tube inserted and feedings started.

One month later, the still unresponsive Mrs. Floral is being cared for at home by her family with the supervision of the local hospice/home-health-care program. She is off all IV medications; however, she is receiving some medications, a commercially prepared feeding, and water through the feeding tube. Some of the family members are beginning to question whether they did the right thing by insisting that everything be done and wished to remove the feeding tube so that Mrs. Floral could die a peaceful and dignified death, rather than just hanging on for months. Other family members feel that if they give permission for the tube's removal, they would be killing their mother and could not live with the guilt.

The hospice nurse in charge of the case had discussed the issue with the family. She too believes that once a feeding tube has been placed, it should not be removed, even if all the family agrees on its removal. She feels that it's not an issue a family can "just change their minds about." Although she is in frequent contact with Mrs. Floral's physician, she has not mentioned that the family is thinking about removing the feeding tube in fear that the physician might agree.

Is the hospice nurse correct in her belief about the removal of the feeding tube? When do tube feedings stop being beneficial to clients? Is there a right to death with dignity? What ethical rationales could be used for removal of the feeding tube in this case?

Nurses need to play an active role in helping to formulate policies concerning the issues that they face daily.

THE RIGHT TO DIE

The right-to-die issue is an extension of the right to self-determination issue discussed in Chapter 8. It also overlaps with the dilemma of **euthanasia** and assisted suicide. Health-care providers often become involved in the decision-making process when clients are irreversibly comatose, vegetative, or suffering from a terminal disease. The choices

that the families of such clients often face are death or the extension of life using painful and expensive treatments.

One of the difficulties in resolving right-to-die issues is understanding the terminology used. Often a client who has a **living will** states that he or she wants no extraordinary treatments if he or she should become comatose or unable to make decisions involving health care. But what actually constitutes extraordinary treatments? A general definition of ordinary treatments includes any medications, procedures, surgeries, or technologies that offer the client some hope of benefit without causing excessive pain or suffering.[3] Using this definition, extraordinary treatments (sometimes called heroic measures) become those treatments, medications, surgeries, and technologies that offer little hope for curing or improving the client's condition. Although these general definitions provide some guidelines for making decisions about ordinary and extraordinary treatments, discerning the nature of the specific modalities remains difficult. For example, a ventilator is a machine that assists a client's breathing. In intensive care units (ICUs), it is a common mode of treatment for many types of clients, including postoperative clients, clients with cardiac and respiratory diseases, and victims of trauma. Does its widespread and frequent use make the ventilator an ordinary mode of treatment? Many would say yes, whereas others would say it is still extraordinary because of its invasive nature and complicated technology (see Box 7.1).

Another issue often included in the right-to-die debate is that of "codes" and "do-not-resuscitate" (DNR or no code) orders. Cardiopulmonary resuscitation (CPR) is widely taught to both health-care providers and the general public. It is often used to treat clients who have suffered heart attacks and have gone into cardiac arrest as well as clients suffering from electrical shock, drowning, and traumatic injuries. In the hospital setting, the nursing staff is obligated to perform CPR on all clients who do not have a specific DNR order. This leads to situations where terminally ill clients may be subjected to CPR resuscitative efforts several times before they die.

> " " *As useful as advance directives are in helping the client decide on future care, clients often are unable to anticipate all the possible types of treatments used.*

As an issue of self-determination, it is essential that the client's wishes about health care be followed. All client communication to the nurse about desires for future care should be documented. If at all possible, the client should be encouraged to designate an individual to act as a moral surrogate, a designated decision maker, should the client become unable to make his or her own decisions. The expressed desires about future medical care are known as advance directives. They are the best means to guarantee that a client's wishes will be honored.

Advance directives, in the form of a living will or durable power of attorney, can and should specify which extraordinary procedures, surgeries, medications, or treatments can or cannot be used. These directives are often in the form of formal documents that need to be witnessed by two individuals who are not related to the client. As useful as advance directives are in helping the client decide on future care, clients often are unable to anticipate all the possible types of treatments used. For example, an elderly client with a long history of cardiovascular disease specified in his living will that he did not want CPR performed and did not want a ventilator. When his heart developed a potentially lethal dysrhythmia that rendered him unresponsive, his physician made the decision to cardiovert* the client using the electric cardioverter because this mode of treatment was not specifically forbidden by the client's living will. Strictly speaking, the physician did not violate the letter of the living will, but did he violate its spirit?

---

*Cardioverting is a procedure in which electrical shock is used to change the heart rhythm from ventricular tachycardia or other rhythms to normal sinus rhythms.

**Treatments Not Specifically Listed in the Living Will:
The Ethical Dilemmas**

Joseph T. Catalano

PART 1: THE ETHICAL CASE

Because of publicity regarding living wills and laws on required request, the number of patients with them has increased. Consequently, related ethical dilemmas are also becoming more common. One example of such an ethical dilemma occurs when a living will fails to describe the current patient situation. The following case illustrates this type of problem, one which critical care nurses are likely to encounter more often over the next few years.

Sharon has worked as an RN in the 15-bed medical intensive care unit (MICU) of a rural 250-bed hospital for 5 years. She is concerned with the ethical and legal obligations of nurses who care for patients with living wills. During her tenure at this facility, several patients entered the hospital with living wills. Recently, however, Mr. K. was admitted to the MICU with congestive heart failure, and he brought along his living will. The presence of the living will created problems for Sharon, Mr. K.'s primary nurse, and the MICU staff.

Mr. K. was 72 years old and had a long history of smoking and emphysema. He had recently developed congestive heart failure and angina. Because of his poor pulmonary function, his condition was inoperable. Mr. K. was one of the MICU's "regulars"; he was admitted to the unit whenever he had an exacerbation of his pulmonary condition, usually once or twice a year. He chose to be treated aggressively with medications and respiratory therapy, excluding the use of a ventilator. Mr. K. usually responded well to treatment and was generally discharged within 1 week of admission.

Mr. K.'s family consisted of three adult children by a first wife, his current wife, their two adult children, plus several elderly brothers and sisters. His extended and immediate family were actively involved with his care and were aware of the living will he had executed 2 years previously after one of his hospitalizations. Based on Mr. K.'s living will, the physician classified him as a "no code" upon his most recent admission.

His living will was one of the general, standard form documents consistent with the laws of his home state. The living will stated that should Mr. K. become unable to make decisions about his care, he should be allowed to die and not be kept alive by artificial means.

The only specific stipulation in the living will was, "I am not to be placed on a ventilator." He had talked with Sharon, his primary nurse, several times about his fear of being kept alive on a ventilator when there was little or no hope of survival, or when he would be unable to return to his prior level of functioning. Mr. K.'s living will did not, however, address tube feedings, cardiopulmonary resuscitation (CPR), or life-sustaining medications.

Upon Mr. K.'s most recent admission to the MICU for acute respiratory distress and chest pain, the electrocardiogram showed changes that might indicate a myocardial infarction, but the enzyme studies were inconclusive. He responded well to the prescribed treatments and medication therapy, and on the evening of his second day after admission Sharon helped Mr. K. into a chair. Shortly thereafter, however, he suffered a sustained run of multiform ventricular tachycardia. During the dysrhythmic event, he became unresponsive and cyanotic. Four family members who were visiting at the time came running out of the room yelling, "Do something, Daddy's passed out!"

Simultaneously, one of Mr. K.'s physicians was making his evening rounds in the unit. The physician and Sharon quickly went into the room. The nurse quietly reminded the doctor that Mr. K. had a living will and was ordered to be a "no code." The physician ordered that a code be initiated anyway. Mr. K. was returned to his bed, intubated with an oral endotracheal tube, and resuscitated, including full CPR, electrocardioversion, and chemical resuscitation using lidocaine and dopamine. The code produced a life-sustaining cardiac rhythm, blood pressure, pulse, and spontaneous respirations, but Mr. K. remained unresponsive and intubated for 2 more days, connected to a T-tube at 60%. His prognosis was extremely poor, and Mr. K. lived only 1 day after extubation.

After the code, the nurse asked the physician why they had resuscitated Mr. K. when he had a living will and was classified as a "no code"? The physician answered that a patient in Mr. K.'s condition was highly unlikely to file a law suit for violating the living will, whereas the family members might easily file a suit for wrongful death, especially if Mr. K. had been allowed to die in the chair before their eyes. He also said that the spirit of the living will was followed by not placing Mr. K. on a ventilator. The physician stated that Mr. K.'s living will was more oriented towards respiratory problems than cardiac dysrhythmias.

PART 2: ETHICAL ANALYSIS

Advance directives, which include living wills, are now a required part of the health care of all patients. The Omnibus Budget Reconciliation Act of 1990 requires that all hospitals, nursing-care facilities, home-health-care agencies, and care givers ask patients about advance directives and provide information concerning living wills and durable power of attorney (DPOA) to help patients make informed health-care decisions. However, the federal law mandates only the requirements and not the directives to implement the law. The actual implementation of the law is left to the individual states. Because of the vagueness of the law, a great deal of confusion exists, particularly with regards to living wills.

Nurses play an important role in ensuring that patients understand the implications of their choices pertaining to decisions that may prolong their lives during medical emergency. Because of their "front-line" position as care givers within the health-care system, nurses must understand this role, specifically as it pertains to living wills.

This case study illustrates some of the difficult issues that nurses encounter when they care for patients with living wills. Some difficult legal and ethical questions need to be considered, for example:

- Dilemma 1: What legal or ethical implications do living wills have if families or physicians act against the patient's expressed wishes?
- Dilemma 2: Does the nurse have any ethical obligation to refuse to participate in the case of resuscitation efforts that are inconsistent with the patient's living will?
- Dilemma 3: If the physician had not been present to initiate the code, should the nurse have allowed Mr. K. to die in the presence of his emotionally involved family?

Ethical Considerations

The questions formulated above address many practical concerns related to the execution of a living will. The living will, however, covers only very specific instances. There are always gray areas in ethically complex situations, such as the one presented here, that make a living will alone inadequate or that it is unable to address.

Identifying the Ethical Issues

Living wills are generally defined as "a directive from a competent individual to medical personnel and family members regarding the treatment he or she wishes to receive when he or she is no longer able to make the decision for himself or herself."[1] Although living wills have been present in the health-care setting, in one form or another, for as long as 20 years, they first attained the status of a legal document in 1976 when California passed the Natural Death act.[2] Since that date, 44 states have adopted a Natural Death Act in some form, although it varies widely from state to state. Also, the form that the living will may take varies, and no single form is acceptable in all states.[3] Some living wills are very specific as to what treatments are included, other living wills are general and nonspecific about treatments. Each state has its own particular regulations determining the exact format and number of signatures required to make a living will valid.[1]

The nurse needs to be able to identify potential problems in the living will and get ethical analysis before situations like the one above occur. Look closely at the patient's living will to identify some of the key components (Fig. 7–1). If the will is not signed, not witnessed or notarized, or is very old, be sure to call that to the attention of the patient and/or ethics committee. If the will is not clear on the types of treatments to use or not, ask the patient what he or she meant by certain sections or requests in the will and record his or her comments.

The concept of and need for living wills developed during the late 1960s as a response to the rapid advances in bioscience technology that allowed nurses

➤ Figure 7-1A

Checklist for evaluating a patient's living will document.

✔ 1. Statement of intention states the document was written freely when the patient was competent.

✔ 2. Statement of when the document goes into effect. This is usually when the patient is no longer able to make decisions for him/her self.

✔ 3. A section specifies general health care measure to be excluded from care.

✔ 4. Open section for specific measures (ventilators, pacemakers, etc) and any other specific instructions concerning care.

✔ 5. Proxy statement (sometimes called Durable Power of Attorney) which is optional, but a strong addition. Allows another person to make decisions in situations that may not have been anticipated in the living will. (Check your state law concerning details of proxy selection.)

✔ 6. Substitute proxy. This section is optional. Specifies who can make decisions, if first choice proxy is not available.

✔ 7. Legal statement that the proxy(s) may make decisions.

✔ 8. Witness selection statement. Many states require that witnesses not be related nor members of the health care team.

✔ 9. Signature and date. Must be signed and dated by the patient. Some states have very specific regulations concerning how long the will is valid. It may range from a few months to 5 years.

✔ 10. Legal signatures of witnesses are required.

✔ 11. Notary seal, if required by state law. State laws differ on notary seal requirement. It is usually required, if a proxy is selected.

➤ Figure 7-1*A*

Key elements in most living wills. (*A*) Checklist of items the nurse should look for in a patient's living will. State laws vary concerning advance directives, but the elements listed here are common and should be present in most states' living wills.

Continued on following page

and other health-care personnel to artificially prolong the lives of patients who would otherwise have died naturally.[4] This technology has progressed even further in the past 15 years. However, both the legal and ethical systems have not been able to keep pace with these technological advances. For some patients, the technology available for resuscitation and prolonging life does result in their active return to society as productive persons who are able to function at their

PENNSYLVANIA DECLARATION

I, _____, being of sound mind, willfully and voluntarily make this declaration to be followed if I become incompetent. This declaration reflects my firm and settled commitment to refuse life-sustaining treatment under the circumstances indicated below.

I direct my attending physician to withhold or withdraw life-sustaining treatment that serves only to prolong the process of my dying, if I should be in a terminal condition or in a state of permanent unconsciousness.

I direct that treatment be limited to measures to keep me comfortable and to relieve pain, including any pain that might occur by withholding or withdrawing life-sustaining treatment.

In addition, if I am in the condition described above, I feel especially strongly about the following forms of treatment:

I ( ) do ( ) do not want cardiac resuscitation.

I ( ) do ( ) do not want mechanical respiration.

I ( ) do ( ) do not want tube feeding or any other artificial or invasive form of nutrition (food) or hydration (water).

I ( ) do ( ) do not want blood or blood products.

I ( ) do ( ) do not want any form of surgery or invasive diagnostic tests.

I ( ) do ( ) do not want kidney dialysis.

I ( ) do ( ) do not want antibiotics.

I realize that if I do not specifically indicate any preference regarding any of the forms of treatment listed above, I may receive that form of treatment.

Other instructions:

➤ Figure 7-1 *B continued*

Sample advance directive. Because the laws on advance directives vary widely from state to state, there is no standard advance directive whose language conforms exactly with all states' laws. (Part *B* reprinted with permission of Choice in Dying, formerly Concern for Dying/Society for the Right to Die, 200 Varick Street, New York, NY 1–14, 212-3665540).

Surrogate decision making:

I ( ) do ( ) do not want to designate another person as my surrogate to make medical treatment decisions for me if I should be incompetent and in a terminal condition or in a state of permanent unconsciousness.

PRINT THE
NAME, ADDRESS
AND PHONE
NUMBER OF
YOUR
SURROGATE

Name: _____

Address: _____

Phone: _____

Name and address of substitute surrogate (if surrogate designated above is unable to serve):

PRINT THE
NAME, ADDRESS
AND PHONE
NUMBER OF YOUR
ALTERNATE
SURROGATE

Name: _____

Address: _____

Phone: _____

I made this declaration on the _____ day of _____.
                                            (*day*)   (*month, year*)

Declarant's signature: _____

Declarant's address: _____

The declarant, or the person on behalf of and at the direction of the declarant, knowingly and voluntarily signed this writing by signature or mark in my presence.

Witness's signature: _____

Witness's address: _____

Witness's signature: _____

Witness's address: _____

Courtesy of Choice in Dying   1/94
200 Varick Street, New York, NY 10014 1-800-989-WILL

PAGE 2

➤ Figure 7-1*B continued*

prior state of health. For many patients, however, resuscitation methods and advanced life support technology merely extend the physiologic existence of the person even though his or her cognitive or conscious activity is diminished.

The key ethical issue that nurses need to be aware of when involved with living wills is the principle of autonomy, the person's right to self-determination. Living wills protect the patient's right to self-determination by clearly stating what the person desires while he or she is competent to decide. This document communicates patient preferences should that person become incompetent and therefore unable to make his or her own decisions.[2]

Nurses need to be aware of a second important ethical issue that is closely related to self-determination in the execution of a living will; this is the person's right to refuse treatment. In general, if a person is determined to be competent, then that person has a right to refuse any and all treatments.[5] From this particular viewpoint, a living will can be seen as a directive for the refusal or withdrawal of treatment at some future time. However, the principle of self-determination does have societal limitations. For example, if a person refuses treatment for a highly contagious disease, that person poses a threat to the needs of society as a whole. Consequently, public health agencies are required by law to report and treat communicable diseases such as sexually transmitted diseases, hepatitis, and tuberculosis.

Ethical Difficulties of Living Wills

While a living will seems to be a simple solution to a complex care situation, there are some ethical difficulties inherent in their use that nurses need to know about. Primary among these ethical difficulties is the question of the person's level of knowledge of potential and future health-care problems at the time the will was formulated. Because living wills are often formulated long before they are to be used, there may later be serious questions about how informed the person was about the disease states and treatment modalities that might later affect care. If there is any indication that the person did not understand the full implications of future therapies or potential medical problems, then the validity of the living will is in question.[2]

A second ethical difficulty for nurses encompasses the principles of beneficence and nonmaleficence. The principle of beneficence states that a health-care professional's primary duty is to benefit or do good for the patient. The principle of nonmaleficence states that the patient should be protected from harm by health-care providers.[6] It is sometimes difficult to determine if the primary duty is to produce benefit or prevent harm. Generally, most health-care providers think that the duty to avoid harming the patient outweighs the concerns for providing benefit. When evaluated from the beneficence and nonmaleficence viewpoints, living wills seem to violate the principle of providing benefit to the patient. This perception makes many health-care providers ethically uncomfortable. In some situations, the implementation of a living will might actually involve the termination of some modes of treatments already in use. Termination seems to constitute actual harm to the patient. In either case, respecting a living will might often appear to health-care providers to be a violation of their duty to help patients and preserve life.

Nurses, as well as other health-care providers, often experience a sense of frustration when they are not allowed to use all the skills they have learned to preserve life. In the case of Mr. K., the physician obviously felt that intubation and clinical resuscitation were consistent with his living will, while the nurse perceived the situation in a different light.

A third difficulty nurses and other health-care workers may have with living wills is their formulation and legal enforcement. In general, the language used in the standard living will document is broad and vague. Living wills are often not specific enough to include all the forms of treatments that are possible for the many types of illnesses that might render a person incompetent to make decisions. Health-care providers may have little direction as to the care they are to give if the circumstances at the time the living will is to be honored are significantly different from the declared wishes of patient.[1]

Furthermore, unless the particular state has enacted into law a special type of living will called a natural death act, the living will has no mechanism of legal enforcement.[1] Currently, 44 states plus the District of Columbia have natural death laws.[8] In states without this legislation, there is no obligation to accept the living will as a valid legal document.

Even in some states that do have a natural death act, it is considered only advisory and the physician has the right to comply with the living will or treat the patient as the physician deems most appropriate. There is no protection for nurses or other health-care practitioners against criminal or civil liability in the execution of living wills in states without a natural death act. Once a valid living will exists, it only becomes effective when the person who formulated it meets the qualifications for the natural death act. In most states, the individual must be diagnosed as having a terminal condition where the continuation of treatment and life-support would only prolong the patient's dying process.[2] But, there is no clear consensus on the definition of "terminal condition."

Despite all these difficulties, living wills are still a good way for a patient to make health-care wishes known to health-care providers. Documents that are specific about treatment modalities, are written in a "legal" format, and signed by two or more witnesses tend to be treated with an increased level of respect by health-care providers.

Case Discussion

These principles regarding living wills can be used to analyze the ethical dilemmas in this case. Here are discussions of the three dilemmas introduced previously.

Dilemma 1
Living wills have more ethical implications than legal weight. Although many states have statutes that recognize living wills, the regulations are variable and

even in states with "strong" living will legislation, the final decision as to whether to honor a living will is often left up to the physician and/or patient's family.

Ethically, there is a fairly strong obligation for nurses and other health-care workers to carry out the patient's wishes as a part of that patient's right to self-determination. However, because patients often do not understand all the implications of "not being kept alive by artificial means" or the various levels of the many treatments available, there is almost always some question about the validity of the living will based on the principles of informed consent. Given the circumstances of the situation involving Mr. K., the physician may have believed that he followed the only reasonable option of action available to him. "No code" order status varies considerably from hospital to hospital. Mr. K.'s primary physician wrote the "no code" order on the basis of the requests in Mr. K.'s living will. More detailed delineation of the aspects of the "no code" order and how the decision is made would be helpful in clarifying its meaning.

Dilemma 2

Nurses always have a right and even an ethical obligation to refuse to perform procedures that they firmly believe to be unethical or harmful to patients. However, there are several factors that must be considered when refusing to carry out procedures requested by physicians. Although Mr. K.'s living will was not specific about the kind of resuscitation, intubation, and ventilation desired, performing a code on him seems to be a violation of his wishes. If the ventricular tachycardia had been terminated quickly with lidocaine or a precordial thump, Mr. K. might have recovered without requiring further treatment or suffering any long-term complications.

Patients with living wills, like Mr. K., are not automatically "no codes." Living wills that make reference to specific treatments, such as "no ventilator," do not necessarily mean that the patient is not to be resuscitated. It is important to discuss exactly what the patient with a living will wishes to have done in a variety of circumstances.

It is also important to clarify these wishes with all the physicians involved in the case. The family members also need to be informed of the patient's wishes. The nurse needs to support the family while simultaneously carrying out the patient's wishes.

Another consideration that the nurse needs to keep in mind in refusing to carry out a physician's request is the consequences of that refusal. A nurse who refuses to act in an emergency situation such as a code, with a physician standing there giving orders, is at risk for a variety of punitive if not legal consequences. If it could later be determined that the nurse failed to meet a standard of care by not following the physician's direct order, then the nurse might be open to a malpractice suit.[7]

Most likely, other nurses on the unit would have responded to the code so that any specific nurse's refusal to conduct the code would not have substantially changed the final outcome of the situation, but a blatant refusal to act in a code situation is unacceptable. However, if the nurse's ethical convictions about performing a code on a specific patient are so strong that he or she is unable to function, then the nurse should remove himself or herself from the situation.

While the family involvement complicates decision making, such as the decision to perform the code on Mr. K., a nurse's first obligation is to meet the needs of the patient. Although they might have been aware of the living will, Mr. K.'s family did not seem to understand the full consequences of the decisions it required. The death of a loved one is always a powerful emotional experience for family members, so powerful that it usually clouds rational decision making. It is even more difficult to actually watch a loved one die, particularly if that patient seems to be on the road to recovery.

Similarly, there are very few nurses who are not affected by the death of a patient, but the education nurses receive helps place that event in a more rational context. The nurse needs to support the family emotionally while carrying out the wishes of the patient as stated in the living will. Education of the family members concerning the important aspects of the living will, prior to the time when the terms of the living will go into effect, may help prevent the type of response demonstrated by Mr. K.'s family.

Dilemma 3

Refusing to initiate a code on Mr. K. is the ethically correct choice of action because the nurse is following his wishes as outlined in the living will. However, not initiating the code is difficult in a situation where a group of hysterical family members are demanding some type of action. Other possible courses of action might include gently but firmly ushering the family members out of the unit to a waiting room while Mr. K. was returned to bed and allowed to expire without a code; allowing the family to stay in the room and attempting to explain what a living will really means while Mr. K. expires in their presence; or calling a code but not pursuing it with a great deal of enthusiasm.

Also, a discussion between the physician, nurse, clergy, ethics committee, and other members of the health-care team to clarify the meaning of "no code" status and how to better uphold the patient's wishes may be valuable.

Understanding Terminology

Defining terminology becomes important when executing living wills. The word "artificial," for example, is likely to have a much different meaning to the patient than it does to the nurse. In the strictest sense, any type of technology or equipment, including intravenous infusions (IVs), monitors, antibiotics, feeding tubes, catheters, and even oxygen delivery equipment is *artificial*.[4,8] Members of the health-care community use artificial technology so frequently that it is accepted as an ordinary part of patient care. Few patients are admitted without having IVs, oxygen, and some type of monitoring equipment attached to them. For health-care providers, the key term becomes "extraordinary" technology used to maintain life. Equipment such as ventilators, intra-aortic balloon pumps, external pacemakers, intracranial pressure monitors, and vasoactive pharmacologic agents may qualify as "extraordinary means." In some tertiary care settings, however, these advanced technologies may be classified as "ordinary means" for maintaining life.

The important question the nurse needs to ask concerning Mr. K.'s living will is did he mean "artificial" or did he say "artificial" but mean "extraordinary"? By allowing "aggressive treatment" (which likely included several "artificial" technologies, such as antibiotics, bronchodilators, intermittent positive pressure breathing treatments, and oxygen therapy) for his acute respiratory distress episodes, it seems that he meant "extraordinary" rather than "artificial" in the strictest sense of the word. Intubation, using an oral or nasal endotracheal tube, is always an "artificial" mode of treatment. Also, this mode of intubation is usually considered an "extraordinary" mode of treatment due to its highly invasive nature and potential for complications. This particular treatment modality would seem to be a clear violation of Mr. K.'s wishes as expressed in his living will, even if he did not understand the nuances of the terminology used. If Mr. K.'s resuscitation could have been accomplished through the use of a manual resuscitator and a mask and not an endotracheal tube, it is less clear that it would be a violation of his wishes as stated in his living will.

Summary

Because of the limitations inherent in living wills, critical care nurses should ask about the patient's personal preferences, values, and choices. Nurses need to ask about specific items that are life sustaining or life-saving. Most importantly, nurses must document any patient statements or discussions that clarify these wishes. Asking patients if they have a living will or advanced directive is not enough. As professionals, nurses must educate patients in the available treatments and help them communicate what measures they do or do not want. This will help prevent the problem of resuscitating patients who really do not want it.

Clinical Research Questions

There are several questions still needing research in this area including:

How do critical care nurses feel about having patients in their units who have a living will or are designated "no code"?

How do critical care nurses feel about conducting codes on patients who have a living will or have been designated "no code"?

Do patients who enter the critical care unit have a full understanding of the therapies that are possible and what they involve?

What teaching methods used by critical care nurses are most effective in educating patients about living wills?

References
1. Guido, GW: Legal Issues in Nursing. Appleton & Lange, E. Norwalk, Conn, 1998.
2. Campbell, G: Ethical principles must guide us. AACN News 15(1):1–12, 1998.

3. Catalano, JT: Ethical and Legal Aspects of Nursing. Springhouse Corporation, Springhouse, Pa, 1991.
4. Davis, AJ, and Aroskar, MA: Ethical Dilemmas and Nursing Practice. Appleton-Century-Crofts, New York, 1997.
5. Frank, L: The ethical imperative to treat pain in infants: Are we doing the best we can? Critical Care Nurse 17(5):80–89, 1997.
6. Menzel, L: Is it worth it? Balancing the benefit of extended life with the cost of suffering during critical illness. Critical Care Nurse 18(4):67–73, 1998.
7. New law requires hospitals to ask about living wills. Medical Ethics Advisor 7(1):1–16, 1991.
8. Nurses Legal Handbook. Springhouse Corporation, Springhouse, Pa, 1992.

The names and insignificant characteristics of this case have been changed for confidentiality; any resemblance to a real person is coincidental. The views expressed in this ethical analysis article are those of the author and not necessarily that of DCCN, the publisher, or editors. The article is published to highlight some of the ethical controversies in practice and is not legal advice. For ethical/legal dilemmas, contact your institution's ethics committee, risk manager, and/or legal counsel for review of your particular situation.

From Catalano, JT: Treatments not specifically listed in the living will: The ethical dilemmas. Dimensions of Critical Care Nursing 13(3):142–150, 1994. Copyright Springhouse Corporation.

Nurses can help clients plan ahead for their care should they become unable to make decisions for themselves. Although the nurse should not make the decisions for the client, the nurse can provide important information about the various treatment modalities that the client is considering. The nurse can also help clients clarify their wishes and guide them through the process in formulating an advance directive.

EUTHANASIA AND ASSISTED SUICIDE

The term *euthanasia* generally means killing or refusing to treat a client to allow a painless or peaceful death. A distinction is often made between passive and active euthanasia.

Passive euthanasia usually refers to the practice of allowing an individual to die without any extraordinary intervention. Under this umbrella definition, practices such as DNR orders, living wills, and with-drawal of ventilators or other life support are usually included. **Active euthanasia,** on the other hand, usually describes the practice of hastening an individual's death through some act or procedure. This practice is also sometimes referred to as mercy killing and takes many forms ranging from use of large amounts of pain medication for terminal cancer clients to use of poison, gun, or knife to end a person's life.

Assisted suicide—brought to public attention by Dr. Jack Kevorkian, a Michigan physician who has publicly practiced it for many years—can be considered a type of active euthanasia or mercy killing. The central issue that has been publicized by Dr. Kevorkian is whether it is ever ethically permissible for health-care personnel to assist in taking a life. In most states the practice is illegal; however, Dr. Kevorkian has been tried three times under Michigan's assisted suicide laws and has not been convicted, although he openly admits to helping more than 130 clients to commit suicide. The definition of homicide—bringing about

What Do You Think?

Do you have an advanced directive? Why not? Make up a sample advanced directive for yourself. What would you include?

✎ _____

_____

_____

_____

_____

_____

_____

_____

_____

_____

_____

_____

_____

_____

a person's death or assisting in doing so—seems to fit the act of assisted suicide. There is still a great deal of hesitation on the part of the legal system to prosecute persons who are involved in assisted suicide or juries to convict physicians who participate in the activity.

In the fall of 1998, Dr. Kevorkian raised the legal and ethical stakes. On a nationally broadcast network news show, "60 Minutes," he not only admitted to administering a lethal medication to a client without the client's assistance, but he also made and played a videotape that showed the whole episode. The client, who had Lou Gehrig's disease (amyotrophic lateral sclerosis), had requested that Dr. Kevorkian kill him. The client had signed a **consent** form and release and was even given an extra 2 weeks to "think about it." The client waited only for 3 days before making his final request for the lethal medication. Under Michigan law, Dr. Kevorkian could have been charged with **manslaughter** or even first-degree murder. Dr. Kevorkian admitted that his **motivation** for the act was to be tried under these laws as a test case for active euthanasia. He was arrested 2 weeks later on a charge of first-degree murder; however, he felt very strongly that a jury will not convict him. Many health-care professionals think that mercy killing like this is always ethically wrong.

The fundamental ethical issue in these situations is the right to self-determination. In almost every other health-care situation, a client who is mentally competent can make decisions about what care to accept and what care to refuse. Yet, when it comes to the termination of life, this right becomes controversial. Supporters of the practice of assisted suicide believe that the right to self-determination remains intact, even with regard to the decision to end one's life. It is the last act of a very sick individual to control his or her own fate. Many believe that medical personnel should be allowed to assist these clients in this procedure, just as they are allowed to assist clients in other medical and nursing procedures.

Those who oppose assisted suicide find these arguments unconvincing. Legally, ethically, and morally, suicide in U.S. society has never been an accepted practice. Health-care staff go to great lengths to prevent suicidal clients from injuring themselves. In addition, it would seem that individuals in the terminal states of a disease, who are overwhelmed by pain and depressed by the thought of prolonged suffering, might not be able to think clearly enough to give informed consent for assisted suicide. Also, because the termination of life is final, it does not allow for spontaneous cures or for the development of new treatments or medications.

Nonmaleficence is the term that describes the obligation to do no harm to clients. Whether assisting in or causing the death of a client is a violation of this principle is most likely to be an issue that will continue to be debated for some time. Several states have passed laws permitting assisted suicide, but these states have very strict guidelines. The American Nurses Association (ANA) and other nurses' organizations oppose assisted suicide as a policy and believe that nurses who participate in it are violating the code of ethics.

HUMAN IMMUNODEFICIENCY VIRUS AND ACQUIRED IMMUNO-DEFICIENCY SYNDROME

Human immunodeficiency virus (HIV) and acquired immunodeficiency syndrome (AIDS) have evoked strong emotions both in the public and in the medical community. Nurses, who for years held strongly to the ethical principle that all clients regardless of race, sex, religion, age, or disease process should be cared for equally, are now questioning their obligation to take care of clients who have AIDS.

Several ethical issues underlie the AIDS controversy. One of the most important is the right to privacy. Although there is a general requirement to report infection with HIV/AIDS to the Centers for Disease Control and Prevention (CDC), many states have strict laws regarding the confidentiality of the diagnosis. Revelation of the diagnosis of HIV/AIDS brings the possibility of a lawsuit against the health-care provider or institution. However, the right to privacy is not absolute. Diseases such as tuberculosis, gonorrhea, syphilis, and hepatitis, which are highly contagious and sometimes fatal, must be reported to public health officials.

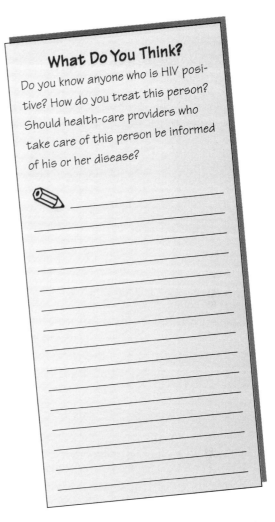

What Do You Think?

Do you know anyone who is HIV positive? How do you treat this person? Should health-care providers who take care of this person be informed of his or her disease?

If the right to privacy can be violated when the public welfare is at stake, does AIDS represent this type of threat? Is it unjust to ask health-care providers to care for clients with this disease without knowing that the client has it? Is it just to violate a client's privacy when the disease carries with it a potential for social stigma and isolation? Does the client have a right to know that a health-care provider is infected with HIV/AIDS?

Another important ethical issue is the right to care. Can a nurse refuse to care for a client with AIDS? Obviously, a fundamental right of a client is to receive care, and a fundamental obligation of a nurse is to provide care. The first statement of the ANA Nurses Code of Ethics states that a nurse must provide care unrestricted by any considerations. Surely, though, there are some exceptions, for example if the nurse is pregnant, or is receiving chemotherapy, or has had other immunity problems. In most situations, however, the nurse is obligated to provide the best nursing care possible for all clients, including those with AIDS.

What about the tremendous cost involved in treating individuals who have AIDS? Studies estimate that the medical cost of treating a client with AIDS from the time of diagnosis to the time of death will be approximately $900,000.[4] In the face of this crisis, governmental agencies, which bear the brunt of paying for AIDS treatment, will have to make some difficult decisions concerning this issue. With more than 2 million people already infected with this disease, the cost to society is astronomical. Nurses have the obligation to care for all clients, including those with AIDS, but ought physicians, hospitals, or governmental agencies also be held to this same precept? Should our society regard health care as a right or a privilege?

ETHICS INVOLVING CHILDREN

Although children are universally acknowledged as the hope of the future, many children remain poorly fed, clothed, housed, and educated and are in dire need of all types of health care, even in affluent countries such as the United States. In the past few years, there has been a marked increase in incidents of child neglect and abuse by parents.

Our society generally acknowledges the tremendous decision-making power that parents have on behalf of their children; however, there are limits to how parents may decide to act. These limits are sometimes obvious, such as in cases of physical abuse and cruelty to children; however, they may also be less conspicuous, such as in the cases of neglect or decisions about withholding medical care for religious reasons. Health-care professionals often find themselves trying to make decisions about the appropriateness of a parent's actions toward a child.

The legal and ethical factors surrounding the decisions that health-care providers must make about child health issues are complicated and sometimes contradictory, ranging from laws about reporting suspected abuse to obtaining permission for treatment. This section focuses on child abuse and the ethical issues that it creates for nurses and also the issues of informed consent as it pertains to children.

> **" "** *Health-care professionals often find themselves trying to make decisions about the appropriateness of a parent's actions toward a child.*

Although issues involving children have always been an important consideration in our society, recent political campaigns have re-emphasized this as a major concern. Whereas the political attention seems to focus on education, drug and alcohol abuse, and child health-care issues, ethical concerns in **pediatrics** are never forgotten and often serve as the unspoken basis for the more visible issues.

Child health ethical issues are numerous and diverse, ranging from mass screening for diseases to withholding permission for treatment.

Child Abuse

Case Study

Emily, who is 8 months old, is brought to the hospital by her 17-year-old unemployed mother who stated that the baby refused to eat at home and vomited a lot. Emily was very small for her age and was below the growth curve for weight. She was also neurologically introverted and showed little interest in her surroundings. She slept a great deal of time. She was admitted to the hospital with a diagnosis of Nonorganic Failure to Thrive. During her stay in the hospital, Emily ate well and gained a significant amount of weight. Her neurological status also improved. One nurse suspected that this was a case of neglect (a form of child abuse) and suggested to the physician that child protective services be notified to evaluate the case. The physician resisted because there was not enough evidence to make a definitive case and thought that it was unfair to the parents to make such a claim. The other nurses felt that by reporting the case they would lose the trust of the mother and cause her to avoid health care for Emily in the future. They also cited a case in which nurses and the hospital were sued when they reported a teenage mother for neglect. The accusation later proved to be false.

Emily was sent home after 3 weeks but was re-admitted 1 month later with the same complaints of poor feeding. She had lost weight since her discharge from the hospital and she was again neurologically withdrawn. The physician still refused to notify child protective services because of the lack of hard evidence. He thought that an investigation and possible removal of the child from the home was too extreme based on the data available. The nurse still believed that the mother should be reported based on suspicions that could be substantiated legally.

Ethical Principles Relating to Child Abuse

There is a general legal requirement in most states that suspected child abuse must be reported by health-care providers as well as by anyone who suspects that child abuse

What Do You Think?

What would you do if you were this nurse? What ethical and legal factors would enter into your decision?

_____
_____
_____
_____
_____
_____
_____
_____
_____
_____
_____

has occurred. Abuse is more obvious when the child has physical injuries that do not fit the medical history or are atypical for the age group. However, in cases of neglect, the evidence may be very minimal or even nonexistent. Often nurses and physicians who specialize in the care of children rely on their experience in making decisions about reporting or not reporting suspected abuse.

Decisions about reporting suspected child abuse or neglect rest on the underlying ethical principles of beneficence and protection of the best interests of the child. It is always difficult to decide how far ranging these concerns for "best interest" should be. Physicians tend to focus on solving the immediate problem. Nurses hold a more holistic viewpoint and tend to see the child in relationship to his or her environment as well as the environment of the parents. Nurses also tend to think of themselves as saviors, protecting the unfortunate or disadvantaged from a malignant social system and often making value judgments about the lifestyles of others from their middle-class vantage point.

A conflicting ethical principle that is sometimes forgotten in the reporting of suspected child abuse is the family's right to privacy and self-determination. It is an equally fundamental right that Emily's parents be allowed to live their lives according to their own values, free from intrusions. However, when the child is a client in the hospital, beneficence usually outweighs fidelity and veracity.

Resolution of the Dilemma

How is the nurse going to resolve this dilemma? Should she report the case and go against the physician's decision? Should she just agree with the physician and defer to his greater experience and better judgment? Should she submit the problem to the hospital ethics committee? Are there any other possible options for action in this case?

It is likely that the physician was correct in his decision about this case, although his ethical reasoning may leave something to be desired. Legally, it is unlikely that there would be sufficient proof to remove the infant from the mother because home monitoring could achieve the same results. Therefore, how can the ethical obligations for the best interest of the child be met?

One very plausible solution is to monitor the child closely through frequent follow-up either at the physician's office or at the local health department. In addition, a follow-up and home evaluation could be arranged through a home-health-care agency, which could also make available other community resources to help in Emily's care. If the infant continued to fail to gain weight, or if it was later determined that Emily's mother

> **" "** *A conflicting ethical principle that is sometimes forgotten in the reporting of suspected child abuse is the family's right to privacy and self-determination.*

was indeed unable to care adequately for her, the case could then be referred to child protective services.

The role of the nurse who cares for the very young or abused child is one of client advocate. These children need help and protection, and at times, for their very survival, must be taken out of an abusive home setting. Nurses need to be aware of and use all the assets available in these situations, including the police, child protective services, welfare, and home-health-care agencies.

Informed Consent and Children

Case Study

Peter, one of a pair of 7-year-old identical twins, developed a severe bilateral glomerulonephritis after a strep throat infection. The renal involvement was so severe that it did not respond to any medical treatment, and both of his kidneys had to be removed. Paul, Peter's identical twin, was evaluated for kidney donation and, as expected, matched on all six antigens as well as blood type and size. Paul seemed to understand what had happened to his brother and agreed to donate one of his kidneys to keep his brother alive.

However, the children's parents were having some trouble agreeing on whether Paul should donate a kidney to Peter. The twins' mother felt that the donation and transplant should be permitted because it would indeed help keep Peter alive and would also make Paul feel like he was an important part of the process. She argued that if Peter ever did die, Paul would be overcome with guilt knowing that he could have saved his brother but did not. The twins' father was not as certain about the transplant procedure. He thought that Paul was too young to make a truly free decision of that type and that he did not really understand the serious nature of a kidney removal operation. He thought that Paul, because he was so young, might have been unduly influenced by subtle, yet powerful pressures from his family. No one had directly told Paul that he *must* donate one of his kidneys, yet the fact that his brother's survival may well depend on his decision could have had a major effect on his willingness to donate. Because Peter was being maintained on dialysis and seemed to be doing fairly well, the twins' father thought that he should be put on the transplant list to see whether a suitable nonrelated donor could be found.

The nurses on the unit where Peter was being cared for were equally divided about whether the transplant should be performed. At various times during Peter's lengthy stay in the hospital, they had all been asked by the parents, usually one parent at a time, whether or not they should go ahead with the transplant.

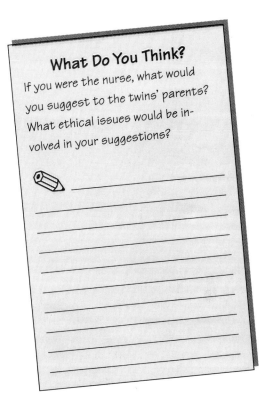

What Do You Think?

If you were the nurse, what would you suggest to the twins' parents? What ethical issues would be involved in your suggestions?

Case Study Analysis

The question, as related to the case study, is: "Does a 7-year-old child have sufficient rational decision-making ability to decide to donate a kidney to his brother?" If, after assessing the child carefully, the answer is "yes," then under the "rights-in-trust" doctrine, the right to self-determination can be turned over to the child and he can make his own decision. If the answer is "no," then the child should not be permitted to donate the kidney.

But there are other ethical principles that can be brought to bear on this decision. From a utilitarian viewpoint, the child should be allowed to donate the kidney, because it would provide the greatest good or happiness for the greatest number of people. Similarly, love-based ethics, or the Golden Rule system of ethical decision making, would also support the donation on the grounds that Paul identifies closely with his brother and appears to understand the issues involved in donation. However, from an egoistic or beneficent viewpoint, because the transplant has little benefit for the donor and will surely cause pain and place him at risk for postoperative complications, the operation should not be permitted.

As with many ethical dilemmas, there is no perfect answer to this situation. The best that can be done is to ensure that the parents and children have as much of the necessary information as possible and support their decisions.

By recognizing the rights of children as individuals, their importance to society is also recognized. However, parents and health-care professionals also have the duty to nurture, support, and guide children as they grow into adolescence and adulthood. Nurses who work with children are challenged to support the independence of the

Issues

Case Study on How to Determine the Greatest Good

Sherry is an RN who works for a rehabilitation center that deals mainly with developmentally delayed children. For several years, Sherry has been following the case of Margie N., who is now 8 years old and has Down syndrome and moderate retardation. Margie has made steady, if slow, progress in achieving basic motor and cognitive skills but still requires close supervision of all activities and care for all basic hygiene needs. Margie is still not advanced enough to participate in group activities at the center's day clinic.

Mrs. N., Margie's mother, a 42-year-old widow, has been providing a high level of care for Margie at home as well as meeting the child's demands for love and attention. Recently, Mrs. N. has been diagnosed with systemic lupus erythematosus (SLE), which has displayed as its primary symptoms severe joint pain and stiffness. During the past several months, Mrs. N. has been finding it increasingly difficult to care for Margie because of the progressive nature of the SLE.

Mrs. N. is trying to make a decision about long-term care for Margie. She trusts Sherry's judgment completely and often relies on the information and teaching given by the nurse to make changes in Margie's care. Sherry is uncertain about what advice she should give. She recognizes that the high level of care and comfort provided by Mrs. N. have been an essential part in the advances Margie has made up to this point, but she also recognizes that Mrs. N. may soon reach a point at which that care can no longer be provided. It seems that to do what is good for Mrs. N. (i.e., placing Margie in an institution) would be harmful to Margie, whereas doing what is good for Margie (i.e., leaving her at home) would be harmful to Mrs. N. What is the best course of action in this situation? Are there any alternative solutions to this dilemma?

child by encouraging the child to be responsible for and participate in his or her own health care.

Ethical Principles Regarding Children

One important difference between adults and children that always needs to be included in ethical decisions about child health issues is that children are dependents. As dependents, they generally are not attributed the right to self-determination that is fundamental to adult decision making. Whenever there is an ethical dilemma involving child health-care issues, a three-way relationship develops involving the child, the health-care professional, and the parents. Generally, the parents have the primary role in deciding health-care issues for their underaged, dependent children based on what they consider to be in the child's best interests.

7.2 When Is a Client Incompetent?

In the current health-care environment, nurses may encounter elderly clients who function independently at home and have not officially or legally been declared incompetent, but whose behavior might indicate that they are unable to make rational decisions about their care. Consider the following situation:

A 74-year-old client, Buster Mack, had been a long-haul truck driver for most of his life and was still driving his big rig into his 60s. He had been in relatively good health until 5 years ago when he was diagnosed with lung cancer. A lobectomy was performed at that time, and he was treated with follow-up radiation and chemotherapy, but the cancer had slowly metastasized to the bone. His current hospitalization was due to a syncopal episode witnessed by a neighbor in the front yard of Mr. Mack's home, where he lives by himself.

During the admission assessment, the nurse observed that Mr. Mack had trouble focusing on the questions, and often the answers were unrelated to the question, or in the form of long rambling accounts of something that happened many years ago. Although he knew he was in some hospital (he could not remember the name), he had no idea where it was or what the date was. His demeanor was cooperative and pleasant, and he laughed easily when the nurse joked with him. He could not remember whether he had any family left living, although the name and address of a son in a distant city were listed on the old records.

Mr. Mack signed all the admission papers and consent forms placed in front of him for a number of neurological tests. His physician was fearful that the cancer might have spread to his brain, and wanted to do an MRI, spinal tap, and brain scan. The MRI and brain scan showed a small tumor in an area of the brain where it could be removed rather easily. Mr. Mack's physician, in consultation with a neurosurgeon, felt that an immediate craniotomy with removal of the tumor was required. After explaining the procedure to Mr. Mack, the physicians placed the consent to operate form on his overbed table and gave him a pen. He promptly signed it, and gave it back.

Later on that day during her shift assessment, the nurse checked on Mr. Mack. The neighbor who had found him unconscious was visiting at the time. When the nurse asked Mr. Mack whether he was ready for the surgery scheduled for the next morning, he had a blank look on his face. On further questioning, the nurse concluded that Mr. Mack had no idea about what was going to happen to him the next day. The neighbor, who helped Mr. Mack with his bills and other paper work at home, stated: "He'll pretty much sign anything that you put in front of him." At this point the nurse felt that Mr. Mack was incapable of making an informed decision about the craniotomy.

The nurse called both the primary physician and the neurosurgeon about her observations. She was told bluntly that the consent had been signed and that they were going to operate on Mr. Mack the next day for his own good. If she wanted what was best for the client, she would just drop the issue.

Should the nurse just drop the issue? Is there anything she could do to resolve the problem? What ethical principles are involved with this situation?

Current routine child health practices reinforce this principle. Young children are given immunizations and medications, have blood drawn for tests, and even have operations such as tonsillectomies or myringotomies, all without asking for their permission. This exemption to the principle of self-determination in children is based on the belief that the young children do not yet have the capacity to make fully rational decisions. Yet, the final expectation for children is that at some point in their lives they develop the capacity to make informed, correct decisions. The primary questions then become: When do they develop this capacity for rational decision making? and How should they be treated until they develop this capacity?

The legal system has fixed the age for rational decision making at age 18. Children who are younger than 18 years of age, with a few exceptions, require the permission of the parent for any and all medical procedures. Children older than 18 years of age can make their own decisions about health care. The difficulty with "fixing" an age is that it is arbitrary and does not reflect the reality of the individual child's development. From experience it can be observed that many children who are 9 or 10 years old exhibit rather advanced and "adult-like" decision-making skills, whereas other children who may be 18 or 19 years of age display a marked lack of this ability.

The more serious question, however, is how should underaged children be treated? One solution is to deny, because of their age, that they have rights and then treat them as being incompetent by bringing to bear paternalistic "best interest" interventions (Box 7.2). Another approach is to say that they do have the same rights as adults except that these rights are temporarily suspended until the child is sufficiently mature to exercise them. This is called "rights-in-trust," and the rights are turned over to the child at the appropriate time. The question then becomes, when is the appropriate time?

One approach is to turn over all the rights to the child at the same time, for example, when he or she reaches 18 years of age. Another approach is to gradually release individual rights as the child grows older and is prepared to exercise them. In either case, appropriate adults, including nurses, have the role of safeguarding the child's rights and act as guardians, protectors, and advocates of the children under their care.

Conclusion

Ethical issues are a factor in the daily practice of all nurses. Any time that a nurse comes in contact with a client, a potential ethical situation exists. In today's world, with rapidly advancing technology and unusual health-care situations, ethical dilemmas are proliferating. Nurses can be prepared to deal with most of these dilemmas if they keep current with the issues and are able to follow a systematic process for making ethical decisions. At some point, difficult decisions must be made, and we should not avoid making them. One of the worst elements of ethical decision making is that it is very unlikely that everyone involved in the dilemma will be happy with the decision. However, if the decision is made after the situation has been analyzed and if it is based on sound ethical principles, it can usually be defended.

Name _____

Course _____

Instructor _____

Date _____

Critical Thinking Exercises

Analyze the following case study using the ethical decision-making process:

Ms. Sally Jones, RN, a public health nurse for a rural health department, was preparing to visit Mr. Weems, a 58-year-old client who was recently diagnosed with chronic bronchitis and emphysema. Mr. Weems was unemployed as a result of a farming accident and had been previously diagnosed with hypertension and extreme obesity. Ms. Jones was making this visit to see why Mr. Weems had missed his last appointment at the clinic and whether he was taking his prescribed antibiotics and antihypertensive medications.

As Ms. Jones pulled up the driveway of his house, she noticed Mr. Weems sitting on the front porch smoking a cigarette. She felt a surge of anger, which she quickly suppressed, as she wondered why she spent so much of her limited time teaching him about the health consequences of smoking.

During the visit, Ms. Jones determined that Mr. Weems had stopped taking both his antihypertensive and antibiotic medications and rarely took his expectorants and bronchodilators. He coughed continuously, had a blood pressure of 196/122, and had severely congested lung sounds. Mr. Weems listened politely as Ms. Jones re-explained the need to stop smoking and the importance of taking his medications as prescribed. She also scheduled another appointment at the clinic in 1 week for follow-up.

As she drove away to her next visit, Ms. Jones wondered about the ethical responsibilities of nurses who must provide care for clients who do not seem to care about their own health. Mr. Weems took little responsibility for his health, refused to even try to stop smoking or lose weight, and did not take his medications. She wondered whether there was a limit to the amount of nursing care a noncompliant client should expect from a community health agency. She reflected that the time spent with Mr. Weems would have been spent much more productively screening children at a local grade school or working with mothers of newborn infants.

✔ What data are important in relation to this situation?

✔ State the ethical dilemma in a clear, simple statement.

✔ What are the choices of action and how do they relate to specific ethical principles?

✔ What are the consequences of these actions?

✔ What decisions can be made?

References

1. Blatt, R, Murray, KL, and Reilly, P: Ethical issues in the age of genetics. Nurse Pract 1(9):28–38, 1998.
2. Fineman, R, Francomano, C, and Ribble, JG: Accessing genetics resources. Nurse Pract 1(9):39–48, 1998.
3. Menzel, L: Is it worth it? Balancing the benefit of extended life with the cost of suffering during critical illness. Critical Care Nurse 18(4):67–73, 1998.
4. Burkhardt, MA, and Nathaniel, AK: Ethics and issues in contemporary nursing. Delmar Publications, Albany, NY, 1998.

BIBLIOGRAPHY

American College of Physicians: Ethics Manual, ed 4. Ann Intern Med 128:576–594, 1998.

American Nurses Association: Code for Nurses with Interpretive Statement. American Nurses Association, Kansas City, 1985.

Brown-Saltzman, K: Living with ethical dilemmas: The art of compromise. AACN News 15(10):2, 1998.

Campbell, G: Ethical principles must guide us. AACN News 15(1):1–12, 1998.

Catalano, JT: Critical care nurses and ethical dilemmas. Critical Care Nurse 11:16–21, 1991.

Catalano, JT: Systems of ethics. Critical Care Nurse 12:91–96, 1992.

Catalano, JT: The ethics of cadaver experimentation. Critical Care Nurse 14:82–85, 1994.

Catalano, JT: Ethical decision making in the critical care patient. Critical Care Nursing Clinics of North America 9(1):45–52, 1997.

Crego, PJ, and Lipp, EJ: Nurse's knowledge of advanced directives. Am J Crit Care 7(3):218–223, 1998.

Curtin, L: Ethics, discipline and discharge. Nursing Management 27(3):51–52, 1996.

Davis, AJ, et al: Ethical dilemmas and nursing practice, ed 4. Appleton & Lange, E. Norwalk, Conn., 1997.

de Tornyay, R: Reconsidering nursing education: The report of the Pew Health Professions Commission. J Nurs Educ 13:296–301, 1992.

Eakes, GG, and Lewis, JB: Should nurses be required to administer care to patients with AIDS? Nurse Educator 16:36–38, 1991.

Fiesta, J: Legal update, Part 1 1995. Nursing Management 25(5):22–24, 1996.

Frank, L: The ethical imperative to treat pain in infants: Are we doing the best we can? Critical Care Nurse 17(5):80–89, 1997.

French, PA: The Spectrum of Responsibility. St. Martin's Press, New York, 1991.

Fromer, MJ: Ethical Issues in Health Care. CV Mosby, St. Louis, 1981.

Howell, JH, and Sale, WF (eds): Life Choices: A Hasting Center Introduction to Bioethics.

Georgetown University Press, Washington, DC, 1995.

Joel, LA: Hungry for the truth. Am J Nurs 96(3), 1997.

Mappes, TA, and Zembaty, JS: Biomedical Ethics, ed 3. McGraw-Hill, New York, 1991.

Mohr, WK: Values, ideologies and dilemmas: Professional and occupational contradictions. J Psychosoc Nurs 33(1):29–34, 1995.

Munro, NL: Apply the rules of people ethics. AACN News 15(11):2–15, 1998.

Nicoll, LH: Nurses' Guide to the Internet, ed 2. JB Lippincott, Philadelphia, 1998.

Perdew, S: Facts About AIDS: A Guide for Health Care Providers. JB Lippincott, Philadelphia, 1990.

Thompson, JE, and Thompson, HO: Bioethical Decision Making for Nurses. Appleton-Century-Crofts, E. Norwalk, Conn., 1985.

Trought, EA, and Moore, F (eds): Guidelines for the Registered Nurse in Giving, Accepting or Rejecting a Work Assignment. Florida Nurses Association, Orlando, Fla., 1989.

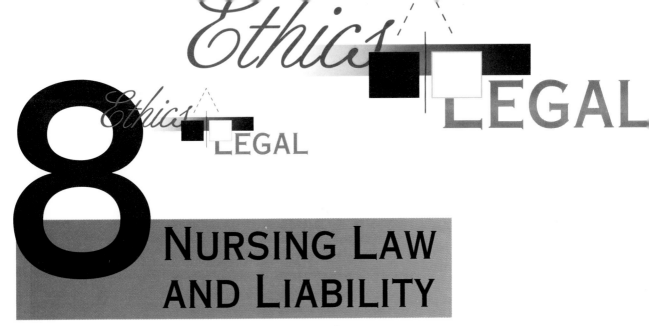

8

NURSING LAW AND LIABILITY

➤ *Mary Evans and*
Tonia Aiken

Learning Objectives

After completing this chapter, the reader will be able to:

1. Distinguish between statutory law and common law.
2. Differentiate civil law from criminal law.
3. Explain the legal principles involved in:
   a. Unintentional torts
   b. Intentional torts
   c. Quasi-intentional torts
   d. Informed consent
   e. Do-not-resuscitate (DNR) orders
4. Describe the trial process.
5. List methods to prevent litigation.
6. Identify the elements in delegation.

For many nurses, the mere mention of the word lawsuit provokes a high level of anxiety. At first glance, the legal system often seems to be a large and confusing entity whose intricacies are designed to entrap the uninitiated. Many nurses feel that even a minor error in client care will lead to huge settlements against them and loss of their nursing license. In reality, even though the number of lawsuits against nurses has increased greatly since the early 1990s, the number of nurses who are actually sued remains relatively small.

It is important to remember that the legal system is just one element in the totality of the health-care system. Laws are rules to help protect people and to keep society functioning. The ultimate goal of all laws is to promote peaceful and productive interactions between and among the people of that society.

An understanding of basic legal principles will augment the quality of care that the nurse delivers. In our litigious society, it is important to comprehend how the law affects the profession of nursing and the individual nurse's daily practice.

SOURCES OF LAW

There are two major sources for laws in the United States—statutory law and **common law.** The majority of the laws that govern nursing are state level statutory laws because licensure is a function of the state's authority (Box 8.1).

Statutory Law

Statutory law consists of laws written and enacted by the U.S. Congress, the state legislatures, and other governmental entities such as cities, counties, or townships. Legislated laws enacted by the U.S. Congress are called federal **statutes.** State-drafted laws are called state statutes. Individual cities and municipalities have legislative bodies that draft **ordinances,** codes, and regulations at their respective levels.

The laws that govern the profession of nursing are statutory laws. Most of these laws are written at the state level, because licensure is a responsibility of the individual states. These laws include the Nurse Practice Act, which establishes the State Board of Nursing, individual licensure procedures, and schedule of fees for the state.

Common Law

Common law is different from statutory law in that it has evolved from the decisions of previous legal cases that form a **precedent.** These laws represent the accumulated results of the judgments and decrees that have been handed down by courts of the United States and Great Britain through

8.1 Division and Types of Law

I. Statutory Law
  A. Criminal Law
    i. Misdemeanor
    ii. Felony
  B. Civil Law
    i. Tort Law
      a. Unintentional tort
      b. Intentional tort
      c. Quasi-intentional tort
    ii. Contract Law
    iii. Treaty Law
    iv. Tax Law
    v. Other
II. Common Law
  A. Criminal Law
    i. Misdemeanor
    ii. Felony
  B. Civil Law
    i. Tort Law
      a. Unintentional tort
      b. Intentional tort
      c. Quasi-intentional tort
    ii. Contract Law
    iii. Treaty Law
    iv. Tax Law
    v. Other

the years. Common law often extends beyond the scope of statutory law. For example, no statutes require a person who is negligent and causes injury to another to compensate that person for the injury. Court decisions that have addressed the same legal issues over and over, such as negligence, however, have repeatedly ruled that the injured person should receive compensation. The way in which each case is resolved creates a precedent, or pattern, for dealing with the same legal issue in the future. The common laws involving **negligence** or **malpractice** are most frequently encountered by the nurse.

Common law or case law is law that has developed over a long period. The principle of *stares decisis* requires a judge to make decisions similar to those that have been handed down in previous cases if the facts of the cases are identical. Common law decisions are published in bound legal reports. Generally speaking, common law deals with matters outside the scope of laws enacted by the legislature.

DIVISIONS OF LAW

In the U.S. legal system, there are many divisions in the law. A major example of such a division is the difference between **criminal law** and **civil law,** either of which may be statutory or common in origin.

Criminal Law

Criminal laws are concerned with providing protection for all members of society. When someone is accused of violating a criminal law, the government at the county, city, state, or federal level imposes punishments appropriate to the type of **crime.** Criminal law involves a wide range of **malfeasance,** from minor traffic violations to murder.

> 66 99 *The most common violation by nurses of the criminal law is through failure to renew nursing licenses. In this situation, the nurse is in effect practicing nursing without a license, which is a crime in all states.*

Although most criminal law is regulated and created by the government through the enactment of statutes, a small portion falls under the common law. Statutes are developed and enacted by the legislature (state or federal) and approved by the executive branch, such as a governor or the President. Criminal law is further classified into two types of offenses: (1) **misdemeanors,** which are minor criminal offenses, and (2) **felonies,** which are major criminal offenses.

In the criminal law system, an individual accused of a crime is called the defendant. The prosecuting attorney represents the people of the city, county, state, or federal jurisdiction who are accusing the individual of a crime. A **criminal action** is rendered when the person charged with the crime is brought to trial and convicted. Penalties or sanctions are imposed on the violators of criminal law and are based on the scope of the crime. They can involve a range of punishment from community service work and fines to imprisonment and death.

Nurses can become involved with the criminal system in their nursing practice in several ways. The most common violation by nurses of the criminal law is through failure to renew nursing licenses. In this situation, the nurse is in effect practicing nursing without a license, which is a crime in all states. Nurses also become involved with the illegal diversion of drugs, particularly narcotics, from the hospital. This is a more serious crime, which may lead to imprisonment for the nurse. Recent cases involving intentional or unintentional deaths of clients and assisted suicide cases have also led to criminal action against nurses.

Civil Law

Nurses are much more likely to become involved in civil lawsuits than in criminal violations. Civil laws generally deal with the violation of one individual's rights by another individual. The court provides the forum that enables these individuals to have their disputes resolved by an independent third party, such as a judge or a jury of the defendant's peers. The individual who brings the dispute to the court is called the **plaintiff.** The formal written document that describes the dispute and the resolution sought is called the complaint. The individual against whom the complaint is filed is called the defendant, who, in conjunction with his attorney, prepares the **answer** to the complaint. In civil cases, the **burden of proof** rests with the plaintiff.

Civil law has many branches, including contract law, treaty law, tax law, and **tort** law. It is under the tort law that most nurses become involved with the legal system.

Tort Law

A tort is generally defined as a wrongful act committed against a person or his or her property independent of a contract. A person who commits a tort is called the **tort-feasor** and is **liable** for **damages** to those who are affected by the person's actions. The word tort, derived from the Latin *tortus* (twisted), is a French word for injury or wrong. Torts can involve several different types of actions, including a direct violation of a person's legal rights or a violation of a standard of care that causes injury to a person. Torts are classified as unintentional, intentional, or quasi-intentional.

Unintentional Torts

Negligence is the primary form of **unintentional tort.** Negligence is generally defined as the commission or **omission** of an act that a reasonable and prudent person would perform in a similar situation, or something a reasonable person would not do in that situation. **Nonfeasance** is a type of negligence that occurs when a person fails to perform a legally required duty.[1]

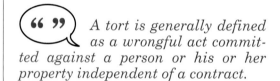

> " " *A tort is generally defined as a wrongful act committed against a person or his or her property independent of a contract.*

Malpractice is a type of negligence for which professionals can be sued (professional negligence). Because of their professional status, nurses are held to a higher standard of conduct than the ordinary lay person. The standard for nurses is what a reasonable and prudent nurse would do in the same situation: "A registered nurse is charged with utilizing the degree and skill and judgment commensurate with his or her education, experience, and position."[2] For instance, it is reasonable and prudent that the nurse put the side rails up on the bed of a client who had just received an injection of a narcotic pain medication, because the drug causes drowsiness and sometimes confusion. If the nurse gave an injection of a narcotic medication but forgot to put the side rails up, and the client falls out of bed and fractures his hip, the nurse can be sued for the negligent act of forgetting to put the side rail up.

Four elements are required for a person to make a claim of negligence: (1) a duty was owed to the client (professional relationship); (2) the professional violated the **duty** and failed to conform to the standard of care (breach of duty); (3) the failure to act by the professional was the **proximate cause** of the resulting injuries (causality); and (4) actual injuries resulted from the breach of duty (damages).

If any of these elements is missing from the case, then the client will probably not be able to win the lawsuit.

Consider the following situation:

Mr. Fagin, a 78-year-old client, was admitted from a nursing home for the treatment of a fractured tibia after he fell out of bed. After the fracture was reduced, a fiberglass cast was applied, and Mr. Fagin was sent to the orthopedic unit for follow-up care. While making her 0400 rounds, the night charge nurse (a registered nurse [RN]) discovered that Mr. Fagin's foot on the casted leg was cold to touch, looked bluish-purple, and was swollen approximately 1½ times normal size. The nurse noted these findings in the client's chart and relayed the information to the day shift nurses during the 0630 shift report. The charge nurse on the day shift promptly called and relayed the findings to Mr. Fagin's physician. The physician, however, did not seem to be concerned and only told the nurse to "Keep a close eye on him, and don't bother me again unless it is an absolute emergency." A short time later, Mr. Fagin became agitated, complained of severe pain in the affected foot, and eventually began yelling uncontrollably. The charge nurse called the emergency room (ER) physician to come to check on the client. The ER physician immediately removed the cast and noted an extensive circulatory impairment that would not respond to treatment. A few days later, Mr. Fagin's leg was amputated. His family filed a malpractice lawsuit against the hospital, the physician, and both the night and day charge nurses.

Are all the elements present in this case for a bona fide lawsuit? What could have been done to prevent this situation from happening? How should nurses deal with reluctant or hostile physicians?

Malpractice is more serious than mere negligence because it indicates professional misconduct or unreasonable lack of skill in performing professional duties. Malpractice suggests the existence of a professional standard of care and a deviation from that standard of care. A professional **expert witness** is often asked to testify in a malpractice case to help establish the standard of care to which the professional should be held accountable.

What Do You Think?

Do you know anyone who has filed a malpractice suit or a health-care provider who was the defendant in a malpractice suit? What was the situation that brought the case? How was it resolved? If you have never been involved with a malpractice suit or do not know anyone who has, how would you feel if a lawsuit were to be brought against you?

A 1988 case in South Dakota presents an example of nursing malpractice. The nurse failed to question the physician's order to discharge a client when she discovered that the client had a fever. In this case, a supervisory nurse provided expert testimony and reported to the judge that the general standard of care for nurses is to report a significant change in a client's condition, such as an elevated temperature. It is the nurse's responsibility to question the physician's order as to appropriateness of discharge. The records on this case indicated that the client's elevated temperature was charted after the physician had completed his rounds. The nurse did not notify the physician of the client's fever; and the client was subsequently discharged. The client was readmitted a short time after discharge and died in the hospital. The nurse was found negligent. The court held that negligence can be determined by failure to act as well as by the commission of an act.

Many other types of actions by nurses can produce malpractice lawsuits. Some of the more common actions include:

> 66 99 *Punitive damages are more likely to be assessed against the nurse in intentional tort cases, and some intentional torts may fall under the criminal law if there is gross violation of the standards of care.*

- Leaving foreign objects inside a client during surgery
- Failing to assess and observe a client as directed
- Failing to obtain a proper informed consent
- Failing to report a change in a client's condition, such as vital signs, circulatory status, and level of consciousness
- Failing to report another health-care provider's **incompetency** or negligence
- Failing to take actions to provide for a client's safety, such as not cleaning up a liquid spill on the floor that causes a client to fall
- Failing to provide a client with sufficient and appropriate education before discharge

If a nurse is found guilty of malpractice, several types of actions may be taken against the nurse. The nurse may be required to provide monetary compensation to the client for general damages that were a direct result of the injury, including pain,

suffering, disability, and disfigurement. In addition, the nurse is often required to pay for special damages that have resulted from the injury, such as all involved medical expenses, **out-of-pocket expenses,** and wages lost by the client while he or she was in the hospital. Optional damages, including emotional distress, mental suffering, and counseling expenses that were an outgrowth of the initial injury, may be added to the total settlement. If the client is able to prove that the nurse acted with conscious disregard for the client's safety or acted in a malicious, willful, or wanton manner that produced injury, then an additional assessment of punitive or exemplary damages may be added to the award.

Intentional Torts

An **intentional tort** is generally defined as a willful act that violates another person's rights or property. Intentional torts can be distinguished from malpractice and acts of negligence by the following three requirements: (1) the nurse must intend to bring about the consequences of the act, (2) the nurse's act must be intended to interfere with the client or his property, and (3) the act must be a substantial factor in bringing about the injury or consequences.

The most frequently encountered intentional torts are **assault, battery, false imprisonment,** abandonment, and intentional infliction of emotional distress. With intentional torts, the injured person does not have to prove that an injury has occurred, nor is the opinion of an expert witness required for adjudication. Punitive damages are more likely to be assessed against the nurse in intentional tort cases, and some intentional torts may fall under the criminal law if there is gross violation of the standards of care.

Assault and **Battery.** Assault is the unjustifiable attempt to touch another person or the threat of so doing. Battery is actual harmful or unwarranted contact with another person without his or her consent. Battery is the most common intentional tort seen in the practice of nursing.

For a nurse to commit assault and battery, there must be an absence of consent on the part of the client. Before any procedure can be performed on a competent, alert, and normally oriented client, the client must agree or consent to the procedure being done. Negligence does not have to be proved for a person to be successful in a claim for assault and battery.

A common example of an assault and battery occurs when a nurse physically restrains a client against the client's will and administers an injection against the client's wishes.

> 66 99 *A common example of an assault and battery occurs when a nurse physically restrains a client against the client's will and administers an injection against the client's wishes.*

False Imprisonment. False imprisonment occurs when a client is confined or restrained with intent to prevent him or her from leaving the hospital. The use of restraints alone does not constitute false imprisonment when they are used to maintain the safety of a confused or disoriented client. In general, mentally impaired clients can be detained against their will only if they are a threat to injure themselves or others. The use of threats or medications that interfere with the client's ability to leave the facility can also be considered false imprisonment.

Intentional Infliction of Emotional Distress. Intentional infliction of emotional distress is another common intentional tort encountered by the nurse. To prove this intentional tort, the following three elements are necessary: (1) conduct exceeds what is usually accepted by society, (2) the health-care provider's conduct is intended to cause mental distress, and (3) the conduct actually does produce mental distress (causation). Any nurse who is charged with assault, battery, or false imprisonment is also at risk for being charged with infliction of emotional distress.

A 1975 case is an example of infliction of emotional distress. In *Johnson v. Women's Hospital,* a mother wished to view the body of her baby who had died during birth. After she made the request, she was handed the baby's body floating in a gallon jar of formaldehyde.[1] The Johnson case epitomizes the lack of respect that was shown to the mother. If the mother in this delicate situation had been treated with dignity and respect, the situation would have been avoided.

Quasi-Intentional Torts

A **quasi-intentional tort** is a mixture of unintentional and intentional torts. It is defined as a voluntary act that directly causes injury or distress without intent to injure or to cause distress. A quasi-intentional tort does have the elements of volition and causation without the element of intent. Quasi-intentional torts usually involve situations of communication and often violate a person's reputation, personal privacy, or civil rights.

Defamation of Character. Defamation of character, which is the most common of the quasi-intentional torts, is harmful to a person's reputation. Defamation injures a person's reputation by diminishing the esteem, respect, good will, or confidence that others have for the person. It can be especially damaging when false statements are made about a criminal act, an immoral act, or false allegations about a client's having a contagious disease. In *Schessler v. Keck* (1954), a nurse was found liable for defamation of character when she told a friend that a caterer for whom she was caring was being treated for syphilis. Even though the statement was false, when the information became public, it destroyed his catering business.[1]

Defamation includes **slander,** which is spoken communication in which one person discusses another in terms that harm a third person's reputation. **Libel** is a written communication in which a person makes statements or uses language that harms another person's reputation. To win a defamation lawsuit against the nurse, the client must prove that the nurse acted maliciously, abused the principle of **privileged communication,** and wrote or spoke a lie.

> " " *Medical record documentation is a primary source of defamation of character.*

Medical record documentation is a primary source of defamation of character. Through the years, the client's chart has been the basis of many defamation lawsuits. Discussion about a client in the elevators, cafeteria, and other public areas can also lead to lawsuits for defamation if negative comments are overheard.

Invasion of Privacy. Invasion of privacy is a violation of a person's right to protection against unreasonable and unwarranted interference with one's personal life. To prove that invasion of privacy has occurred, the client must show (1) the nurse intruded on the client's seclusion and privacy, (2) the intrusion is objectionable to a reasonable and prudent person, (3) the act committed intrudes on private or published facts or pictures of a private nature, and (4)

public disclosure of private information was made.[3] Examples of invasion of privacy include using the client's name or picture for the sole advantage of the health-care provider, intruding into the client's private affairs without permission, giving out private client information over the telephone, and publishing information that misrepresents the client's condition.

Breach of Confidentiality. Confidentiality of information concerning the client must be honored. A breach of confidentiality results when a client's trust and confidence are violated by public revelation of confidential or privileged communications without the client's consent. Most breach of confidentiality cases involve a physician's revelation of privileged communications shared by a client. Nurses who overhear privileged communication or information, however, are held to the same standards as a physician with regard to that information.

Privileged client information can only be disclosed if it is authorized by the client. Most health-care facilities have specific guidelines dealing with client information disclosure. Disclosure of information to family members is also not acceptable unless the client gives permission to do so. For instance, a client may not wish to disclose to a family member a specific diagnosis, such as cancer. If this is the case, the nurse should honor this request; otherwise, it could be considered a violation of that client's privacy.

Use of computerized documentation and telemedicine have led to several lawsuits based on breach of confidentiality and malpractice. (See Chapter 15 for examples.) The legal system has lagged behind in its attempts to keep pace with the use of computers and electronic record keeping. To date, there are no state codes that systematically deal with all the issues raised by computerization. Cases exist where medical records have been lost because of computer failure. Other issues, such as correction of errors in **charting,** are complicated by use of the computer. In the paper charts, health-care providers had to draw a line through the erroneous entry, initial the entry, and date it. With computerized charting, simply hitting the delete button will completely erase all evidence of a mistaken entry. Understandably, the legal system is very concerned about this practice.

FACING A LAWSUIT

Because of the rapid proliferation of lawsuits during the past decade, there is now a higher probability that a nurse, at some time in his or her career, will be involved either as a witness or as a party to a nursing malpractice action. Knowledge of the litigation process increases the nurse's understanding of the way in which the nurse's conduct is evaluated before the courts.

> **❝ ❞** *Issues, such as correction of errors in* **charting,** *are complicated by use of the computer.*

Statute of Limitations

A malpractice suit against a nurse for negligence must be filed within a specified time. This period, called the **statute of limitations,** generally begins at the time of the injury or when the injury is discovered and lasts until some specified future time. In most states, the limitation period lasts from 1 to 6 years, with the most common duration being 2 years. If the client fails to file the suit within the prescribed time, the lawsuit will be barred.

The Complaint

Filing the suit (also called the complaint) with the court begins the litigation process. The written complaint describes the incident that initiated the claim of negligence against the nurse. Specific allegations, including the amount of money sought for damages, are also stated in the **legal complaint.** The plaintiff, who is usually a client or a family member of a client, is the alleged injured party, and the defendant (i.e., the nurse, physician, or hospital) is the person or entity being sued. The first notice of a lawsuit occurs when the defendant (nurse) is officially notified or served with the complaint. All defendants are accorded the right of **due process** under constitutional law.

The Answer

The defendant must respond to the allegations stated in the complaint within a specific timeframe. This written response by the defendant is called the answer. If the nurse had liability insurance in force at the time of the negligent act, the insurer will assign a lawyer to represent the defendant nurse. In the answer, the nurse can outline specific defenses to the claims against him or her.

The Discovery

After the complaint and answer are filed with the court, the discovery phase of the litigation begins. The purpose of discovery is to uncover all information relevant to the malpractice suit and the incident in question. The nurse may be required to answer a series of questions that relate to the nurse's educational background, emotional state, the incident that led to the lawsuit, and any other information the plaintiff's lawyer deems important. These written questions are called **interrogatories.**

In addition, the plaintiff's lawyer may seek requests for production of documents. These are actual documents related to the lawsuit, including the plaintiff's medical records, **incident reports, Kardex,** the institution's policy and procedure manual concerning the specific situation, and the nurse's job description. The plaintiff is also required to disclose information as part of the discovery process that includes the plaintiff's past medical history.

The Deposition

The next step in the process is the taking of a deposition from each party to the lawsuit, as well as any potential witnesses, to assist the lawyers in the trial preparation. A **deposition** is a formal legal process that involves the taking of testimony under oath and is recorded by a court reporter. These are usually wide-ranging in scope and often include information not allowed in a trial, such as **hearsay** testimony. In some cases, videotaped depositions may be used. Nurses can prepare for a deposition by keeping some key points in mind (Box 8.2).

The deposition **testimony** is reduced to a written document for use at trial called an **affidavit.** If a witness during the actual trial changes testimony from that given at the deposition, the deposition can be used to contradict the testimony. This process is called impeaching the witness. Impeaching a witness on a specific issue can create doubt about that witness's credibility and can thus weaken other areas in the witness's testimony. In some situations, witnesses can later be charged with **perjury** if it is proved that they gave false testimony under oath.

BOX

8.2 Preparing for a Deposition

1. Do not volunteer information.
2. Be familiar with the client's medical record and nurse's notes.
3. Remain calm throughout the process and do not be intimidated by the lawyers.
4. Clarify all questions before answering; ask the lawyer to explain the question if not understood.
5. Do not make assumptions about the questions.
6. Do not exaggerate answers.
7. Allow at least 5 seconds after a question is asked before answering it to allow objections from other lawyers.
8. Tell the truth.
9. Do not speculate about answers.
10. Speak slowly and clearly, using professional language as much as possible.
11. Look the questioning lawyer in the eye as much as possible.
12. If unable to remember an answer, simply state "I don't remember" or "I don't know."
13. Think before answering any question.
14. Bring a resume or curriculum vitae to the deposition in case it is requested.
15. Request a break if tired or confused.
16. Avoid becoming angry with the lawyers or using sarcastic language.
17. Avoid using absolutes in the answers.
18. If a question is asked more than once, ask the court recorder to read the answer given previously.
19. Be sure to read over the deposition just before the trial.

Aiken, TJ and Catalano JT: Legal, Ethical and Political Issues in Nursing. F.A. Davis: Philadelphia 1994.

The Trial

The actual **trial** often takes place years after the complaint was filed. Once **jurisdiction** is determined, the *voir dire* process, more commonly called jury selection, begins. After jury selection, each attorney presents opening statements. The plaintiff's side is presented first. Witnesses may be served with **subpoenas** that require them to appear and provide testimony. Each witness or party is subject to direct examination, cross-examination, and redirect examination. Direct examination involves open-ended questions by the attorney. Cross-examination is performed by the opposing lawyer, and questions are asked in such a way as to elicit short, specific responses. The redirect examination consists of follow-up questions to address issues that were previously raised during the cross-examination. After both parties have presented their case, the lawyers deliver their closing arguments. The case then goes to a jury or a judge for deliberation. If the facts are not in dispute, the judge may render a **summary judgment.** The decision or ruling made about the case can be appealed if either party is not satisfied. The party appealing the decision is called the **appellant.**

Possible Defenses to a Malpractice Suit

Contributory Negligence versus Comparative Negligence

Damages awarded vary from one state to another and also with the types of injuries sustained. In a state with contributory negligence laws, clients are not allowed to receive money for injuries if they contributed to that injury in any manner. For example, the nurse forgot to raise the bed rail after administering an injection of a narcotic pain medication to a client who had an operation but instructed the client to turn on the call light if he wanted to get out of bed. The client fell while attempting to go to the bathroom; however, because he did not use the call light, he had contributed to his own injuries and thus could not receive compensation.

In a state with comparative negligence laws, the awards are based on the determination of the percentage of fault by both parties. For example, in the aforementioned case, if $100,000 was awarded by the jury, it may be determined that the nurse was 75% at fault and the client was 25% at fault. In that case, the client would receive $75,000. In general, if the client is 50% or more at fault, no award will be made. As can be seen, determination of these types of awards is highly subjective and an **appeal** is often made to a higher court about the decision. Consider the following case:

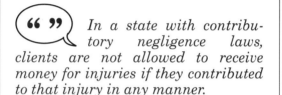

In a state with contributory negligence laws, clients are not allowed to receive money for injuries if they contributed to that injury in any manner.

Ms. Gouge, a 44-year-old client who weighs 307 lb, was admitted to a large university medical center ER with complaints of chest pain and disorientation and a blood pressure of 208/154. She also displayed aphasia, hemiplegia, and loss of sensation and movement on her right side. After a magnetic resonance imaging (MRI) scan of the head, it was discovered that she had a nonoperative cerebral aneurysm. In addition to appropriate medical treatment for blood pressure and circulation, her family physician told her that she had to lose a significant amount of weight.

The nurse in the physician's office instituted a weight loss teaching plan for Ms. Gouge, planned out a calorie-restricted low-fat diet, and gave her a large amount of information about healthy diet and also a videotape of low-impact aerobic exercises. At a follow-up visit 1 month later, Ms. Gouge weighed 315 lb. Six months later, Ms. Gouge's aneurysm ruptured, leaving her in a vegetative state.

Ms. Gouge's family filed a lawsuit against the physician and his office nurse claiming that they had failed to institute proper and appropriate preventative measures and that they had failed to inform the client of the seriousness of her condition.

Did the nurse's decisions or actions contribute to the filing of this suit? Is there any contributory negligence? What is the nurse's role in defending against this suit? What might the nurse have done to prevent the suit in the first place?

Assumption of Risk

When the client signs the informed consent form for a particular treatment, procedure, or surgery, it is implied that he or she is aware of the possible complications of that treatment, procedure, or surgery. Under the assumption-of-risk defense, if one of those listed or named complications occurs, the client has no grounds to sue the health-care provider. For example, a common complication from hip replacement surgery is some loss of mobility and range of motion of the affected leg. Even if a client, after having a hip replaced, is able to walk only using a walker, he still does not have any grounds for a lawsuit.

> 66 99 *A health-care professional who provides care in an emergency situation cannot be sued for injuries that may be sustained by the client if that care was given according to established guidelines*

Good Samaritan Act

Health-care providers are sometimes hesitant to provide care at the scene of accidents, in emergency situations, or disasters because they fear lawsuits. The **Good Samaritan Act** is designed specifically to protect health-care providers in these situations. A health-care professional who provides care in an emergency situation cannot be sued for injuries that may be sustained by the client if that care was given according to established guidelines and was within the scope of the professional's education. For example, a nurse who finds a person in cardiac arrest administers cardiopulmonary resuscitation (CPR) to revive the person. In the process, she fractures several of the client's ribs. The client would not be able to sue the nurse for the fractured ribs if the CPR was administered according to established standards.

Good Samaritan laws do, however, have some limitations. They do not cover nurses for grossly negligent acts in the provision of care or for acts outside the nurse's level of education. For example, in the case of a person choking on a piece of meat, the nurse initially attempts the Heimlich maneuver but without success. As the person loses consciousness, the nurse decides to perform a tracheostomy. The client survives but can sue the nurse for injuries from the tracheostomy, because this is not a normal part of a nurse's education.

Unavoidable Accident

Sometimes accidents happen without any contributing causes from the nurse, hospital, or physician. For example, a client is walking in the hall and trips over her own bathrobe. She breaks an ankle. There were no puddles on the floor or obstacles in the hall, and the client was alert and oriented. Because no one is at fault, there are no grounds for a lawsuit.

Defense of the Fact

This defense is based on the claim that the actions of the nurse followed the standards of care, or that even if the actions were in violation of the standard of care, the action itself was not the direct cause of the injury. For example, a nurse wraps a dressing too tightly on a client's foot after surgery. Later, the client loses his eyesight and blames the loss of vision on the nurse's improper dressing of his foot.[4]

Going through the litigation process can produce high levels of anxiety. Placing every aspect of the nurse's conduct under scrutiny in a trial is very stressful. All aspects of the alleged negligent act will be examined and re-examined. Every word of the nurse's notes and the medical record will be analyzed and questioned. Nurses can survive the litigation process with the help of a good attorney, and by being honest and demonstrating that they were acting in the best interest of the client. From this viewpoint, it is easy to see the importance of carrying nursing liability insurance.

ALTERNATIVE DISPUTE FORUMS

Although most lawsuits against nurses are settled through the court system, there are other methods of settling them. Because of the large number of cases and the resultant overload of the judicial system, other methods of resolving disputes have become increasingly popular. These alternative forums of dispute resolution (ADR) are being used for many types of conflicts and are seen more frequently in the area of torts, contracts, employment, and family law mat-

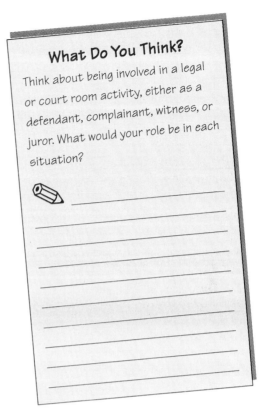

ters. **Mediation** and arbitration are the most commonly used alternatives to trial.

Mediation

Mediation is a process that allows each party to present his or her case before a mediator, who is an independent third party trained in dispute resolution. The mediator listens to each side individually. This one-sided session is called a caucus. The mediator's role is to find common ground between the parties and encourage resolution of the disputed matters by compromise and negotiation. The mediator aids the parties in arriving at a mutually acceptable outcome. The mediator does not act as a decision maker but rather encourages the parties to come to a "meeting of the minds."

Arbitration

Arbitration, in contrast, allows a neutral third party to hear both parties' positions and then make a decision or ruling based on the facts and evidence presented. Arbitration, by agreement or by statutory definition, can be binding or nonbinding. **Arbitrators** or mediators can be, and frequently are, retired judges who work on an hourly-fee basis. They are often attorneys. In the family law areas, they are frequently social workers or specially trained mediators. Negligence and malpractice issues are frequently resolved through arbitration and mediation.

COMMON ISSUES IN HEALTH-CARE LITIGATION

Informed Consent

Informed consent is both a legal and ethical issue. Informed consent is the voluntary permission by a client, or by the client's designated proxy, to carry out a procedure on the client. Clients' claims that they did not grant informed consent prior to a surgery or invasive procedure can and does form the basis of a small percentage of lawsuits. Although these lawsuits are most often directed against physicians and hospitals, nurses can become involved when they provide the information but are not performing the procedure. The person who is performing the procedure has the responsibility to obtain the informed consent. However, some physicians have gotten into the habit of giving nurses the consent forms and saying "Get the client to sign this." Informed consent can only be given by a client after the client receives sufficient information on:

1. Treatment proposed
2. Material risk involved
3. Acceptable alternatives
4. Outcome hoped for
5. Consequences of not having treatment

The physician should provide most of this information. Nurses can reinforce the physician teaching and even supplement the information but should not be the primary or only source of information for the informed consent. It is often difficult to draw a clear distinction between where the physician's responsibility ends and that of the nurse begins.

Exceptions to Informed Consent

There are two exceptions to informed consent:

1. In emergency situations when the client is unconscious, incompetent, or otherwise unable to give consent.
2. In situations where the health provider feels that it may be medically contraindicated to disclose the risk and hazards because it may result in illness, severe emotional distress, serious psychological damage, or failure on the part of the client to receive life-saving treatment.

Delegation versus Supervision

The health-care system's headlong rush to managed care has increased nurses' liability for lawsuits in the area of supervision and delegation. In the search for cost-effective client care, current managed care strategies attempt to make optimal use of relatively expensive RNs by replacing them with less costly and less educated personnel. As more and more health-care facilities move toward restructuring, the use of less-educated unlicensed assistive personnel (UAP) who have minimal education and experience will continue to increase. Although RNs have always been responsible for the delegation of some tasks and the supervision of less-qualified health-care providers, it is now one of the primary functions of RNs in today's health-care system.

Although delegation and supervision are closely related concepts, they are different. **Delegation** is recognized as assigning or designating a competent individual the responsibility of carrying out a specific group of nursing tasks in the provision of care for certain clients. Delegation includes the understanding that the authorized person is acting in the place of the RN and may be carrying out tasks that generally fall under

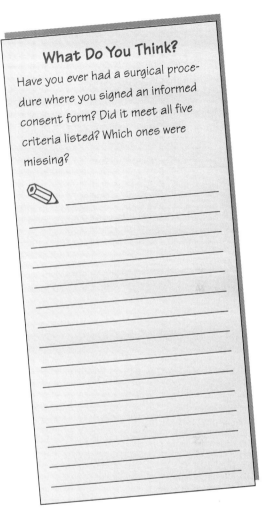

What Do You Think?

Have you ever had a surgical procedure where you signed an informed consent form? Did it meet all five criteria listed? Which ones were missing?

the RN's scope of practice. Supervision, on the other hand, is the initial direction and periodic evaluation of a person performing an assigned task to ensure that he or she is meeting the standards of care. Although delegation almost always requires supervision, it is possible to have supervision without delegation. When nurses delegate nursing tasks to nonnurses, the RNs are always legally responsible for supervising that person to ensure that the care given meets the standards of care. However, if the facility, or the state board of nursing, or some other official body has a predesignated list of tasks that nonnursing personnel may undertake in the care of clients, then the RN is responsible only for supervising them to make sure the tasks are carried out safely.

Legally, the power to delegate is restricted to professionals who are licensed and governed by a statutory practice act. RNs are considered professionals and can delegate independent nursing functions to other personnel. Most state practice acts do not give delegatory authority to **dependent practitioners** like licensed practical nurses/licensed vocational nurses (LPNs/ LVNs) or UAP. In addition, professionals who delegate specific tasks retain accountability for the proper and safe completion of those tasks as well as responsibility for determining whether the assigned personnel are competent to carry out the task. One exception is when the person who is assigned a task also has a license and the tasks fall under that person's scope of practice. Then, again, the RN is responsible only for supervision of the other licensed person; this is often seen in situations where there are LPNs/LVNs assigned to client care.

The delegation and supervision responsibilities of RNs have been and continue to be a major concern for the nursing profession, both ethically and legally. The Code for Nurses states, "The nurse exercises informed judgment and uses individual competence and qualifications as criteria in seeking consultation, accepting responsibilities, and delegating nursing activities to others."[5] From the ethical view, RNs have an obligation to refuse assignments that they are not competent to carry out and also to refuse to delegate tasks to individuals whom they believe are incapable of or unprepared to perform particular nursing tasks.

> 66 99 *Professionals who delegate specific tasks retain accountability for the proper and safe completion of those tasks as well as responsibility for determining whether the assigned personnel are competent.*

The legal side of the delegation issue has also been addressed by the American Nurses Association (ANA) in a publication *ANA Basic Guide to Safe Delegation.*[6] This document makes a distinction between direct delegation, which is a specific decision made by the RN about who can perform what tasks, and indirect delegation, which is a list of tasks that certain health-care personnel can perform that is produced by the health care facility.[6] The **consensus** among many experts is that indirect delegation is really a form of covert institutional licensure. Lists of activities from the facility allowing nonnursing personnel who do not have the education of the RN to carry out professional nursing functions is a de facto permission to practice nursing without a license. Indirect delegation places RNs in a precarious legal position.

Basically, indirect delegation takes away much of the authority of the RN to assign personnel tasks, yet the RN remains accountable for the safe completion of the tasks under the doctrines of **respondent superior** and **vicarious liability.** Although some states are beginning to address the UAP and delegation issues in their nursing practice acts, many states either have no official standards for UAP delegation or include UAP standards under the medical practice act.

Before delegating any task, RNs should give careful consideration to the condition of the client, his or her health-care needs, the availability of staff, and the education and competency levels of the personnel to be assigned. The RN needs to know both the institution's official position description for the UAP as well as the UAP's actual abilities. For example, the position description may state that the UAP can care for postoperative clients who have multiple wound drains. However, when the RN assigns a specific UAP to such a postoperative client, he or she discovers that the UAP has worked only in the newborn nursery for the past 5 years and has no knowledge of how to care for complicated postoperative clients. If the RN assigns this UAP anyway, and some major complication develops with the client as a result of the UAP's lack of competence (even though the position description states that this is an appropriate function for the UAP), the RN is held legally responsible for the poor outcome (Box 8.3).

RNs who delegate are also responsible for educating the UAP about the task that is to be done. The RN is required to demonstrate how the tasks or procedures are performed and then document the training. Education also includes telling the UAP what is expected in the completion of the task and which possible complications to watch for and report to the RN. The ANA suggests that the RN watch the UAP perform the designated task at least initially, then make periodic observations throughout the shift to ensure safe and competent care for the client. Furthermore, the RN must always be available to answer questions and help the UAP whenever assistance is required.[6] Consider the following situation:

> " " *The ANA suggests that the RN watch the UAP perform the designated task at least initially, then make periodic observations throughout the shift to ensure safe and competent care for the client.*

Elsie Humber, RN, is the evening charge nurse on a busy oncology unit of the county hospital. On one particularly busy evening, she discovers during shift report that one of the scheduled LPNs has called in sick, and there are no other LPNs available to take her place. Ms. Humber assigns the LPN's duties and clients, including a heat lamp treatment for a decubitus ulcer, to a UAP who has worked on the unit for several months. The UAP protests the assignment, but Ms. Humber rebukes her saying: "I have no one else. If you don't care for these clients, they won't get any care this shift." In setting up the heat lamp treatment, the UAP knocks the lamp over and burns the client. Because of his suppressed immune system from chemotherapy and generally debilitated condition, the burn does not heal and develops into an infection. The client later sues the hospital for malpractice. The hospital in turn attempts to shift the legal responsibility for the burn to Ms. Humber. Who is legally responsible for the incident? Does the client have grounds for a successful case?

It is important to remember that when nurses delegate nursing tasks they are *not* delegating nursing. Professional nursing practice is both a science, based on a unique body of knowledge, and an art, guided by the nursing process. It is not merely a collection of tasks. Of all health-care workers, professional nurses are the most qualified to provide holistic care of the client by promoting health and treating disease. Nurses' education and experience provide them with the skills and knowledge to coordinate and supervise nursing care and to delegate specific tasks to others. The long-term effect of the growing trend to delegation on the quality of client care remains to be seen. However, the knowledge and judgment of the professional nurse will remain essential elements in any health-care system reforms, including clinical integration, case management, outsourcing practices, **total quality management (TQM)**, and **continuous quality improvement (CQI)**.

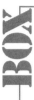

BOX

8.3 Delegate With Care

by Pamela Copeland

WORKING WITH UNLICENSED ASSISTIVE PERSONNEL? BE SURE YOU KNOW THE LEGAL RISKS

Unlicensed personnel have assisted registered nurses in the delivery of patient care throughout their professional history. In recent years, with economic pressures increasingly driving the current healthcare delivery system, the use of unlicensed assistive personnel (UAP) has expanded considerably.

What are some of the risk considerations and legal consequences? Can registered nurses minimize the risk of harm to patients, ensure professional and ethical standards and minimize allegations of professional liability? What can UAPs do to insure quality patient care and minimize allegations of negligent care or practicing nursing without a license?

REGISTERED NURSE LICENSURE

The legislature of each state enacts laws that govern the practice of nursing. The purpose of licensing law is to ensure that the public is protected from unqualified practitioners by developing and enforcing regulations that define who may practice in the profession, the scope of that practice and the level of education for the profession.

A fundamental premise of nursing practice is that a professional nurse is personally responsible for all acts or omissions undertaken within the scope of practice. The American Nurses Association defines delegation as "the transfer of responsibility for the performance of an activity from one person to another while retaining accountability for the outcome."[1] Additionally, the nurse is responsible for the adequate supervision of a delegated task to a subordinate. Failure of the nurse to delegate appropriately or supervise adequately and any injuries resulting from the acts of the subordinate may result in licensure ramifications. The state licensing board may take disciplinary actions.

YOU MAKE THE CALL

Nancy Nurse, RN, is team leader on a busy adult medical-surgical unit. There are 22 patients on the unit. On a particular shift, staffing includes one RN and one LPN and two nurses' aides. Fannie Aide, NA, is in school to become a registered nurse. She is assigned to work with Nancy Nurse. One of Fannie Aide's patients complained about a painful IV site. Fannie Aide assessed the site and reported the matter to Nancy Nurse. Nancy was in the midst of suctioning a patient who had just been resuscitated, and informed Fannie that she was too busy and would tend to the patient later. Fannie informed the patient that Nancy was tied up, upon which the patient began to cry and writhe in pain as she threatened to call the hospital administrator if she did not get immediate attention. Fannie reported the patient's concerns to Nancy and suggested that she pull the IV out as she had training in her registered nurse clinical program. Nancy agreed to Fannie's suggestion and instructed her to "be careful" when pulling out the IV. Fannie informed the patient that she would remove the IV and cut the patient's skin with the scissors (using suture removal scissors) while cutting through the tape. She removed the catheter, and applied a small bandage over the site, but the patient continued to bleed unbeknownst to Fannie.

Approximately four hours later Nancy Nurse went to assess the patient and noted that she was still oozing blood from the IV site, and the sheets were soaked with blood. The IV site was puffy. Immediately Nancy applied a pressure dressing to the IV site, called the physician and obtained an order for a stat hemoglobin and hematocrit (H&H). The H&H dropped from 12 to eight and 32 to 28, respectively. Within 24 hours, the patient spiked a temperature to 101; blood cultures revealed the patient had staph aureus growing in the blood. Within 48 hours, the patient became unresponsive and was diagnosed as having meningitis.

Based on this scenario, see if you can answer these questions:

1. Nancy Nurse correctly delegated the task of removing the IV to Fannie Aide. True or False
2. Nancy Nurse committed malpractice when she allowed Fannie Aide to remove the IV. True or False
3. Fannie Aide committed negligence in removing the IV. True or False
4. The state may revoke Fannie Aide's license because of this incident. True or False
5. Nancy Nurse demonstrated adequate supervisory skills when she instructed Fannie Aide to "be careful" in removing the IV. True or False.
6. The patient may take legal action for contracting meningitis against:
   a. the hospital
   b. Nancy Nurse
   c. Fannie Aide
   d. All of the above

7. Nancy Nurse assessed that the patient's complaint of pain at the IV site was an emergency. Additionally, she was in an emergency situation herself. Therefore, she was correct in directing Fannie Aide to remove the IV. True or False

Answers
1. **False.** The fact pattern did not list Fannie Aide's responsibilities. Unless a specific task is clearly identified and the UAP has had training and has been determined to be competent in performing it, the task should not be assigned.
2. **True.** Nancy Nurse has a duty to provide safe care to her patients. That duty was breached when she directed Fannie Aide to remove the IV. Fannie had not been determined to be competent to remove the IV and removed it in an unsafe manner. Nancy failed to supervise Fannie when the IV was removed. The patient sustained an infection that could probably be attributed to the manner in which the IV was removed. In summary, Nancy could be found to have committed malpractice, because she inappropriately delegated a task for which she was responsible and she failed to properly supervise Fannie.
3. **True.** Fannie Aide had the responsibility and duty to remove the IV in a safe manner. When an individual performs a professional task she will be held to the standard of a licensed experienced professional, regardless of the individual's training, skill or expertise. The court will not be lenient with Fannie because she is a UAP or a nursing student.
4. **True.** The state is responsible for ensuring licensed professionals practice in a safe manner. Once the state be-

comes aware that a practitioner may have committed an act that puts the public at risk, the state is obligated to investigate the matter. If the state makes a determination that the practitioner is guilty the state may revoke or suspend the practitioner's license.

5. **False.** Appropriate supervisory skills require more than giving directives. Appropriate supervision requires an assessment of the needs of the situation, evaluation of the competency and skill of the supervised individual and ensuring the task is performed in a safe manner.

6. **D.** All of the above. The hospital may be held liable under an agency theory. Nancy and Fannie are hospital employees; the hospital is responsible for their actions. Nancy Nurse may be held liable, as she inappropriately delegated the task of having the patient's IV removed, and negligently supervised Fannie Aide. And Fannie herself can be held liable, because she performed a task that exceeded the scope of responsibility and removed the IV in a negligent manner.

7. **False.** Emergency situations must be true emergencies—an immediate threat to life and limb. The patient complained of having severe pain and threatened to contact the hospital administrator. The situation should have been personally assessed by a licensed professional and another nurse could have been called to assist. This scenario was not an emergency.

Malpractice Considerations

Nursing malpractice is based on the legal premise that a nurse can be held legally re-

sponsible for the personal injury of another individual if it can be proven that the injury was the result of negligence.[2] Nursing malpractice is based upon four elements: 1) duty, 2) breach of duty, 3) causation (the "but for" test), and 4) damage or injury.

Inappropriate work assignment and inadequate supervision are a breach of duty and could be the basis for finding a nurse's actions to be negligent. Failure or breach of duty to delegate is established by proving that a reasonably prudent nurse would not have made a particular assignment or delegated a certain responsibility, or that supervision was inadequate under the circumstances.

The act of improper delegation of tasks or inadequate supervision must be evaluated in light of the "but for" test related to the injury. If the person who performed the injurious act had not been assigned or delegated to perform the task, or had been adequately supervised, the injury could have been avoided. Consequently, the nurse is not being held liable for the negligent act of her subordinate, *but for the lack of competence in performing the independent duties of delegation and supervision.*

Factors to Be Considered When Delegating

Remember that nursing is a knowledge based, processed oriented profession that provides patient care through patient assessment, nursing diagnoses, outcome identification, planning, evaluation or the use of nursing judgment.[3]

When delegating to UAP, the licensed nurse should consider the following:

1. Ensure that policies and procedures concerning delegation and supervision

are consistent with the state nurse practice act.

2. Be sure that registered nurses receive education and demonstrate knowledge and skills of delegation.
3. Do not include patient care responsibilities that require a license to perform them in UAP job descriptions, whether the license required is in nursing or another area (e.g., physical or respiratory therapy).[4]
4. Determine the level of preparation and education of UAP required to perform the delegated task.[5]
5. Delineate in UAP position descriptions and job duties which patient care activities they can perform.[6]
6. Confirm that UAP have demonstrated competency for each patient care activity that will be delegated to them.[7]
7. Provide the appropriate numbers of licensed nurses to supervise and coordinate the performance of patient care activities that may be delegated to UAP.[8]
8. Establish and implement a mechanism for the regular evaluation of UAPs by nursing staff members.

For their part, the UAP must consider the following:

1. Know your job description and do not exceed the scope of responsibilities.
2. Ask for assistance or clarification whenever you are not clear about a task or assignment.
3. Promptly report any and all findings to the licensed nurse.
4. Become certified in your role as an assistant care provider, through your healthcare agency, employer or the state.

Off-site Consideration

Registered nurses who practice in public health, community or home care settings must rely frequently on written or telephone communication when delegating patient care duties to assistive personnel. The nurse who must supervise from off site has a particular duty to assess the knowledge, skills and judgment of the assistive personnel before assignments are made. Regular supervisory visits and impeccable documentation will help the registered nurse ensure that care provided by assistive personnel is adequate.[9]

Conclusion

Registered nurses are responsible for providing patient care that conforms with their state practice act. The core of the nursing process requires specialized knowledge, judgment, competence, and skill. These activities include performing patient assessment, making nursing diagnoses, making nursing interventions, and evaluating a patient's progress.

It is inappropriate to delegate nursing activities to a UAP that compromises the nursing process. If patient injury occurs because a nursing function has been inappropriately delegated, the licensed nurse may have licensure ramifications and liability for professional negligence for the UAP's alleged negligent care. Matters like this may be avoided when policy and procedures that reflect state nurse practice acts determine the scope of the UAP's delineation of tasks. Additionally, nurses must understand the legal significance of delegation and supervision pursuant to the state nurse practice act. Finally, orientation, training, and competency assess-

8.3 Delegate With Care *(continued)*

ments must be provided to all members of the healthcare team to ensure a safe environment for the patient and the people that service them.

We all can get along when we know our roles and responsibilities.

Notes

1. American Nurses Association. The American Nurses Association position statement on registered nurse utilization of unlicensed assistive personnel. *American Nurse,* February 6–8, 1993.
2. Pozgar G., *Legal Aspects of Health Care Administration,* Fifth ed., Gaithersberg, MD, Aspen Publications, 1993.
3. Dawes, B, Delegation of Patient Care Responsibilities to Unlicensed Assistive Personnel, *AORN Journal 1992,* Vol. 66, No. 138, 141.
4. Blouin, A, Brent N, Unlicensed Assistive Personnel Legal Considerations, *JONA,* Vol. 25, No. 11, 1995, 7, 8, 21.
5. AORN Center for Nursing Practice, Research, and Health Policy, *Top 10 Most Frequently Asked Questions, Unlicensed Assistive Personnel,* 1996, 1997.
6. Ibid.
7. Ibid.
8. Ibid.
9. Ibid, at 4.

Pamela Copeland, RN, BSN, Esq, ARM, is currently employed as Director of Risk Management and Associate General Counsel at Greater Southeast Community Hospital in Washington, DC.

From Copeland, C: Delegate with care. Minority Nurse, Winter/Spring 1988, 32–34. Reprinted from Minority Nurse, Winter/Spring, 1997–1998.

Patient Self-determination Act

The Patient Self-Determination Act of 1990, sponsored by Senator John Danforth, is a federal law that requires that all federally funded institutions inform clients of their right to prepare advance directives. The advance directives seek to encourage people to discuss and document their wishes concerning the type of treatment and care that they want (i.e., life-sustaining treatment) in advance, so that it will ease the burden on their families and providers when it comes time to make such a decision (Box 8.4).

There are two types of advance directives: the living will and medical durable power of attorney. The living will is a document stating what health care a client will accept or refuse after the client is no longer competent or able to make that decision. The medical durable power of attorney, or health-care proxy, designates another person to make health-care decisions for a person if the client becomes incompetent or unable to make such decisions.

Each state outlines its own requirements for executing and revoking the medical durable power of attorney and living wills.

Incompetent Client's Right to Self-determination

The courts are protective of incompetent clients and require high standards of proof before allowing a physician to terminate any life-sustaining treatment for that client.

Nancy Cruzan was 30 years old and in a persistent vegetative state. She had a gastrostomy feeding and hydration tube inserted to assist with the feedings, which was consented to by her husband. Her parents, however, petitioned the court for

BOX

8.4 Common Questions Asked About Advance Directives

Q. Which is better—a living will or a medical durable power of attorney for health care or health-care proxy?

A. The documents are different and allow the nurse to do two different things. The living will states what health care procedures a client will accept or refuse after the client is no longer competent or able to make that decision. The medical durable power of attorney or health-care proxy allows you as a client to designate another person to make health-care choices for you.

Q. If I change my mind and have a living will, can I cancel the living will or durable medical power of attorney?

A. Yes, each state has ways that your advance directives can be cancelled or negated. Most states require an oral or written statement, destruction of the document itself, or notification to certain individuals, such as the physician. Again, each state's statute should be checked for the specific details required.

Q. If I have a living will in one state, is it good in all states?

A. It may or may not be, depending on the requirements for the living will. It is important that you have your living will checked by an attorney in order to determine whether or not it may be effective in the states in which you are traveling or working.

Q. If I have a living will and have medical durable power of attorney who should get copies?

A. Copies should be given to your next of kin, your physician, and your attorney so that more than one person has a copy and knows what your intentions are. Some states will allow you to register your living will with certain state agencies such as the Secretary of State. Also there are national groups that will allow you to register your living will with them so that there is access to it.

---

removal of the tube. In the Cruzan case, the court held that the state had the right to err on the side of life. The U.S. Supreme Court recognized that a living will would have been sufficient evidence of Cruzan's wishes to sustain or to remove her feeding tube.

The issue before the U.S. Supreme Court was whether the state of Missouri could use its own standard of clear and convincing proof for removal of the tube or whether there was a 14th Amendment due process guarantee of a "right to die" that would override the state statute. It was decided

that the constitutional right would not be extended and the state procedural requirement would be allowed, at which time the burden of proof was put on Cruzan's family to show that she would not have wanted to continue living in this manner.

The Nurse's Role in Advance Directives

Nurses must know the laws of the state pertaining to advance directives, clients' rights, and the policies and procedures of the institution in which they work. Nurses must inform clients of their right to formulate advance directives and to realize that not all clients can make such decisions. It is important for the nurse to establish trust and rapport with a client and the client's family so that the nurse can assist them in making decisions that are in the client's best interests. Nurses must also teach about advance directives and document all critical decisions, discussions with the client and client's family about such decisions, and the basis for the decision-making process. Discrimination must be also prevented against clients and their families based on their decisions regarding their advance directives. It is also important that nurses determine whether or not the client has been coerced into making advance directive decisions against his or her will. Nurses need to become involved in ethics committees at hospitals or nursing specialty groups at local, state, or national levels to better help clients make decisions about advance directives.

> **" "** *Nurses must also teach about advance directives and document all critical decisions, discussions with the client and client's family about such decisions, and the basis for the decision-making process.*

Do-Not-Resuscitate (DNR) Orders

Although a DNR instruction may be included in an advance directive, DNR orders are legally separate from advance directives. For the health-care professional to be legally protected, there should be a written order for a "no code" or DNR order in the client's chart. Each hospital should have a policy and procedure that outlines what is required with regard to a client's condition for a DNR order. The DNR order should be reviewed, evaluated, and reordered. Different facilities have established different time periods for these reviews. Nurses must also know whether there is any law that regulates who should authorize a DNR order for an incompetent client who is no longer able to make this decision. Hospitals often have policies and procedures describing what must be done and which clients fit the requirements for a DNR order. The ANA has published a position statement on nursing care and DNR decisions.

Nurses face many legal dilemmas when dealing with confusing or conflicting DNR orders. For example, it may be difficult to interpret a DNR order when it has been restricted, for instance, "do not resuscitate except for medications and defibrillation" or "no CPR or intubation." Often a lack of proper documentation in the medical records indicating how the DNR decision was reached can be an important and crucial issue if a medical malpractice case is involved and it is disputed whether or not the client or family actually gave consent for a DNR order.

Many facilities have developed DNR decision sheets for recording information about DNR discussions; or the sheets are dated and signed by the client and those family members who took part in the discussion. It then becomes a permanent part of the medical record. It is very important that nurses not stigmatize clients by the use of indicators for DNR orders, such as dots on the wristband or dots over the bed. Health-care providers' attitudes often change because they feel that the client is "going to die anyway." This abandonment can jeopardize the care of a client designated with a DNR order. However, it is also important for the nurses and staff to know whether an order is to be honored and what the policies and procedures are with regard to transfer clients and DNR orders that accompany the incoming client. Information about the DNR status of a client should be obtained during shift report. If there has not been a periodic review, is the order still in effect? If a client is transferred from one facility to another but has a DNR order that is time-limited and has not been reordered, what should a nurse do?

Standards of Care

Standards of care are the yardstick that the legal system uses to measure the actions of a nurse involved in a malpractice suit. The underlying principle used to establish standards of care is based on the actions that would likely be taken by a reasonable person (nurse) who was placed in the same or similar circumstances. The standard usually includes both objective factors (e.g., the actions to be performed) and subjective factors, including the nurse's emotional and mental state. Specifically, a nurse is judged against the standards that are established within the profession and specialty area of practice. The ANA and specialty groups within the nursing profession, such as the American Association of Critical Care Nurses (AACN), publish standards of care that are updated continually as health-care technology and practices change.

Both external and internal standards govern the conduct of nurses. External standards include nursing standards developed by the ANA, the State Nurse Practice Act of each jurisdiction, criteria from accrediting agencies such as the Joint Commission on Accreditation of Healthcare Organizations, guidelines developed by various nursing specialty practice groups, and federal agency regulations. Nurses are encountering an increasing number of incidents where conflicts occur between institutional and professional standards, for example in staffing ratios. These conflicts are difficult to resolve and

> 66 99 *A nurse is judged against the standards that are established within the profession and specialty area of practice.*

may require deliberation and decisions from institutional committees. As a general rule, where a conflict exists, it is safer legally to follow professional standards.

Internal standards include nursing standards defined in specific hospital policy and procedure manuals that relate to the nurse in the particular institution. The nurse's job description and employment contract are examples of internal nursing standards that define the duty of the nurse.

The rationale for advancing standards of care for the nurse is to ensure proper, consistent, and high-quality nursing care to all members of society. When nurses violate their duty of care to the client as established by the profession's standards of care, they leave themselves open to charges of negligence and malpractice. Until recently, nurses were held to the standards of the local community. National criteria have now replaced most **locality rule standards of care.** Individual nurses are held accountable not only to acceptable standards within the local community but also to national standards as well.

Although standards of care may appear to be specific, they are merely guidelines for nursing practice. Because every client's situation is different, the appropriate standard of care may be difficult to identify in a specific case. More than one course of nursing action may be considered appropriate under a proper standard of care. The final decision must be guided by the nurse's judgment and understanding of the client's needs.

The Nurse Practice Act

The Nurse Practice Act defines nursing practice and establishes standards for nurses in each state. It is the most definitive legal statute or legislative act regulating nursing practice. Although nurse practice acts vary in scope from one state to another, they tend to have similar wording based loosely on the ANA model published in 1988. The Nurse Practice Act provides a framework for the court on which to base decisions when determining whether a nurse has breached a standard of care.

Most state nurse practice acts define scope of practice, establish requirements for licensure and entry into practice, and create and empower a board of nursing to oversee the practice of nurses. In addition, nurse practice acts identify grounds for disciplinary actions such as suspension and revocation of a nursing license.[4]

The judicial interpretation of the Nurse Practice Act and its relationship to a specific case provide guidance for decisions about future cases. Many state legislatures have responded to the expanded role of the nurse by broadening the scope of their nurse practice acts. For example, the addition of the term *nursing diagnosis* to many states' nurse practice acts reflects the legislature's recognition of the expansion of the nurse's role. In addition, occupational roles such as nurse practitioner, **nurse clinician,** and clinical nurse specialist are beginning to be included in nurse practice acts. It is important to remember that as the nurse's role expands, so does the legal accountability of the role itself.

PREVENTION OF LAWSUITS

What can the nurse do to avoid having to go through the stressful, sometimes financially and professionally devastating process of litigation? The following guidelines provide some ways to avoid a lawsuit.

Medical Record

The medical record is the single most frequently used piece of objective evidence in a malpractice suit. In preparation for the trial, the lawyers attempt to reconstruct the events surrounding the incident in a minute-by-minute time line. The client's chart is the most important source for this time line. Maintaining an accurate and complete medical record is an absolute requirement. The old adage "if it isn't written, it didn't happen" remains true in most situations; however, recent court trials have recognized some exceptions. Some judges and juries have begun to recognize that "charting by exception" is a valid form of health-care record keeping. Charting by exception, very closely related to problem-oriented charting, was developed initially to save busy nurses time and to save the facility money by reducing the volume of documents created and stored. In institutions where charting by exception is used, the nurse charts only those elements of client care that are abnormal or unusual or that constitute a health-care problem. If the client is stable and recovering as expected, there may be very little written in the chart about his or her physical or mental assessments.

Trying to recall specific events from 2 to 6 years previously without the benefit of written notes is almost impossible. In general, the client record should *not* contain personal opinion, should be legible, should be in chronological order, and should be written and signed by the nurse. Although opinions have a relatively low value in legal proceedings, the documentation should indicate the nursing judgments made by the nurse. An entry should never be obliterated or destroyed. If a nurse questions a physician's order, record must be made that the physician was contacted and the order clarified.

> 66 99 *The medical record is the single most frequently used piece of objective evidence in a malpractice suit.*

Charting: What You Need to Know

It would be difficult to find nurses who enjoy charting. In general, nurses view charting and most other kinds of paper work as a necessary evil that should be, if not avoided completely, at least put off for as long as possible. From a legal standpoint, however, it is one of the most important activities that nurses undertake. The following is a list of considerations that improve charting and help make it a valuable element of patient care.

1. Be accurate, because a client's condition changes throughout the shift. The time at which you performed a nursing action, as well as the time and nature of the client's response, can be very important when you are defending yourself from a lawsuit. When 2 or 3 years have elapsed after the action, the chart is the only hard evidence of what happened. From a legal viewpoint, if it was not charted, it was not done.
2. Demonstrate the priority of nursing actions. It is important that the chart reflect not only that an action was taken but also why it was taken. Showing that you treated a client's most serious, life-threatening problems first is essential to demonstrate that the actions you took are based on sound nursing judgment.
3. Incorporate standards of care. In any lawsuit, nurses are held to the applicable standards of care. If these standards are violated in the provision of care, it becomes difficult to defend yourself against a lawsuit. Charting should demonstrate that the overall nursing care was planned according to an acceptable standard of care. Charting should reflect any deviations from this plan as valid nursing judgments made within the scope of practice, for example, normal growth and development. Make sure to include the rationales for the deviation in plan based on the client's changing condition.
4. Chart all communications with physicians. A major element in many lawsuits is the failure of the physician to communicate with the nurse. Any telephone conversations, orders from the physician, and verbal exchanges while the physician is on the unit should be documented. If these exchanges involve information that has the potential to provoke a lawsuit, they should be charted in more detail.
5. Be careful with a physician's orders. Always check charts for new orders after physicians have handled them. When taking orders off, make sure that a line is drawn after the last order in such a way that the physician cannot add any orders on that sheet. Prewritten order sheets should be timed and dated when they were received by the nurse. Always read back verbal or telephone orders to the physician to doublecheck what was said. Misinter-

pretation of a physician's orders is a frequent source of lawsuits against nurses.

6. Never change, recopy, or white out any part of a record. Obvious changes in medical records are a red flag to lawyers, indicating that someone is trying to hide something. If a part of a chart needs to be recopied because it has become soiled or illegible, the original should remain with it.

7. Keep advance directives on the chart. Living wills, durable powers of attorney, or other documents that describe the client's wishes if clients are no longer able to make decisions about their care should be readily available in the chart. In situations where a client goes into cardiac or respiratory arrest, it is much easier for the health-care providers to make decisions about what actions to take if this information is at hand. In addition, family members will be more comfortable with the actions taken if they can see the advance directives.

8. Record interactions with the family and client. Because of the stress on both client and family during a serious illness, misinterpretations of information often occur. Charting what was said to the client and family and their responses to the information is a good method to protect yourself from legal actions that may occur years later. Note any hostility or anger expressed by the family, but chart it in a nonjudgmental manner using direct quotes as much as possible. It is better to chart: "Client's husband states: 'You nurses are really stupid in this hospital—nobody seems to know what is going on'" rather than "Client's husband seems hostile and angry." Angry families are more likely to sue than satisfied ones.

9. Be as descriptive as possible. Even if you do not know the exact medical term for what you are observing, try to describe it as clearly as possible. You may have forgotten that anasarca is the term that describes generalized body edema, but stating "+2 to +3 pitting edema of arms, hands, legs, feet, and torso" accomplishes the same goal. Avoid charting opinions and avoid the use of the words "seems" or "appears."

Despite universal distaste for it, charting is an important part of client care. It allows you to take credit for the care you have given and demonstrates your knowledge of the important patient responses to be evaluated. If you are ever sued for malpractice, the chart, if done well, will become your most important ally.

From Calfee, BE: Tips for better charting. Nursing 94:32–33, 1994.

Rapport with Clients

Establishing a rapport with the client through honest, open communication goes a long way in avoiding lawsuits. Treating clients and their families with respect and letting them know that the nurse really cares about them may well prevent a lawsuit. Many people are willing to forgive a nurse's error if they have good rapport and a trusting relationship with a nurse who they believe is interested in their well-being.

Current Nursing Skills

Keeping one's nursing knowledge and skills current is vital to prevent errors that may lead to lawsuits. It is better to refuse to perform an unfamiliar procedure than to attempt it without the necessary knowledge and skills. Taking advantage of in-service training, workshops, and continuing nursing education classes is an important part of maintaining the nurse's skill level. Nurses must practice within their level of competence and scope of practice.

Knowledge of the Client

Recognizing the client who is lawsuit-prone can help reduce the risk of litigation. Some common characteristics of this type of client include constant dissatisfaction with the care given, constant complaints about all aspects of care, and negative comments about other nurses. This client often complains about the poor care given by nurses on the previous shift. This client may also have a history of lawsuits against nurses.

> **" "** *Some hospitals have liability insurance policies for the nurse as a part of the nurse's employment package with the institution.*

Being direct, solving problems with the client, and helping the client become involved in his or her care are helpful to diffuse this negative behavior. Also, even more careful documentation of the care provided and the client's responses to the care can be helpful if a lawsuit is later filed.

Liability Insurance

Maintenance of proper liability insurance is a necessity. Nurses who do not carry liability insurance place themselves at high risk. The nurse's personal assets as well as the nurse's wages may be subject to a judgment awarded in a malpractice action. Even if the client does not win at the trial, the litigation process including hiring a lawyer and paying the costs of experts can be financially devastating.

A professional liability insurance policy is a contract with an insurer who promises to assume the costs paid to the injured party in exchange for payment of a premium. There are two types of malpractice policies: claims-made and occurrence. Claims-made policies protect only against claims made during the time the policy is in effect. Occurrence policies protect against all claims that occurred during the policy period, regardless of when the claim is made. Generally, the occurrence type of liability insurance offers more protection. Claims-made policy coverage can be broadened by purchasing a tail that is a separate policy that extends the time of coverage.

Some hospitals have liability insurance policies for the nurse as a part of the nurse's employment package with the institution. This hospital policy may be limited to claims arising from nurse's employment and might not apply in a situation in which a nurse renders care outside the institution, for instance, at an automobile accident site. It is preferable to have liability insurance coverage that includes all situations in which the nurse may be involved. Individual **indemnity insurance** coverage independent of the facility's policy is recommended for all nurses. With passage of the **Federal Tort Claims Act,** and similar state laws, nurses who were formally protected from lawsuits by working at federal or state health-care facilities can now be sued for malpractice like nurses at any other facility.

REVOCATION OF LICENSE

One of the most drastic punishments that a nurse can experience is revocation of the li-

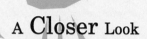

A **Closer** Look

WHAT TO LOOK FOR IN AN INSURANCE POLICY

The following factors should be reviewed in order to determine what is the best policy for your type of nursing practice:

1. *Type of insurance policy (claims-made or occurrence basis)*
2. *Insuring agreement*

   The insurance company's promise to pay in exchange for premiums is called the insuring agreement. The insurance company agrees to pay a money award to a plaintiff who is injured by an act of omission or commission by a health-care provider who is insured by the company.
3. *Types of injuries covered*

   The language must be scrutinized to determine whether it is broad or limiting. Some companies will agree to pay only if the insured nurse is sued for damages, which means the nurse must be sued for a money amount or award. If the nurse is sued for a specific performance lawsuit or an injunctive relief action, which means that the nurse will either have to perform something or discontinue doing something, that particular insurance policy may not be adequate. Also, most insurance policies will not cover the nurse for disciplinary actions.
4. *Exclusions*

   Items that are not covered by a policy are called exclusions. It is important to review the exclusions. Some of the more common exclusions include sexual abuse of a client, injury caused while under the influence of drugs or alcohol, criminal activity, and punitive damages. Punitive damages are used to punish the defendant for egregious acts or omissions.

Who Is Covered Under the Policy

The purchaser is the named insured and can be an individual, institution, or a group. Others who may be covered by the policy are nurses, employees, agents, and volunteers, among others.

Limitations and Deductions

In exchange for payment of the premium, the insurance company agrees to pay up to a certain amount on behalf of the insured. This amount is called the limit of liability. It is usually expressed in two ways: the amount that can be paid per incident (per occurrence), and the amount that will be paid for the entire policy year. For example, if you have a policy that states $1,000,000/$3,000,000, it means that the company will pay up to $1 million per incident and a total of $3 million per policy year.

The insurance industry relies on the A. M. Best Company to evaluate both the financial size and relative strengths of insurance companies. An A. M. Best rating of A– or better should be a prerequisite for purchase of any policy.

The Right to Select Counsel

Some insurance companies will allow nurses to select their own attorneys to represent them in a medical negligence claim. Others will retain attorneys or law firms, and the nurse will not have the opportunity to make that selection.

The Right to Consent to Settlement

Some policies will allow the nurse to decide whether or not a case should be settled or go to trial, whereas others will not.

cense to practice nursing. The nursing profession is responsible for monitoring and enforcing its own standards through the state licensing board. These actions may or may not be related to tort law, contract law, or criminal charges. Each state's licensing board is charged with the responsibility to oversee the professional nurse's competence.

The state's nursing board receives its authority to grant and revoke licenses from specific statutory laws. The underlying rationale for establishment of a licensing board is to protect the public from uneducated, unsafe, or unethical practitioners. If a nurse fails to adhere to the standards of safe practice and exhibits unprofessional behavior, he or she can be disciplined by the state nursing licensing board. One of the remedies that these boards can use is suspension or revocation of the nurse's license.

A disciplinary hearing is held to review the charges of the nurse's unprofessional conduct. This hearing is less formal than the trial process, and the nurse is allowed to present evidence and be represented by legal counsel at the hearing. Due process requires that the nurse be notified in advance of the specific charges being made. The question of what constitutes unprofessional conduct is an issue frequently dealt with at the disciplinary hearing. Each respective state's nurse practice act provides guidance with regard to the specifics of unprofessional conduct.

Unprofessional conduct can be reported by a nursing peer, supervisor, client, or a client's family. Many cases are dismissed before the hearing takes place if the board finds there is no support for the allegation being made against the nurse. If a hearing is necessary, it is in the best interest of the nurse to seek legal counsel because of the potential risk of license revocation.

License revocation is a serious consequence for the nurse because it removes the nurse's right to practice. Drug abuse, administering medication without a prescription, practicing without a valid license, and any singular act of unprofessional or unethical conduct can constitute grounds for losing a nursing license.

Conclusion

The legal system and its effects on the practice of nursing are ever-present realities in today's health-care system. Nurses need to be aware of the implications of their actions but should not be so overwhelmed by fear that it reduces their ability to care for the client. The more advanced and specialized the nurse's practice becomes, the higher the standards to which the nurse is held. Nurses will be challenged throughout their career to apply legal principles in the daily practice of nursing. An awareness of what constitutes malpractice and negligence will aid in the prevention of litigation.

Critical Thinking Exercises

Consider the following case: *Thomas v. Corso* (Md. 1982)

The client was brought to the hospital emergency room (ER) after being involved in an automobile accident. The ER nurse assessed and recorded the client's vital signs and a complaint of numbness in his right anterior thigh. The client was able to move the right leg, and there was no discoloration or deformity. After he was given meperidine (Demerol) for his pain, his blood pressure (B/P) dropped to 90/60 and the nurse notified the ER physician of the change. The physician ordered the nurse to arrange for admission to the hospital, which she did.

The client was transferred to a medical/surgical unit, but he could not be placed in a room because of an influenza epidemic. Rather, the client was placed in the hall next to the nurses' station for close observation. A nurse checked the client's vital signs about 20 minutes after the transfer and noted that the B/P was now 70/50, respiratory rate 40, and pulse 120. His skin was cool and diaphoretic, his breathing was deep and rapid, and he was asking for a drink of water. The client also complained of pain in his leg, but the nurse did not give him more pain medication because of his blood pressure.

The nurse assessed him about 30 minutes later and found his skin warmer, although he still complained of pain and thirst. The nurse also noted a strong odor of alcohol on the client's breath. An assistant supervisor also assessed the client's condition but refused to give him any water because he had obviously been drinking alcohol. She had been told about the low blood pressure by the client's nurse but attributed it to the alcohol and pain medication combination. The nurse checked his vital signs again and found a B/P of 100/89. Thirty minutes later it was 94/70, pulse 100, and respirations 28. When the nurse next assessed the client an hour later, he had a Cheyne-Stokes respiratory pattern, no pulse, and no blood pressure. She started cardiopulmonary resuscitation (CPR) and called a "code blue," but after a lengthy attempt at resuscitation, the client died.

An autopsy was performed and showed that the client had a lacerated liver and a severe fracture of the femur with bleeding into the tissues. The coroner determined that traumatic shock, secondary to the fractured femur and lacerated liver, was the cause of death. His family sued the nurses for poor judgment, and the hospital for malpractice, and won.

✔ What mistakes were made by the nurses in this case?

✔ What legal liability did the nurses incur by their actions?

✔ How can the nurses best prepare for trial in this case?

✔ What actions could the nurses have taken to prevent a lawsuit with this client?

✔ What are your feelings toward inebriated clients? Did the nurses' attitudes about inebriation affect their judgments?

✔ Why are clients who are drunk at higher risk for injury and poor medical outcomes than other clients?

References

1. Guido, G: Legal Issues in Nursing: A Source Book for Practice, ed 2. Appleton & Lange, E. Norwalk, Conn., 1997.
2. Louisell, D, and Williams, H: Medical Malpractice. Matthew Bender, New York, 1990.
3. Fiesta, J: Legal update, 1995, Part 2. Nursing Management 27(6):24–25, 1996.
4. Aiken, TD: Legal, Ethical, and Political Issues in Nursing. FA Davis, Philadelphia, 1994.
5. American Nurses Association: Code for Nurses with Interpretive Statements. American Nurses Association, Washington, DC, 1985.
6. American Nurses Association: ANA Basic Guide to Safe Delegation. American Nurses Association, Washington, DC, 1995.

BIBLIOGRAPHY

American Nurses Association: Policy Series: Regulation of Unlicensed Assistive Personnel. American Nurses Association, Washington, DC, 1996.

Carroll, V, and Morin, K: Workplace violence affects one-third of nurses. American Nurse 30(5):15, 1998.

Copeland, P: Delegate with care. Minority Nurse Winter/Spring, 1997–1998, 32–35.

Crego, PJ, and Lipp, EJ: Nurse's knowledge of advanced directives. Am J Crit Care 7(3):218–223, 1998.

Creighton, H: Law Every Nurse Should Know, ed 5. WB Saunders, Philadelphia, 1986.

Curtin, LL: Your license or mine. Nursing Management 26(12):7–8, 1995.

Cushing, M: Nursing Jurisprudence. Appleton & Lange, E. Norwalk, Conn., 1988.

Davis, AJ, Aroskar, MA, and Liaschenko, J: Ethical Dilemmas and Nursing Practice, ed 4. Appleton & Lange, E. Norwalk, Conn., 1997.

Feutz-Harter, S: Nursing and the Law, ed 5. Professional Education System, New York, 1993.

Fiesta, J: The Law and Liability: A Guide for Nurses, ed 2. John Wiley, New York, 1988.

Fiesta, J: Legal update, 1995, Part 1. Nursing Management 27(5):24–25, 1996.

Hudson, SA: Are you confused about restraints? Oklahoma Nurse 43(3):28, 1998.

Keepnews, D: Emerging issues in licensure and regulation. Am J Nurs 96(10):70–72, 1996.

Louisell, D, Hazard, G, and Colen, T: Pleading and Procedure, ed 5. The Foundation Press, New York, 1983.

Lynn, R: Jury Trial Law and Practice. John Wiley, New York, 1986.

Marullo, G: Criminal prosecution for med errors does not address system problems or prevent recurrences. American Nurse 29(6):6, 1998.

Monarch, K: Insurance portability. Oklahoma Nurse 43(1):11, 1998.

Murchison, I, Nichols, T, and Hansen, R: Legal Accountability in the Nursing Process, ed 2. CV Mosby, St. Louis, 1982.

Nawar, M: Workplace violence: One nurse's night of fear. American Nurse 30(5):15, 1998.

Nicoll, LH: Nurses' Guide to the Internet, ed 2. JB Lippincott, Philadelphia, 1998.

Rhodes, A, and Miller, R: Nursing and the Law. Aspen Systems, Rockville, Md., 1984.

Rodgers, B: Is health care a risky business? American Nurse 29(5):5, 1997.

Slattery, M: Caring for ourselves to care for our patients. American Nurse 30(5):12–13, 1998.

Stewart, M: Managed care law blocks quality care to indigent patients. American Nurse 29(6):12, 1997.

Sullivan, TJ: Collaboration: A Health Care Imperative. McGraw-Hill, New York, 1998.

Wlody, GF: Assisted suicide: Recent judicial decisions and implications for critical care nurses. Critical Care Nurse 17(5):71-79, 1997.

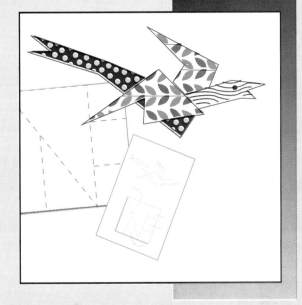

Making the Transition: From Student to Professional

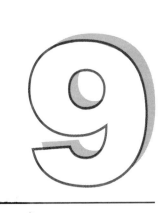

9

➤ *Joseph T. Catalano*

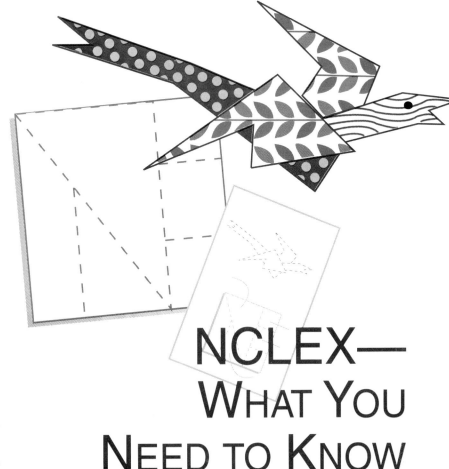

NCLEX—
WHAT YOU
NEED TO KNOW

Learning Objectives

After completing this chapter, the reader will be able to:

1. Describe the NCLEX-RN, CAT test plan.
2. Discuss the NCLEX-RN, CAT test format.
3. Analyze and identify the different types of questions used on the NCLEX-RN, CAT.
4. Select the most appropriate means for preparing for the NCLEX-RN, CAT.
5. Apply key test-taking strategies to help improve examination grades.

The primary purpose of licensure examinations is to protect the public from unsafe or uneducated practitioners of the profession. When nurses pass the National Council Licensure Examination (NCLEX), it indicates that they have attained the minimal level of competency deemed necessary by the state in order to practice nursing without injury to clients. Licensure is a legal requirement for all professions that deal with public health, welfare, or safety.

All examinations produce anxiety in those who are about to take them. The more important the examination, the higher the anxiety levels. Anxiety is sometimes defined as fear of the unknown. This chapter presents information about the NCLEX test plan, tips for improving the score on multiple choice examinations, and some suggestions for study. It is hoped that this information will help lower the student's anxiety levels about the NCLEX. There are also several sample practice questions included to give you an idea of how the NCLEX asks about different types of nursing information. Try to answer these questions as you read the chapter. The answers and rationales are found at the end of the chapter.

NATIONAL COUNCIL LICENSURE EXAMINATION TEST PLAN

The NCLEX is a computerized, **criterion-referenced examination** that is taken after graduation from a school of nursing. Unlike a **norm-referenced examination** that establishes a passing score based on how others fare in the examination, criterion-referenced examinations compare the test taker's knowledge to a pre-established standard. The examination measures nursing knowledge of a wide range of material. With computerized adaptive tests, such as the NCLEX, the computer selects questions in accordance with the examination plan and how well the graduate answered the previous question.

In April, 1998, several substantive changes were made in the National Council Licensure Examination—Computerized Adaptive Testing for Registered Nurses NCLEX-CAT RN test plan. The changes included reorganization of the test plan into three primary components: (1) client needs, (2) level of cognitive ability, and (3) integrated concepts and processes. The third component was expanded to include nursing process, caring, communication, cultural awareness, documentation, self-care, and teaching/learning.

Client Health Needs

The NCLEX examination asks questions about four general groups of material called client health needs:

- Safe and effective care environment
- Physiologic needs
- Psychosocial needs
- Health promotion and maintenance needs

Safe and Effective Care Environment

a. Management of care . . . 7%–13% of NCLEX questions
b. Safety, infection control . . . 5%–11% of NCLEX questions

Total questions in this category make up between 13% and 24% of the total questions on the NCLEX examination. These questions deal with overt safety issues in client care, such as use of restraints, medication administration, safety measures to prevent injuries (like putting up side rails), preventing infections, isolation precautions, safety measures with pediatric clients, and special safety needs of clients with psychiatric problems.

This needs category also includes questions about laboratory tests, their results, and any special nursing measures associated with them; legal and ethical issues in nursing; a small amount of nursing management; and quality assurance issues. Questions on these issues are interspersed with other questions throughout the examination.

Physiologic Integrity

a. Basic care and comfort . . . 7%–13% of NCLEX questions
b. Pharmacologic/parenteral therapies . . . 5%–11% of NCLEX questions
c. Reduction of risk potential . . . 12%–18% of NCLEX questions
d. Physiologic adaptation . . . 12%–18% of NCLEX questions

> **" "** *The NCLEX examination asks questions about four general groups of material called client health needs.*

The physiologic integrity needs are concerned with adult medical and surgical nursing care, pediatrics, and **gerontology.** This category comprises the largest groups of questions, with about 50% to 55% of the total number of questions on the NCLEX. The more common health-care problems, both acute and chronic conditions, that nurses deal with on a daily basis include:

- Diabetes
- Cardiovascular disorders
- Neurological disorders
- Renal diseases

There are also questions about nursing care of the pediatric client, including such topics as:

- Growth and development
- Congenital abnormalities
- Child abuse
- Burn injury
- Fractures

Psychosocial Integrity

a. Coping and adaptation . . . 5%–11% of NCLEX questions
b. Psychosocial adaptation . . . 5%–11% of NCLEX questions

Psychosocial integrity needs are those health-care issues that revolve around the client with psychiatric problems. This material also deals with coping mechanism for high-stress situations such as acute illness and life-threatening diseases or trauma. These clients do not necessarily have any psychiatric disorders. This category com-

> **" "** *Health promotion and maintenance needs deal with pregnancy, labor and delivery, the care of the newborn infant, growth and development, and contagious diseases, particularly sexually transmitted diseases. This section constitutes approximately 15% of the total examination.*

prises approximately 15% of the examination and includes questions about the care of clients with anxiety disorders, depression, schizophrenia, and organic mental disease. Also included in the psychosocial needs section are questions about therapeutic communication, crisis intervention, and substance abuse.

Health Promotion and Maintenance

a. Life span growth and development . . . 7%–13% of NCLEX questions
b. Prevention/early detection of disease . . . 5%–11% of NCLEX questions

Health promotion and maintenance needs deal with pregnancy, labor and delivery, the care of the newborn infant, growth and development, and contagious diseases, particularly sexually transmitted diseases. This section constitutes approximately 15% of the total examination. Teaching and counseling are important parts of the nurse's care during pregnancy, and knowledge of diet, signs and symptoms of complications, fetal development, and testing used during pregnancy is necessary.

Levels of Cognitive Ability

The level of cognitive ability is a component of the NCLEX that measures how information has been learned and how it can be used by the nurse. For the NCLEX, knowledge is tested at three different levels.

Level 1

Level 1 consists of knowledge and comprehension questions. Only approximately 15%

of the questions are at this level. These questions involve recalling specific facts and the ability to understand those facts in relationship to a pathophysiologic condition and cover knowledge of specific anatomy and physiology, medication dosage and side effects, signs and symptoms of diseases, laboratory test results, and the elements of certain treatments and interventions. Being able to remember and understand information is the most basic way of learning. Although this type of knowledge is important and underlies the other levels of knowledge, it is not itself sufficient to ensure safe nursing care. An example of a level 1 question is:

1. A client is admitted to the medical unit with respiratory failure. Which of the following is the normal range for the Po_2?
   ○ a. 10–30 mm Hg
   ○ b. 35–55 mm Hg
   ○ c. 10–20 cm H_2O
   ○ d. 70–100 mm Hg

Level 2

Level 2 consists of questions that ask the nurse to analyze and apply the memorized information to specific client care situations. Analysis and application questions are more difficult to answer because they require the nurse to do more than simply repeat the information he or she has learned. Analysis requires the ability to separate information into its basic parts and decide which of those parts are important. Application requires that the nurse be able to use that information in client care decisions. Some examples of this type of question are the interpretation of electro-

cardiographic (ECG) strips, interpretation of blood gas values, making a nursing diagnosis based on a set of symptoms, or deciding on a course of treatment. These questions provide a better indication of the nurse's ability to safely care for clients. An example of a level 2 question is:

2. A client is becoming progressively short of breath. The results of his arterial blood gas (ABG) tests are pH, 7.13; Po_2, 48; Pco_2, 53; and HCO_3, 26. These values indicate:
   ○ a. Uncompensated metabolic acidosis with moderate hypoxia.
   ○ b. Respiratory alkalosis with hypoxia.
   ○ c. Uncompensated respiratory acidosis with severe hypoxia.
   ○ d. Compensated respiratory acidosis with normal oxygen.

Level 3

Level 3, synthesis, judgment, and evaluation, takes the process a step further. Approximately 85% of the questions are at either level 2 or level 3. Questions at the synthesis and judgment level ask the nurse to make decisions about client care. One factor that adds to the difficulty of answering this type of question is that there is often more than one correct answer. The nurse is asked to choose the best, or highest priority, answer from among several correct answers. Questions at this level often ask about the priority of care to be given, the priority of nursing diagnosis formulated, how to best evaluate the effectiveness of care that has been given, and the most appropriate nursing action to be taken.

> **" "** *Being able to remember and understand information is the most basic way of learning. Although this type of knowledge is important and underlies the other levels of knowledge, it is not itself sufficient to ensure safe nursing care.*

It is believed that the ability of the nurse to make decisions about nursing care at these higher levels is the best indication of the thought processes expected of a nurse demonstrating safe nursing care. An example of a level 3 question is:

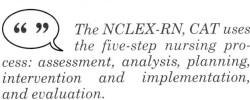

> **66 99** *The NCLEX-RN, CAT uses the five-step nursing process: assessment, analysis, planning, intervention and implementation, and evaluation.*

3. A client has become cyanotic and is having Cheyne-Stokes respirations. The best action for the nurse to take at this time is:
   - ○ a. Call a code blue and begin cardiopulmonary resuscitation.
   - ○ b. Call the physician and report the condition.
   - ○ c. Make sure the client's airway is open and begin supplemental oxygen.
   - ○ d. Give the ordered dose of 200 mg aminophylline intravenous piggyback (IVPB) now.

Integrated Concepts and Processes

The integrated concepts and processes component includes the following:

- Nursing process
- Concepts of caring
- Therapeutic communication
- Cultural awareness
- Documentation
- Self-care
- Teaching/learning

These concepts will be integrated throughout the examination and included as elements in the four needs categories.

Nursing Process

The nursing process has traditionally been a very important part of the NCLEX.

The NCLEX-RN, CAT uses the five-step nursing process: assessment, analysis, planning, intervention and implementation, and evaluation. Each of the questions that the graduate answers falls into one of these five categories. It is important that the graduate keep in mind the steps of the nursing process when answering questions. Often questions that ask "What should the nurse do first?" are looking for an assessment type answer because that is the first step in the nursing process. Questions on the nursing process are equally divided on the examination (approximately 20% in each category).

Assessment. The assessment phase primarily establishes the database on which the rest of the nursing process is built. Some components of the assessment phase include both subjective and objective data about the client, significant history, history of the present illness, signs and symptoms, environmental elements, laboratory values, and vital signs. Often the examination will ask the nurse to distinguish between appropriate and inappropriate assessment factors. An example of an assessment phase question is:

4. A client's respiratory status continues to worsen. Which of the following signs and symptoms would be most indicative of a deterioration of respiratory status?
   - ○ a. Increased restlessness and changes in level of consciousness
   - ○ b. Bradycardia and increases in blood pressure
   - ○ c. Complaints of chest pain and shortness of breath
   - ○ d. Rapidly dropping P_{CO_2} and pH

Analysis. The analysis phase of the nursing process involves developing and using nursing diagnosis for the care of the client. The NCLEX uses the North American Nursing Diagnosis Association (NANDA) nursing diagnosis system. Questions concerning nursing diagnosis often ask the graduate to prioritize the diagnoses. An example of an analysis phase question is:

5. A client is admitted to the unit with a diagnosis of bronchitis, congestive heart failure, and fever. The nurse assesses him as having a temperature of 101.8°F, peripheral edema, dyspnea, and rhonchi. The following nursing diagnoses are all appropriate, but which one has the highest priority?
   ○ a. Anxiety related to fear of hospitalization
   ○ b. Ineffective airway clearance related to retained secretions
   ○ c. Fluid volume excess related to third spacing of fluid (edema)
   ○ d. Ineffective thermoregulation related to fever

Planning. The planning phase of the nursing process primarily involves setting goals for the client. Included in the planning phase are such factors as determining expected outcomes, setting priorities for goals, and anticipating client needs based on the assessment. An example of a planning phase question is:

6. A client is found to be in respiratory failure and is placed on oxygen. Which of the following goals has the highest priority for this client?
   ○ a. Walk the length of the hall twice during a nurse's shift.
   ○ b. Complete his bath and morning care before breakfast.
   ○ c. Maintain an oxygen saturation of 90% throughout the shift.

○ d. Keep the head of the bed elevated to promote proper ventilation.

Intervention and Implementation. The intervention and implementation phase of the nursing process involves identifying those nursing actions that are required to meet the goals stated in the planning phase. Some of the material in the intervention and implementation phase includes:

• Provision of nursing care based on the client's goals
• Prevention of injury or spread of disease
• Therapy with medications and their administration
• Giving treatments
• Carrying out procedures
• Charting and record keeping
• Teaching about health care
• Monitoring changes in condition

An example of an intervention/implementation phase question is:

7. When the nurse ambulates a client who has been on bed rest for 3 days, he suddenly becomes very restless, displays extreme dyspnea, and complains of chest pain. Which of the following would be the most appropriate nursing action?
   ○ a. Call a code blue.
   ○ b. Continue to help the client walk, but at a slower pace.
   ○ c. Give the client an injection of his ordered pain medication.
   ○ d. Return the client to bed and evaluate his vital signs and lung sounds.

Evaluation. The evaluation phase of the nursing process determines whether or not the goals stated in the planning phase have been met through the interventions. The evaluation phase also ties the nursing process together and makes it cyclic. If the goals were achieved, it is an indication that the plan and implementation were effective, and new goals need to be established. If the goals were not met, then the nurse has to go back and find the difficulty. Were the assessment data inadequate? Were the goals defective? Was there a deficiency in the implementation? Evaluation is a continual process. Material in the evaluation phase includes comparison of actual outcomes to expected outcomes, verification of assessment data, evaluation of nursing actions and client responses, and evaluation of the client's level of knowledge and understanding. An example of an evaluation question is:

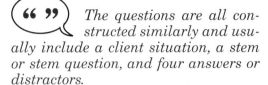

> *The questions are all constructed similarly and usually include a client situation, a stem or stem question, and four answers or distractors.*

8. A client is being prepared for discharge. He is to take theophylline by mouth at home for his lung disease. The nurse will know that her teaching concerning theophylline medications has been effective if the client states:

    ○ a. "I can stop taking this medication when I feel better."

    ○ b. "If I have difficulty swallowing the time-released capsules, I can crush them or chew them."

    ○ c. "If I have a lot of nausea and vomiting or become restless and can't sleep, I need to call my physician."

    ○ d. "I need to drink more coffee and cola while I am on these medications."

NCLEX EXAMINATION FORMAT

The NCLEX is a multiple-choice test taken on a personal computer. The questions are all constructed similarly and usually include a client situation, a stem or stem question, and four answers or distractors.

All the questions on the NCLEX stand alone, although a similar situation may be repeated. Occasionally a single question may be included without a case situation.

The graduate is asked to select the best answer from among the four possible choices. No partial credit is given for a "close" answer; there is only one correct answer for any particular question. The questions are totally integrated from the content areas previously discussed in the approximate percentages identified. Each question carries an equal weight or value toward the final score.

The graduate may take between 75 and 265 questions. There is a time limit of 5 hours for the entire examination, although there is no minimum time limit. The test is graded on a statistical model that compares the graduate's responses with a pre-established standard. The graduate who demonstrates a knowledge level consistently above that standard passes the examination.

Because the NCLEX-RN examination is given by computerized adaptive testing (CAT), the increase in the passing standard does not necessarily require a higher number of items to be answered correctly by the graduate. However, it does require that the graduate answer questions correctly at a slightly higher difficulty level than last year's graduates. Questions are assigned a difficulty value on a 7-logit (unit) scale called the NCLEX-RN logistic scale, ranging from the easiest (-3), which all graduates should answer correctly, to the most difficult ($+3$), which almost all graduates would be expected to miss (Box 9.1). The difficulty level of the questions is determined by the question writers and question reviewers.

The National Council again revised the passing standard of the NCLEX-RN CAT in 1998. The new passing standard is -0.35 on the NCLEX-RN logistic scale, 0.07 logit (unit) above the previous standard of −0.42. This increase is similar to past increases in the difficulty level that occurred in 1995 (0.06-logit increase) and in 1992 (0.04-logit increase).

The new passing standard was established by a nine nurse member panel that included diverse representation (regional, nursing specialty, minority, educator, new RNs) in conjunction with the results of a survey of nursing professionals such as nursing administrators of all types of facilities, and directors of nursing. After consideration of all the data, including current trends in health care, the National Council Board of Directors determined that safe entry level practice for RNs required a higher level of knowledge, skills, and abilities than was required in 1995. The passing standard and test content will again be evaluated in 2001 to maintain the current 3-year cycle of revision.

The NCLEX is given at Sylvan Learning Centers. After the graduates have completed the nursing program, they apply to the state board of nursing. Appointments at the examination sites are made on a first-come, first-served basis. The centers are required to schedule the examination within 30 days from the time the graduate applies. Each state establishes its own time interval for application after graduation, generally within 1

year. There are both morning and afternoon sessions of 5-hour duration. Depending on the size of the center, between 8 and 15 graduates may be accommodated at one time.

The computer skills required are minimal. After the graduate types in his or her name, address, and identification number, the only two keys that are used are the space bar and the enter key. All other keys are locked. The computer screen is split with the situation and stem question on the left side and the answers on the right (see example in Box 9.2). The space bar highlights a different answer each time it is pushed. When the graduate decides which answer is correct, he or she pushes the enter key. A message comes on the screen asking the graduate whether

BOX

9.2 Example of Computer Examination Question

A client is being prepared for discharge. He is to take theophylline by mouth at home for his lung disease. The nurse will know from her teaching that theophylline medications have been effective if the client states:

a. "I can stop taking this medication when I feel better."

b. "If I have difficulty swallowing the time-released capsules, I can crush them or chew them."

c. "If I have a lot of nausea and vomiting or become restless and can't sleep, I need to call my physician."

d. "I need to drink more coffee and cola while I am on these medications."

that is the desired answer. If yes, the enter key is pushed again. The question is replaced with another question and answers. No question is ever repeated, nor is the graduate able to change the answer once it has been selected.

The NCLEX is graded on a pass-fail basis. If the student has failed the examination, the entire examination must be taken again. The National League for Nursing (NLN) requires a 90-day waiting period before repeating the examination, and first-time takers are given preference over those who are repeating the examination. The results are sent to the graduate 7 to 10 days after the examination has been completed.

STUDY STRATEGIES

There are several ways to prepare for the NCLEX. To attempt to take the examination with an attitude of "if I don't know it by now, I never will" is to court failure. Carefully directed study and preparation will considerably increase the chances of passing the examination.

Review Books

The material covered by review books is the key material found on the NCLEX. These books usually follow the NCLEX Test Plan very closely. A review book is, however, just that; it reviews the material that graduates should already know. Reviewing is important to reinforce learning and recall unused information.

Review books are not really designed to present any new information about key material. If a graduate is totally unfamiliar with the material in a particular section of the review book, then reading a more complete textbook on that particular subject area will be necessary.

Another important function that a review book serves is to point out areas of weakness. If the graduate finds sections that seem to contain "new" material, it is important to investigate that particular section in more detail. If graduates find most of the material familiar and easy to grasp, then they are probably prepared for the NCLEX examination.

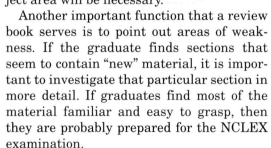
Review books are not really designed to present any new information about key material.

Group Study

Group study can be an effective method of preparation for an examination such as the NCLEX examination. To optimize the results of group study sessions, there are several rules that should be followed.

Rule 1. Be very selective when choosing the members of the study group. They should have a similar frame of mind and orientation toward studying. They should be nurses who are also going to be taking the NCLEX. The ideal size for a study group is between four and six people. Groups larger than six become difficult to organize and handle. After the group has been formed and has begun its study sessions, it may be necessary to ask an individual to leave the group for not participating or for being disruptive to the study process or displaying negative attitudes about the examination.

Rule 2. Have each individual prepare a particular section for each group study session. Study groups generally meet once or twice a week. For example, if next week the group is going to study the endocrine system, assign group member #1 the anatomy and physiology of the system, #2 the pathologic conditions, #3 the medications used for treatment, and #4 the key elements of nursing care. When the group comes together, have each individual present his or her prepared section. This type of preparation prevents the "What are we going to study tonight?" syndrome that often plagues group study sessions.

By following this process, the study group is organized and allows for more in-depth coverage of the topic. It also permits the members of the group to ask questions of the other members, thereby reinforcing the information being discussed.

Rule 3. Limit the length of the study session. No single study session should be longer than between 90 and 120 minutes. Sessions that go for longer tend to get off the topic and foster a negative attitude about the examination. Try to avoid making group study sessions into party time. A few snacks and refreshments may be helpful to maintain the energy level of the group, but a real party atmosphere will detract significantly from the effectiveness of the study session.

Individual Study

No matter what other study and preparation methods are used, individual preparation for the NCLEX is a necessity. This preparation can take several forms.

As previously discussed, use of a review book is valuable to indicate areas of deficient knowledge. Reading and studying the appropriate textbooks and study guides can be helpful if it is approached correctly. It is important that the graduate mentally organize the information being read into a format similar to that found in the NCLEX. After reading each page of a textbook or study guide, the graduate should be able to ask three or four multiple-choice questions about that information. These questions can be asked silently or actually written out, and should answer the question "How might the NCLEX test my knowledge of this material?"

A second and extremely effective method of individual study is to practice answering questions similar to those found on the NCLEX itself. When practice questions are answered, several important mental processes occur. First, the graduate is becoming more familiar with and therefore more comfortable with the format of the examination. In research, this process is termed the practice effect; it must be accounted for when analyzing the results from pretest/posttest-type research projects. Individuals will have better results after a test even without any type of intervention because of having practiced answering questions on the pretest. Similarly, the score on the NCLEX may increase by as much as 10% through answering practice questions.

A second result of answering practice questions is that it reinforces the information already studied. Although it is unlikely that a question on the NCLEX examination will be identical to a practice question, there are many similarities in the questions. Realistically, only a limited number of questions can be asked about any given subject. After a while, the questions will begin to sound very similar.

A third advantage of answering practice questions is that it reveals subject areas that will require more study. It is relatively easy to say, "I understand the renal system pretty well." It is quite another to answer correctly 10 or 15 questions about that system. If the questions are answered correctly, then the graduate can move on to the next topic. If the majority of the questions are missed, however, then further review is required.

In order to obtain the optimal benefit from working practice questions, it is probably best to spend 30 to 45 minutes each day working 10 to 20 questions rather than trying to do 100 questions on 1 day during the week.

After the questions are answered, the student reviews them and compares them with

> **" "** *An extremely effective method of individual study is to practice answering questions similar to those found on the NCLEX itself.*

the answers the study book provides. The student should also look at the rationales and the categories into which the questions fall.

Formal NCLEX Reviews

The NLN does not endorse or sponsor any review courses for the NCLEX directly, but many companies offer reviews shortly after graduation. However, the National Council of State Boards of Nursing began an online comprehensive review course for the NCLEX-RN examination in the spring of 1999 (http://www.nclex.com). These review courses range from 2 to 5 days and basically cover the information found in review books. They are rather expensive, and the quality of NCLEX reviews varies. In general they are only as good as the people who are presenting the material. Also, look at the reported pass rate of the graduates after they take the review. Those with higher pass rates are probably better.

> " " *Even though there may be client situations somewhere else in the examination that are similar to the one currently on the screen, avoid returning mentally to these previous items for help.*

TEST-TAKING STRATEGIES

The multiple-choice question test format is one of the most commonly used. Some individuals seem always to do well on multiple-choice question tests, whereas others seem to have problems with that test format. The individuals who always do well are not necessarily more intelligent; rather, they most likely have intuitively mastered some of the strategies or "tricks" necessary to do well on multiple-choice tests. Fortunately, once graduates become aware of these strategies and master them, they also will be able to score well on this type of examination format.

Knowing how to take a multiple-choice examination and optimizing the selection of the correct answers is a skill that can be mastered. When mastery of this skill is combined with knowledge of the key material, the probability of passing the NCLEX increases greatly. The following section lists and describes these important test-taking strategies.

Strategy 1. Read the client situation, stem question, and answers carefully. Many mistakes are made on this type of examination because the person taking the test did not read all parts of the question carefully. As you read the question and answers, try to understand what knowledge the question is asking for. As you did when reading the stem question, look for any key words, qualifiers, or statements that may help select the correct answer or eliminate the incorrect ones.

Strategy 2. Treat each question individually. Use only the information that is provided for that particular question in answering. Even though there may be client situations somewhere else in the examination that are similar to the one currently on the screen, avoid returning mentally to these previous items for help. You should also be careful about reading into a question information that is not actually provided. There is a tendency to recall exceptions or unusual clients that the nurse may have encountered. By and large, questions on the NCLEX examination ask for "textbook" levels of knowledge of the material.

Strategy 3. Monitor the time. Although the examination is not strictly speaking

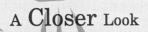

A Closer Look

A NEW GRADUATE'S PERSPECTIVE

I remember sitting in my first nursing class, listening to the Director of Nursing describe to what we were committing for the next 4 years of our life. She stood so confident, almost intimidating, as she described an overview of what we were expected to learn as nursing students. I experienced absolutely horrifying fear. As a result, one question kept coming to mind: "What am I going to do?" I considered running to the advisor's office and changing my major to Spanish, but I remembered why I wanted to be a nurse.

One evening I had to take my roommate to the emergency room. While I thumbed through a magazine in the waiting room, a man with a gaping wound in his forehead sat down next to me. Over it he held a small gauze pad, which a nurse had given him. I became curious: Couldn't that nurse have done something more for him? What other options were available? What would I have done in this situation? Sure that there was more to nursing than this, I enrolled myself in the Tulsa University nursing program.

Looking at the 4 demanding years of nursing school I have just completed, I have a better understanding of our director's confidence. After only three semesters of lectures and clinical practice, I felt very overwhelmed with the knowledge I was "supposed" to have. As a hands-on learner, I couldn't quite grasp the concepts our instructors tried to convey. I focused on practicing skills and learning techniques in clinical. I became a technician instead of a nurse until the day I had no choice but to become a nurse.

On that day, the reporting nurse stated that my patient had suffered a cerebrovascular accident (CVA) with right-sided weakness but was able to communicate her needs. She was to have an assessment done as well as an enema performed. I mentally planned how I would efficiently perform my skills in 4 hours, and set out for her room. Aphasia! Why hadn't I considered this in my plan? She motioned for me to come closer and began pointing to the phone. "Beer, beer, beer, beer," she said, as she pointed to the phone, the window, and then the phone again. I asked her if someone was going to call her, and she shook her head "no." She began pointing again, and as we both started to get frustrated, I told her I would return shortly.

I went to my instructor with tears in my eyes. "I can't understand!" I cried. She patted me on the shoulder and encouraged me to try. I returned, and after an hour of pointing and guessing, we succeeded. My patient wanted to call her daughter and wish her a happy birthday! I was excited that I finally understood what she was communicating, and she seemed grateful that I had tried. I confidently left clinical that day with a new understanding of what it meant to be a nurse.

As a new graduate, I realize that spending 1 hour communicating with a patient is an unrealistic goal for a nurse with 10 to 12 patients to care for within 8 hours. I have learned that balance is a key to safe, efficient, holistic nursing care. With the possibility of health-care reform approaching rapidly, flexibility in nursing will be vital. I am excited to learn all I can about future changes and growth in the nursing field to expand my current knowledge. Utilizing this knowledge base and my experiences as a student, I plan to continue delivering holistic care with confidence.

From Deming, Stacia: A new grad's perspective. The Oklahoma Nurse, April–June 1995, p. 16. Reprinted with permission.

timed, the graduate is never sure how many questions will need to be answered. If the graduate plans on taking all 265 questions in 5 hours, he or she will need approximately 70 seconds per question. Actually, most individuals who take this type of test average approximately 45 seconds per question, thus it is likely that the student will be finished well before the time limit is reached. Take a watch along to the examination. If any question takes more than 2 minutes, put an answer down and move on. Theoretically, the graduate could sit in front of the computer screen for 5 hours with the same question.

Strategy 4. An educated guess is better than no answer at all. There is no penalty for guessing on the NCLEX. If the graduate is unable to make any decision at all about the correct answer, he or she should just select one and move on. There is at least a one-in-four chance of choosing the correct answer. Statistically, answer *b* has about a 30% higher probability of being correct than any other. Wild guessing for large numbers of questions, of course, will have a negative effect on the total score.

Strategy 5. Use the process of elimination to select the correct answer. Usually there are one or more of the answers that can easily be identified as being incorrect. By eliminating these from the possible choices, the graduate will be better able to focus attention on the answers that have been identified as having some chance of being correct. Go back and read the stem question over again to try to determine exactly what type of information is being figured. If you are still unable to decide which of the remaining two answers are correct, select one and move on. Using this method increases the probability of choosing the correct answer to 1 in 2.

Strategy 6. Look for the answer that has the broader focus. Another method that may be used when the choices have been narrowed down to two is to examine the answers and try to determine whether one answer may include the other. The answer that is broader, that is to say includes the other answer, is the correct one. An example of this type of question is:

9. A client has been diagnosed as having Wolff-Parkinson-White (WPW) syn-

drome, type A. In evaluating the electrocardiogram (ECG), the nurse would note which of the following characteristics for this condition:
- ○ a. PR interval less than 0.12 second and wide QRS complex.
- ○ b. PR interval greater than 0.20 second and normal QRS complex.
- ○ c. Delta wave present in a positively deflected QRS complex in lead V_1 and PR interval less than 0.12 second.
- ○ d. Delta wave present in a positively deflected QRS complex in lead V_6 and PR interval greater than 0.20 second.

Strategy 7. Trust intuition. When a question and answers are read for the first time, an intuitive connection is made between the right and left lobes of the brain. The end result is that the first answer selected is usually the best choice. When a question is read too many times, the graduate may start to read into it elements that are really not there.

Strategy 8. Look for qualifying words in the question stem. There are some important words that can help determine what type of information is being elicited in the answer. Some of these words are:

First
Best
Most
Initial
Better
Highest priority

When words like these appear in the question stem, it is an indication that more than one of the choices are correct. The task then becomes to select the one answer that should be first or the answer that ought to receive the highest priority. An example of a "first" type of question is:

10. A 62-year-old client has a history of coronary heart disease. He is brought into the emergency room (ER) complaining of chest pain. The initial action taken by the nurse is to:
- ○ a. Give the client nitroglycerin gr 1/150 sublingual now.
- ○ b. Call the client's cardiologist about his admission.
- ○ c. Place the client in an elevated Fowler's position after loosening his shirt collar.
- ○ d. Check his blood pressure and note the location and degree of chest pain.

Strategy 9. Look for negatives in the question stem. Although there are very few negative questions on the NCLEX, negative words or prefixes in the question stem change how the correct answer is selected. Some common negatives include:

Not
Least
Unlikely
Inappropriate
Unrealistic
Lowest priority
Contraindicated
False
Except
Inconsistent
Untoward
All but
Atypical
Incorrect

In general, when a negative question is asked, it indicates that three of the choices are correct and one is incorrect. The incorrect choice is the answer. When a negative question appears, the test taker needs to ask: "What is it they don't want me to do in this situation?" An example of this type of question is:

11. A client is admitted to the medical unit. He is still having some mild chest pain. Which of the following medications would be inappropriate for relief of chest pain?
    ○ a. diltiazem (Cardizem)
    ○ b. propranolol (Inderal)
    ○ c. digoxin (Lanoxin)
    ○ d. meperidine (Demerol)

Strategy 10. Avoid selecting answers that have absolutes in them. Answers that have absolutes in them are almost always incorrect choices. Some absolute words to be aware of include:

Always
Every
Only
All
Never
None

Humans are very complex biochemical entities. Every person is different and almost every rule will have an exception. An example of this type of question is:

12. Which of the following is an accurate statement concerning cardiac chest pain in clients?
    ○ a. This pain is always caused by constriction or blockage of the coronary arteries by fat plaques or blood clots.
    ○ b. True cardiac pain is never relieved without treatment.
    ○ c. This type of pain is only relieved by nitroglycerin.
    ○ d. Clients often attribute the pain to indigestion.

Strategy 11. The answer that seems different is usually incorrect. The NCLEX is difficult because the material itself is difficult, but the examination is not designed to

be "tricky" or difficult for the sake of confusing the test taker. On the other hand, the test question writers are not going to make the correct answer completely obvious. Therefore, if one answer is much longer or shorter than the other three, it is probably not the correct choice. Be wary of answers that sound like they are trying to rationalize the correct choice by using a lot of explanation. Such answers are probably incorrect. You should also avoid answers that are different from the other three because of measurements or the way in which they are presented. An example of this type of question is:

13. A client has developed congestive heart failure. Which of the following would be the correct loading dose of digoxin (Lanoxin) for an adult client?
    ○ a. 0.75 mg divided into three doses every 8 hours.
    ○ b. 0.75 g divided into four doses every 8 hours.
    ○ c. 10 mg because the client is from a Native-American background and is a very large man, thus causing slow absorption of the medication.
    ○ d. 0.25 mg.

Strategy 12. Avoid selecting answers that refer the client to the physician. The NCLEX is for nurses and deals with conditions and problems that nurses should be able to resolve independently. The answer that refers a client to the physician is usually incorrect and can be eliminated from the choice selection.

Strategy 13. Avoid looking for a pattern in the selection of answers. The questions and answers on the NCLEX are arranged in a random fashion without any particular pattern. If something appears to be in a pattern, ignore it. Any pattern is just coincidental. For example, if question 6 had answer *a*, question 7 had answer *b,* question 8 had answer *c,* question 9 had answer *d,* question 10 had answer *a,* and question 11 had answer *b,* you might expect that question 12 would require answer *c.* This is probably not the case. Here is another example of a pattern-type situation that sometimes occurs with answers on this type of test. Questions 22 to 29 all have *c* as their correct answers. The answer to question 30 also seems to be *c,* but the tendency may be to not select it because of all the other choice *c* answers on the previous questions. The correct answer may very well be *c,* and if that is the best choice, go ahead and select it. It is important that each question be treated individually.

Strategy 14. *Do not panic* if a totally unfamiliar question is encountered. Examinations such as the NCLEX are designed so that it is very difficult, if not impossible, for anyone to answer all of the questions correctly. As a result, there are questions that are very complex, which deal with disease processes, medications, and laboratory tests that may be unfamiliar to the graduate. Questions like this may be encountered no matter how much review or study has been done.

Nobody knows everything! When encountering these types of questions, it is important to avoid panic. It is just one question out of many. Use some of the strategies already discussed in this chapter to select the best answer. Remember that nursing care given is very similar in many situations even though the disease processes themselves may be quite different. Select the answer that seems logical and involves general nursing care. Common sense can go a long way on this type of examination.

An example of this type of question is:

14. A 33-year-old African-American male client has been diagnosed as having a pheochromocytoma. Appropriate initial nursing care would involve:

○ a. Administering large doses of xylometazoline to help control the symptoms of the disease.
○ b. Monitoring his vital signs closely, particularly his blood pressure.
○ c. Preparing the client and family for the client's imminent death.
○ d. Having the family discuss the condition with the physician before informing the client about the disease, because of the protracted recovery period after treatment.

Strategy 15. When answers are grouped by similar concepts, activities, or situations, select the one that is different. If three of the four choices have some common element that makes them similar, and the fourth answer lacks this element, the different answer is probably correct. An example of this type of question is:

15. A female client has been treated for severe chronic emphysema for several years using bronchodilators and relatively high doses of prednisone (Deltasone). Which of the following activities would pose the least risk for this client in relation to the side effects of prednisone therapy?
○ a. Shopping at the mall on Saturday afternoon.
○ b. Spring-cleaning her two-story house.
○ c. Attending Sunday morning church services.
○ d. Serving refreshments at her 6-year-old son's school play party.

Strategy 16. Be positive about the examination! Motivational research has shown that people who have a positive attitude about an examination will score higher on the examination than people who are negative about it.

Conclusion

Taking and passing the NCLEX-CAT, RN is a necessary step in the process of becoming a professional registered nurse. Like all licensure examinations, its purpose is to protect the public from undereducated or unsafe practitioners. The examination is comprehensive and includes material from all areas of the graduate's nursing education. Although most graduates have some anxiety about taking this examination, knowledge about its format and content and strategies for taking the examination can lower anxiety to an acceptable level.

In addition, many of these test-taking strategies can be applied to the student's course examinations during the nursing program. Although nothing is as effective for passing an examination as paying attention in class, good note taking, and thorough study, awareness of these important test-taking strategies may improve the student's overall score.

Critical Thinking Exercises

✔ Obtain an NCLEX-RN, CAT review book. Analyze the questions in the practice examination for type, cognitive level, and level of difficulty.

✔ Identify three to five other students in your class with whom you would feel comfortable working in a study group. Organize a study group session before the next major course examination.

✔ When you get the results of your next course examination, identify why you missed the questions you did and what strategies might have been used to answer those questions correctly.

Answers to Questions in the Chapter

1. The correct answer is *d*. You either have or do not have the knowledge for this particular laboratory test.

2. The correct answer is *c*. Not only does the nurse have to know the normal values for each of the blood gas components given, he or she must also be able to use that information in determining the underlying condition.

3. The best answer to this question is *c*. Choices *b* and *d* are also actions that should be carried out, but at this particular time opening the airway and oxygenating the client must receive highest priority. Not only does this question require that the nurse know some specific facts (definitions of "cyanotic" and "Cheyne-Stokes respirations"), but it also requires that a decision be made about the seriousness of the condition (analysis) and a selection of the type of care to be given from several correct options (judgment).

4. The correct answer is *a*. The brain is one of the first organs to be affected by a decrease in oxygenation. Restlessness and changes in level of consciousness indicate this decrease. All the other choices are assessments for other conditions.

5. The correct answer is *b*. Nursing diagnoses that deal with airway always have highest priority.

6. The correct answer is *c*. Choice *a* is unrealistic for this client; choice *b* is not client-centered; and choice *d* is a nursing intervention, not a goal. Maintaining an oxygen saturation of 90% is realistic and within normal limits.

7. The correct answer is *d*. These are symptoms of a pulmonary embolism, which is a common complication of prolonged bed rest.

8. The correct answer is *c*. Answer *c* lists some side effects of theophylline medications that may indicate the onset of toxicity. The physician needs to know about these so that the theophylline level can be determined and the dosage adjusted accordingly. Other instructions that the client could be given when taking theophylline medications include to avoid excessive amounts of caffeine, never to suddenly stop taking the medication, to take it with a full glass of water and a small amount of food, and to watch for interactions with over-the-counter (OTC) medications.

9. The correct answer is *c*. Answer *a* may also be correct, but answer *c* includes the information in answer *a* and adds additional information. Again, reading all the answers carefully is essential before making a choice. Just reading answer *a* and selecting it without reading the rest of the answers would have led to an incorrect choice.

10. The correct answer is *d*. It is important to remember that when asked for an "initial" or "first" action to think of the nursing process. The first step in the nursing process is always assessment. If there was not an assessment-oriented choice, then look for a planning choice, and so forth. The other three answers provided for this question are also correct and should be done at some point, but in this particular situation, the first need is to assess his chest pain to determine whether it is indeed cardiac. Many other conditions can also cause chest pain.

11. The correct answer is *c*. Digoxin is a positive inotropic medication, which increases contractility and the oxygen demands of the heart. It is likely it would actually increase chest pain in this client. The other three medications all

relieve chest pain by somewhat different mechanisms. But notice that if the question was not read carefully and the reader missed the *in-* prefix of inappropriate, then certainly *c* would not have been selected.

12. The correct answer is *d*. The answers to this question very obviously demonstrate the "avoid the absolute" strategy. Coronary-type chest pain can also be caused by spasms of the coronary arteries as in variant angina (*a*). Chest pain sometimes can go away by itself, although it will probably return later (*b*). A number of medications will relieve chest pain besides NTG (e.g., morphine and narcotics, calcium channel blockers, and beta blockers) (*c*).

13. The correct answer is *a*. The loading dose for digoxin is usually three times the maintenance dose (0.25 mg) divided over 24 hours. Choice *b* is in a different measurement form (grams instead of milligrams); choice *c* should be avoided because it exemplifies the longer-than-average answer; and choice *d* is much shorter than any of the others. Look for one of the average-length answers to be the correct choice.

14. The correct answer is *b*. A pheochromocytoma is a tumor of the adrenal medulla that increases secretion of epinephrine and norepinephrine. One important result of having this type of tumor is that a hypertensive crisis may occur in some individuals. Monitoring the blood pressure would be an important nursing care measure. Assessment is also the first step of the nursing process and fits well with the qualifying word, *initial*, as used in the question stem.

15. The correct answer is *b*. In choices *a, c,* and *d,* there is the common element of groups of strangers. Because of suppression of the immune system, clients need to be protected from exposure to potential infections when they are taking steroid medications. Spring-cleaning her house, although strenuous, poses the least exposure to infection.

BIBLIOGRAPHY

Alfaro-LeFevre, R: Applying Nursing Process: A Step by Step Guide, ed 4. JB Lippincott, Philadelphia, 1998.

American Association of Colleges of Nursing: The Baccalaureate Degree in Nursing as Minimal Preparation for Professional Practice. AACN, Washington, DC, 1996.

Beeken, JE, et al: Teaching critical thinking skills to undergraduate nursing students. Nurse Educator 22(3):37–39, 1997.

Delegate assembly approves implementation of new NCLEX-RN test plan. Issues. National Council of State Boards 18:1–5, 1997.

Konradi, D, and Stockert, P: Preparing for the NCLEX-RN. Imprint 40(1):6–9, 1993.

McCloskey, JC, and Bulechek, GM: Nursing Interventions Classification (NIC), ed 2. CV Mosby, St. Louis, 1996.

National League for Nursing: Nursing Data Reviews. Division of Research, NLN, New York, 1995.

Passing standards revised for the NCLEX-RN examination. National Council of State Boards 18:5, 1997.

Update on NCLEX using computerized adaptive testing (CAT). Issues. National Council of State Boards 16:1–4, 1995.

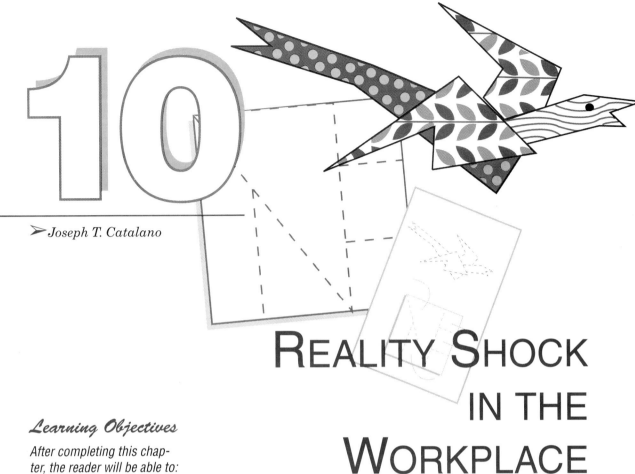

10

➢ *Joseph T. Catalano*

REALITY SHOCK IN THE WORKPLACE

Learning Objectives

After completing this chapter, the reader will be able to:

1. Describe the concept of reality shock.
2. Define burnout and list its major symptoms.
3. Discuss the key factors that produce burnout.
4. List the important elements in personal time management.
5. Analyze how the nurse's humanity affects nursing practice.
6. List at least four health-care practices nurses can use to prevent burnout and to improve their professional performance.

Most nursing students, if asked what they wanted most in the world, would likely answer, "to graduate and practice real nursing in the real world." To some extent, they are correct in assuming that the world of nursing school and education is not the real world. Although nursing school is demanding physically, mentally, and emotionally and raises the anxiety levels of nursing students a great deal, it is also a place where the student is sheltered from the realities of the workplace and provided with relatively clear goals for advancement. Students are given a constant stream of reinforcement and always have someone to turn to if they have a question. Things are different in the "real world." The transition from nursing student to registered nurse is referred to as transition shock or reality shock.

MAKING THE TRANSITION FROM STUDENT TO NURSE

At any point in their lives, most people fulfill several different roles simultaneously. For a nursing student, the biggest role conflict might occur during the transition from student to registered nurse. The roots of the conflict may lie in integrating three distinct aspects of any given role: the **ideal role image,** the **perceived role image,** and the **performed role image.**

In the academic setting the student is generally presented with the ideal of what a nurse should be. The ideal role projects society's expectations. It clearly delineates obligations and responsibilities as well as the rights and privileges that those in the role can claim. Although the ideal role presents a clear image of what is expected, it is often static and somewhat unrealistic to believe that everyone in this role will follow the expected patterns of behaviors.

The ideal role of nurse might require someone with superhuman physical strength and ability and unlimited stamina and also one who possesses superior intelligence and decision-making ability, yet remains kind, gentle, caring, and able to communicate with any client at any time. Ideal nurses function independently, know more than the physician, and are able to prevent the physician from making grievous errors in client care while continuing to be responsive to client requests and to carry out any physician's order with unerring accuracy and absolute obedience. Some perceptive students, early in their clinical experiences, may begin to suspect that this ideal role of nurse is not the way that it actually is in the real world.

The perceived role is an individual's own definition of the role, which is often more realistic than the ideal role. When individuals define their own roles, they may reject or modify some of the norms and expectations of society in establishing the ideal role. Intellectually, though, the ideal role is often used as the yardstick against which the perceived role is measured.

After a minimal amount of clinical experience, the nursing student may realize that nurses do not possess extraordinary physical strength or intellectual ability but may continue to cling to the idea. Many students accept unconditionally, as part of their perceived role, that nurses must be kind, gentle, and understanding at all times with all clients. The perceived role is the role with which the nursing student usually graduates.

Reality shock occurs when the ideal or perceived role comes into conflict with the performed role. The performed role is defined as what the practitioner of the role actually does. Many new graduate nurses soon realize that the accomplishment of role

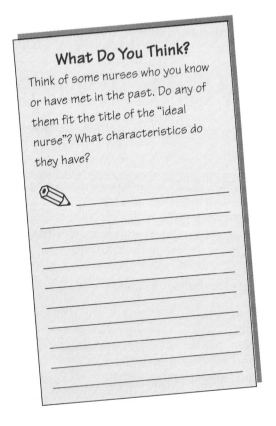

What Do You Think?

Think of some nurses who you know or have met in the past. Do any of them fit the title of the "ideal nurse"? What characteristics do they have?

expectations depends on many factors other than their perceptions and beliefs about how nursing should be performed. The environment has a great deal to do with how the obligations of the role are met.[1]

In nursing school, where students are assigned to care for one or two clients at a time, there is plenty of time to practice therapeutic communication techniques; to provide completely for the physical, educational, and emotional needs of the client; and also to develop an insightful care plan. The realities of the workplace may dictate that a nurse be assigned to care for six to eight clients at a time. In this situation, the perceived role of the nurse as an expert communicator may have to be set aside for the more realistic performed role of the nurse as expert task organizer. Meeting all the client's physical and emotional needs becomes impossible, and the care plan may be forgotten.

Such situations can produce what is called cognitive dissonance in many new graduate nurses; that is, they know what they should do and they know how they should do it, yet the circumstances do not allow them to carry it out. The end result is increased anxiety. High levels of anxiety, left unrecognized or unresolved, can lead to various physical and emotional symptoms. When these symptoms become severe enough, a condition called burnout may result.

The reality shock that new graduates often experience can be reduced to some extent. Recently, some schools of nursing have instituted a **preceptor** clinical experience during the last semester of the senior year. The main goal of this type of clinical experience, which occurs just before graduation, is

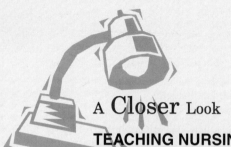

A Closer Look

TEACHING NURSING IN THE NEIGHBORHOODS—
THE NORTHEASTERN MODEL

Since September of 1991, the College of Nursing at Northeastern University has been actively developing educational partnerships with inner city neighborhoods in Boston. Students, teachers, health-care providers, and consumers collaborate in the development of mutually desired goals and objectives. Clinical interventions are conceived and developed to provide programs that benefit all participants. The philosophical foundation underlying the program is that client-centered health care, developed in this collaborative process, empowers both the nursing students and the residents of the neighborhood.

Why Should a Student's First Clinical Experience Be in the Community?

Because most nursing care takes place outside the hospital setting, students must learn to provide care within a variety of settings with patients, their families, and neighborhood members assuming a major responsibility for continuity of care. The education required to prepare students to provide this type of care requires the participation of both providers and recipients of care.

To successfully prepare for this level of practice, students must not only become capable of developing a process for continually learning throughout their careers but they must also be able to critically analyze their own experiences. Their learning process and clinical application must be grounded in reality.

When students have their first clinical experience in a neighborhood setting, it socializes them into a profession that regards health, not disease, as the paramount concern. During the first clinical course, health teaching and counseling are equally valued and promoted along with health assessment and the fundamentals of technical care. In subsequent courses, students continue to integrate advocacy, education, and counseling into their practice even as the required technical skills of patient care become more complex.

Assigning students to a neighborhood at their clinical site initiates the process of reality orientation as they begin to develop their skills in nursing care. Most students define what is normal and what they expect from patients by referring to their own experiences. Students who are provided with the proper tools and the opportunity to interact with residents and providers from different backgrounds are able to broaden their knowledge and insight.

The commitment of neighborhoods to this type of partnership is serious, yet at the same time, tenuous. A collective memory of prior incidents of exploitation by members of academia has left some suspicious. To demonstrate their genuine concern for the neighborhood and its residents, faculty, administrators, and students participate in a variety of activities such as community meetings, holiday parties, fund-raising activities, and food or clothing drives.

Structure of the Program

During the first clinical course, each neighborhood accepts up to eight new nursing students. After their first course, students return to the same neighborhood for subsequent clinical experiences. A neighborhood that stays with the partnership soon has students functioning at every level of the educational program. Each time students return, they offer more advanced nursing skills. Residents and providers within each neighborhood set high standards and take pride in the professional growth and development they observe in "their" nursing students.

By the time the students finish the program, they will have provided 50% of their clinical care in a specific neighborhood and 50% in Boston hospitals. Their concurrent professional development in both arenas of care enables students to identify and facilitate a continuum of care for their patients and their families.

What are the Outcomes of the Model?

The neighborhood/college of nursing partnerships have led both groups to develop a sense of mutual responsibility and ownership for providing quality health care and developing professional nurses. Although there is an acknowledged difference in motivation, each has a vested interest in the success of this joint venture. Participants share their joys and concern, while at the same time, negotiating grounds for continued participation.

Community residents and health-care providers are valuable sources of information for what students must know to provide quality care within their neighborhood. Then the clinical faculty develops teaching methods that meet both the learning needs of the students and the health-care needs of the neighborhood.

Students interact with residents as individuals, families, and groups, in homes, places of work, school, or worship and as residents conduct their business at laundromats, libraries, courthouses, and social clubs. Each interaction provides an opportunity for the practice of professional nursing.

Clinical nursing faculty and providers from a variety of disciplines working in the neighborhood assist students. Within a clinical course and across the curriculum no two students will have the same experiences, but each will have the opportunity to meet their educational objectives. Students are also encouraged to identify and develop specialized skills in areas of client need.

Value to the Residents

In just one neighborhood, during the past 6 years, students have had more than 17,000 client contacts. How that has influenced the health status of the residents is now being analyzed. Early indications are positive.

Clients have reported that their work helping students to identify and evaluate health-care needs and resources in the neighborhood has led to their increased self-esteem. They have developed a sense of pride as they learn that they have a unique knowledge to offer nursing students.

Value to the Student's Professional Development

Because of their increased understanding of their clients' living situations, students are prepared to ask realistic questions before they discharge a patient. Questions such as, "Will you have access to clean running water when you change this dressing?" and "How will you obtain your supplies and where will you store them?" have special relevance for a homeless person or family.

Students learn what it means to encourage a client to take a daily brisk walk and eat lots of fresh fruits and vegetables after they have walked with clients through high crime areas and understand there may be no grocery store closer than three bus transfers away.

Students experience frustration and understand the value of persistence when advocating for social services for their clients over the telephone. And student opinion is valued by staff and hospital educators who have enlisted them to provide information on topics such as the Women, Infants, and Children (WIC) nutrition program.

When students reach the senior level community nursing course, they come with experiences and skills that enable them to provide a level of care that was formerly expected only of graduate students. By the time they graduate, students have the opportunity to choose employment either in the community or in the hospital.

Value to the Clinical Faculty

Faculty have developed new colleagues both within and outside the university. Many unique opportunities for students have resulted from the shared responsibility for developing clinical sites within the neighborhoods. Guiding, teaching, and role modeling continue across disciplines and reinforce to students that lifelong learning is required of all professionals.

Some collaborative relationships have led to the clinical-based research projects with shared responsibility among community and university participants. Other projects have promoted interaction between faculty, graduate, and undergraduate students regarding a specific community issue or program.

Foundation for the Program

Nursing students learn about the many aspects of a neighborhood by building relationships with residents and their health-care providers and returning to the same area for clinical work across the curriculum.

- The collaboration between neighborhood residents and health-care providers and the college of nursing enriches the students' education.

- The collaborative process facilitates the opportunity for community residents and academic participants to learn more about each other's lives.
- Students learn to view health and illness in context, as part of the total experience of their clients' lives.

Clinical Scenarios

These scenarios portray three examples of nursing students' response to the directive to bring health care to every neighborhood, family, and individual. These cases document only a portion of the care provided by nursing students who are in the fifth week of their first clinical nursing course. Often this level of community-based nursing care is expected of students who are almost at the end of their educational programs.

Scenario 1

Allison is working with a nurse in the pediatric clinic of a neighborhood health center. One of the clients seen the previous day was Jeff, a 7-year-old boy with asthma. His mother expressed uneasiness with Jeff's condition. Allison calls the mother to make an appointment for a home visit today.

During the visit, Allison explores the mother's concerns, fills knowledge gaps, reviews Jeff's prescriptions and his use of them, assesses the home for possible asthma triggers, and develops a plan with the mother to put her more at ease about her son's condition. Allison receives permission from the mother to visit Jeff's school to continue the assessment. Before leaving, Allison makes an appointment with the mother to return in 1 week.

Allison returns to the health-care center and reviews the assessment data: the inhalers in the home are out of date, and Jeff has a cat. The mother's main concern is that Jeff will have an asthma attack while playing soccer or participating in some other activity and that he will die. The mother does not know who would take care of Jeff if he had difficulty at school.

Allison calls Jeff's school and makes an appointment to visit that afternoon. She schedules her visit so that she will have an opportunity to observe Jeff in the playground, meet with the principal to learn the protocol for care of children with asthma, and review the medications kept for Jeff's use at school. After school she talks with Jeff to learn how he feels about the asthma, whether he knows how and when to use the inhalers, and if he understands his mother's concerns. She also asks him what he thinks Allison might do to help.

Scenario 2

Jodi comes to work at the health-care center. She is obviously sick due to a head cold. Although she appears more miserable than she feels, she realizes that direct contact with patients might compromise their health status.

Jodi learns that one of the community organizers is meeting with a committee of local ministers concerned with violence in the neighborhood. She asks to accompany him to a meeting to represent health-care providers. During the meeting, the group discusses how they might successfully convince an international company to change the name of their latest product from Run and Gun to something less supportive of a violent interpretation. Strategies are developed; tasks are assigned; and the group meets again in 1 week to review their progress. Two weeks after the initial meeting, the group is notified by the corporation's lawyers that even though it will cost the company more than 1 million dollars to redesign the product and the advertising campaign, the name has been changed.

Scenario 3

Eliza is providing a series of range of motion classes to a group of older citizens at Day Activity Program. While talking with the clients, she reviews other aspects of their health. She learns that many of them will not be receiving flu shots because the local bus route does not travel to the site. When she asks the participants if they would get the injection if it were offered at the day program, she receives a positive response.

After the exercise program, Eliza calls the state department of Public Health to arrange for the necessary supplies for the flu clinic. She sets a date and time that fits the schedule of the seniors and then starts a publicity campaign. Flyers are made up in each of the five languages spoken in the neighborhood and distributed throughout the neighborhood. Pastors of the local churches are contacted and asked to encourage their parishioners to attend.

The nearest health-care center agrees to send a nurse to give the immunizations. On the day of the clinic more than 100 neighborhood residents appear. They enjoy drinks and cookies while the nurse explores other health-care needs with them. After the session ends, Eliza returns to each of the places that the flyer has been posted and removes it. This last activity demonstrates her respect for the environment of her clients.

Conclusions

Since starting this process 7 years ago, the members of the partnership have learned a great deal. One of the joys has been to watch the development of a model that has affected and enriched all participants in many more ways than we first envisioned. Yet, it remains a work in progress as new participants join the partnership. The basic concept of responding to real health-care needs means that the implementation part of the model is open to change. We may never sit back and say, "It is finished."

Is this an easy model of nursing education to develop and implement? No. Is it necessary to do all this? Yes, if we are going to prepare students to provide realistic and effective care in the developing health-care system.

Many educational institutions and communities have expressed an interest in obtaining our help to implement this model in their area. While responding to these requests, we continue to learn information that can be applied within our program.

to produce a type of anticipatory socialization into the role of registered nurse, in which the student is allowed to fill the requirements of an employment situation before actually graduating.

In the preceptor clinical experience, the student is assigned to one registered nurse for supervision for most of the semester. The student, who practices the role of the registered nurse, works the same hours and on the same unit as the nurse to whom he or she is assigned. As the role expectations of the workplace are absorbed by the student during the preceptor experience, the student's perceived role expectations also change, allowing movement from the student role to that of practicing professional with less anxiety and stress.

Internships are available to students between the junior and senior years at some hospitals. Internships allow the students to work in a hospital setting as nurses' aides, while permitting them to practice, with a few restrictions, at their level of nursing education. These experiences are invaluable for gaining practice in skills and for becoming socialized into the professional role.

EMPLOYMENT IN TODAY'S JOB MARKET

The health-care industry is currently in an upward trend in the employment of RNs that will continue for at least the next 10 years.[2] However, employers are still looking for the best of the best for the positions that they have available. In addition, **employers** are looking for graduates who can function independently, require little retraining or orientation, and can supervise a variety of less educated and unlicensed employees.

Although these requirements may seem daunting, some strategies can be used to increase the chance of being hired. Students should take advantage of preceptor and "extern" experiences in their senior year and attempt to meet their clinical obligations in the institution where they desire employment. In this way the student can evaluate the hospital closely and observe its working conditions and the type of care provided to clients. The hospital, on its part, has the opportunity to examine closely the student's knowledge, skills, personality, and ability to relate with clients and staff. The hospital benefits by getting **employees** who are familiar with the hospital before employment starts, thus decreasing the overall time of paid adjustment (referred to as "orientation").

Resumes

In today's job market, the **resume** is often the institution's first contact with the nurse seeking employment, and it has a substantial effect on the whole hiring process. First impressions are important. Preparing a neat, thorough, and professional-looking resume is worth the time and effort. If you have access to a computer, a good-looking resume can be prepared at almost no cost. If a computer is not available, it is a good idea to spend a few dollars to have the resume professionally prepared and reproduced.

The goal of a resume is to provide the hospital with a complete picture of the prospective employee in as little space as possible. It should be easy to read and visually appealing and have flawless grammar and spelling. Although various formats may be used, all resumes should contain the same information. There are many books available in local bookstores that can serve as a guide in organizing the information for a resume. This information includes the following:

> 66 99 *Although a friendly, rambling letter might provide insight into a prospective employee's underlying personality, most personnel directors or directors of nursing are too busy to read through the whole document.*

- Full name, current address (or address where the person can always be reached), and a telephone number (including area code).
- Educational background (all degrees), starting with the most recent first, naming institution, location, dates of attendance, and degrees awarded.
- Former employers, again starting with the most recent. Give dates of employment, title of position, name of immediate supervisor, supervisor's telephone number, and a description of the job responsibilities.
- Describe any scholarships, achievements, awards, honors, or activities that have been received, starting with the most recent.
- List professional memberships, offices held, dates of the memberships.
- List any publications. If both books and journal articles were published, list the books separately, starting with the most recent.

- Include an "Other" category to describe any unpublished materials produced (e.g., an internal hospital booklet for use by clients), research projects, **fellowships,** grants, and so forth.
- Provide professional license number and annual number for all states where licensed, along with the date of license and expiration date.

Each area of information should have a separate heading. References should be included on a separate sheet of paper. Most institutions require three references. After obtaining permission from the individuals listed as references, the nurse preparing the resume should make sure to have accurate titles, addresses, and telephone numbers. When selecting individuals for references, it is important that the individual know the applicant well, either in a professional or personal capacity, have something positive to say about the applicant, and be in some type of position of authority. It is best not to list relatives, unless the hospital is asking for a specific personal reference (Fig. 10-1).

A cover letter should be sent with every resume. Like the resume itself, it should be neatly typed without errors and should be short and to the point. Although a friendly, rambling letter might provide insight into a prospective employee's underlying personality, most personnel directors or directors of nursing are too busy to read through the whole document. The letter should be written in a business letter format and should include the name and title of the person who will receive the letter. Letters beginning "To Whom It May Concern" do not make a favorable impression. The statement of interest and the name of the position should constitute the opening para-

Mary P. Oak

100 Wood Lane, Nicetown, PA 22222   *   Telephone (333) 555-1234 (H)

Objectives

Obtain an entry-level position as a Registered Nurse; deliver high-quality nursing care; continue my professional development.

Skills

- Good organizational and time management skills
- Communication and supervisory ability
- Sensitivity to cultural diversity

Education

Mountain University, Nicetown, PA
Bachelor of Science in Nursing, May, 2001

Experience

Supercare Hospital, Hilltown, PA
Nursing Assistant, 1996 to present
  Responsibilities: Direct client care, including bathing, ambulation,
  daily activities, feeding paralyzed clients, assisting nurses with procedures,
  charting vital signs, and entering orders on the computer.

Big Bob's Burgers, Hilltown, PA
Assistant Manager, 1993–1996
  Responsibilities: Supervised work of six employees; counted cash-register
  receipts at end of shift; inventoried and ordered supplies.

Awards

Nursing Student of the Year, 1998
Mountain University, Nicetown, PA

Pine Tree Festival Queen, 1994
Hilltown High School, Hilltown, PA

Professional Membership

National Student Nurses Association, 1999 to present
Mountain University, Nicetown, PA

➤ Figure 10-1

Sample resume.

graph of the letter. The prospective employee should mention where he or she heard about the position. This should be included in this first paragraph as well as a date when the applicant would be able to begin working.

The second paragraph should give a brief summary of any work experience or education that qualifies the applicant for this position. Newly graduated nurses will have some difficulty with this part, but they should include their graduation date, the name of the school that they graduated from, and the director of the program. This paragraph should also state which shifts the applicant is willing to work.

What Do You Think?

Have you ever been on a job interview? What were some of the mistakes you made? How can you correct these mistakes in the future?

The third paragraph should be very short. It should express thanks for consideration of the nurse's resume and a telephone number. Both the letter and the resume should be sent by first-class mail in a 9″ by 12″ envelope so that the resume will remain unfolded, thus making it easier to handle and read (Fig. 10-2).

Waiting for a reply can be the most difficult part of the whole process. Resist the urge to call the hospital too soon. Because most health-care institutions recognize the high anxiety levels of new graduates, they return calls within 1 or 2 weeks after receipt of the application. If no response is given after 3 weeks, the nurse should call the hospital to see whether or not the application was received. Mail does get lost. If the application has been received, the applicant should make no further telephone calls. Harassing the personnel director or director of nursing about a job is not usually an effective employment strategy.

Interviews

The next important step in the process is the interview. The interview allows the institution to obtain a first-hand look at the applicant, as well as an opportunity for the applicant to obtain important information about the institution and position requirements. The interview often produces high levels of anxiety in new graduates, who are interviewing for what might be their first real job.

Again, first impressions are important. The interview starts from the moment that the applicant enters the office. Conservative business clothes that are clean, neat, and well pressed are recommended. Similarly, a conservative hairstyle and a limited amount of accessories, jewelry, and makeup produce the best impression. Smoking, chewing gum, biting fingernails, or pacing nervously do not make good first impressions. The interviewer recognizes that interviews are stress producing and will make

Mary P. Oak
100 Wood Lane
Nicetown, PA 22222

May 30, 2001

Mr. Robert L. Pine
Director of Personnel
Doctors Hospital
Gully City, PA 44444

Dear Mr. Pine:

I am interested in applying for the Registered Nurse position in the General Medical/Surgical unit. I have five years of experience in providing care for a variety of clients with medical/surgical health-care problems as a nursing assistant. I completed my baccalaureate degree in nursing on May 9, and am scheduled to take the NCLEX examination on June 3. Enclosed find my resume.

I believe that my organizational and time management skills will be a great asset to your fine health-care facility. I work well with all types of staff personnel, and having been a nursing assistant for the past five years, I can appreciate the problems involved in their supervision.

Thank you very much for consideration of my resume and application. I will call you within the next few days to arrange a date and time for an interview. Feel free to call me at home anytime (333) 555-1234.

Sincerely,

Mary P. Oak

➤ Figure 10-2

Sample cover letter.

allowances for certain stress-related behaviors. Arriving a few minutes early allows time for last-minute touch-ups of hair and clothes and gives the applicant a chance to calm down. Carrying a small briefcase with a copy of the resume, cover letter, references, and information about the hospital also makes a favorable impression.

Mental preparation is as important to a successful interview as physical preparation. Most interviewers start by asking about the resume, thus a quick review just before the interview is helpful. Expect questions about positions held for only a short time (less than 1 year), gaps in the employment record (longer than 6 months), employment outside the field of nursing (waitress, clerk), educational experiences outside the nursing program, or unusual activities outside the employment setting. Answer the questions honestly but briefly. Most personnel directors or directors of nursing are busy and do not appreciate long, detailed, chatty answers. Applicants can anticipate being asked:

* Why do you want this position?
* Why have you selected this particular facility?
* Why do you think that you are qualified for the position?
* What unique qualifications do you bring to the job to make you more desirable than other applicants?

Because of the emphasis placed on discrimination issues in recent lawsuits, there are a number of areas that prospective employers are not supposed to discuss, but sometimes do anyway. These include questions about sexual preferences or habits, age, race, plans for a family, personal living arrangements, **significant others,** and religion or political beliefs. If these questions are asked, the applicant needs to consider the implications of not answering them. Although there is no legal obligation for the applicant to answer, refusal to do so or pointing out that the question should not have been asked in the first place may be unwise. If these personal questions that violate an individual's right to privacy or seem discriminatory are answered by the graduate and then the graduate does not get the position, there may be grounds for some type of legal action.

At some point in the interview, usually toward the end, applicants are asked whether they have any questions. Although most do have questions, many applicants are afraid to ask. In fact, asking questions can be seen as a demonstration of independence, initiative, and intellectual curiosity, all traits that are highly valued by health-care providers. It is important that the first questions are not about salary, vacations, and other benefits. Questions that indicate interest in the institution would inquire about:

> **" "** *Asking questions can be seen as a demonstration of independence, initiative, and intellectual curiosity, all traits that are highly valued by health-care providers.*

* Responsibilities involved in the position
* Other staff or personnel involved in the area
* The client-to-staff ratios
* Requirements for rotating shifts, weekend obligations, and floating
* Opportunities for continuing education, **clinical ladder,** advancement, or movement to other departments
* Facility policies for employee health and safety

After these questions have been answered, the applicant may want to ask, in passing, about salary, raises, vacations, and other benefits. The applicant should also ask for written material on the nurse's contract

Issues

Powdered Latex Gloves: Rx for Disability

All employers are required to provide a safe and hazard-free environment for their employees. But what happens when a measure taken to protect the employee itself becomes a hazard to the employee's health?

With the discovery of human immunodeficiency virus (HIV) and recognition of its mode of transmission, health-care workers were required to wear latex gloves as part of the universal precautions taken to prevent the transmission of pathogens transmitted by blood and body fluids. However, as the use of latex gloves has grown, more and more nurses are becoming sensitized to the allergenic proteins in the latex. To compound this growing problem is the lack of knowledge many nurses have about latex allergies and their tendency to dismiss the symptoms they have as a simple skin rash, or hay fever, and self-treat it with lotion or creams.

Latex allergy follows a predictable progression of symptoms that will continue as long as the person is in contact with the allergin. The symptoms usually begins as a local irritation and itching on the skin of the hands. The irritation gradually progresses to hives and open lesions. Repeated exposure to the allergen then leads to asthma, watery eyes, and recurrent sinusitis and may eventually produce anaphylactic shock with continued exposure.

The initial allergy-producing culprit seems to be the latex-laden powder in the gloves rather than the gloves themselves. This powder contains microscopic particles of the latex protein, which over time and with continued exposure enter the pores of the skin and are absorbed into the body where the immune system reacts to them. Once there has been a primary immune reaction to the latex powder, further exposure to any type of latex triggers an ever-increasing immune response that can eventually produce the massive release of histamine causing the condition known as anaphylactic shock. Unless treated quickly and aggressively, anaphylactic shock often causes respiratory arrest and can be fatal.

A secondary problem only recently recognized is that once a person develops a latex allergy, exposure to even the microscopic particles of latex powder that become airborne whenever a coworker puts on or takes off a pair of powdered gloves can trigger a severe reaction. This powder can be carried through the ventilation system in the hospital, and circulate to parts of the building where gloves are not being used. Sensitized persons in these areas distant from the actual glove use can have severe reactions.

Although it is likely that there will always be some individuals who develop latex allergies, industry-wide limitation on the use of powdered gloves is an important step in preventing the initial allergy development. Also, early recognition of the symptoms of latex allergy is vital to the prevention of the progression of symptoms. Nurses who develop these symptoms should be referred by the employee health services to allergists who have experience in treating latex allergies. After nurses have been diagnosed with latex allergy, it is essential that they not wear latex gloves and that their coworkers not wear powdered latex gloves that release the latex particles into the air.

As with many workplace issues, it is essential that nurses become involved and take an active part in changing practices that put them at risk. Although slightly more expensive, most glove manufacturers now make low-allergen, powder-free gloves that provide as much protection as the cheaper latex gloves. Nurses have many possible avenues to change hospital policies and promote the use of these safer gloves. All health-care facilities have policy and procedures committees, safety committees, administrative committees, and so forth. If nurses become active members of these committees, and speak with a united voice, they can force the facility to change policies that in the long run will improve client care.

Data from Toland, P: ONA intensifies campaign against hazardous powdered latex gloves. American Nurse September/October 1997, p 13; Rodgers, B: Is health care a risky business? American Nurse September/October 1997, p 5; and Gritter, M: The latex threat. Am J Nurs 98(9):26–34, 1998.

with the agency, including benefits and job descriptions. Often the interviewer will provide this information without being asked in the course of answering some of the other questions.

It is appropriate to close the interview by asking for a tour of the facility. This allows first-hand evaluation of the workplace and a chance to observe the staff and clients in a real work setting. The interviewer may not be able to provide a tour at that time and so may ask another individual (e.g., a secretary) to take the applicant on the tour. It would also be wise to inform the interviewer of the dates scheduled for the National Council Licensure Examination (NCLEX) so that arrangements can be made for time off.

As with the resume, making frequent calls about the results of the interview is unwise. It is, however, appropriate for the applicant to send a letter within 1 week after the interview to thank the interviewer for his or her time and express how appreciative he or she is to be considered for the position. The applicant should also acknowledge how much it would mean to him or her to become a member of the staff at such a fine agency or hospital. If the position is offered, a formal letter of acceptance or refusal should be sent to the institution. Hospitals will not hold positions indefinitely, and failure to accept the position formally may cause the hospital to offer it to someone else. In today's health-care system, many applicants are often in search of a few positions.

ISSUES AFTER EMPLOYMENT

Burnout

Although it has existed for many years, the **burnout syndrome** has only recently been recognized as a problem that can be reduced or even prevented. A widely accepted definition of burnout is a state of emotional exhaustion that results from the accumulative stress of an individual's life, including work, personal, and family responsibilities. Although the term is not often applied to students, many of the symptoms of burnout can be observed in these aspiring nurses.

The people who are most likely to experience burnout tend to be more intelligent than average, hard-working, idealistic, and perfectionist. There are certain categories of jobs and careers that tend to produce a higher incidence of burnout: situations and positions in which there is a demand for consistently high-quality performance, expectations are unclear or unrealistic, there is little control over the work situation, and the financial rewards are inadequate. These jobs or careers tend to be very demanding and stressful, with little recognition or appreciation of what is being done. Also, jobs in which there is constant contact with people (customers, clients, students, or criminals) rank high on the burnout list.

Even with the most superficial knowledge of nursing, it is easy to see that many of these elements are present in the nurse's work situation. It is possible to recognize nurses who are in the early stages of burnout by identifying some classic behaviors (Box 10.1).

One of the earliest indications is the attitude that work is something to be tolerated, rather than eagerly anticipated. Nurses in the early stages of burnout often are irritable, impatient, cynical, pessimistic, whiny, or callous toward coworkers and clients. These pre-burnout nurses take frequent sick days, are chronically late for their shifts, drink too much, eat too much, and often are not able to sleep. Eventually, as their idealism erodes, their work suffers. They become careless in the performance of their duties, uncooperative with their colleagues, and unable to concentrate on what they are doing, and they display a general attitude of boredom and **apathy.** If allowed to continue, burnout may lead to feelings of helplessness, powerlessness, purposelessness, and guilt.[3]

BOX 10.1 Symptoms of Burnout

- Extreme fatigue
- Exhaustion
- Frequent illness
- Overeating
- Headaches
- Sleeping problems
- Physical complaints
- Alcohol abuse
- Mood swings
- Emotional displays
- Anxiety
- Poor-quality work
- Anger
- Guilt
- Depression

What Do You Think?

Do you have any of the symptoms of burnout either from school or your job? List the symptoms. How are you dealing with this problem?

Despite this bleak picture, nurses do not have to fall victim to the burnout syndrome. There are many nurses who practice their profession for many years, manage to deal with the stress, and find great personal satisfaction in what they do. These satisfied and motivated nurses have developed ways to deal with the stress of their careers while maintaining their goals and purpose as nurses.

The first step in dealing with burnout is to be able to recognize its signs. Many nurses who are burning out use denial and rationalization to block recognition of burnout, because it is just too painful for them to think that they put so much time, money, and effort into preparing for a career that they no longer want or enjoy. It is important to realize that it is not the career that is producing the burnout, but rather the difficulty in coping with the stresses the career is producing. Although it may not be possible to change the requirements of the profession significantly, it is possible to learn how to cope more effectively with stress.

Managing Stress and Time

Although there are many schools of thought about stress and time-management techniques, several common threads run through many of these theories. These views include setting personal goals, identifying problems, and using strategies for problem solving.

Setting Personal Goals

Goals and goal setting are an important part of client care. Nursing students—and by extension, practicing nurses—are highly proficient in the planning stage of the nursing process, in which goal setting is the primary task. They know that a good set of goals should be client centered, time oriented, and measurable and that they should write these goals with every care plan they prepare.

In their personal lives, however, these nurses may rush full-tilt into one erratic day after another, subordinating their own needs to the needs of others, working long, hard hours, but without accomplishing very much and feeling frustrated about it. What is the problem here? Very simply, nurses can prepare realistic, beneficial goals for their clients, but they seem to be unable to do the same for themselves.

Personal goals should include both long-term and short-term goals. Typically, personal long-term goals look into the future at least 10 years and include a statement about what the nurse wants to achieve during his or her lifetime. Some examples are going back to school to obtain an advanced degree, becoming a director of nursing, or even writing a book about nursing. Practicing nurses who are caught up in the whirlwind of everyday life find it difficult to formulate statements about the future. One other important characteristic of long-term

> ## What Do You Think?
> List your short-term and long-term personal goals. Are they realistic? How are you going to achieve them?

goals is that they need to be flexible. As life circumstances change, modifications are required.

Short-term goals are those that the nurse expects to accomplish in 6 months to 2 years. These goals should be aimed primarily at making the nurse's professional or personal life more satisfying and fulfilling. Like long-term goals, they do not need to be related to work. Perhaps visiting a foreign country, a skiing trip in the mountains, even learning how to paint a picture or play the piano may be achievable in a relatively short time. In the professional realm, joining a professional organization, becoming a head nurse, or changing an outdated hospital policy all are goals that can be achieved in a short time. The fact that everyone ages over time cannot be altered, but that time can also be used to achieve personal satisfaction in life and increase knowledge and accomplishments.

Although goal setting is an important first step in dealing with the stress that leads to burnout, any good nurse recognizes that a plan without implementation is useless. As difficult as goal setting may be for nurses, carrying it out may be even more difficult. Although goal achievement requires a degree of hard work and personal sacrifice, when people are working toward something they really want, the effort that it takes to achieve the end actually becomes enjoyable. At first glance, this process may seem like a lot of work (and it is), but it actually becomes an exciting adventure in its own right.

> **" "** *Although goal setting is an important first step in dealing with the stress that leads to burnout, any good nurse recognizes that a plan without implementation is useless.*

Identifying Problems

Another important step in dealing with burnout is to identify the actual problems that are producing the stress. Again, nurses are taught as students that they need to identify client problems so that they can work toward solving them. Formulation of a nursing diagnosis is nothing more than precisely stating a client's problem. One thing that nurses realize early in the learning process is that what may appear to be an obvious problem may in reality not be a problem at all (Box 10.2). And, conversely, something that may only be mentioned in passing by a client may turn out to be the real source of the client's nursing needs. Perhaps nurses should look at their own lives and attempt to formulate nursing diagnoses that deal with their stress-related problems (setting the North American Nursing Diagnosis Association list aside).

For example, a new graduate has just completed a shift where he has been assigned to eight complete-care clients. He has had to supervise two badly prepared nurses' aides and has put in 55 minutes of overtime (for which he will not be paid) to complete the charting. This nurse is feeling tired, frustrated, and even a little bit guilty because of an inability to provide the type of care that he was taught in nursing school. What is the problem? A possible nursing diagnosis might be: Alterations in personal satisfaction related to excessive workload, evidenced by sore feet, headache, shaky hands, feelings of guilt, frustration, and small paycheck.

Now that the problem has been identified, goals and interventions can be introduced to solve the problem. The goals may range from organizing time better to refusing to take care of so many complete-care clients. Interventions, depending on the goals, can include activities such as attending a time management seminar, talking to the head nurse, or changing a policy in the policy and procedure book.[3] Nurses already

BOX

10.2 It Isn't Always What It Seems to Be

My heart sank. The list of assignments for my clinical section was posted, and next to my name was "Room 234—Paulo Simonetti, 72—CHF." As the only male nursing student in a class of 58 students, I had become used to being assigned difficult, very large or highly hostile clients, or any combination thereof. My fellow students had been discussing Mr. Simonetti that morning before classes, and the general conclusion was that he was a demanding "dirty old man" who liked to fondle the young female nurses. I tried to think back to where this topic was covered in my course work, but couldn't remember it ever being discussed.

I carefully went through his chart gathering the appropriate data for my care plan. Then I went to visit him to obtain some of the subjective assessment data that can only be gotten through a direct interview. The gods smiled on me that day.

He was asleep, and his nurse admonished me not to wake him because of his weakened state. A reprieve.

The next day dawned clear and cold. I hardly noticed. That night had been one of the longest in my life—stretched by little sleep and lots of worry about what I was to face the next day. The little "call-in-sick" voice of my subconscious was starting to get very loud, but my instructor's admonition that the only excuse for not coming to clinical was death (mine) with a 48-hour prior notification outweighed that temptation.

Change-of-shift report that morning seemed much too short, and then I was out on the floors. Let's see, I need to check my medications, look through the chart for any changes in physician orders or lab results, make sure the care plan and kardex are current.

My instructor wants to know why I've been out of report for 30 minutes and haven't checked on my patient yet. "I was just on my way" seemed like a good answer.

When I walked into his room, his bed was empty. Another reprieve? Hardly. His roommate said he was in the bathroom and should be out any time now. I wanted to run. I wanted to hide. I wanted . . . the door to the bathroom began to open. I took a deep breath and said, "Hi, Mr. Simonetti, my name is Don and I am going to be taking care of you today."

Without a word, he walked over to me, wrapped his ample arms around me and gave me a bear hug. Then he said in heavily accented English, "Thank you, I'm happy to meet you."

A bit surprised, I responded, "I thought you were only supposed to hug the girls?"

He replied, "I hug everybody!"

At that point, it became clear to me where Mr. Simonetti's reputation had originated. In his Italian background, greeting people with hugs and the physical demonstration of affection were a natural part of his behavior. In our more aloof American culture, actions that would be a natural part of his behavior could be easily misinterpreted as sexual advances. Coupling that with the fact that his English language skills were limited would only deepen the misunderstanding.

The nurses would respond to his behavior by avoiding him. His response to the nurses' avoidance was to put his call light on frequently. The call light often went unanswered for long periods of time. Mr. Simonetti's response to the unanswered call lights was to yell loudly for a nurse. Thus a reputation is born.

10.2 It Isn't Always What It Seems to Be *(continued)*

My day with Mr. Simonetti was very pleasant, hugs included. I never was able to get all the background data for the subjective portion of the care plan because of the language difference, but the communication was sufficient for the normal daily care activities. I even convinced one of my more adventurous female classmates to come in and get a hug.

Probably the most important lesson I learned that day was that you need to form your own opinion about clients based on your own observations. Client behavior, like all human behavior, is very complex and often defies simple explanations. Appreciation of a client's culture and their ways of expression is essential in providing high-quality nursing care.

know the nursing process as a client problem-solving technique. Why not apply the same knowledge and skills to personal problems? The stress level only increases if problems are left unsolved.

Strategies for Problem Solving

Although specific problems may require specific solutions, several widely accepted methods exist to deal with the general stresses produced by everyday work and personal life. Included in these methods are activities such as recognizing that nurses are only human, improving time-management skills, practicing what is preached, and decompression.

Improving Time-Management Skills. In modern life there is often not enough time to do everything that needs to be done. The key to time management is setting priorities. In the world of nursing and client care, nurses are often required to do many tasks. Multitasking, the process of doing several tasks at the same time, tends to fragment the nurse's attention and concentration. Nurses need to recognize that only some nursing activities are essential to the safety and well-being of clients. These include ensuring that the clients get their medications on time, that their comfort needs are met,

and that accidental injuries are prevented. Beyond these actions, nurses really have a great deal of discretion in what they can do when providing care to clients.

Burnout results mainly from personal and professional dissatisfaction. If nurses feel fulfilled in what they are doing, burnout is much less likely to occur. Activities that may increase nurses' satisfaction include spending time talking with clients, learning new skills, and decreasing the anxiety of families through teaching and listening. After such activities have been identified, time should be set aside for them during the shift. The real secret in using time management to prevent burnout is for the nurse to use the time left for those nursing activities that bring the most professional and personal satisfaction.

Several skills need to be developed to be able to allow time during a shift for these preferred activities. First, the nurse must learn to delegate by letting the licensed practical nurses (LPNs) or aides do those tasks that they are supposed to be able to do. Many nurses graduate from nursing school with the attitude that if you want it done right, you need to do it yourself. After becoming familiar with the LPN and nurse's aide job descriptions, nurses need to give others a chance to prove themselves.[3]

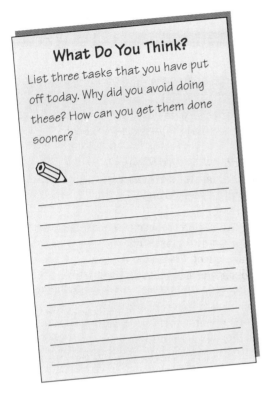

What Do You Think?

List three tasks that you have put off today. Why did you avoid doing these? How can you get them done sooner?

Another necessary skill is overcoming procrastination. Most people have a natural tendency toward procrastination, particularly when unpleasant or difficult tasks are involved. The primary reasons that people postpone or delay doing something is because they either do not want to begin or do not know where to begin the task. More time and energy are expended in inventing excuses for putting off tasks than would actually be taken in doing the task.

The best way to overcome procrastination is by starting the task, even if it is only a small step. An effective method is to select the most distasteful task to be done that day and to commit just 5 minutes to it. After 5 minutes are over, the task can be either set aside or continued. It is very likely that once the task is started and momentum builds, the task will be carried to completion.

Tasks can be prioritized by listing them in three categories. Category A tasks (e.g., passing out medications, treatments, and dressing changes) are those that need to be completed on time. Category B tasks (bath, linen change, lunch break, charting) can be postponed until later in the shift. Category C tasks (cleaning up the room, attending to personal grooming tasks other than those that are absolutely required) are tasks that can wait until the next day.

For daily tasks, both pleasant and unpleasant, the best time to do them is immediately. If achievement of the plan requires delegation, then it needs to be done at the beginning of the shift, not at the middle or end of the shift. Often nurses have a built-in fear of taking chances; as a result, they avoid doing things where there is a chance for failure in the hope that somehow the problem will resolve itself. Any time that an important decision is made, there is a chance that someone will disagree or that the decision will be incorrect. These types of situations need to be viewed as a challenge or an opportunity, rather than life-altering risk to be avoided. Although mistakes in health care do have the potential to be fatal, learning from mistakes is one of the most fundamental ways of increasing knowledge.

Time management, like other skills, requires some practice. Once a nurse masters this skill, his or her life becomes more satisfying.

Practicing What Is Preached. Because nursing is oriented toward keeping people healthy as well as curing illness, nurses spend a large amount of their time teaching clients about eating well; getting enough sleep; going for regular dental, eye, and physical examinations; avoiding too much drinking and smoking; and exercising regularly. It might make an interesting project for a student taking a nursing research course to have nurses rank themselves on how well they have incorporated these health maintenance activities in their own lives. The results would probably indicate a low overall score on the "practice what you preach" scale.

Nurses know all about the food pyramid, but they do not translate that knowledge into feeding themselves properly. In reality, there are going to be some busy days when it is impossible to eat right. But it should be possible, at least occasionally, to follow a diet that will promote health and reduce the buildup of fat plaques in the arteries.

It is important to get enough sleep to avoid chronic fatigue. People can adjust to a state of fatigue, but it tends to decrease the enjoyment that they find in life, as well as make them irritable, careless, and inefficient. Most people need between 5 and 8 hours of good-quality sleep each night. It also probably would not hurt for nurses to take a short nap during the afternoon on their day off.

Many nurses feel that they get enough exercise during their busy shifts. And, in truth, the average staff nurse will walk between 2 and 5 miles during each 8-hour shift. Unfortunately, this type of walking does not qualify as the type of aerobic exercise recommended for an improved cardiovascular condition. Exercise, in order to be beneficial, must be done consistently and must raise the heart rate above the normal range for an extended period. The short sprint-type walking involved in client care does not accomplish this goal.[4]

Walking 1 or 2 miles a day outside the hospital is a beneficial, simple exercise that will improve health. Nurses can also use a wide variety of exercise equipment for those days when walking outside is undesirable. The important requirement is that the exercise be done consistently and frequently. Regular exercise not only improves the cardiovascular system but also helps improve stamina, raise self-image, and promote a general sense of well-being.

Decompression. *Nurses Need Time to Decompress.* The profession of nursing is stressful, even under ideal circumstances. Nurses are required to deal with other people constantly and to carry out numerous tasks that are potentially dangerous. At the end of any shift, even the most skilled and best-organized nurse has a sense of internal tension. This tension must be released or it will eventually cause a major explosion or (if turned inward) produce anxiety.

Establish a Daily Decompression Routine. It may take a little time for an individual to discover, through trial and error, what works to reduce the tension built up during the shift. Some effective techniques include setting aside approximately 30 minutes of private, quiet time during which the nurse can dream and reflect about the day's activities. Perhaps relaxing in a tub of hot soapy water or sitting in a favorite reclining chair might meet the nurse's need for decompression. Relaxation activities, such as swimming, shopping, or even going for a drive, can

What Do You Think?

How do you feel after a busy day at school or work? What type of tension-lowering activities do you participate in?

10.3 Prayer: A Potent Factor in Healing

Science and religion have come full circle. Many ancient cultures believed that disease and illness could be cured by prayer. As mankind took a more rational viewpoint, knowledge and science looked for a medical cure for disease and illness and came to view prayer as a meaningless ritual. In his book, *Healing Words: The Power of Prayer and Medicine,* Larry Dossey, MD, demonstrates that prayer is a potent force in producing healthy physiologic changes in clients.

Although many in the examination professions are hesitant about mixing prayer and medicine, evidence indicates that prayer can improve and sometimes even cure a client's condition. These positive results do not necessarily occur as a result of the client's own beliefs, faith, or hopes that healing will occur. In double-blind studies conducted by Dr. Dossey, clients receiving prayer who did not know they were being prayed for had higher rates of improvement. This evidence seems to eliminate the factors of positive thinking and placebo effects as elements in the clients' improved conditions.

Nurses find the data about prayer and cure fascinating and view it as a way to enhance recovery in clients in critical care units and to increase the healing rates of wounds and other disease states. Nurses also recognize the important part prayer can play in their own lives in dealing with the stress of a physically, mentally, and spiritually demanding career. Quiet periods of meditation, even if only a few minutes each day, can help the nurses avoid the burnout syndrome and rejuvenate their professional dedication.

From Dossey, L: Healing Words: The Power of Prayer and Medicine. Harper, San Francisco, 1993, as printed in AACN News, February 1995, p 1.

---

help reduce tension and act as a time for decompression. Of course, stress-management techniques learned at seminars (e.g., self-hypnosis or meditation) can be used by those who have developed these skills (Box 10.3). Finally, meeting with a nurse support group can help the nurse to vent feelings and make constructive plans for solving problems.

Nursing Shortage/Oversupply Cycle

The lack of qualified nurses has been present in the health-care system for so long that the term *nursing shortage* has become a truism. However, as recent history has demonstrated, the demand for nurses increases and decreases with changes in the health-care system. In addition, the demand for nurses is to some extent regional. Some areas of the country will have a sharp demand for registered nurses, and other areas have an oversupply, with few available jobs. However, studies about employment opportunities project that there will be a shortage of nurses well into the twenty-first century.[2]

This variability in the demand for nurses has placed high-school counselors and employment agencies in an uncertain position. Encouraging young people to enter nursing schools increases enrollment. However, recently there has been a downward trend in all types of nursing school enrollment, which is reflected by decreased numbers of applicants and fewer graduates. Although disappointing to nurse educators, this drop in enrollment has been seen in the past when the economy was strong. Simply stated, when the economy is strong, there are more opportunities outside of the traditional female employment areas for young women to pursue. Also, overall enrollment in higher education also decreases during periods of strong economic growth.

There are many reasons for the decrease in professional nursing positions that occurred in the past. The primary reason is increased concern for cost reduction in the health-care system. Although no comprehensive **national health insurance** or health-care reform bills have ever been passed, the writing is on the wall. Health care is going to have to become more efficient and to reduce the cost of operations. One of the most obvious places to cut costs is in personnel. Although a reduction in nursing positions may greatly reduce the costs in the short term, health-care facilities are finding that the long-term effects to the quality of health care are devastating. It is obvious that exchanging qualified nurses for lower-paid unlicensed technicians will eventually have an effect on the quality of client care.[5] When quality of client care goes down at a facility, so does the number of clients seeking care there (Box 10.4).

Certain groups of nurses are in higher demand than ever, such as nurses who can practice independently in several different settings, **multi-skilled practitioners,** home care nurses, community nurses, and hospice nurses.[6] A major trend in health care today is to move the care out of the hospital and into the community and home settings. Provision of nursing services in these settings often requires that a nurse have at least a bachelor's degree or even higher education. Fewer than 50% of all new graduate nurses today are graduating from bachelor's degree programs.[7]

Another area of health care in which there is no oversupply of nurses is in the realm of the nurse practitioner. Advanced practice nurses are able to provide various services that were traditionally kept within the physician's scope of practice.

Although most nurse practitioners are currently based in community clinics, there is an ever-expanding opportunity for them to become involved in the care of hospitalized clients. A key element in many of the proposed health-care reform plans is that clients would be required to be evaluated by a primary health-care provider before they could be referred to secondary health-care providers or specialists. The advanced-practice education of nurse practitioners would make them eminently qualified to fill this role of primary health-care provider.

Certain specialty areas (e.g., intensive care units, neonatal units, and burn units) are always seeking nurses. As with community nurses, nurses who provide care in specialty units must be able to work independently and to draw from a large base of theoretical knowledge.

Although an oversupply of nurses may at first glance appear to be harmful to the profession, it can also be considered as an opportunity to improve the quality of the nursing profession. During periods of nursing shortage, there was, and continues to be, a great impetus to turn out more nurses with less and less education, even though advances in technology and changes in society require that nurses have more education. When an oversupply occurs, this situation may offer nursing a chance to regroup, reorganize, and regain the professional status that it has long been seeking. It may also lead to expanded roles for nurses in the future.

Nursing education must pay attention to these trends and prepare nurses for ex-

 Although an oversupply of nurses may at first glance appear to be harmful to the profession, it can also be considered as an opportunity to improve the quality of the nursing profession.

BOX

10.4 'Magnet Hospitals' Tout Nursing Quality

Hackensack University Medical Center in North Jersey flies green-and-yellow flags to broadcast the nursing seal of approval it has won.

Robert Wood Johnson University Hospital in New Brunswick, N.J., which also earned the distinction last month, is mounting an advertising campaign to showcase the nurses.

The two hospitals are among the first in the nation to meet new voluntary quality nursing standards drawn up by a division of the American Nursing Association (ANA). They have earned the designation of "magnet hospital" for outstanding nursing care.

The standards, which measure everything from how much time nurses spend with patients to how many patients get bedsores, come at a time when cost cutting by hospitals is leaving both health-care workers and patients wondering whether quality is on the decline.

Each time there's an announced layoff, like at Allegheny University Hospitals earlier this fall, nurses are quick to warn that care could surely suffer.

"Nurses feel hospitals are being gutted," said Linda H. Aiken, director of the Center for Health Services and Policy Research at the University of Pennsylvania.

The ANA hopes that its nursing seal of approval will come to be recognized as a credible measure of quality, reassuring patients and making hospitals more accountable.

Jennifer Mathews, who oversees the ANA's American Nurses Credentialing Center, said studies show that patients fare better and are more satisfied at hospitals with the type of care her group is promoting.

At ANA-credentialed hospitals, nurses "are empowered to give old-fashioned hands-on care," Mathews said. Patients "are guaranteed to have a listener and someone who responds."

But some experts are skeptical, questioning whether the ANA's credentialing program is merely a veiled attempt to protect nursing jobs.

In recent years as hospitals adapted to the cost-conscious managed-care environment, the average nurse has become responsible for more patients, Aiken said. Instead of adding more nurses, hospitals often assign less-skilled workers to tasks once done by nurses, such as tube feedings and getting patients out of bed after surgery.

Many nurses say the changes are bad, but hospital executives say they are delivering good medical services while adjusting to the new economic realities.

"Clearly, we would be concerned if the motivation behind this [credentialing process] was something unrelated to patient-care issues and was more related to locking into place particular standards of nursing care," said Andrew Wigglesworth, president of the Delaware Valley Healthcare Council.

"Whether or not they are necessarily the most impartial organization to review nursing care in hospitals is obviously a question."

Other experts say the ANA's standards will simply pose more paperwork and add new costs for hospitals, which already must comply with numerous standards—including nursing—set by government agencies, managed-care firms, and other medical organizations.

"The last thing a hospital needs is more oversight," said Gerald Katz, a health-care consultant in Plymouth Meeting. "It is not productive."

10.4 'Magnet Hospitals' Tout Nursing Quality *(continued)*

Still, more than 70 hospitals have asked the ANA's credentialing center for applications for the voluntary program. So far, seven of 15 hospitals that have formally applied have passed the review process. None is in the Philadelphia area.

Depending on its size, a hospital will spend between $1,000 and $7,500 to have its application reviewed. As part of the process, the hospital undergoes a two-day site visit.

The standard setting represents "an important countermovement in nursing," said Donald Light, a professor of comparative health care at the University of Medicine and Dentistry of New Jersey.

"Identifying hospitals of nursing excellence is a way to assure that patients get excellent nursing care," he said, "and assure the nursing profession that its professional status does not get diluted" by changing job descriptions.

The ANA's program is one of several new efforts to assess whether the changing health system is giving good care. The American Medical Association just launched an accreditation program that it hopes will become the national standard of physician quality. And the ANA's credentialing body plans to expand the program to long-term care facilities.

"The public has grown increasingly apprehensive," said Ron Pollack, executive director of Families USA, a national group for health-care consumers. "The expansion of managed care and the fears generated by economic incentives, which now focus on withholding care as opposed to providing care, have made the public far more sensitive to quality issues."

But, he said, the many measures to distinguish between good and bad are "really in their infancy." And the public, he said,

has trouble understanding much of the information already available.

The concept of credentialing hospitals based on nursing care had its origin in the 1980s, when there were nursing shortages. Nursing groups studied why some hospitals could recruit and retain nurses and others could not. They discovered that nurses were attracted to so-called magnet hospitals, where they had more time with patients and more control over resources.

Subsequent studies showed that those magnet hospitals had fewer patient deaths, a lower nurse-burnout rate, and higher patient satisfaction, said Aiken, the author of several of the studies. In 1993, the American Nurses Credentialing Center used the findings to start developing standards.

"One of the hallmarks of a magnet hospital is that every patient has a defined, specific nurse who is responsible for their care over the entire admission," Aiken said. "The case management is what leads to better outcomes."

In considering a hospital's application, the credentialing group assesses whether nurses are among the executive leadership, can update their education, have a low turnover rate, and are given enough resources to do their jobs. The standards also look at specific indicators of good nursing care, such as lower rates of infections and bedsores.

In a 1992 study of 20 hospitals, Aiken said, the average cost of caring for a patient was not any greater at hospitals that had the kind of nursing called for by the new standards.

"It is a positive example of how hospitals can organize within their existing resources to provide the best possible care," she said.

Hospital officials say having ANA-approved status tells the community that a hospital is somehow different. And officials are not shy in bragging about it. After Inova Fairfax Hospital in Virginia won approval earlier this year, it took out a full-page newspaper ad that listed the names of its 1,700 nurses.

Since Hackensack University Medical Center earned the designation two years ago and began to market it with colorful flags, more than a dozen of its competitors have inquired about how to acquire magnet status, according to officials at the ANA's credentialing center.

But nurses say it isn't all show.

"You would hear patients say, 'The care here is different,'" said Vickie Mullins Moore, chief nursing executive at St. Joseph's Hospital of Atlanta, which earned the nursing seal of approval in 1996. "I feel people care about me and whether I get well or not. I am not a case or on an assembly-line production."

From Uhlman, M: Magnet hospitals tout nursing quality. The Philadelphia Inquirer, December 6, 1997, p A-1. Reprinted with permission from The Philadelphia Inquirer.

panded roles in the community. Professional nurses who are not employed in the community will most likely find challenging and meaningful careers in the specialty units of large urban hospitals. The few nurses who are employed in community hospitals will likely be in positions in which they are supervising a number of unlicensed workers. Many of the other jobs currently filled by nurses will be taken over by lower-paid technicians.

Conclusion

Although transition shock and burnout are realities of the nursing profession, they can be reduced or even avoided altogether. Nurses should be able to recognize the causes and early symptoms of transition shock and burnout in order to prevent them from developing into a problem. Therefore, nurses should use techniques to prevent these disorders from becoming insurmountable obstacles. In doing so, nurses will be able to practice their profession proficiently and gain the satisfaction that only nursing can provide.

Critical Thinking Exercises

✔ Make a list of the characteristics that would be found in the "perfect nurse." Make a second list of characteristics found in nurses observed in actual practice. Discuss how and why these lists differ from each other.

✔ Outline a plan for implementing a preceptor clinical experience for the senior class of a nursing program. Make sure to include how many hours of practice are required, criteria for the selection of preceptors, student objectives from the experience, and methods of evaluation.

✔ Write at least three long-term and five short-term personal or professional goals. Develop a realistic plan and time frame for achieving these goals. Make sure to include what is required to achieve these goals.

✔ Complete this statement, using as many examples as possible. "I feel most satisfied when I am done with my shift in knowing that. . . ." Analyze these answers and discuss how they can be implemented in everyday practice.

✔ Think of at least three situations in which you were asked to do something that you really did not want to do. How did you handle these situations? How could they be handled in a more assertive manner?

References

1. Gardiner, DL: Conflicts and retention of new graduate nurses. West J Nurs Res 14:76–85, 1992.
2. American Association of Colleges of Nursing: Issues Bulletin: With Demand for RNs Climbing, and Shortening Supply, Forecasters Say What's Ahead Isn't Typical Shortage Cycle. AACN, Washington, DC, February 1998.
3. Chenevert, M: Pro-Nurse Handbook. CV Mosby, St. Louis, 1993.
4. Kramer, M: Reality Shock. CV Mosby, St. Louis, 1979.
5. Buerhaus, PI: Is a nursing shortage on the way? Nursing 98 98:34–35, 1998.
6. Hegner, BR, and Caldwell, E: Nursing Assistants: A Nursing Process Approach. Delmar, New York, 1995.
7. Gray, BB: Another nursing shortage? You can bet on it. Nurse Week/Health Week. http://www.nurseweek.com/97428/shortage.html. 1998.

BIBLIOGRAPHY

Al-Assaf, AF: Executive stress: An ounce of prevention. Nursing Management 23:69–72, 1992.

Anderson, H: Hospitals seek new ways to integrate health care. Hospitals 66:26–36, 1992.

Blegen, MA, Gardner, DL, and McCloskey, JC: Who helps you with your work? Am J Nurs 91:26–31, 1992.

Bradlby, M: Status passage into nursing: Another view of the process of socialization into nursing. J Adv Nurs 15:1220–1225, 1990.

Hunt, R, and Zurec, EL: Introduction to community based nursing. Lippincott-Raven, Philadelphia, 1997.

Jamieson, EM, Sewall, MF, and Suhrie, EB: Trends in Nursing History. WB Saunders, Philadelphia, 1968.

Kalisch, PA, and Kalisch, BJ: The Advance of American Nursing, ed 3. JB Lippincott, Philadelphia, 1995.

Keepnews, D: The national sample survey of RNs: What does it tell us. American Nurse 30(3):11, 1998.

Kirkwood, C: Your Services Are No Longer Required: The Complete Job Loss Recovery Book. Plume Books, New York, 1993.

Lelis-Grice, D: Loving, human touch helps family cope with loss. AACN News 15(9):4–6, 1998.

Lindquist, KD: Finding the perfect match: Health Care Trends Transition 1:6–8, 1989.

Loscalzo, F: The essence of nursing is touching another soul. AACN News 15(10):3, 1998.

Maffeo, R: Divorcing the UAP: Heresy or solution? American Nurse 30(1):5, 1998.

Marks, D: Nurse-managed health centers gain recognition for innovation. American Nurse 29(4):10, 1997.

McKinley, M: Collaboration is an effective tool. AACN News 15(10):2, 1998.

Morgan, A, and McCann, JM: Problems in nurse-physician relationships. Nursing Administration Quarterly 7:28–32, 1983.

Nawar, M: Workplace violence: One nurse's night of fear. American Nurse 30(5):15, 1998.

Nicoll, LH: Nurses' Guide to the Internet, ed 2. JB Lippincott, Philadelphia, 1998.

Rode, D, et al: The therapeutic use of technology. Am J Nurs 98(12):32–35, 1998.

Sindul-Rothschild, J: Where have all the nurses gone? Am J Nurs 96(11):63–70, 1996.

Stewart, M: Health care community faces the year 2000. American Nurse 29(6):24, 1997.

Strategies advance family-centered care philosophy. AACN News 15(10):5, 1998.

Welton, RH, Morton, PG, and Amig, A: How to succeed in job interviewing. Critical Care Nurse 18(1):68–73, 1998.

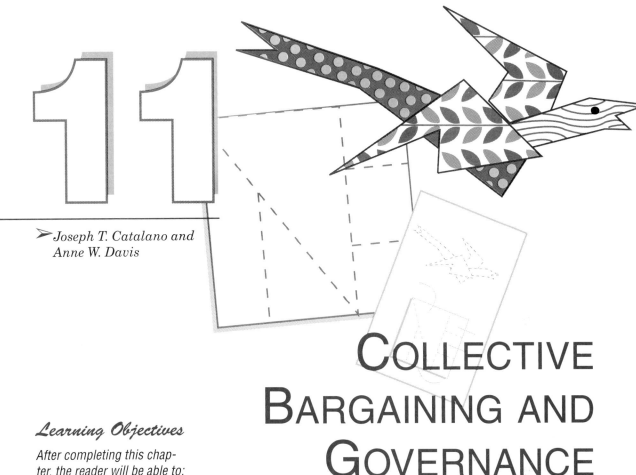

➤ *Joseph T. Catalano and*
Anne W. Davis

COLLECTIVE BARGAINING AND GOVERNANCE

Learning Objectives

After completing this chapter, the reader will be able to:

1. Define collective bargaining.
2. Analyze the key issues that concern nurses in collective bargaining.
3. Identify the steps in the contract negotiation process.
4. Distinguish between a mediator and an arbitrator.
5. Delineate the important elements in a contract.
6. Name alternative forms of governance.
7. Analyze the effect governance has on collective bargaining.

As nursing moves toward achieving its full status as a profession, the issue of collective bargaining becomes more important. Since the early 1960s, the number of nurses who have joined unions has increased steadily, yet the question remains: Is professionalism compatible with membership in a union? Union members still have the image of male workers in blue-collar, heavy industry jobs. However, not only are registered nurses (RNs) joining unions at a faster pace than most other categories of workers, they are also more militant and aggressive in their demands.[1]

Throughout its early history of developing into a profession, nursing practices have often been defined and controlled by other groups, such as physicians and hospital administrators. These groups saw the potential power of an organized large group of well-educated and dedicated nurses and feared the time when they would become independent. Even today, most hospital management reacts to any unionization attempts on the part of nurses with hostility and resistance. As nurses begin to accept the independence, authority, and responsibility of the profession, they need to consider whether or not joining a union will help them reach their goal of full professionalism. Without a doubt, this is one of the most highly charged issues that a nurse might face in professional practice.

The image of nursing has always been one of dedication, service to clients, and selflessness. In the past, nurses' pay and working conditions were often secondary considerations, and many nurses felt that too much emphasis on money demeaned the profession. In today's society, nurses are beginning to realize that professionals with a career should have a say in matters that affect their practice, including working conditions, staffing patterns, benefits, and income (Box 11.1). They need to be able to express these concerns without loss of status or reputation with the general public and other health-care professionals.

PERSPECTIVE ON COLLECTIVE BARGAINING

Collective bargaining is the uniting of employees for the purpose of increasing their ability to influence their employer and to improve working conditions.[2] Collective bargaining is based on the principle that there is greater strength in large numbers. Its primary goal is to equalize the power between labor and management. The primary collective bargaining unit is the union.

Unions were initially formed to protect workers from exploitation by greedy and insensitive employers. Although confronted with much opposition, they did accomplish their goals and became very powerful entities themselves. Recently, unions have received a more negative image because of the use of destructive and sometimes illegal practices in the quest for additional power. The end result is that the union movement itself is now in a fight for survival because of decreasing membership.[3] For some, unions and collective bargaining arouse images of picket lines, rowdy strikes, and violence. Many professionals, including nurses, do not regard this as an activity that professionals should be involved in and tend to reject the idea of union membership outright.

Legislative Development of Collective Bargaining

Although the informal roots of collective bargaining can be traced back to the middle 1800s, formal collective bargaining in this country was first legally recognized in 1935 with passage of the National Labor

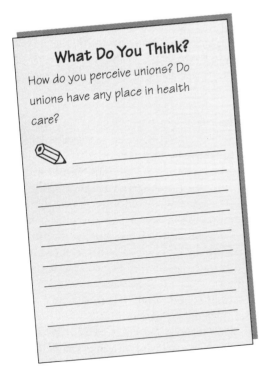

What Do You Think?

How do you perceive unions? Do unions have any place in health care?

BOX

11.1 Patient Care: Twelve Hours in the Life of a Big-City Nurse

Reprinted with permission from *The Philadelphia Inquirer,* Dec. 28, 1997.

It was oddly quiet in the predawn, artificial light of the hospital as nurse Sandy Pincik arrived for work. As usual, she came 15 minutes early, so she could organize a little before things really took off at 7.

Doctors huddled with nurses in the hall, discussing the day's treatment plans. Soon, they would head for their offices or operating rooms, and then the floor would belong mostly to nurses like Pincik.

Pulling a flowered smock out of her bag, she put it on over her white T-shirt and draped a purple stethoscope around her neck. She grabbed a pile of pens, a clipboard and a box of supplies and put them on a movable writing stand in the corridor.

A low-key woman with wavy, light-brown hair and magenta nail polish, Pincik would be responsible for five beds—four patients so far this day—and would help out with five others.

She and Jean Smyth, another registered nurse, worked as a team to cover 10 beds on Thomas Jefferson University Hospital's 7 North, a unit that treats people recovering from urologic surgery, kidney or liver transplants, or problems of dialysis.

Pincik's day would revolve around making sure those patients got everything they needed, from fresh ice and new sheets to CPR. It would be a day filled with a thousand small duties, tasks few would notice—unless they didn't get done.

Complaints about modern, cost-conscious medicine are everywhere these days.

Patients are warned that their doctors, their hospitals and their insurance companies make more money by providing less

treatment. They read about hospital layoffs and dire predictions of more to come and wonder if enough people will remain to take care of them.

Nurses, who have been among the most vocal critics, argue loudly that hospitals have compromised care by increasing nurses' workloads and replacing them with cheaper, lesser-skilled employees, a trend they derisively call "deskilling."

A national survey of 7,500 nurses last year by Boston College nursing professor Judith Shindul–Rothschild found that more than a third would not recommend that a family member receive care in their institutions. Plus, nearly 70 percent reported having less time for basic nursing care and nearly 75 percent less time to comfort patients. Nonetheless, only 14 percent rated the quality of the places where they worked as poor or very poor.

Nursing employment statistics do little to clarify the debate. The American Hospital Association says the number of RNs working in hospitals has continued to rise, even as the number of patients has fallen.

Linda Aiken, a University of Pennsylvania nurse researcher who has studied the AHA statistics, said the number of RNs working in inpatient care has declined in recent years. But when the number of patients, their length of stay, and the severity of their illnesses were taken into account, she noted, the number of nurses remained relatively constant, at least through 1994.

The number of other caregivers, meanwhile, fell significantly, Aiken said. That may account for the perception among nurses that they are working much harder.

The quality of hospital care, according to early research, has shown on decline. Still, it is common to hear former patients complain that their nurse seemed harried, that he or she took forever to come when the call button was pressed. These patients may be well now, but they feel bad about their hospital stay, they say.

Most patients have little idea what the nurse is doing when not with them, and few have had enough hospital experiences to compare today's care with that given before costs were such an issue.

Jefferson, saying its nursing care is as good or better than ever, welcomed a request to have a reporter follow one of its nurses. Several other hospitals refused.

Sandy Pincik's day, therefore, may not be typical of what nurses in other hospitals experience. But it is a window into what life is like for a nurse at a major teaching hospital in 1997. And it reveals the pivotal role of employees, who as Pincik puts it, do "everything."

By 7:20 A.M., the night nurse was filling Pincik in on the status of her patients.

Mark Pannapacker, a young man recovering from a kidney-stone operation, thought he had passed another stone overnight.

Jerry Singleton, a dialysis patient admitted with fluid around his heart, was being prepared for surgery the next day.

Pincik would have to draw blood from Kevin Margaret Scharff, a post-transplant patient who had come in with pneumonia.

And the fourth patient would be going home if tests showed him to be free of infection.

Though, for most of this day, Pincik's primary responsibility was only four patients—she usually has five and sometimes as many as eight—she would spend as much of her eight-hour shift on paperwork and the phone as she would in their rooms. In a modern hospital, hands-on time at bedside is only part of a nurse's workday.

Pincik began her day zipping from patient to patient, from phone to computer to patient file. Most of the tasks were short, but she rarely finished one without being interrupted by a phone call or questions from nursing students helping on the floor.

She drew blood from the still-sleeping Scharff, then dropped it off in a pneumatic tube that would take it to the lab. She called a doctor to see whether the dialysis staff could take a blood sample from Singleton, saving him a needle stick. She took vital signs. She checked Pannapacker's pain medication orders and called dietary to stop his breakfast tray, on orders from his doctor. She asked a student to change Pannapacker's dressing. She made Singleton's bed and checked how much he had had to eat and drink (fluid balance is important in dialysis patients). She talked with her colleague Smyth about a post-op patient due in later in the day.

The desk clerk told her that the alarm on Scharff's IV was beeping, so she went in to fix it. She brought Scharff a regular Coke instead of the Diet Coke that dietary had sent her by mistake. In one chart or another, she wrote down virtually everything she did, even the Coke.

There was just time for a friendly "How ya doing?" in most of the rooms. She asked Scharff if she felt more like eating today. She asked Pannapacker, who worked for a medical case-management company, if he thought he might need a nurse when he returned home, and he said he thought that would be unnecessary and expensive. She asked Singleton about his scheduled trip to the OR, so that his dialysis could again work properly.

The conversations were brief and to the medical point, no chitchat about the weather or the holidays.

Brief as her contact with them was, her patients seemed satisfied with their care. There were no long waits for attention, and no one seemed to want more hand holding.

By 8:45, Pincik thought she had things well enough under control to start doing the little things that make her feel good about being a nurse.

She began going from room to room, making sure that everyone had fresh ice, a task that might also be done by a nursing assistant.

Seeing that Smyth was busy, she ducked into 24, Daisy Lake's room. Lake, a friendly 57-year-old from Glassboro, was one of Smyth's patients. She had had kidney stones removed, a relatively routine operation, a few days earlier but was a complicated patient because she was paralyzed from the waist down.

She wanted coffee, so Pincik hurried to the pantry down the hall to fetch it. Getting coffee may seem a mundane task for a woman only months from a master's degree, but Pincik liked doing it and knew that every contact with a patient might tell a nurse something important.

She filled the cup and headed back to Lake's room. What happened next is why critics say de-skilling is a bad idea.

Pincik gave Lake the coffee and handed her a spoon.

"Can you put it in there for me?" Lake asked, motioning toward the coffee cup. "I'm afraid to move."

She told Pincik that her arm hurt. In an instant, Pincik switched from waitress to nurse. This was a clue that something was wrong, the kind of clue, nursing advocates say, lesser-trained employees might miss.

Pincik looked at Lake's IV arm. It was swollen. She touched the puffy skin. It was warm. She turned off the IV pump. No blood drained back into the tube. The IV had come loose.

"I'll be right back," Pincik said as she went to get supplies to start a new IV.

Lake had been getting fluids and antibiotics through the tube. Failure to fix it not only would keep her from getting the treatment she needed but could lead to a badly swollen and painful arm.

When Pincik returned, Lake worried that the nurse would not be able to find a vein for the new IV. Pincik looked carefully at the smooth skin on the underside of Lake's other arm.

"I see a couple of prospects here," she said.

Concentrating, Pincik pressed her index finger on Lake's skin until she found a vein. She slowly pushed a large needle into the skin, poking it around beneath the surface for several seconds, then, finally, pushing it all the way in.

"Did you get it?" Lake asked.

"Yep," Pincik said. "Sure did."

"Bless you," Lake said.

Pincik, 34, became a nurse in 1986, during the nursing shortage, when some hospitals were offering signing bonuses and lots of other perks to attract RNs. In a few years, though, everything had changed.

Big employers had grown exasperated by skyrocketing health-insurance costs. They demanded cost control and got it from HMOs and other managed-care insurers, who began scrutinizing health expenses like never before. Insurers pressured hospitals to send patients home more quickly, leaving empty beds and unwieldy payrolls.

Between 1986 and 1992, the length of the average hospital stay fell from 7.1 to 6.5 days. Before long, the hospitals that had fought to attract nurses were making headlines with layoffs or transferring staff to new home-care departments.

At the same time, medical improvements were allowing doctors to save older, critically ill patients. That, combined with the shorter hospital stays, left hospitals with sicker and sicker patients. As Penn's Aiken put it, hospitals have become "giant intensive-care units."

All these changes were making nurses feel more harried.

Two years ago, like most hospitals in the city, Jefferson looked at its declining admissions and the projections of more to follow and decided to "restructure" its staff. Its goal was to reduce its $500 million budget by $75 million within four years, CEO Tom Lewis said.

Although it has retained a heavier emphasis on RNs than many hospitals, Jefferson reduced its nursing staff by attrition. Broader responsibilities for nurses allowed it to reduce staff in other areas, such as respiratory therapy and phlebotomy. Since then, staffing has increased as the hospital lured several high-volume physician practices.

Jefferson also has a slightly smaller percentage of RNs caring for patients. In the 1980s, RNs, who make about $45,000 a year, would have provided 100 percent of the nursing care in ICUs and intermediate units. Today, they make up 90 percent of the staff in ICUs and 85 percent in intermediate units. On acute-care general units, they make up 80 percent of the staff, 5 percent less than before. Licensed practical nurses, nursing assistants, and techs make up the difference.

On this day, along with Smyth and Pincik, an LPN was on the unit, as were several nursing students. A nursing assistant had called in sick.

After Pincik finished with Lake, she returned to her own patients, ping-ponging between rooms and charts, moving so quickly that she could disappear into a room or around a corner in the time it took to glance over a shoulder and back.

At least half of her working day was spent with paper rather than patients. Unpleasant as it is, paperwork has always been a significant part of nurses' jobs, Pincik and nursing leaders said. With so many different caregivers involved with only one patient, the charts and other forms are the primary means of communication.

The paperwork also is important when hospitals seek accreditation, a key hurdle for prestige and insurance reimbursement. Increasingly, in the era of managed care, it is used to justify bills or longer hospital stays.

Standing at the portable desk in the hall, Pincik explained a new discharge planning form to Smyth. Then she filled out forms describing in detail the treatment the man in Room 21 was getting. He had been evicted, and she wanted the people at the shelter where he was going to know how to care for him.

By 12:15, Leonard Polidor, a patient with a history of heart problems who had just had a hernia operation, arrived. Pincik's beds were now full.

In the old days, a patient like Polidor might have been admitted the night before surgery. Now Pincik often sees patients for the first time while they are still groggy from anesthesia. She does not know what their normal color looks like or how clearly they normally think.

Nurse advocates say this change has made nursing more difficult, but Pincik says she can get the information she needs from the patient's records and from the assessment she does when she meets him.

Pincik grabbed a thermometer and went into the room ahead of the gurney. Smyth and Sue Horter, the LPN, went in, too. They asked Polidor to scoot from the gurney to the bed. Pincik stuck the thermometer in his mouth. Horter took his pulse. Pincik got the blood-pressure cuff.

"My name's Sandy," she said. "I'm going to be your nurse today, OK?"

Looking tired and still a little dazed, Polidor said nothing.

Soon, Pincik was out in the hall, grabbing Singleton's chart, so it could go with him to dialysis.

She was hungry. It would be another half-hour before she could run to the cafeteria.

Pincik, her knife and fork poised to touch her Caesar salad, sat at a table in the break room at 1:08 P.M.

The unit clerk called her to the phone. The facility that was taking the patient in 21 had questions.

Then her new patient asked for pain medicine. Just as she finished getting the medicine, the nurse-call light went on outside Lake's door. Pincik knew Smyth was eating, so she answered it.

The nephrostomy tube in Lake's back was leaking. Her sister had noticed the bed was wet. Pincik got Lake a new gown.

She changed her dressing and slipped clean absorbant pads under her.

Just as Pincik finished, Lake soiled the new pad. Now, finished with her lunch, Smyth came to help replace the pads and clean up Lake, who lay quietly on her side.

Lake disliked this, but it had become part of her life since the car accident that paralyzed her. The nurses worked quickly, without embarrassment or judgment. They had done this countless times. It was part of being a nurse.

When they finished, Pincik went back to her salad.

As Pincik ate, a student nurse gave Pannapacker his discharge instructions. Another student had talked with the patient in 21. He, too, would be going soon. Scharff, who was feeling much better, also wanted to go home. Pincik thought she would have to wait another day.

Pincik's day was winding down. In a few minutes, Smyth would get a new patient, a man who had just finished penile-prosthesis surgery. Another patient, who had had his bladder removed, was due in Pannapacker's room.

Pincik stripped the beds in her two empty rooms and emptied urinals. (The housekeeping staff doesn't touch human wastes.) She checked on Scharff and Polidor. Singleton was still in dialysis.

At 3, she turned her patients over to the night nurse. For the most part, her patients said they were satisfied with their care.

But Pincik didn't leave. Working a 12-hour shift this day, she spent the next four hours helping other nurses and working on scheduling and other paperwork.

It was night when she left the hospital for the dark streets outside and the trip home.

1. What recent changes in the health-care industry affect the quality of care nurses provide daily?
2. Identify the situations described in the article where Ms. Pincik's nursing skills made a difference.
3. How would you rate the quality of care provided by Ms. Pincik? What personal or professional qualities did she display that figured in your assessment of her?
4. How does this portrayal of nursing compare with other stories or images you have seen in the media?

From Burling S: Patient care: Twelve hours in the life of a big-city nurse: in an age of cost-cutting, RNs and LPNs find they can't cut back on TLC. The Philadelphia Inquirer, December 28, 1997.

Relations Act (NLRA). This act granted employees the right to self-organization and to form, and help in the organization of, labor unions that could then bargain collectively through representatives. The representatives would be appointed by the union and bargain with management for the purpose of collective bargaining, mutual aid, and protection.[4] Under NLRA, the National Labor Relations Board (NLRB) was established to supervise the implementation of the act.[1]

Originally, the NLRA included nonprofit hospitals and other health-care providers under its authority. In its attempt to protect unions, the NLRA prevented some employers from reducing wages in hopes that higher paid workers would spend more and decrease the severity of the depression. One negative result of NLRA was that many employers who did not have enough income to pay the higher wages went bankrupt. The NLRA was amended in 1947 by the Taft-Hartley Act, also called the Labor Management Relations Act (LMRA), with the goal of restoring equality between the unions and management. Taft-Hartley excluded nurses in nonprofit hospitals from coverage under the NLRA, legally preventing nurses from organizing collective bargaining units and going on strike. It was not until 1974 that the Taft-Hartley Act was amended to cover nurses in nonprofit hospitals, thus allowing nurses to form collective bargaining units.[5]

In April of 1991, the U.S. Supreme Court ruled that the NLRB had the authority to define bargaining units for health-care providers in all settings, including acute care hospitals. Under this ruling, the NLRB defined eight separate bargaining units that were appropriate for use in hospitals.[6]

1. Nurses
2. Physicians
3. All professionals except nurses and physicians
4. All technical employees
5. All skilled maintenance employees
6. All business office clerical employees
7. All guards
8. All other nonprofessional employees

Ultimately, this ruling by the Supreme Court permitted "all registered nurses (RNs) bargaining units" to be formed so that work issues important to professional nurses could be addressed. The current major representative for nurses is the Service Employees International Union, which represents almost 500,000 nurses and health-care providers nationwide. The American Nurses Association (ANA) has been active in the support of collective bargaining throughout its history.

Although the ANA does not serve as a bargaining agent, it does support the State

Nurses Associations (SNAs) to function as bargaining agents. As early as 1944, the ANA ruled that the SNAs could engage in collective bargaining. In response to the attempt to regulate nursing from the outside, the ANA presented a position paper in 1946 that stated the importance for nursing to assume responsibility for advancing the social and economic security of its practitioners rather than leaving it to organizations outside the profession.[7] Today the SNAs represent approximately 140,000 RNs in some 840 individual bargaining units across the United States. Since the ruling by the Supreme Court in 1991, there has been an increased interest in organizing additional bargaining units.[8] The Workplace Advocacy Initiative was also initiated in 1991 to help RNs improve the work environment and gain more control over professional practice.

Goals of Collective Bargaining

Although the basic goal of collective bargaining is to equalize power between management and employees, the inequality of power between the two groups is not so great as it initially appears. Although the majority of employees in most organizations are near the bottom of the power structure hierarchy, the management relies on these employees to carry out the work of the organization. Employees are vital to the growth, development, and even the survival of the organization. Employees also far outnumber individuals in management. Collective bargaining takes advantage of these two factors when attempting to produce change in the organization. An individual employee is highly vulnerable when attempting to force the employer to change.

The main area of concern of collective bargaining is basic economic issues such as salaries and benefits. In some hospital settings, nurses are paid less than other individuals in the hospital who have less education and fewer responsibilities. Collective bargaining attempts to balance these inequities.

Other concerns of collective bargaining include shift differentials, overtime pay, holidays, personal days off, the number of hours required in a work week, sick leave, maternity and paternity leave, uniform reimbursements, lunch and coffee breaks, health insurance, pension plans, and severance pay.[2] These elements all are found in the employment contract and may vary greatly depending on the hospital and the power of the bargaining unit.

One of the most important goals of a bargaining unit is to protect the employee against arbitrary treatment and unfair labor practices. These can be anything from working five weekends in a row to being fired because a physician felt the nurse was acting in an insubordinate manner. Other issues that might be considered unfair labor practices include being passed over for promotion without an explanation, unreasonable staffing and scheduling policies, excessive demands for overtime, rotating shifts, unfair on-call time, transfers, layoffs, seniority rights, and failure to post job openings. The collective bargaining unit establishes a grievance procedure by means of which the employee can bring a complaint against management without fear of reprisals. These grievance procedures also allow a mechanism for the employee to follow up on the complaint to a satisfactory conclusion.

An important goal of collective bargaining is to maintain and promote professional practice. Often overlooked by management, this goal is one way nurses can keep and increase control over their own professional practice. For example, some nurses' bargaining units have been able to

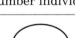 *An important goal of collective bargaining is to maintain and promote professional practice.*

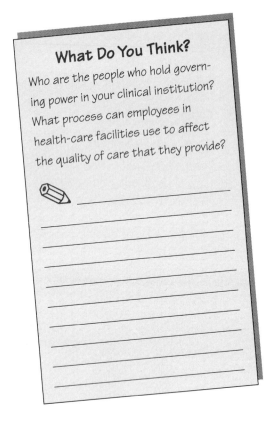

What Do You Think?

Who are the people who hold governing power in your clinical institution? What process can employees in health-care facilities use to affect the quality of care that they provide?

include the entire ANA Code of Ethics into the contract with the hospital. Other units have been able to address issues such as staffing, standards of care, and quality of care in the contract negotiations.

Nurses' Questions About Collective Bargaining

Although large numbers of RNs have successfully unionized, there remain some fundamental questions about collective bargaining. These questions are at the heart of what makes collective bargaining an ethical issue for many nurses.

Is It Unprofessional?

Nurses have a great deal of difficulty in adjusting their image to that of a union member or a striker. It just does not seem to be professional. For many nurses it seems that there must be other ways to achieve the same goals without collective bargaining.

Organizers of collective bargaining units stress that many other professionals, such as pilots, teachers, and even physicians, are members of unions. The NLRB defines nurses as professionals because their work requires advanced and specialized education and skills. They also make critical judgments that affect the health and well-being of others. Union organizers contend that it is even less professional to accept low pay and poor working conditions than it is to join a union to improve these elements. They also feel that collective bargaining will give nurses control over their practice, which is one of the keys to professionalism.

Is It Unethical?

One of the major beliefs of nurses is the priority of the clients' health and well-being over the personal needs and gains of the health-care provider. This concern conflicts with the methods commonly used by collective bargaining units, such as strikes or work slowdowns. There is a feeling among many health-care providers that these types of actions constitute abandonment of their clients and therefore violate the code of ethics. Those who support collective bargaining stress that poor or intolerable work conditions are as much a threat to that client's health and well-being as the work actions taken to correct these conditions. The ability of nurses simply to threaten to strike, even though it may never materialize, is often powerful enough to bring about change.[9] Law requires that there must be a 10-day notice given before a strike takes place. This gives the hospital a chance to prepare for the strike and to make changes to ensure client safety, such as transferring critical care clients to another hospital,

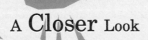

A Closer Look

DECIDING TO GO ON STRIKE

Sharon S., RN, was completing her charting on another busy 3 P.M. to 11 P.M. shift. While she was walking down the hall toward the time clock, she wondered who would be taking her place for the rest of the week. Like most of the other nurses at the Medical Center, she had decided to go on strike starting with the 7 A.M. to 3 P.M. shift the next day. The decision to strike had not been an easy one and had only been reached after much discussion (arguments?), many hours of meetings and conferences with the hospital negotiators, and animated discussion among the nurses' negotiating team.

Sharon could see both positive and negative sides to a strike. On the positive side, increased salaries, better fringe benefits, and improvements in working conditions and staffing would be a plus for all the nurses and clients at the Medical Center. Sharon herself had felt increasingly stressed during the past year because of the hospital's measures to reorganize. From what Sharon was able to see, reorganization meant saving money by cutting professional staff and partially replacing them with less trained, unlicensed individuals. This pattern of restaffing had led to longer hours, increased responsibilities for the RNs, and fewer support services. She also felt that the overall quality of care had decreased noticeably.

On the negative side, Sharon was experiencing a real ethical and emotional dilemma about going on strike. The quality of care was sure to deteriorate even further because of the reduced services caused by the strike. Was it really fair to decrease the services and care for clients who had nothing to do with the issues that brought on the strike? Of course, during the past 3 days, the clients who had been well enough were sent home early in anticipation of the strike. Some whose conditions were too complicated for them to be cared for at home were sent to other facilities. The hospital had severely restricted admissions, reducing the census to an all-time low.

Yet there were several clients who were too ill to transfer or send home. Mrs. Anderson, a 78-year-old client with renal failure, congestive heart failure, and a recent colostomy for a bowel obstruction, came to mind. Mrs. Anderson and a number of other clients like her, who had no family nearby and few resources, were highly dependent on the nursing staff to meet their needs of care. Mrs. Anderson was just beginning to be taught how to care for her colostomy. Even if she was discharged to a nursing home, there was no way to ensure that she could receive the teaching needed for her eventual self-care.

Although there was to be a skeleton crew of nurses left in the facility, they would be stretched very thin in trying to care for the remaining clients.

Sharon also thought about the ANA Code for Nurses she had been taught in nursing school, particularly the passage that stated "the nurse participates in the profession's effort to establish and maintain conditions of employment conducive to high-quality nursing care." The reason for the strike was to bring about improved working conditions that would benefit future clients in the hospital. But should these measures be carried out when nursing services were already operating at a reduced level of care and at a minimal level of safety? Didn't that somehow contradict the first statement in the Code, that "the nurse provides services with respect for human dignity"? When Mrs. Anderson was admitted to the hospital 4 days before, she came with the expectation of the best possible care under any circumstances. The Code seemed to have a split personality on strikes. While calling for service to the profession to maintain high standards and quality of care, the Code also insisted that the health, welfare, and safety of the clients should be the nurses' first consideration.

What should Sharon do? Does the overall welfare of the profession ever supersede the obligation to provide client care?

eliminating elective surgeries, and refusing to admit new clients.

In the few times when nurses have gone on strike, client safety and well-being have not been affected. The institutions involved were always given enough lead time to discharge or transfer the majority of the clients. The few remaining clients were cared for by management personnel who are not covered by unions.

Is It Divisive?

Does the process of collective bargaining set nurse against nurse? The process of collective bargaining is adversarial by nature. It sets two groups, management and employees, against each other. Although this relationship can result in conflict, it allows the staff nurses to be heard and to initiate changes that affect the practice of nursing. Nurses have been attempting for years to improve working conditions in the health-

care setting, and to achieve **comparable worth.** Administrators pay little attention to an individual nurse or to a small group of concerned nurses. When a collective bargaining unit speaks for all of the nurses, however, administration will listen.[1]

Different collective bargaining units have different requirements for membership, which are often included in the negotiations. Many unions negotiate a *closed shop* or *agency shop* clause in the contract. A closed shop institution requires that all of the employees pay membership dues whether they belong to the union or not. The rationale behind the closed shop approach is that because all of the employees benefit from the union's negotiations, they should all pay for it. It also encourages employees to join the union because they are already paying the dues. However, many states have *right to work* laws that make closed shop contracts illegal. In these states the *open shop* collective bargaining model is used, and only those employees join the union, pay dues, and desire to be members. There is more chance for nurse-to-nurse conflicts in open shop institutions because of the divisions between those who belong to the union and those who do not. Collective bargaining does not have to be adversarial, and in facilities where administration is open to change and the collective bargaining unit is realistic in its requests, the process can be very smooth and amicable.

Is There a Threat to Job Security?

Although the main goals of collective bargaining are improvement of working conditions and protection from unfair labor practices, it can itself pose a threat to job security. In some cases employees who are active in the collective bargaining process become well known to management and may become the targets for reprisals, particularly if the collective bargaining fails. Facilities sometimes suggest that granting RNs higher wages and benefits will cause bankruptcy and closure of the facility or that the higher RN wages will at least drain the organization's resources so much that it has to cut back the number of other employees. In reality, recent changes in contract law have resulted in job losses. Nurses can be replaced during strikes, and even if a settlement is reached, they are hired back only after new employees leave or openings occur. If no settlement is reached, striking nurses may never be hired back.

Taking an action always carries risk. Nurses involved in collective bargaining have to weigh the risk-to-benefit ratio before they take action. Are the working conditions so poor and the pay so inadequate that they overshadow the risk of possible job loss? The first attempts at organizing a collective bargaining unit are usually the most dangerous in terms of job security. Initial attempts at organizing nurses are usually made outside the hospital between rep-

What Do You Think?

What are some other objections to unionization of nurses that you can think of or have heard? How might you respond to these objections?

resentatives of the SNA and the union. This type of activity prevents any individuals from becoming targets of management's anger and makes management's reprisals more difficult. In addition, there are also some legal protections for nurses who organize collective bargaining. There are grievance procedures that can be followed under the unfair labor practices rules that vary somewhat from state to state.

The Contract

After a collective bargaining unit has been selected, the next important step is to develop or negotiate a contract between the nurses and the hospital. The contract is a legal document that is binding for both management and the union.[2] Contracts can be very specific and include just a few items, or very broad and include many. Contracts often contain requirements for union mem-

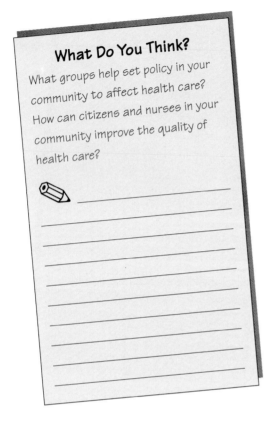

What Do You Think?

What groups help set policy in your community to affect health care? How can citizens and nurses in your community improve the quality of health care?

bership by the employees and set the cost of dues for that membership.

Negotiating teams are selected by both management and employee groups. One member of each of these teams is designated as the spokesperson who will be the main representative for the group. Before negotiations start, each team meets separately to decide on its position on various issues and on what they are willing to compromise. A list of demands is exchanged by the two sides; it should include everything each might possibly want.

Generally, management is reluctant to give up power or relinquish money. The employees' group tries to gain some of management's power and gain benefits for its members. Often many meetings between the two groups are required before they discover the key issues and determine where compro-

mise is possible. Posturing and showmanship play a big part in the initial negotiations. Later, when serious issues are discussed and dealt with, final agreements may be reached behind closed doors.

The law requires that each side bargain in good faith. Good faith bargaining requires that both parties must agree to meet at reasonable times, to send individuals to the negotiations who can make binding decisions, and to be willing to bargain with the other side.[2] A lack of willingness to negotiate is not bargaining in good faith.

When the sides are unable to reach a settlement, a stalemate occurs. Stalemates are sometimes resolved through mediation, in which a neutral third party provided by the Federal Mediation and Conciliation Service meets with each side. After determining the nature of the conflict, the mediator brings the two sides together to attempt to work out a settlement. Both sides must work with the mediator, but they are not required to accept the mediator's recommendations.

If mediation fails, the Federal Mediation and Conciliation Service may appoint a fact-finding panel to investigate the conflict and to make recommendations. The panel's report is made public and can exert pressure on both sides to accept the recommendations of the mediator.

In some situations, an arbitrator with binding power may be appointed. This person is a neutral third party who, like the mediator, investigates the conflict, meets with both sides, and makes a recommendation for settlement. Unlike that of the mediator, however, the arbitrator's recommendation must be accepted by both sides. Both labor and management try to avoid binding arbitration because it limits their negotiating powers and they may lose something gained during previous negotiations.

When all else fails, the final step in the contract negotiation process is work slowdowns or stoppages (strikes). Although

Site Seeing

American Nurses Association
http://www.ana.org/
http://www.nursingworld.org/
Contact: mail to:webfeedback@ana.org

GlobalRN Website
http://nurseweb.ucsf.edu./www/globalrn.htm
Contact: Chuck Pitkofsky
chuckp@itsa.ucsf.edu

Healthcare Information Systems Directory
http://www.health-infosys-dir.com/
Contact: mail to:hisd@health-infosys-dir.com

Health Organizations
http://www.social.com/health/nhic/data/index.html

National League for Nursing
http://www.nln.org/
Contact: mail to:nlnweb@nln.org

NURSE WWW Information Server
http://medsrv2.bham.ac.uk/nursing/
Contact: Denis Anthony
mail to:cudma@csv.warwick.ac.uk

NURSEWEEK
http://www-nurseweek.webnexus.com
Contact: chriss@healthweek.com

Revolution: The Journal of Nurse Empowerment
http://ideanurse.com/advon
Contact: Laura Gasparis Vonfrolio
adeduprn@aol.com

Student Nurse Information Center
http://glass.toledolink.com/~ornrsg/
Contact: mail to:ornrsg@toledolink.com

What Do You Think?

Have you ever been involved in a strike or work action or know someone who went on strike? How did it affect the individual? Was the strike worth it in the long term?

strikes are usually the tool used by employees to gain power, management can use a form of enforced strike called a lockout, whereby employees are not permitted to enter the work facility.

The prospect of a strike is usually accompanied by more intense negotiations that may lead to a last-minute settlement. Strikes are detrimental to both sides. Employees lose pay and benefits during a strike, and management loses income. In addition, the overall public image of strikes is negative, and they have little support. Some collective bargaining units have developed alternative ways of achieving their goals without a strike. Methods such as disruption of services on a random basis or boycott of an organization can achieve the same effects as a full-blown strike without damaging the image of the union.

After a settlement has been reached, the contract must be ratified. The collective bargaining unit takes the contract back to the employees, who must approve it. Once it is

Collective Bargaining and Governance:
A New Model for Collective Bargaining

Traditionally, collective bargaining has been viewed as a struggle between two groups, one (usually employees) attempting to gain more power and another (usually management) attempting to retain power. This type of struggle often resulted in hurt feelings or impasses in negotiations. In 1995 the Minnesota Nurses Association (MNA) ratified a contract with 12 Twin Cities–area hospitals using a new collective bargaining technique called interest-based bargaining.

Interest-based bargaining, also called mutual gains, win-win, and best-practice bargaining, is based on the idea that the way to achieve a mutually beneficial contract is to create an environment in which all parties can openly discuss all issues to the fullest extent. In interest-based bargaining, a highly structured six-step process is followed: (1) selection of issues; (2) discussion of interests; (3) generation of options; (4) establishment of standards to measure the options; (5) measurement of the options; and (6) development of solutions. This step-by-step process prevents the parties involved in the bargaining from reverting to the traditional power struggle. All steps are done jointly, and even the 2-day training session that precedes negotiations requires participation by both management and labor.

Central to the contract negotiations by the MNA was ensuring that the role of the registered nurse as the primary assessor and planner of care be maintained. The contract included specific language stating that only RNs will assess, plan, and evaluate a client's nursing care needs. In order to guarantee this aspect of the contract in the future, the MNA negotiated greater participation by RNs in the hospital committees that establish priorities for labor-management relations, nurse staffing, client-care standards, and health and safety policies. This partnership between nurses and hospital administrators allowed for joint decision making when issues of nursing practice and delivery of care were involved.

Interest-based bargaining may be the trend for the future, particularly in the health-care industry. Traditional collective bargaining methods are primarily adversarial and often leave the parties involved with deep-seated feelings of hostility toward each other. The old methods sometimes result in strikes or other types of work actions that harm the reputations of both nurses and the hospitals. Interest-based bargaining allows participants an opportunity to negotiate without hostility and to develop a more positive relationship after the contract has been agreed on.

Traditional Bargaining versus Interest-Based Bargaining

Traditional Bargaining	Interest-Based Bargaining
Adversarial in nature	Collaborative
Victory-oriented goals	Multiple-gain goals
Negotiation process	Problem-solving process
Compromise on decisions	Consensus on decisions
Predetermined position	No prejudgment on issues
Controlled communication	Brainstorming
Limit information given	Open exchange of information

From Himali, U: MNA ratifies ground-breaking multi-employer contract. American Nurse 271:10, 1995.

approved by a majority of the employees, the contract becomes legally binding for both management and the employees.

A good contract should contain the following elements:

- A statement outlining the objectives of both management and the employees
- A description of the official collective bargaining group
- A description of the benefits included in the contract, such as wages and salary, overtime pay, holiday pay, shift differentials, differentials for advanced education or certifications
- A description of other benefits, such as health insurance, life insurance, retirement, legal benefits, among others
- A description of acceptable in-house labor practices, such as transfers, promotions, seniority, lay-offs, **grievance** procedures, and work schedules
- A description of the procedure to be used when employees have disciplinary problems or when there is a **breach of contract**
- A description of the grievance procedures and the due process to be followed
- A description of what is expected of the professional, including standards of care and codes of ethics[3]

CONCERNS FOR PROFESSIONAL NURSES

Representation

One of the most difficult decisions that nurses have to make is who shall represent them as a collective bargaining unit. It is reasonable to conclude that only a professional organization, such as State Nurse's Association (SAN), that understands the complex and varied needs of the profession will be able to represent that profession in a collective bargaining situation.

Over the years, SNAs have developed into skilled representatives who are able to negotiate contracts with considerable success. However, nonprofessional unions have years of experience with negotiations and large sums of money to spend on developing skilled individuals whose only job is negotiating contracts. The union must be able to convince the group of nurses that it is able to represent the interests of the nurses more effectively than the SNA.

Union groups who attempt to represent nurses soon find that nurses have difficulties in forming a consensus concerning problems and issues. Individuals outside the nursing profession have difficulty understanding issues such as quality and standards of care, ethical dilemmas, or even the different levels of nursing education.

Nurses should also be concerned about the public image of the collective bargaining unit they select to represent them. Some nurses' groups have been represented by a machinists' union, a teamsters' union, or even a meat cutters' union. Although these unions are highly proficient at negotiating contracts to gain benefits for their members, some feel the image of nursing is tarnished in the process.

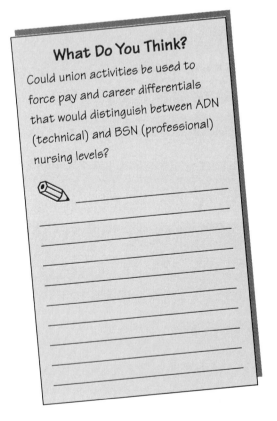

What Do You Think?

Could union activities be used to force pay and career differentials that would distinguish between ADN (technical) and BSN (professional) nursing levels?

Nursing Supervisors—Employees or Management?

Everyone is familiar with the idea of the traditional nursing supervisor. This is the older, more experienced nurse who guides the less experienced nurses. Nursing supervisors make sure staffing is adequate for their assigned shifts, resolve problems that are beyond the skills of the staff nurse, act as mediators between physicians and nurses, and use their higher skill levels to assist the staff nurses with code blues or complicated procedures. The term *nursing supervisor* also includes nurse educators, directors of nursing, head nurses, unit supervisors, assistant head nurses, and sometimes even charge nurses on the 3 P.M. to 11 P.M. or 11 P.M. to 7 A.M. work shifts.

Under the amendments to the Taft-Hartley Act of 1974, a supervisor was defined as any individual with authority to hire, transfer, suspend, lay off, promote, assign, reward, or discipline another employee.[2] From this legal viewpoint, nursing supervisors were no longer employees but really members of the management. Management cannot be involved in collective bargaining activities and is therefore prevented from joining units. A careful reading of the definition of a supervisor as presented in the Taft-Hartley Act makes the category of supervisor open to interpretation. Anybody who assigns a task to another nurse could be considered a supervisor.

Management has sometimes used this provision in the Taft-Hartley Act in the attempt to control the organization and function of collective bargaining units. Management, if so inclined, can use this distinction to induce tension between nursing staff and supervisors, thus reducing the cohesion of the group. Supervisors often serve on important hospital committees to develop standards of care, foster professional recognition, and support nurse advancement.

When contracts are negotiated, the supervisors are on the opposite side of the table from the staff nurses. Often in the heat of negotiation, things are said that foster negative feelings. After the negotiations have ended, it is difficult to re-establish that sense of unity that contributes to high-quality client care.

Attempts have been made by some health-care institutions to categorize all of their RNs and LPNs as supervisors, thus preventing any of them from organizing into a collective bargaining unit.

1994 Supreme Court Decision

In a 5-to-4 vote, the Supreme Court of the United States supported the decision that licensed practical nurses (LPNs) at the Heartland Nursing Home in Urbana, Ohio, should be considered supervisors because they directed the work of nurses' aides "in the interest of the employer." Under this ruling, these LPNs were not protected under the NLRA. This ruling has been of great concern to all nurses, but particularly to the ANA's Department of Labor Relations and Workplace Advocacy committee.

The implications of this decision are far-reaching and pose a direct threat to the ability of RNs to pursue collective bargaining. Employers have already begun to use this ruling to fight nurses in collective bargaining units from Alaska to Washington, DC. The ANA has been working toward developing language that would follow the description of a supervisor as found in the NLRA and the Taft-Hartley Act (see earlier discussion). Since the passage of the NLRA, nurses who provide client care have been considered to be acting within the professional nature of nursing and not in the interests of the employer (as a supervisor would primarily be).

Under the ANA's proposed revisions, the scope of the definition of supervisor would be narrowed to include only employees of health-care institutions. This change would allow the NLRB to continue to determine, on a case-by-case basis, whether nurses were supervisors or professional or technical employees. This legislation, introduced to Congress in 1996, was initially tabled; but it is scheduled for re-introduction some time in the near future.

GOVERNANCE

The term *governance* has a variety of meanings in different contexts. In general, the term describes the arrangement of the hierarchy of power within an organization and

What Do You Think?

Consider the Taft-Hartley definition of "supervisor" carefully. One of the realities of today's health-care system is that RNs assign and direct the care of a wide number of other employees. Why shouldn't they be considered supervisors? How does delegation differ from supervision?

how that power flows through the organization. In relationship to nursing, governance has been defined as "the establishment and maintenance of social, political, and economic arrangements by which nurses maintain control over their practice, their self-discipline, their working conditions, and their professional affairs."[10] The traditional structure of authority in the health-care industry has been based on the triad of the board of directors, the administrator, and the medical staff.

Authority is a type of power that has its origins in the position that an individual holds within an organization.[2] This individual has this power only because others are willing to accept the decisions made by the person in that position. This allows relatively few people in the organization's hierarchy to control large number of employees as well as the directions and functions of the rest of the organization.

At the top of the governance hierarchy is the board of directors, also called the trustees or governors. The board of directors is usually composed of influential business people who are considered community leaders. Although they retain the ultimate legal and ethical responsibility for the operation of the organization, generally the day-to-day operation is delegated to the administrator. The board's main function is to set general policies and to plan for the long-range development of the organization. Most boards become directly involved in the facility's operations only when there is a crisis, such as a financial shortfall or a major lawsuit.

The administrator is usually the highest ranking member of the hierarchy who actually becomes involved in the daily operation of the facility. The administrator has the education and knowledge required to direct the highly complex and technologically advanced elements that are an essential part of today's health-care system.

In most health-care facilities, the medical staff also exerts a great deal of control over the governance structure. The medical staff also has its own internal governance structure with higher- and lower-level members. Traditionally, the physicians in a facility had a great deal of influence in the facility because they were neither employed nor controlled by the facility. However, the advent and spread of managed care has markedly altered the traditional physician–institution relationship in many facilities. In a managed care setting, physicians are hired and salaried employees just like nurses, housekeepers, administrators, or security personnel. Their practice and productivity are monitored and evaluated, and they can be terminated from the facility for poor performance.

> " " *The traditional structure of authority in the health-care industry has been based on the triad of the board of directors, the administrator, and the medical staff.*

Nurses' Role in Governance

In the recent past, nurses had little say in the governance of their facility or agency. Because of their traditional ideology of professionalism, nurses were more oriented toward loyalty and respect than autonomy of practice and independent decision making about the quality of care.[1] Nurses often accepted the work hours assigned to them without question, withstood disrespect and abuse from physicians and administrators as part of the work environment, and were satisfied with the meager salaries paid to them because theirs was a profession of caring and dedication. This situation has, however, changed drastically since the 1970s.

Self-governance is a concept that is important to all professions. The most powerful professional groups are those that maintain a strong sense of self-governance over their members. The American Medical Association (AMA) is a classic example of the power that an organized group can exert. Much of the physicians' power to affect institutional governance, and even broader issues such as managed care, comes from the AMA. Membership in a powerful organization can be an alternative to unions. Up to this time, the ANA has split its activities and focus between self-governance and collective bargaining. It has been successful in most of its efforts at collective bargaining but somewhat limited in its success for self-governance.

As nursing responsibilities increased with advancing technology and changes in the health-care system, nurses began to recognize that their responsibilities far exceeded their authority to influence their practice. They started to view professional autonomy, authority, and accountability as essential elements in high-quality client care. One approach to gaining these elements was to change the organizational structure of the health-care facilities where they were employed.

Nurses have challenged the traditional governance structure at a number of levels with varying amounts of success. Nursing service administrators are the leaders of the largest single group of health-care professionals in most health-care organizations—generally about 50% of all the employees.[2] Because of their education and experience, many nursing administrators have moved into positions of power in the health-care system and are no longer willing to accept the traditional role to which nurses were relegated. As middle managers, nursing administrators are often caught in the middle of conflicting expectations. For example, the chief administrator may want to cut the budget by reducing staffing, whereas the nurses on the units recognize that they can no longer provide high-quality nursing care because the staffing levels are already too low.

What Do You Think?

What are some reasons that nurses have had little power in relation to governance? How can nurses gain power in governance?

Staff RNs often view themselves as located at the bottom of the hierarchy with very little power. This is rarely the case. Depending on the organization of the facility, RNs have positional authority over LPNs, nursing assistants, and individuals from the laboratory and radiology department.

Nurses have gained greater control over their practice by fostering change in the organizational structures of health-care facilities and agencies. The changes include decentralization of authority, identification of professional nurses as peers, agreement on the philosophy and goals of nursing care, and increased responsibility for directing and planning the care given to clients while they are in the facility.[11]

Alternative Models for Governance

In an attempt to redistribute power and authority within health-care organizations, several alternative forms of governance have been developed. Some of these work better than others, depending on the facility and the willingness of the individuals involved to cooperate.

The Board of Nursing Model

In this model of governance, the nursing staff structure is similar to the medical staff structure. There is a general board of trustees at the top and, immediately below, at the same level, a medical board of directors, a nursing board of directors, a board of directors representing other professionals, and the hospital administration itself.[2] The nursing board of directors deals with such matters as credentials and standards of care and also promotes cooperation between nurses and the other professionals of the facility. Although this type of structure places nurses on an equal administrative footing with the physicians, administration, and other professionals in the facility, it does have the tendency to create a large number of administrative personnel. A tendency for conflicts to arise between the different board members does exist.

Contracting for Nursing Services Model

The **fee for service** model proposes that clients be billed for nursing care as a separate item, much the same way that they are billed for medical care by the physicians. Currently, when a client receives a hospital bill, the care provided by nurses is included in the overall room charge. In order to make this model work, nurses select individual clients for whom they wish to care and then accept responsibility for providing that care. Some type of scale would need to be developed so that the nurse could charge a higher rate for taking care of more seriously ill clients with more complex health-care needs. Nurses would take responsibility for scheduling and for self-management. And as with physicians, there would have to be a **peer review** mechanism to monitor the quality of health care provided.

Although this model supports primary care and the expansion of the nurse's role and responsibility, it would be very difficult to implement. Some of the problems include establishing acceptable pay scales, ensuring adequate staffing, and paying ancillary help such as orderlies and nursing assistants. Probably the most significant single factor that affects the implementation of this model is the hospital administration's loss of control over the nursing staff. If the nurses' pay were to come directly from the client, rather than the hospital, nurses would tend to place the client's needs before the needs of the facility. This model is still unacceptable to most facilities.

The Shared Governance Model

In the shared governance model, power and authority are transferred to the nursing staff rather than being seated primarily in nursing administration. The key to shared governance is decentralization of the nursing administration structure. Its goal is to involve professional nurses in the decision-making process at all levels to ensure that their knowledge and expertise are used to deliver the highest-quality care possible.[5]

> **" "** *In the shared governance model, power and authority are transferred to the nursing staff rather than being seated primarily in nursing administration.*

Shared governance allows the nurse autonomy in decisions about nursing practice, working conditions, staffing levels, standards of care, and other areas. It gives professional nurses the chance to be held accountable and responsible for their clinical judgment and the care they give to clients. It allows their peers a chance to recognize their knowledge and competence as true health-care professionals.

In general, shared governance locates the source of power in the clinical areas rather than in the **administrative** areas. Several different types of shared governance exist.

In the congressional shared governance model, a group of professional nurses is organized into a congress. This congress develops by-laws, elects representatives, and forms committees to govern the activities of the nursing staff.[10] Composed entirely of professional nurses, the committees oversee professional practice, evaluate quality of care, provide continuing education, plan for staffing, conduct research, and discipline errant nurses. Although this is a highly effective method to provide nursing care and to increase the autonomy of nurses, it does require a tremendous initial expenditure of time, effort, and money. Many institutions are not willing to make that commitment.

In the unit-based model, the shared governance is on a smaller scale. Groups of nurses on each unit form councils for professional practice that perform many of the functions that the professional congresses perform. In order to make this model succeed, there must be a real transfer of decision-making power from the head nurse or unit supervisor to the staff nurses. Shared governance is a model that the staff is willing to undertake, rather than being forced into it by the administration. Unfortunately, many facilities that profess a shared governance structure really are using a traditional hierarchy structure with somewhat more open lines of communication. The test of a true shared governance model quickly becomes evident when difficult decisions have to be made. For example, if the staff nurses decide that more staffing is needed for their unit, but the administration refuses to make money available for new

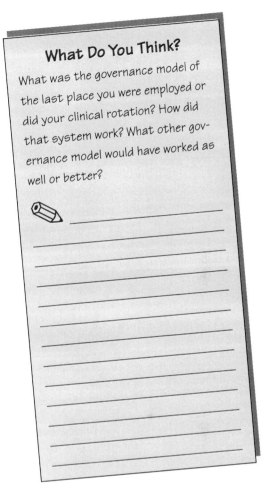

nurses, then it is not a true shared governance model.

Governance and Collective Bargaining

Forms of governance directly affect which issues are likely to be involved in nurses' collective bargaining. Although salary and benefits are important considerations in professional nursing, issues of autonomy, accountability, and control of practice are gaining importance for many nurses. In a health-care facility with a form of governance that allows nurses to have a relatively large degree of control over their practice, the issues discussed at the bargaining table are more likely to revolve around a professional agenda. In facilities with a rigidly structured hierarchy of authority that gives nurses little autonomy, accountability, or control over their practice, collective bargaining is more likely to center on control and power issues.

Nurses are highly educated professionals. They recognize that they can practice autonomously and can make sound decisions about client care. They also recognize that an increased understanding of the governance process requires many of the same skills used in collective bargaining. Key elements in both processes require an understanding of negotiation, compromise, and consensus building to attain one's goals. Changes in methods of governance also will require major changes in the health-care system. Professional nurses have the power to produce those changes and the ability to deal with the future of health-care successfully.

Conclusion

Although few issues elicit such strong emotions among nurses as collective bargaining, it is a reality in today's health-care system. Nurses are beginning to realize that they are not in a strictly altruistic profession, but rather one in which they use their knowledge and skills to provide high-quality services to clients. The knowledge and skills used in client care are gained at the cost of years of expensive education in schools of nursing and of dedication to an often underappreciated profession. Nurses no longer need to apologize or feel guilty about seeking payment for their work on a level commensurate with their knowledge and skills.

Negotiation is the process of give and take between groups with the goal of reaching an agreement acceptable to both sides. Although negotiations may be formal or informal, hostile or friendly, a cooperative atmosphere fostered by both sides that recognizes the similarity of each side's demands will be the most productive in reaching a satisfactory contract.

Although not a new concept for nursing, collective bargaining is an issue that is still hotly debated among professional nurses. Collective bargaining is viewed by some as unprofessional, unethical, divisive, and a fundamental threat to job security. However, the goals of collective bargaining, including improvement of economic benefits, better staffing and scheduling, fair treatment for all nurses, and improved quality of care for clients, are common to all health-care providers. Nurses must decide at some point in their careers whether joining a collective bargaining unit will best help them to achieve these goals. This is not an easy decision to make, and each nurse should gather as much information as possible about the situation before making a decision.

Nurses need to recognize that the time has arrived to elevate the profession to a new level. Change in forms of governance is one method that nurses can use to change the health-care system. Nursing as a profession now has the opportunity to gain tremendous power and take its rightful place as an indispensable force in the health-care system. All that is required is for nurses to become educated in the issues involved and to take an aggressive stance in the shaping of the future.

Critical Thinking Exercises

✔ Develop a position paper either supporting or opposing collective bargaining.

✔ A nurse on your unit states one day: "Membership in the state nurses association is a waste of time and money. They can't help you make a better living!" How would you respond to this nurse?

✔ Develop an ideal contract for nurses. Which elements would receive the highest priority?

✔ Develop a plan for shared governance in a facility you are familiar with. How would the organizational process take place? What are some of the major difficulties in developing this plan?

References

1. Breda, KL: Professional nurses in unions: Working together pays off. J Prof Nurs 13(2):99–109, 1997.
2. Tappen, RM: Nursing Leadership and Management, ed 2. F. A. Davis, Philadelphia, 1998.
3. Snell, J: Danger—bully at work. Nursing Times 93(21):24–27, 1997.
4. Mapel, L: Nursing unions: Are they necessary? Kansas Nurse 71(4):1–2, 1996.
5. Huber, D: Leadership and Nursing Management. WB Saunders, Philadelphia, 1996.
6. Supreme Court okays all-RN unit. American Nurse 20:1, 1991.
7. Tappen, RM: Nursing Leadership and Management. FA Davis, Philadelphia, 1995.
8. Keenan, M: Collective bargaining: The nursing workplace. Kentucky Nurse 45(4):22, 1997.
9. Heally, P: Nurses doing junior doctors work are safe claim unions. Nurs Standard 10:34–35, 1996.
10. Sullivan, TJ: Collaboration: A Health Care Imperative. McGraw-Hill, New York, 1998.
11. Maloney, MM: Professionalization of Nursing, ed 2. JB Lippincott, Philadelphia, 1999.

BIBLIOGRAPHY

American Nurses Association: Nursing's Agenda for Health Care Reform. American Nurses Association, Kansas City, 1992.

Anderson, K: Getting What You Want. Dutton, New York, 1993.

Bazerman, MH: Negotiating Rationally. Free Press, New York, 1992.

Chenevert, M: Pro-Nurse Handbook. CV Mosby, Philadelphia, 1998.

Delegation: Concepts and decision-making process. National Council of State Boards 16(4):1–4, 1995.

Flanagan, L: How collective bargaining benefits nurses. Directions 22:8–22, 1992.

Giovinco, G: When nurses strike: Ethical issues. Nursing Management 24:86–90, 1993.

Johnston, W, and Packer, A: Workforce 2000: Work and Workers for the Twenty-first Century. Hudson Institute, Indianapolis, Ind., 1987.

Hoffman, S: Nurses must unify to bring change for patients and profession. American Nurse 29(6):5–7, 1997.

Lippman, H: Legally speaking: Expect to hear about unions. RN 54:68–72, 1991.

McKinley, M: Collaboration is an effective tool. AACN News 15(10):2, 1998.

Mahony, C: State of the union's union leadership, pay campaign, political lobbying. Nursing Times 92(40):28–31, 1996.

Malone, B: Professionalism: An exercise in stretching. American Nurse 30(3):5, 1998.

Naisbitt, J, and Aburdene, P: Megatrends 200: Ten New Directions for the 1990s. Morrow, New York, 1990.

Nicoll, LH: Nurses' Guide to the Internet, ed 2. JB Lippincott, Philadelphia, 1998.

NLRB to the Supreme Court: Labor law protects nurses. Am J Nurs 96(4):67–72, 1996.

Nicotera, AM: Beyond two dimensions: Handling conflict. Management Communication Quarterly 6:282–306, 1993.

Raelin, JA: Unionization and deprofessionalization: Which comes first? Journal of Organizational Behavior 10(2):101–115, 1989.

Rowden, R: Days of confusion—What exactly are nursing unions trying to achieve in their national pay campaign. Nursing Times 91(29):53, 1995.

Scott, K: SNA representation means increased job satisfaction. American Nurse 24:2, 1993.

Shindul-Rothschild, J, Long-Middleton, E, and Berry, D: 10 keys to quality care. Am J Nurs 97(11):35–43, 1997.

Shindual-Rothschild, J, et al: Where have all the nurses gone? Am J Nurs 96(11):25–32, 1996.

Stone, T: Collective bargaining protects nurses and patients. American Nurse 29(6):5–7, 1997.

Stearly, H: The rise and fall of nursing unions. Revolution Summer, 56–59, 1995.

Strickland, OL, and Fishman, DJ: Nursing Issues in the 1990s. Delmar, Albany, NY, 1994.

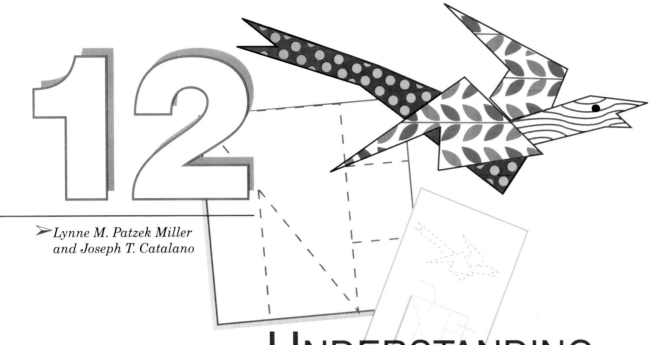

12

➤ *Lynne M. Patzek Miller*
and Joseph T. Catalano

UNDERSTANDING AND DEALING WITH DIFFICULT PEOPLE

Learning Objectives

After completing this chapter, the reader will be able to:

1. Explain the importance of understanding human behaviors.
2. Describe conflict resolution and relationship tools.
3. Identify communications styles.
4. Analyze and apply problem-solving and conflict-resolution tools.
5. Discuss the use of the nursing process in conflict resolution.
6. Formulate coping strategies to handle difficult people.

Good communication skills are often advertised as the answer to many of the problems encountered in everyday life. Television personalities, instructors, and psychologists promote improved communication skills as the answer to parental, marital, financial, and work-related problems. The nursing profession recognizes communication as one of the cornerstones of its practice. Nurses must be able to communicate with clients, family members, physicians, peers, and associates in an effective and constructive manner to achieve their goals of high-quality care.

In today's rapidly evolving health-care system, nurses are called on to supervise a growing number of assistive and unlicensed personnel. One of the keys to good supervision is the ability to communicate to the individual what he or she must do to provide the required care and, often, how the care should be given. It is not always easy. Many of the people whom nurses supervise are poorly trained, lack the theoretical and technical knowledge base of the nurse, and may display attitudes that make them resistant to direction. However, nurse supervisors can be and often are held legally responsible for the actions of those individuals who work under their direction.

FACTORS THAT AFFECT COMMUNICATION

Change

How people deal with change can affect how they respond to the environment and communicate with others. Change is one of the few absolute certainties in today's healthcare system. Change can produce many emotions, ranging from excitement and anticipation to stress, fear, and anxiety. At minimum, change makes most people feel uncomfortable. Any change can be simultaneously positive and negative. During the process of learning new skills, treatments, or techniques, most people feel a sense of accomplishment at the same time as they feel afraid of making mistakes, being judged by others, or being labeled as "slow learners." An example is when a new graduate nurse starts his or her first day at work and is very excited about the new experience and the potential for career development. However, at the same time the nurse is worried about being accepted into the group, being able to practice what was learned in nursing school, and being able to learn the new skills required by the unit. Almost everyone has a sense of dread when moving away from activities with which they have become comfortable. Setting realistic personal goals and timelines for learning new information will help re-duce the fear and stress when making major changes.

Change affects communication in various ways. People may be afraid to ask questions about new procedures or policies because they fear that they might appear "stupid" in front of their colleagues. Fear of being criticized closes individuals off to positive suggestions and new ideas. Others may hesitate in sharing ideas because they are afraid of being labeled as being confrontational. For example, a nurse is reassigned from the medical surgical unit to the intensive care unit (ICU). This nurse will initially be somewhat fearful in the new environment with the highly trained and assertive expert unit nurses who always seem to be in control. A more positive approach would be for the new nurse to utilize the unit nurses' expertise and learn from their example. The new nurse needs to remember that everyone on that unit was a novice at one time. In the current healthcare system, almost everyone is fearful much of the time of making mistakes and of falling short of the high standards of the profession.

Change is not always negative. Often a staff that is initially resistant to a change and fights to prevent it, once they have gone through the process, would never go back to the old way of doing things. All change involves some risk taking, and some people are better at risk taking than are others. Consider the following case study:

After analysis of the needs of the clients and the nursing workload of a busy medical unit, the unit manager decided to change the work shift times. In addition to the standard 7 A.M. to 3 P.M., 3 P.M. to 11 P.M., and 11 P.M. to 7 A.M. shifts, she de-

> " " *People may be afraid to ask questions about new procedures or policies because they fear that they might appear "stupid" in front of their colleagues.*

cided to add a 5 A.M. to 1 P.M. shift to increase coverage during the busiest period of the shift. The RN assigned to the new shift recognized the benefits to the unit and clients, thus she accepted and supported the change with few objections. Also, the change in shift times allowed her to alter her personal schedule so that she could take extra courses toward her master's degree at a local college. For the RN, the change in shifts was a positive experience.

However, the LPN assigned to this new shift was upset with the change. She was a "late sleeper" and did not want to come in so early. She liked the shifts the way that they were and did not see any advantages to changing things needlessly.

After the new shift was initiated, the LPN was usually 15 to 30 minutes late, called in sick frequently, and was "grumpy" and hard to talk to when she did come in to work. For this LPN, the change was negative and unacceptable.

Nurses need to keep in mind that the communication abilities of clients who are experiencing change will be affected in very much the same way as nurses who are experiencing change. As a result of disease, trauma, or surgery, many clients face sudden and major alterations in their bodies, as well as changes in their ability to function and carry out daily self-care activities. For example, a client with a new colostomy must adapt to major physiologic, psychological, and emotional changes. Most clients who have surgical procedures that result in major body function alterations go through the stages of the grief process: denial, anger, guilt, depression, and resolution.

> 66 99 *Nurses need to keep in mind that the communication abilities of clients who are experiencing change will be affected in very much the same way as nurses who are experiencing change.*

Communication with a client in the anger stage of the grief process who is hostile, critical of his care, and verbally abusive will be much different than communication with a client in the depression stage who is withdrawn, reticent, and sleeps most of the time. Recognition of the communication behaviors of each of the grief stages is essential in understanding why clients are acting in a particular way. A decision must then be made regarding the most effective communication technique to use when providing care.

Stress

Stress is produced by many factors and always affects an individual's ability to communicate. Some common causes of stress for health-care workers include institutional restructuring, group interaction and dynamics, unilateral management decisions, or personal issues and experiences. Regardless of the source, stress usually decreases people's ability to interact and communicate and increases the demands on their coping mechanisms. When people are unable to cope with a stressful situation successfully, they may experience an increased state of tension or anxiety; they may develop physiologic symptoms such as nausea, stomach cramps, diarrhea, or palpitations; and, in extreme cases, they may even become paranoid or psychotic. Uncontrolled, high levels of stress on a nursing unit may lead to competition among the nurses that affects their teamwork, productivity, and the quality of the care given.

Physicians who are stressed by worry about a severely ill client or threats to their autonomy, practice, and income by changes in reimbursement policies may become tense and highly critical of or even verbally abusive toward nurses. The hospital management may also experience increased stress owing to the escalating responsibility of maintaining high-quality services with ever-shrinking revenues. Management often deals with its stress by becoming more autocratic, making increased demands on the nursing staff while reducing the control that nurses have over their practice, and becoming closed off to input from nurses and physicians. At some point, one group's stress always affects another group's stress level, whose stress in turn increases another group's stress. The process becomes a destructive circle of cause-and-effect responses that increases the stress levels for everyone in the facility.

Stress in the health-care environment is not just experienced by health-care providers. Stress for clients starts when they first come into contact with the health-care system, peaks when they have to undergo physical examinations, surgery, or invasive treatments, and continues throughout the recovery period. The fear that a nurse may not respond to clients' needs increases clients' stress levels and they sometimes become more demanding of care, which, in turn, increases the nurse's stress levels. If the nursing staff is experiencing high stress levels, clients often sense this subconsciously, and as a result, clients' stress levels will increase also.

Several techniques can be used to reduce clients' stress levels so that they can better communicate and become more receptive ot teaching. Stress reduction techniques range from very simple measures that everyone can use such as distraction with music or simple activities, exercise, or reduction in

> " " *Stress for clients starts when they first come into contact with the health-care system, peaks when they have to undergo physical examinations, surgery, or invasive treatments, and continues throughout the recovery period.*

stimuli to more advanced techniques such as meditation, **biofeedback,** and even anti-anxiety medications.

Nurses need to be able to identify situations that produce stress, recognize the symptoms shown by someone in a stressful situation, know how to reduce stress, and be able to use appropriate communication techniques with someone under stress. Of course, if possible, the best way to reduce stress is to eliminate the stressful situation. For example, the hospital management has just sent a memo to all the hospital units that a new client assessment form they have developed is to be implemented next week. This new form is in addition to the ones that the nurses already fill out each day. The new form is to be completed by RNs only and must be done each shift on every client and then sent to the house supervisor so that management can track acuity. Because of recent facility restructuring and changes in staffing patterns, often there is only one RN on the 3 P.M. to 11 P.M. and 11 P.M. to 7 A.M. shifts to cover a 42-bed unit. This extra, time-consuming, and seemingly redundant paperwork increases the stress of the staff RNs to an unacceptable level. They meet as a group with management and propose that the assessment forms that they already are using be modified so that they include the data that management wants on the new forms. Photocopies of the revised "old" form could then be made by the unit clerk for each shift and given to the supervisors, thus eliminating the new form. Management notes the high stress levels of the RNs, recognizes that increased stress lowers the quality of care, and decides to follow the RNs' proposal, thus eliminating the primary source of the RNs' stress. Although all sources of stress cannot be eliminated completely, in most situations it can be reduced to a manageable level. However, high stress levels should never be used as an excuse for destructive anger and behaviors, failure of communication, or abuse of individuals.

Anger

In addition to being one of the stages of the grief process, anger can be a symptom of personal frustration, lack of control, fear of change, or feelings of hopelessness. Anger is one of the strong primitive natural emotions that helps individuals protect themselves against a variety of external threats. Although everyone experiences anger, how it is expressed often depends on a person's family and ethnic background, life experiences, and personal values. In some cultures, loud and physically expressive outbursts are the norm for the expression of anger, whereas in other cultures, anger is internalized and expressed only as a "controlled rage."

As with most of the other factors that affect communication, anger can be either positive or negative. When anger is used in a positive, productive manner, it can promote change and release tension. Anger can be used positively to increase others' attention, initiate communication, problem solve, and energize the change process. Sensitivity to internal anger can warn individuals that something is wrong either within themselves or with someone or something in the external environment.

However, many individuals have difficulty expressing and using their anger in a positive manner. Anger that is used negatively is very destructive. It hinders communication, makes coworkers fearful, and erodes relationships with others. Anger expressed by abusive behaviors such as pounding on nursing station counters, throwing carts or surgical instruments, verbal outbursts, or even in violent physical contact is never acceptable and may lead to civil or criminal actions against the perpetrator. The negative expression of anger may cause the person who is the object of the anger to retaliate or seek revenge. But probably the most destructive form that negative anger can take is when it is internalized and suppressed. Long-term, suppressed anger has been associated with a number of physiologic and psychological problems ranging from gastric ulcers and hypertension to myocardial infarctions, strokes and even psychotic rage episodes.

Nurses who understand what makes both themselves and others angry are better able to either avoid anger-producing situations or cope effectively with their own anger or with that of others. For example, even new graduate nurses soon learn that there are some situations that will almost always evoke an angry response from hospitalized clients. These include serving meals that are cold or poorly cooked, not answering call lights in a timely manner, waking up soundly sleeping clients at midnight to give them a sleeping pill, or taking 10 attempts to start an intravenous (IV) line. Similarly, unit managers and hospital administrators quickly learn that some of the things that they do will almost always produce angry responses from the staff. These actions include unilateral changes in the work schedule, additional paperwork, reduction in staffing levels, or refusal for requests for vacation or time off.

It is important that nurses understand that anger is a normal human emotion. Once it is recognized, it should be dealt with and then let go. There are times when situa-

> " " *Even new graduate nurses soon learn that there are some situations that will almost always evoke an angry response from hospitalized clients.*

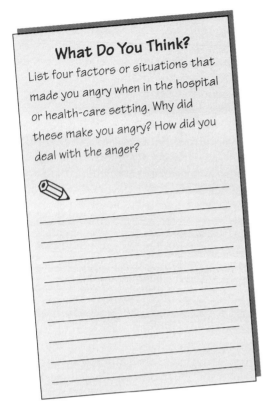

tions are not going to change, no matter how angry the person becomes, and other times when no amount of anger will prevent changes from occurring.

Group Dynamics

The power of the group over an individual's behavior should never be underestimated. Groups establish and exert their power through a set of unique behaviors or norms that their members are expected to follow. These norms may be formal or informal, written or unwritten, promulgated or merely understood. Unfortunately, in most nursing units the norms are often not clearly expressed, yet they may be used as judgment tools or standards for evaluating work behaviors. When new nurses begin work on a particular unit, in order to function effectively they must quickly learn the unwritten unit norms and identify the informal leaders.

As with most elements in communication, group dynamics may be positive or negative. Nurses who do not learn and fail to display the expected group behaviors may be ostracized from the group, thus making the work environment psychologically uncomfortable and perhaps even physically difficult. For example, nonconforming nurses may find that there is no one around when they need help ambulating an unsteady client. Or a particular nursing unit staff may have a strong team approach. If the new nurse is highly independent and prefers to work alone, he or she may not "fit in" and experience hostility or sarcasm from the other nurses on the unit.

Consider the following scenario demonstrating group dynamics:

The ICU has the responsibility for on-call coverage for the recovery room for unscheduled postoperative clients on the evening shifts, night shifts, and all of the weekend shifts. There is no formal written policy, but coverage has traditionally been handled on a voluntary, rotating basis. Because it is "voluntary," one of the ICU nurses has decided that he does not want to take call any more. He is the only member of the ICU staff who does not take call. Soon after he announces his decision, he begins to sense anger and experience alienation from his peers. Although he is very knowledgeable, has highly developed nursing skills, and provides consistently high-quality care to assigned clients on his regular shifts, on his semi-annual peer evaluation, he receives low ratings from his coworkers based on the informal call coverage standard and expectations. The unit nurses feel that he is no longer a team player.

The nurse becomes angry because he feels that the use of unclear, unwritten standards is an unfair way to evaluate his ability as a nurse. He soon finds that the other ICU nurses accidentally "forget" to invite him to group functions. He also seems to be assigned the most difficult and largest number of clients during any given shift, seemingly to compensate for not taking call.

Group dynamics involves many factors, including methods of communications, professional behaviors, professional growth, flexibility, problem solving, participation, and competition. The ability to understand and use the elements of group dynamics has a direct relationship on the behaviors, cooperation, and effectiveness of the team. Often, when a team labels an individual member as "difficult," it most likely means that the individual is not following one or more of the informal, unwritten group norms.

Competition

Competition can be a very powerful element in group dynamics and communication. Depending on how it is channeled, expressed, and used, competition can be a positive or negative force within the group. The various forms of competition can be individual, team, or unit focused. A common expression of competition in the group setting is peer evaluations. For peer evaluations to be a positive form of competition, the unit must decide ahead of time on the norms and expectations that they value and then design an objective measurement tool to evaluate whether the individual is meeting the norms. Also, each individual being evaluated must be aware of the criteria before the evaluation is conducted. The evaluation team must be educated on evaluation techniques and must be as objective and professional as possible.

In the health-care setting, it is important for all professionals, unit groups, and management to promote competition in a positive, progressive, and supportive environment. When competition is channeled positively, it leads to new and creative ideas, better programs, increased growth, more productive interactions, and higher quality client care. When the competition is negative, it often produces failures, depression, sabotage, unit turf conflicts, decreased productivity, and lower quality care. For example, the competition on a nursing unit turned negative when the nurses on the 7 A.M. to 3 P.M. shift began competing with the nurses on the 3 P.M. to 11 P.M. shift in order to appear more knowledgeable about client care to the nurse manager. In order to "look better," the nurses on the 7 A.M. to 3 P.M. shift intentionally withheld selected client laboratory test results during shift report. As a result of this action, several tests scheduled for the 3 P.M. to 11 P.M. shift were not done, angering the physicians, potentially threatening the safety of the clients, and making the nurses on the 3 P.M. to 11 P.M.

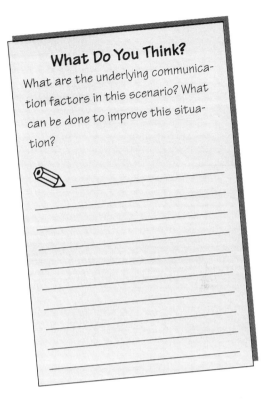

What Do You Think?

What are the underlying communication factors in this scenario? What can be done to improve this situation?

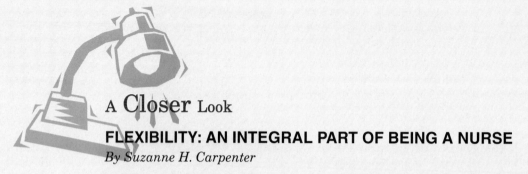

A Closer Look

FLEXIBILITY: AN INTEGRAL PART OF BEING A NURSE

By Suzanne H. Carpenter

I graduated from nursing school with many definite, black-and-white, inflexible options. I knew how things were supposed to be done, and that if you were not doing things by the book, it must be wrong. However, after 14 years in nursing, I have learned that the ability to be flexible is an integral part of nursing. It does not mean compromising values or patient care. It means being a patient advocate, always working to empower the patient in the face of the "organized chaos" of any healthcare system. It also means being able to take care of the immediate, acute, physiological needs of patients while remembering to acknowledge their emotional and spiritual needs.

Mrs. C immediately comes to mind when I think about my role in empowering patients. She suffered an acute cerebral vascular accident 2 days after coronary artery bypass surgery. Once an active tennis player, she was now faced with right hemiparesis. She was right-handed. Surprisingly, at 75 years of age, she weaned easily from mechanical ventilation and was extubated without incident.

In shift-to-shift report one day, it was communicated that the physicians had discussed Mrs. C's case with her son, a staff physician, and it was decided that, because of her poor prognosis, for a "full recovery," she would be made a "no code." Within 1 week all IVs, antibiotics, and wall nebulizers were discontinued. I was uneasy with these decisions, which had been made so quickly and without any conversation with Mrs. C.

During the 7-to-7 shift one night, Mrs. C was awake, restless, and having difficulty coughing. I enlisted the help of the respiratory therapist to dangle her in an effort to assist her in coughing. While I supported her body on her weak side, the respiratory therapist began to splint her chest in an effort to ease pain and facilitate a productive cough.

What happened next is burned in my memory. Mrs. C looked up into my eyes and said, "Please don't let me die. I am not ready to die yet." I reassured her that I was there to help her during this postoperative period. A knot formed in the pit of my stomach as I recalled the earlier shift-to-shift report. I decided it was time for me to talk to Mrs. C. I asked her what she knew about what had happened to her since surgery. She said she did not know anything, but that she was frightened and wanted to make sure we knew she was not ready to die. I explained why she had the paralysis of her right side. I acknowledged that this loss of the use of her right arm and leg must be exceptionally difficult because of her love for tennis. I remember a single tear on her cheek when she responded that she was not sure how she felt about the possibility of not being able to play tennis. I spent some quiet moments with Mrs. C as she cried, letting her grieve her loss, and reassured her that I was there for her.

I knew that I had to document what Mrs. C had confided to me in the nurse's notes, and in report. I had to be her voice, the advocate who empowered her by making her wishes known. After documenting and quoting Mrs. C's plea not to let her die, I shared the events of the night with the attending surgeon and asked him to read my nursing notes. He read them, took a deep breath, and said, "Thank you for doing what I wish I had done—listen to the patient." When the son called to check on his mother that morning, I spoke to him about my conversation with his mother and asked him to read my nursing notes, which documented what his mother had stated.

What happened next brings a memory of sorrow as well as joy. The sorrow came when her son read my note and furiously reported me to the nursing supervisor for "going beyond the scope of where a nurse should go." The joy came when the nursing supervisor supported my actions, stating that a nurse was a patient advocate, and that what I had done was indeed what a nurse should be doing.

Within 24 hours the attending surgeon had consulted with other physicians on the case. Antibiotic therapy, respiratory treatments, and IV therapy were reinstated. Physical therapy was also consulted. Within 2 weeks Mrs. C became stable enough to be discharged. The last report I received on her was that she was doing some gardening at home and was able to walk with a cane. This experience confirmed for me that, whereas being a patient advocate is not always the easiest thing to do, it is indeed the only right thing to do. It is the essence of nursing.

As I write about patient advocacy and caring practices, distinct memories of other patient situations flood my mind. There was Nellie, described in the report I received as a "screaming, crazy woman." I wondered what I could do with this patient who did nothing but cry, moan, and yell loudly, "Why me, oh Lord?" Most of the staff tried to stay away from her. I sat next to her bed and said, "Tell me about what you've been through." She told me about her diabetes, how her doctors wanted to cut off her leg, and her feelings of isolation and loneliness. As she spoke, her moans and loud screaming subsided. She wept softly, and I listened. She asked me to pray with her. I shared a copy of *A Mother's Topical Bible,* which I kept in my pocket. She read it quietly until she fell asleep. The staff kept peeking in the room to make sure she was still there. They asked, "What on earth did you do with her?" I answered, "I listened."

Then there was Ann, who was admitted to the medical ICU with an overdose of a propranolol blocking agent. She had taken the whole bottle because, she said, "I knew it would stop my heart and I wanted to die." While tending to her nasal-gastric tube, Foley catheter, frequent vital signs, and cardiac monitoring, I made a point to hold her hand and say, "You must have been through a lot tonight to have tried to end your life." She began to cry and related a story of personal pain and rejection—of her attempts to call hospital mental health crisis lines, only to be told that they could not help her because she did not have the right insurance. She sobbed that, after attempting suicide, she was so angry that not one emergency medical service or emergency room physician or staff member had even acknowledged her attempt at suicide. Everyone kept telling her how lucky she was and how she was stable, cardiacwise. She cried, "You are the only person who has acknowledged that I tried to kill myself." I continued to listen. I asked if she wanted to talk to our hospital social worker. I documented her desires to see a social worker and to visit with pastoral care. In the morning, I communicated these findings to her physician and we worked on ensuring these referrals. A psychiatric referral was also made. Two weeks later I received a lovely letter from the hospital chaplain, who thanked me for being there for this girl when no one else was. I smiled. I felt warm inside. I love nursing.

I also remember Richard, the "no code" who needed haloperidol (Haldol) intermuscular injections round the clock, according to the information I received in report. By this time I was a nursing instructor and my freshman student needed experience in giving an IM injection. I assigned this patient to the student, who later appeared distraught. She said, "He won't let me touch him." I went to the room to find a frightened patient. He was trying to sit up in bed, his ears and lips were dusky, there was scant dark urine in the catheter, his respiratory rate was 40, and he had diffuse rhonchi bilaterally and distended neck veins. A staff member on the previous shift had placed him in restraints, which I promptly removed. I elevated his head and called respiratory therapy for an 02 saturation. I put my mouth close to his ear and told him that I was there for him. I told him in a calm tone that he was not producing much urine and that his lungs had some fluid in them. I told him I would see that his doctor was notified so that medication could be ordered. His respiratory rate slowed a little as he clutched my hand. My student notified the charge nurse, who called the physician. We got this patient an order for 40-mg Lasix (furosemide) intravenously, an arterial blood gas, oxygen, and a chest x-ray. The man held my hand, looked into my eyes, and said, "I'm dying, you know." I asked him if he would like to see his own minister or someone from our pastoral care department. He nodded he would. His daughter was at the bedside with us. Whatever I explained to him, I also explained to her. She said that she too would like to see a priest from pastoral care. We had the priest paged. By this time our shift was over and my student reported off. We had a wonderful postclinical conference, sharing these events with the clinical group. I found out that 2 days later the patient died peacefully after having said a prayer with a priest and his family. You see, he was a "no code," not a "no care." My student learned much more than how to give an injection. I love teaching students how to care.

SUZANNE H. CARPENTER, RN, MSN, CCRN
Assistant Professor of Nursing
Our Lady of the Lake College of Nursing
Baton Rouge, LA

Reprinted with permission from AACN News 14(9):5, 10, 1997.

shift appear incompetent. In addition, the nurses on that shift had to complete several incident reports on the errors that occurred on their shift. One informal component of the staff nurses' performance evaluations used by the unit manager is the number of incident reports that a nurse must file. The more incident reports, the poorer will be the nurse's performance evaluation. To the unit manager, the nurses on the 7 A.M. to 3 P.M. shift appear to be more competent because of the seemingly poor care, indicated by a large number of incident reports, that is being given on the 3 P.M. to 11 P.M. shift. However, when the nurses on the 3 P.M. to 11 P.M. shift discovered what really happened, they devised several ways to "get even" with the nurses on the 7 A.M. to 3 P.M. shift.

Working Environment

The delivery of health care is currently in a rapid transition from a fee-for-service to a managed care environment. Health care is shifting from acute, inpatient care to long-term outpatient care and from being illness based to a prevention and wellness focus. The changes produced by this transition are creating a high degree of stress at all levels of the health-care system. As discussed earlier, both change and stress are major barriers to effective communication.

What Do You Think?

Have you ever been in a situation where others have intentionally sabotaged your work? What was the situation? How did you feel? How did you deal with it? Did you try to retaliate?

One measure that can be taken to both alleviate some of the stress caused by the current changes in health care and improve unit communication is to encourage all members of the health-care team to participate in the renovation of their work environment. Through active participation, workers have an opportunity to have an impact on and direct the changes that are being made. Some people mistakenly believe that if they do not become involved, the changes will not happen. Unfortunately, when people are not actively involved in the restructuring process, others who are probably less qualified will make the changes anyway.

Increased fear, high stress levels, angry outbursts, and feelings of insecurity all are potential results of a work environment where the workers do not participate in the change process. Difficult behaviors resulting in unclear communication become more evident during times of change and stress. Ugly rumors, feelings of resentment, and increased insecurity often result when intergroup communications are not clear. An open, interactive work environment increases the probability of successful communication and adaptation to change.

Understanding what motivates a person's behavior permits the individual to design a plan or develop coping mechanisms for communicating based on sound interpersonal techniques. When individuals are able to separate themselves from the difficult situation, they are less likely to take things personally and more likely to begin to focus on the underlying issues causing the problems rather than the other person's difficult behavior. The interaction becomes less judgmental and threatening to the other person. However, understanding the other person's

> **" "** *Increased fear, high stress levels, angry outbursts, and feelings of insecurity are potential results of a work environment where the workers do not participate in the change process.*

motives never excuses unacceptable behaviors such as sarcasm, angry outbursts, and abusive language. Rather, it allows for direct confrontation of the behavior in a more controlled and less emotional way.

All professional nurses need to develop coping mechanisms in order to deal with the behaviors demonstrated by difficult people. The very nature of the profession exposes nurses to a large number of people who are experiencing change, are under stress, and have a wide range of backgrounds and values as well as varying expectations. By understanding communication, using **behavior modification,** developing **assertiveness,** avoiding submissive and aggressive behaviors, and appreciating diversity, the nurse can develop the coping skills required for problem solving, handling conflict in the work setting, and confronting the unacceptable behaviors of difficult people.

UNDERSTANDING COMMUNICATIONS

Communication is an interactive sharing of information. It requires a sender, a message, and a receiver. After the sender sends the message, the receiver has a responsibility to listen to, process, and understand (encode) the information and then to respond to the sender by giving feedback (decoding). The encoding process occurs when the receiver thinks about the information, understands it, and forms an idea based on the message.

Several factors can interfere with the encoding process. On the sender's side, these can be factors such as unclear speech, monotone voice, poor sentence structure, inappropriate use of terminology or jargon, or lack of knowledge about the topic. On the receiver's side, factors that may interfere with encoding include lack of attention, prejudice and bias, preoccupation with another problem, or even physical factors such as pain, drowsiness, or impairment of the senses. For example, a staff nurse is in a mandatory meeting where the unit manager is discussing a new policy that will be starting next month. However, the nurse is thinking about an important heart medication that her client is to receive in 5 minutes. The nurse's primary concern is to get out of the meeting in time to give the medication. After the meeting, the nurse has only a minimal recollection of what was said because she did not encode the information well. The following month when the new policy is started, the staff nurse is confused about what she should do and makes several errors in relationship to the new policy.

There are two primary methods of communication—verbal and nonverbal. Verbal communication is either the written or spoken word and constitutes only about 7% of the communicated message. Nonverbal communication, which makes up the other 93% of communication, is everything else, including body language, facial expressions, gestures, physical appearance, touch, vocal cues (tone, pauses), and spatial territory (personal space). When the verbal and nonverbal messages are congruent, then the message is more easily encoded and clearly understood. If the verbal and nonverbal messages are conflicting, the nonverbal message is probably the most reliable. It is relatively easy for people to lie with words, but nonverbal communication tends to be unconscious and more difficult to control. For example, the nurse suspects that the mother of a newborn infant may be experiencing postpartum depression. The nurse

asks the mother how she feels about her new baby. The mother responds in a low volume, very slow-paced monotone voice: "I'm so happy I have this baby," while looking down at her feet in a slouched-over posture. The message from the mother is conflicting. The words are saying she is happy, but all the nonverbal signs indicate that she is depressed. The nurse concludes that more assessment for depression is required.

Effective communication requires understanding that the perceptions, emotions, and participation of both parties are interactive and have an effect on the transmission of the message. Nurses often encounter situations that require clarification of the information for accuracy and encoding. The following is an example of client teaching requiring a return demonstration: A nurse gives a teaching session to a client who is being sent home with a T-tube after surgical removal of gallstones from the common bile duct. After the nurse finished, she asked the client whether he understood how to empty the drainage bottle and measure the drainage. The client looked very confused, but mumbled "yes," while shaking his head back and forth. The nurse recognized that although the verbal response was positive, the nonverbal responses indicated that he really did not understand. The nurse surmised that further explanation or demonstration was required for proper encoding of the message by this client.

Nurses should recognize the many barriers to clear communication as well as the benefits of clear communication. Once the barriers to communication are identified, they can be overcome and the benefits of clear communication will result. These barriers and benefits that result when they are overcome are outlined in the following table.

> **" "** *Once the barriers to communication are identified, they can be overcome and the benefits of clear communication will result.*

BARRIERS TO CLEAR COMMUNICATION	BENEFITS OF CLEAR COMMUNICATION
Unclear/unexpressed expectations	Clear expectations
Confusion	Understanding
Retaliation	Forgiveness
Desire for power	Recognized leadership
Control of others	Companionship
Negative reputation	Respect
Manipulation	Independence
Low self-esteem	Realistic self-image
Biased perceptions	Acceptance
Inattention	Clear direction
Mistrust	Trusting relations
Anger	Self-control
Fear/anxiety	Comfort
Stress	Motivation/Energy
Insecurity	Security
Prejudice	Increased tolerance
Interruptions	Increased knowledge
Preoccupation	Concentration

COMMUNICATION STYLES

There are two predominant styles of communication—assertive and nonassertive. Nonassertive communication can be either submissive or aggressive. Individuals develop their communication styles over the course of their lives in response to many personal factors. Although most people have one predominant style of communication, they can and often do switch or combine styles depending on the situation in which they find themselves. For example, a unit manager who uses an assertive communication style when supervising the staff on her unit may revert to a submissive style when called into the Director of Nursing's office for her annual evaluation. Recognizing which communication style a person is using at any given time, as well as a person's own style, is important in making communication clear and effective.

Assertive Communication Style

Assertive communication involves interpersonal behaviors that permit people to defend and maintain their legitimate rights in a respectful manner that does not violate the rights of others. Assertive communication is honest, direct, and accurately expresses the person's feelings, beliefs, ideas, and opinions. Respect for self and others constitutes both the basis for and the result of assertive communication. It encourages trust and teamwork by communicating to others that they have the right to and are encouraged to express their opinions in an open and respectful atmosphere. Disagreement and discussion are considered to be a healthy part of the communication process, and negotiation is the positive mechanism for problem solving, learning, and personal growth.

Assertive communication always implies that the individual has the choice to voice an opinion, sometimes forcefully, as well as not to say anything at all. One of the keys to assertive communication is that the individual is in control of the communication and is not merely reacting to another's emotions.

Assessing Self-Assertiveness

Answer the following questions to assess your self-assertiveness:

- Who am I and what do I want?
- Do I believe I have the right to want it?
- How do I get it?
- Do I believe I can get it?
- Have I tried to be assertive with a person I am having difficulty communicating with?
- Am I letting my fears and perceptions cloud my interactions?
- What is the worst that can happen if we communicate?
- Can I live with the "worst"?
- Will communications have a long-term effect?

- How does it feel to be in constant fear of alienation or rejection?

Rules for Assertiveness

Anyone can learn to use an assertive communication style and develop assertiveness. When first developing this skill, people often feel frightened and overwhelmed. However, once individuals become comfortable with assertiveness, it helps to reinforce their self-concepts and becomes an effective tool for communication. There are a few rules to keep in mind while developing an assertive communication style and assertiveness:

- It is a learned skill.
- It takes practice.
- It requires a desire and motivation to change.
- It requires a willingness to take risks.
- It requires a willingness to make mistakes and try again.
- It requires an understanding that not every outcome sought will be obtained.
- It requires strong self-esteem.
- Self-reward for change and positive outcomes is essential.
- Listening to self is necessary for identifying needs.
- Constant re-examination of outcomes helps assess progress.
- Role-playing with a friend prior to the interaction builds skill and confidence.
- Goals for assertiveness growth need to be established beforehand.
- It requires recognition that change is a gradual process.
- Others should be allowed to make mistakes.

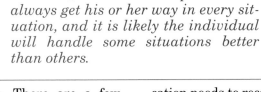

Assertiveness does not mean that a person will always get his or her way in every situation, and it is likely the individual will handle some situations better than others.

Personal Risks of Assertive Communication

There are always personal risks involved in learning any new skills or in attempting to change behavior. Learning assertive communication is no exception. People often fear that they may not choose the "perfect" assertive response. However, even seasoned assertive communicators may err from time to time, because every encounter is unique, involving different people and situations. The person who is new to assertive communication needs to recognize that it is a skill that takes practice.

Assertiveness does not mean that a person will always get his or her way in every situation, and it is likely the individual will handle some situations better than others. Remember that the goal to assertive communication is not to have an "I win, you lose" situation, but rather an "I win, you win" outcome. A "win-win" goal is achieved when both parties have the ability and willingness to negotiate even though they do not get all that they want. However, there may be situations when personal goals are not achieved. Some questions to consider when this occurs are:

1. How do I feel about losing?

_____

_____

2. Did I express my opinion clearly? Why not? How could I make it more clear?

_____

_____

3. Did I do the best I could do? How could I have done better?

_____

_____

4. Was I in control when responding to the situation? When did I lose control? What should I have done to regain control?

_____

_____

5. Did I stay focused on the issues? What side issues distracted me? How could I have avoided distractions?

_____

_____

6. Did I allow the situation to get personal? Did the other person initiate the personal attack? How could I have redirected it away from the personal?

_____

_____

7. Was what I asked for under my control? If not, why did I ask for it? What would have been more realistic?

_____

_____

12.1 Rights and Responsibilities of Assertiveness

- To act in a way that promotes your dignity and self-respect
- To be treated with respect
- To experience and express your thoughts and feelings
- To slow down and make conscious decisions before you act
- To ask for what you want
- To say "No"
- To change your mind
- To make mistakes
- Not to be perfect
- To feel important and good about yourself
- To be treated as an individual with special values, skills, and needs
- The right to be unique
- To have your own feelings and opinions
- To say "I don't know"
- To feel angry, hurt, frustrated
- To make decisions regarding your life
- To recognize your needs are as important as others

Reviewing these questions and analyzing the answers will help when attempting to be assertive in future communications. For example, if the answer to question 6 was yes, then during the next communication, a special effort can be focused on avoiding personal attacks during the encounter. Learning to communicate assertively is a process of continual improvement.

Another risk factor that quickly becomes evident when changing to an assertive communication style is the impact that it has on those who know the person best. Sometimes family, friends, peers, and coworkers become barriers to change. As mentioned earlier, change always produces some degree of stress. Those individuals who are closest to the person trying to initiate changes may feel uncomfortable because they have become accustomed to the old communication styles and behaviors over a long time. They can no longer anticipate and depend on the person responding and reacting in the usual way. In addition, they will have to develop new communication patterns of their own to match the changes caused by assertive communication. Sometimes family, friends, peers, and coworkers become so uncomfortable that they may try to sabotage the person's attempts at assertive communication. It is important to recognize why and when these sabotage efforts occur and also to remember that assertiveness is an internal, personal process. Everyone has a right to change, and it must be respectfully communicated to others that their support for these changes is important.

It is also important to know and periodically review the rights and responsibilities of assertiveness to help reinforce the assertive communication process. The rights and responsibilities of assertiveness are listed in Box 12.1.

Practice and reinforcement of assertiveness skills may be required, especially when preparing for an anticipated conflict negotiation or a confrontational meeting with another. Although a confrontational situation always produces anxiety, rather than being feared, it should be recognized as having the potential to be highly productive. Box 12.2 lists several behaviors that, if practiced and used, will help increase confidence and assertiveness skills during anticipated confrontational meetings.

Nonassertive Behavior/ Communication

There are two types of interpersonal behaviors that are considered to be nonassertive. These are submissive and aggressive behaviors.

Submissive Behaviors/Communications

When people display submissive behaviors, they allow their rights to be violated by others. When people use submissive behaviors and submissive communications they surrender to the requests and demand of others without regard to their own feelings and needs. Many experts believe that submissive behavior and communication patterns are a protective mechanism that helps insecure persons maintain their self-esteem by avoiding negative criticism and disagreement of others. In other situations it may be a means of manipulation and the basis for passive-aggressive behavior.

Because of their great fear of displeasing others, personal rejection, or future retaliation, submissive communicators dismiss their own feelings as being unimportant. However, at a deeper level, submissive behavior and communication merely reinforce negative feelings of powerlessness, helplessness, and decreased self-worth. Rather than

> **12.2 Assertive Communications Suggestions**
>
> - Maintain eye contact.
> - Convey empathy, stating your feelings does not mean sympathy or agreement.
> - Keep your body position erect, shoulders and back straight.
> - Speak clearly and audibly, be direct and descriptive.
> - Be comfortable with silence.
> - Use gestures and facial expressions for emphasis.
> - Use appropriate location.
> - Use appropriate timing.
> - Focus on behaviors/issues; do not attack the person.

being in control of the communication or relationship, the person is trading his or her ability to choose what is best for the avoidance of conflict. Every communication by a submissive person becomes an "I lose, you win" situation.

Aggressive Behavior/Communication

Sometimes there is only a very fine line separating assertiveness from aggressive behavior and communications. Whereas assertive communication permits individuals to honestly express their ideas and opinions while respecting the rights, ideas, and opinions of others, aggressive communication strongly asserts the person's legitimate rights and opinions with little regard or respect for the rights and opinions of others. Aggressive communication can be used to humiliate, dominate, control, or embarrass the other person or lower the other person's self-esteem and creates an "I win, you lose" situation. The other person may perceive aggressive behavior or communication as a personal attack. Aggressive behavior and communication is viewed by some psychologists as a protective mechanism that compensates for a person's own insecurities. By demeaning another person, aggressive behavior allows the person to feel superior and helps inflate his or her own self-esteem.

Aggressive communications can take several different forms, including screaming, sarcasm, rudeness, belittling jokes, and even direct personal insults. It is an expression of the negative feelings of power, domination, and low self-esteem. Although outwardly the aggressive person may seem to be in control, in reality they are merely reacting to the situation to protect their self-esteem.

> " " *Aggressive communications can take several different forms, including screaming, sarcasm, rudeness, belittling jokes, and even direct personal insults.*

DIVERSITY

Diversity is a multifaceted issue that involves many areas of people's lives, including culture, values, life experiences, instinctual responses, learned behaviors, personal strengths and weaknesses, and native abilities or skills. Each time two people interact, they bring the sum total of all these elements into their communication. In order to communicate effectively, both parties need to first recognize that the other person is different, then understand how these differences affect the communication, and finally accept and build on these differences. Rather than being divisive, diversity, when recognized and used correctly, can promote teamwork, improve communication, and increase productivity. Recognizing diversity helps people better understand each other as well as themselves. The ultimate goal of diversity recognition is to use each individual's strengths rather than emphasizing the weaknesses, to build a stronger, more self-confident, and productive environment. For example, consider the following scenario:

Anne B., RN, is a nurse in your unit who has a reputation as being a "nitpicker." She is constantly judging her peers and criticizing their actions based on her own personal standards. Her judgments of others are not well accepted by her co-workers, who try to avoid her as much as possible.

Betty A., RN, another nurse on the unit, always seems to be coming up with ideas to change things in the unit, but then

What Do You Think?

With this basic understanding of the three types of behavioral/communication styles, complete the self-assessment evaluation below. After reading the statement, select and write in the response column which one of the three behaviors (assertive, aggressive, or submissive) you demonstrated. There are no right or wrong answers to this activity, but note which style is most dominant. This exercise is designed to help you make a personal assessment about your current communication style and where there is room for improvement.

Assertiveness Self-Assessment Evaluation

STATEMENT	COMMUNICATION BEHAVIOR
1. I didn't say what I really wanted to say at the last staff meeting.	
2. I always express my opinion because it is better than everyone else's.	
3. I have the courage to speak up almost all the time.	
4. I wish someone else would speak up at the meetings besides me.	
5. I am not intimidated by the high-pressure tactics of supervisors, physicians, and/or teachers.	
6. I have trouble stating my true feelings to those in authority.	
7. I really put that know-it-all aide in her place last shift.	
8. After the last meeting with my unit director I felt hopeless, resentful, and angry.	
9. I speak up in meetings without feeling defensive.	
10. When I need to confront someone, I avoid the problem because it will usually resolve itself.	
11. When I need to confront someone, I address them directly.	
12. When I confront someone, I let them know in no uncertain terms that they are wrong and need to change their behavior.	
13. When I'm reprimanded, I keep silent even though I'm seething inside.	
14. The last time I was asked to stay over for another shift, I said "no" and didn't feel guilty.	

avoids joining the committees that are formed to put the ideas into practice. When she does join a committee, she quickly gets bored and does not follow through on her responsibilities. The other committee members become angry and frustrated by Betty's behavior. They feel that because it was her idea in the first place, she should work as hard as everyone else to make the change.

You have been selected as the chairperson for a committee that has been formed to design a new client care documentation tool. Both Anne and Betty are on the committee. The other committee members are upset because Anne and Betty are on the committee. Everyone knows about Anne's and Betty's personality quirks. As chairperson of the team, you need to utilize everyone's strengths while recognizing his or her diversities in order to develop a new, comprehensive yet easy-to-use form. If you perform well in your chairmanship role, each team member's self-esteem should be enhanced, and the morale of the group should improve.

At first glance, these may not seem like diversity issues. However, Anne is a detail-oriented person, whereas Betty is a visionary. Although their interests and abilities are very diverse, neither one is right or wrong. Persons who are preoccupied with details are left-brain dominant; creative, visionary individuals are usually right-brain dominant.

Two primary tasks are required to complete the project: *Task 1.* Brainstorming sessions must be conducted with staff members, physicians, and ancillary personnel to develop a general concept of what the documentation should include and how the form should look. *Task 2.* Work with the printshop to design the specific layout and content of the final form.

Plan. *Task 1:* It would be most appropriate to include Betty in the group that directs the brainstorming groups and collects different ideas. She probably has no preconceived form in mind before starting the process and will feel comfortable investigating and researching a variety of different possibilities. Anne would have difficulty with this task. The lack of structure of the brainstorming process would make her feel out of control and would probably frustrate her urge to consider all the details of the project. Anne would most likely already have a good idea of the form she wanted. *Task 2:* Anne would be much better at this task because of her orientation to structure and detail. Working with the printshop, she could focus her attention on each item on the form, decide where it should be placed, how much room it should be given, and how it flows in the document. She would make sure that the form met all the standards and regulatory requirements of the Joint Commission as well as ensuring that it was error free. Betty, on the other hand, would very quickly become bored with this aspect of the project. To her, all the attention given to the details would seem like a waste of time, and she would probably start recommending changes in other unit forms.

Results of committee work. Placing the right person in the right working environment that corresponds with his or her strengths ensures success for the project. The project will be a successful experience for the nurses and will promote positive changes in peer relationships.

For many people, working with diversity can be difficult, especially when individuals feel insecure about their skills or abilities. When people feel insecure, they may revert to submissive or aggressive behavior or communication styles to hide their weaknesses or differences. Because assertive persons recognize that everyone, including themselves, have both strengths and weaknesses, they feel comfortable with diversity and are more likely to accept and support others by recognizing and using their strengths. Focusing on the strengths of people provides them with positive feedback and helps them grow personally and professionally. Focusing on weaknesses and differences tears down an individual's self-esteem, creates an uncomfortable work atmosphere, and makes people defensive and sometimes hostile.

PROBLEM SOLVING

Problem solving is a process that everyone uses all the time. For example, on the way to work, a tire goes flat on a person's car. That is a problem. How the person solves the problem depends partially on critical thinking skills, partially on past experiences, and partially on physical abilities. If the person with the flat tire is a 250-lb 33-year-old male construction worker in good health, he most likely has changed tires before and will probably be physically able to remove the flat tire and put on the spare without difficulty. However, if the person with the flat tire is a 90-lb, 67-year-old female church organist who is unable to distinguish a lug nut from a tire valve, her solution to the problem will likely be different. She will probably call the automobile association and have someone come and change the flat for her.

One of the primary activities for nurses in the work setting is problem solving using the nursing process. It really does not matter whether the problem is client centered, management oriented, or an interpersonal issue, the nursing process is an excellent framework for problem resolution. It focuses on the goals of mutual interaction and communication to establish trust and respect. Using the process of assessment, analysis, planning, implementation, and evaluation helps the nurse organize and structure interpersonal interactions in a way that will produce an "I win–You win" situation.

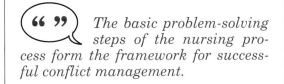

The basic problem-solving steps of the nursing process form the framework for successful conflict management.

The basic problem-solving steps of the nursing process form the framework for successful conflict management. Many people experience less anxiety when practicing personal problem solving than when they are involved in conflict management. Problem solving is often perceived as less emotional and more structured, whereas conflict management is considered to be more emotionally charged with the potential to produce hostility. However, the steps of conflict management are almost identical to those of the nursing process. The one additional element that must be included in conflict resolution is the ability to use assertive behaviors and communication when discussing the issues. Nurses who are good problem solvers using the nursing process also tend to be good at conflict resolution, and nurses who are good at conflict resolution tend to be excellent problem solvers. Rather than avoiding conflict in the work setting, it should be considered as an opportunity to practice and grow in the use of problem-solving skills.

Conflict Management

Everyone experiences conflict at one time or another as a part of daily life. Often people feel more comfortable addressing the conflict that arises in their personal lives rather than the professional conflicts that arise from the job setting. A common situation that causes conflict is when nurses feel overworked or overwhelmed by their assignments. The overloaded nurse might say something like: "I have such a heavy load today, why isn't anyone helping me?" rather than asking a particular individual for help. When the person who is expected to help fails to comply with the implied request for help, the overworked nurse becomes angry and resentful. The other person may not understand where this anger is coming from and often avoids addressing the angry person for fear of making him or her angrier. This type of poor communication and lack of direct, respectful conflict management produces tension among workers, deterioration of working relationships, decreased efficiency, and, ultimately, poor client care.

There are many reasons why individuals are uncomfortable handling or addressing conflict, including:

- Fear of retaliation
- Fear of ridicule
- Fear of alienation of others
- Mistaken belief that they are unable to handle the conflict situation
- Feeling like they do not have the right to speak up
- Past negative experiences with conflict situations
- Family background and experiences
- Lack of education and skills on conflict resolution

There are several different strategies that can be used to resolve workplace conflicts. Depending on a person's communication style and personality traits, different outcomes may occur:

Strategy 1: IGNORE THE CONFLICT

- *Submissive personality:* Person avoids bringing the issue to the other because he or she is afraid of retaliation or

ridicule from others if he or she confronts and expresses honest feelings or opinions.

- *Aggressive personality:* Person has decided not to pursue the conflict because the other person is "too stupid to understand" or it would just be a "waste of their time."

Strategy 2: CONFRONT THE CONFLICT

- *Submissive personality:* Person does not handle the situation directly but refers the problem to a supervisor or to another person for resolution.

- *Assertive personality:* Person sets up a time and place for a one-on-one meeting. At the meeting, the two parties focus on the issues that caused the conflict and negotiate to define goals and problem solve.
- *Aggressive personality:* Person confronts the other loudly, in front of an audience, and attacks the other's personality rather than the issue. Person either walks away before the other can speak or keeps talking without stopping and does not allow the other person to respond. The communication is strictly one-sided and very negative.

Strategy 3: POSTPONE THE CONFLICT

- *Submissive person:* Person keeps "count" of the issues until they reach a critical issue, then dumps all the issues at one time on the offender in a highly aggressive manner. The other person generally has no idea why they are being attacked and may respond with anger or submission.
- *Aggressive personality:* Person waits until he or she can either use the incident as a threat or blackmail or until the conflict can be expressed in front of an audience.

Professional nurses need to be assertive and feel comfortable when handling conflict situations and confronting others. The conflict situations that nurses may encounter range from uncooperative clients and lazy coworkers to hostile, insecure, but influential physicians. Practicing assertiveness skills during confrontational situations will help increase the nurse's confidence in handling daily work-related conflicts and allow the honest but respectful expression of opinion and ideas. Keep in mind that unresolved conflicts never really go away. Ignoring a conflict situation may postpone it, sometimes for a long time, but it will not resolve the issue. Unresolved conflicts often fester until they either reach the boiling point or are manifested in negative behaviors or feelings. Some of the feelings and behaviors that are symptoms of unresolved conflicts include:

- Tension and anxiety manifested as sudden angry outbursts
- Generalized distrust among the staff members
- Gossiping and rumor spreading
- Intentional work sabotage
- Backstabbing and lack of cooperation
- Isolation of certain staff members
- Division and polarization of the staff
- Low-rated peer evaluation reports

Often, when conflict is handled appropriately, it produces much less anxiety than was initially anticipated. An individual who prepares for a confrontational meeting by expecting the worst-case scenario may be pleasantly surprised when the actual meeting and discussion take place. Many conflicts turn out to be merely errors in perception, simple misunderstandings, or misquotes of something that was said. If a situation is cleared up at an early stage, this prevents the development of the symptoms of unresolved conflict (listed earlier) and improves staff relationships. Individuals feel more confident and have better self-esteem when they resolve the conflicts in an adult and productive manner.

Another advantage of good conflict management is the improvement in communication skills. As with any skills, the more these skills are practiced, the easier they will become to use. Some tips for conflict resolution are listed in the Issues in Practice box.

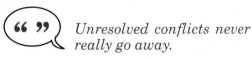 *Unresolved conflicts never really go away.*

Issues

Conflict Resolution Tips

In nursing practice, good communication and conflict management skills are essential. The following tips may help resolve communication problems:

Improve your conflict management skills

- Seminars
- Books
- Mentors

Change your paradigm

- Focus on the positive not the negative.
- Realize that *appropriately* confronting is a risk-taking activity for:
  - Better communication
  - Improved relationships
  - Improved teamwork
  - Mentoring

Understand your values

- Focus on a win-win.
- Be willing to negotiate/compromise.
- Be direct and honest.
- Focus on the issues.
- Do not attack the person.
- Do not make judgments.
- Do not become the third person, encourage peers to go direct.
- Do not spread rumors.

Set personal guidelines

- Confront in private, *never* in front of anyone else.
- Confront the individual, do not report them to their supervisor first.
- Do not confront when you are angry.
- Start with an "I" message.
- Express how you feel and your opinions.
- Allow the other person to talk without interruptions.
- Listen attentively.
- Set goals and future plans of action.
- Let it go!
- Keep it private and confidential.

DIFFICULT PEOPLE

All nurses recognize that obtaining a thorough history and understanding the underlying disease processes better prepares them for the care of their clients. Similarly, when working with difficult people, a knowledge of their backgrounds and understanding of the underlying personality traits better prepare the individual to deal with the important issues. It would seem that nurses should be better at handling conflict and difficult people, because an understanding of cause and effect and the intricacies of human nature are skills that are used daily in the care of clients. By shifting the communication paradigm from one of instinctual response to one that uses the nurse's relationship skills should make dealing with difficult people a much less difficult task. Remember that the behavior displayed by a difficult person is really a symptom of a deeper problem, just as an assessment of shortness of breath is a symptom of a respiratory disease. Identification of the cause of the problem permits the nurse to treat the disease rather than just the symptoms. The problem will not be cured by merely ignoring it or only dealing with the symptoms. In the long term, it usually only makes things worse.

Identifying Difficult People

Most of the time, it is rather easy to identify when a person is being "difficult." However, there are some behaviors of difficult people that may not be evident at first glance. Each type of difficult person requires a different strategy for dealing with their behaviors.

There are four basic behavioral pattern types of communication (1) in control and responsive pattern, (2) in control but unresponsive pattern, (3) uncontrolled and responsive pattern, (4) and the uncontrolled and unresponsive pattern of communication.

Anyone who has been employed in or even associated with the health-care setting for any length of time soon becomes aware of a variety of different personality types among the staff members. These personality types can be identified by their predominant behaviors and also require different strategies for communication. Keep in mind that these are stereotypes that tend to batch individuals into groups based on predetermined characteristics. In reality, people may have an overlapping or combination of characteristics that may require combining the listed strategies for communication.

The various types of characterizations, behavioral patterns, and stereotypes all are

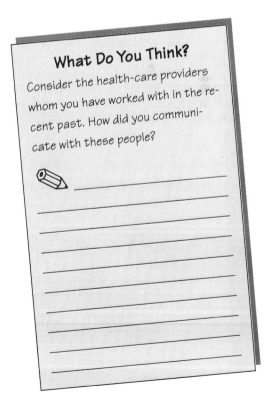

What Do You Think?

Consider the health-care providers whom you have worked with in the recent past. How did you communicate with these people?

interrelated and based on individual communication styles. An increased awareness of the various identifying characteristics and strategies for communication will help develop the coping skills and communication techniques necessary for communicating with difficult people.

DEVELOPMENT OF COPING SKILLS

Just as developing communication skills requires a willingness to change and a lot of practice, so does the development of coping skills. Coping skills can be used to resolve crisis situations, deal with anxiety, and resolve difficult issues of communication. Everyone has at least a fundamental set of coping skills that they have developed during their lives, and these can be used as the foundation for adding to or building new coping skills for future problems. Presented here are some strategies that will help in the development of coping skills to use in communicating with difficult people.

First, separate the person from the problem by focusing on the issues without personally attacking the person. Having the facts about the situation makes people much more receptive to resolution of the problem than attacking their personality. When situations are made into personal attacks, it makes people feel defensive, responsible, or persecuted and either blocks or closes off the communication.

One way to avoid making a conversation into a personal attack is to use "I" rather than "you" messages. Avoid starting a conversation by saying, "*You* made a mistake," or "*You* said this about me," or especially "*You* always do this." People are less likely to perceive a communication as a personal attack when the conversation begins by explaining a personal view of the situation or even how feelings were affected. State-

> 66 99 *First, separate the person from the problem by focusing on the issues without personally attacking the person.*

ments such as "*I* thought it was done this way," or "*I* heard something the other day," or even "*I* feel hurt when people judge me" are a more productive way to begin an exchange of ideas and information. For example:

During shift report on a particular client, the 11 P.M. to 7 A.M. nurse forgot to tell the 7 A.M. to 3 P.M. charge nurse, Gail L., RN, that the client had fallen out of bed during the night shift. Later in the day, both the client's physician and family confronted Gail to find out what happened and why the client was not placed on "fall protocols." Later, when Gail confronts the night nurse about the omission, she has two options for initiating the discussion of the incident with the responsible night nurse. Which approach would the night nurse probably take as a personal attack?

Option 1: Gail: "*I* was taken off guard and unprepared when the family and physician asked me about this client's fall, and I felt unprepared to explain the problem or a solution to them. My lack of knowledge about the fall really made me feel incompetent."

Option 2: Gail: "*You* failed to tell me about his fall last night. Because of *you*, I was not aware of the incident and was not prepared to answer questions. You always make me look like a fool!"

Another way to avoid making issues into personal attacks is to avoid focusing on what a person "should" have done based on a personal standard. This type of statement becomes an arbitrary judgment call. Instead, ask the person for his or her ideas on how the situation could have been handled differently or what other options were available. One should especially avoid becoming personally or verbally abusive.

A second important strategy for developing communication-related coping skills is to be willing to actively listen to and respect the other person's perspectives, ideas, or opinions. Active listening can help minimize the misunderstandings or erroneous perceptions that cause much of the tension seen on nursing units. As mentioned earlier, active listening involves "listening" not only to the words but also to the body language in order to hear the real meaning of the communication and understand the underlying message. When a person is focused in on the communication, he or she is not preoccupied with other issues or preparing mentally a response or a defense. Allowing the other person to say all he or she has to say without interruption before responding provides for an atmosphere where honest and open communication can occur. In some situations, merely allowing a person to ventilate emotions by using active listening will reduce the levels of anger and animosity and will sometimes even solve the conflict situation. Also, when intelligent people are allowed to speak openly and freely, they may be able to develop a new solution to the problem that they had not considered previously.

Before responding to a person, it is important to ask clarifying questions that validate the person's concerns, feelings, and perceptions. Validating will help ensure that the responses address the real issues. Also, avoid reflex type of reactions to hostile or aggressive statements. It is a human instinct to become defensive when one is attacked and to attack the person back. However, this behavior only escalates the anger and tension and blocks effective communication.

A third strategy that is useful in developing communication coping skills is to always make a conscious decision about the importance of the issue that needs to be discussed. When individuals can identify the issues that really matter and focus their efforts on them, they gain credibility among their peers and develop a reputation for caring and realism.

What Do You Think?

Make a list of the problematic issues that you have observed on a nursing unit. Which ones would you consider to be high priority? Which ones are trivial?

Again, it is a very human tendency to become preoccupied with trivial and unimportant issues. If a person is spending a large portion of his or her energy in dealing with trivia, he or she will have little energy left to deal with the major issues when they come along. By establishing and analyzing the outcomes to be attained and by being open to negotiations and compromise, both parties will leave the confrontation with a sense of accomplishment and fair resolution even if they did not get everything they wanted.

Setting the Stage

After a decision is made to deal with a difficult issue or person, it is important to set the stage for a positive experience. The location for the exchange should be private. The format of the meeting needs to be established ahead of time, including an explanation to the other person that each party will take turns expressing his or her opinions and feelings without interruption.

Establishing Trust

An important issue in conflict negotiations is the establishment of trust. In addition to showing respect for the other person's opinions and ideas, trust can be established by talking first and directly to the person about the problem issue rather than everyone else on the unit. Being talked about behind one's back tends to make people resentful and defensive. Trust is reinforced when a person makes it known that all he or she wants is to resolve the issue and then move on. When the threat of retaliation is removed, people are more likely to express themselves honestly, as well as becoming more open to the other side's ideas. Once two people begin to trust each other, even if they disagree about some of the issues, they are much more likely to come to a satisfactory resolution of the problem.

The Actual Exchange

When the actual exchange takes place, it is important to avoid the "I" language and be direct by focusing on the facts and issues. Remember that active listening is a two-way street. A person's own body language, tone of voice, and eye contact can say much more than the actual words. Showing the other person that his or her opinion is respected, even if not agreed with, helps develop that important sense of trust between the two parties.

After each person has had a chance to express himself or herself and validate the communication, they begin to address the issues and develop a solution for the problem. Sometimes there is a need to set goals for, or at least agree on, how the issues are to be approached and settled. It is fairly common that some issues will remain unresolved after the first meeting. A decision about when and where the second meeting will take place needs to be made before leaving the first meeting. Also, before leaving the first meeting, each party should summarize what they agreed to and how they felt about the exchange. This summarization will help clarify any miscommunications and give each party one last chance to introduce any issues that remain unresolved.

Dealing with difficult people and conflict resolution are never pleasant undertakings. However, like most skills, the more it is practiced, the more comfortable the individual will become using the communication techniques discussed. The importance of handling problematic situations in a timely, honest, and caring manner is self-evident. The anxiety and fear provoked by confrontation are part of the price that nurses must pay in order to do their jobs well and provide high-quality client care.

> *The anxiety and fear provoked by confrontation are part of the price that nurses must pay in order to do their jobs well and provide high-quality client care.*

Conclusion

A person's professional and personal life is influenced by communication styles and behavioral patterns. The ability to analyze personal strengths, weaknesses, and communication behaviors is particularly important when dealing with difficult people.

Certain specific communication qualities and skills are essential when interacting with difficult people. First of all, it is important to develop the skill of assertive communication, which allows people to express themselves openly and honestly while respecting the other person's opinions and ideas. Being able to identify submissive and aggressive behavior is also essential when trying to resolve problems, as well as recognizing issues of diversity, which underlie many problems in communication. Difficult situations are ultimately resolved through the practice of conflict management. Because it is an outgrowth and extension of the problem-solving method, nurses should be able to quickly grasp its structure and master its use.

In conjunction with communication skills, the development and use of coping skills are also important. Communication is also enhanced by practicing techniques to avoid making confrontations seem like a personal attack and to establish trust.

Critical Thinking Exercises

Julie H., RN, has been working the 7 P.M. to 7 A.M. shift in a busy, 32-bed surgical unit of a large university hospital since her graduation from a small bachelor of science in nursing (BSN) program 6 months ago. Although Julie was told by the unit director when she was hired that she would have at least a full year of training before she had to work as charge nurse, tonight the other two RNs who usually work the shift called in sick, and Julie was left in charge. The 7 P.M. to 7 A.M. shift is always busy because the unit has to both discharge clients who are ready to go home after surgery as well as admit clients who are going for surgery the next day. The hospital policy requires that the RN make and sign both the discharge and admission assessments.

Although Julie is nervous about this new role as charge nurse, she feels that she can handle the responsibility if she has some additional help. Normal staffing for the unit on this shift is three registered nurses (RNs), three licensed practical nurses (LPNs), and three unlicensed assistive personnel (UAP). Julie calls the house supervisor to see if she can get some help. The only place in the hospital that is not busy that night is the obstetrics (OB) unit, so the supervisor sends two of the OB unit's UAPs to the surgical unit to help Julie.

It was not the help Julie really wanted, but she feels that she can handle the responsibility. However, when Julie begins to make assignments, the older of the OB unit UAPs, Hanna J., informs Julie that she, for the past 15 years, had worked only in the newborn nursery and does not know anything about the care of adult clients who had surgery. In addition, Hanna states that she has a bad back and cannot lift or turn adult clients and is afraid that she might catch some disease from the adults that she would take back to the babies. Julie asks Hanna: "What *do* you feel you are qualified to do on the surgical unit?" In response, Hanna crosses her legs, folds her arms across her chest, puts her head down and mumbles under her breath: "A lot more than a new know-it-all RN like you."

✔ What messages, both verbal and nonverbal, are being communicated?

✔ How should Julie respond to this comment?

✔ What should she do to rectify the situation?

✔ Using the various tables in the chapter, identify the personality type of each of the persons involved in the situation.

✔ How can the RN best communicate with this UAP?

✔ What were some of the communication mistakes that the RN made?

Critical Thinking Exercises

✔ What background, cultural, and diversity factors played a part in this situation?

✔ Develop a strategy for resolution of this conflict.

✔ Make a list of your values and where they came from. Describe how each value affects your work ethic and life.

✔ List your communication strengths and weaknesses. Rank them on a scale of 1 to 10—10 being the highest.

✔ Determine which weaknesses you want to change, and create an improvement plan.

✔ Identify your primary communication style and character type.

✔ Complete this statement, using as many situations or statements as possible:

✔ In a conflict situation, I have difficulty saying _____.

✔ Analyze reasons that prevent you from saying it. What would have been the worst thing that could have happened to you if you had said it?

✔ Create a phrase that you feel comfortable with that you could use the next time you want to say something difficult to the members of your team.

✔ Identify the communication and behavior characteristics of your work group or team. List areas of diversity for each member, including yourself. Identify their strengths and weaknesses.

✔ Identify methods for using the team members' diversity to enhance the team.

BIBLIOGRAPHY

Austin, N, and Phelps, S: The Assertive Woman. Impact Publishers, Calif., 1975.

Bertinasco, L: Strategies for resolving conflict. Health Care Supervisor 8(4):35–39, 1990.

Blanchard, K, and Johnson, S: The One Minute Manager: The Quickest Way to Increase Your Own Prosperity. Berkley Books, New York, 1984.

Broom, C: Conflict resolution strategies: When ethical dilemmas evolve into conflict. Dimension of Critical Care Nursing 10(6):354–363, 1991.

Cornell, D: Say the words: Communication techniques. Nursing Management 24(3):24, 1993.

Covey, S: The 7 Habits of Highly Effective People: Powerful Lessons in Personal Change. A Fireside Book, Simon & Shuster, New York, 1989.

Davis-Funk, J: You Can Conquer Procrastination. Seminar International, Kan., 1991.

Delegation: Concepts and decision-making process. National Council of State Boards 16(4):1–4, 1995.

De Press, M: Leadership is an Art. Dell Trade Paperback, New York, 1989.

Jones, MA, Bushardt, SC, and Cadenhead, G: A paradigm for effective resolution of interpersonal conflict. Nursing Management 24:10, 1990.

Lewis-Ford, B: Management techniques: Coping with difficult people: Nursing Management 24(3):36–38, 1993.

McKinley, M: Collaboration is an effective tool. AACN News 15(10):2, 1998.

Medical Laboratory Observer: Coping with difficult people. 23–42, 1990.

Munro, NL: Apply the rules of 'people ethics.' AACN News 15(11):2–15, 1998.

Nicoll, LH: Nurses' Guide to the Internet, ed 2. JB Lippincott, Philadelphia, 1998.

Prim, R: Communication: Coping with the unspoken dance. Nursing Management 24(3):40–45, 1993.

Puetz, B, and Thomas, D: Don't let difficult people catch you off guard. RN 58(2):24, 1995.

Rowan, R: The Intuitive Manager. Little Brown, Boston, 1986.

Schuller, R: Tough Times Never Last, But Tough People Do! Bantam Books, New York, 1984.

Stewart, J: How to Deal with Anger. Seminar International, Kan., 1996.

Sullivan, TJ: Collaboration: A health care imperative. McGraw-Hill, New York, 1998.

Thomas, G: Assert Yourself. American Business Communication Inc, Kan., 1991.

Weiss, D: How To Deal with Difficult People. American Management Association, New York, 1987.

Zoglio, S: Teams At Work: 7 Keys to Success. Tower Hill Press, Pa., 1993.

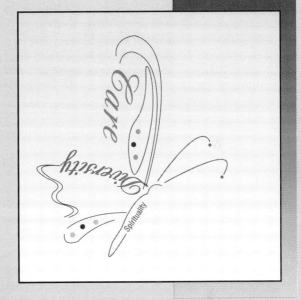

Unit 5

Issues in Delivering Care

13
Cultural Diversity

➤*Joseph T. Catalano*

Culture is a powerful influence on how nurses and clients interpret and respond to health care. It is not unreasonable for both nurses and clients to demand that they should be treated with respect and understanding and that their individuality should be recognized no matter what their cultural origins. Nurses who understand the essential characteristics of transcultural nursing will be able to provide competent and culturally sensitive care for clients from diverse cultural backgrounds.

WHAT IS CULTURE?

There are many definitions of culture and ways that culture is understood. Culture may be seen as a group's acceptance of a set of attitudes, ideologies, values, beliefs, and behaviors that influence the way that the members of the group express themselves.

Cultural expression assumes many forms, including language; spirituality; works of art; group customs and traditions; food preferences; response to illness, stress, pain, **bereavement,** anger, and sorrow; decision making; and even world philosophy. An individual's cultural orientation is the result of a learning process that literally starts at birth and continues throughout the life span wherein behaviors, beliefs, and attitudes are transmitted from one generation to the next. Although expressions of culture are primarily unconscious, they have a profound effect on an individual's response to the health-care system.

Consider the following situation:

> 66 99 *Cultural expression assumes many forms, including language; spirituality; works of art; group customs and traditions; food preferences; response to illness, stress, pain, bereavement, anger, and sorrow; decision making; and even world philosophy.*

Mrs. Sung Gwak, who is 74 years old, is brought into the emergency room (ER) by her family because of "very bad indigestion that won't go away." Three family members (a middle-aged man and woman and a younger woman) accompany the elderly lady. They are discussing her condition in a mixture of English and another language, which the nurse does not recognize. Because the client does not seem to understand any English, the nurse attempts to address the family. The younger woman speaks broken English but manages to explain that the client is her grandmother and she is accompanied by her mother and father, who speak even less English than she does.

By default, the granddaughter serves as the translator. After much prompting, she explains that her grandmother arrived in the United States for a visit only 2 days ago from a small mountain village in Korea where she had lived all her life.

She had been having periodic episodes of "indigestion" for several weeks before the visit and used traditional herbal teas prescribed by the local healer to treat her condition. Based on further assessment and a diagnostic test, it is determined that Mrs. Gwak had an extensive myocardial infarction at least 1 week before her trip and is currently in a mild state of congestive heart failure (CHF).

She is given medications for the chest pain and CHF and is started on anticoagulant medications in the ER. She is then transferred to the coronary care unit (CCU), where she is scheduled to have coronary angiography the next day. The angiogram shows multiple blockages in her coronary arteries and extensive myocardial damage. Because of her age and also the extensive damage to her heart, the physician thinks that it would be too risky to attempt bypass surgery and decides to monitor her closely and treat her medically until she is stable enough to have a balloon angioplasty.

When the cardiac care unit (CCU) nurse assigned to Mrs. Gwak enters the room at the beginning of her shift the day after the angiogram, she finds the client covered with four heavy blankets and a bedspread and sweating profusely. When the nurse attempts to remove the excessive bed covers, the client's daughter protests vehemently in Korean and puts the blankets back on as soon as the nurse leaves the room. The daughter seems to think that her mother is sick because she is too cold and gives the elderly woman hot herbal drinks from a thermos bottle that she had brought from home.

When the granddaughter arrives, the nurse explains to her why excessive heat is harmful to the client's cardiac status and the need to follow the diet restrictions prescribed by the physician. The ingredients of the herbal drinks were unknown, and there may be some serious interactions with the numerous medications that the client was receiving. The granddaughter translated this information to her mother, who seemed to become even angrier with the nurse. Although she outwardly seems to comply with the restrictions, she continues the traditional folk treatments in secret, believing that the Western hospital food is bad for her mother's health.

Mrs. Gwak is very quiet and hardly ever asks for help. When she does talk to her family, the conversation is usually about the airplane flight to the United States and the belief that the high altitude probably caused all Mrs. Gwak's problems.

Her condition gradually deteriorates during her hospitalization, despite all the medical treatment. The nurse and physician tell the family about the client's worsening condition and the likelihood that she will not survive the hospitalization, but they refuse to relay the information to the client.

What Do You Think?

Identify the cultural factors expressed by the client and her family that made it difficult for the ER and CCU nurses to take care of this client. What are some strategies that the nurses might have used to facilitate cultural understanding? Why is the family refusing to tell the client about her worsening condition?

It is important to note that culture is not a monolithic concept. Any individual probably belongs to several subcultures within his or her major culture. Subcultures develop when members of the group do not accept all the values of their dominant culture. Even within a given culture, many variations may exist. For example, it is logical to conclude that people who live in the United States all belong to the American culture and would be very similar in most ways. However, teenagers living in the rural areas of Oklahoma may find it difficult to relate to the teenagers raised in the inner city of Philadelphia. Even though they speak the same language and share some similar interests, they have so many different past experiences that change their perspectives on life that it may be difficult for them to relate to each other.

Culture can be considered to be a type of photocopy machine that makes duplicates of the original document. A society attempts to preserve itself by passing down its values, beliefs, and customs to the next generation. Although some parts of the culture remain very similar, other parts change greatly owing to effects from both within and outside of the group.

Diversity

Diversity is a term that is used to explain the differences between cultures. The characteristics that define diversity can be divided into two groups: primary and secondary. Primary characteristics are those that tend to be more obvious, including nationality, race, color, gender, age, and religious beliefs. Secondary characteristics, such as socioeconomic status, education, occupation, length of time away from the country of origin, gender issues, residential status, and sexual orientation, may be more difficult to identify, even though they may have an even more profound effect on the person's cultural identity than the primary characteristics. When individuals make generalizations about other individuals based on the obvious primary characteristics, and do not take the time to consider the secondary characteristics they are stereotyping the other person. Stereotyping is an oversimplified belief, conception, or opinion about another person (or group) based on a limited amount of information.

> 66 99 *Many individuals who migrate to the United States from other countries now cling tenaciously to their traditional cultural practices and languages, thus producing a phenomenon that is called multiculturalism.*

MELTING POT VERSUS SALAD BOWL

The United States has traditionally been considered a melting pot of world cultures. Early in the history of the United States, most people who came here from distant lands were eager to be assimilated into American culture. Many people Americanized their names; they shed their traditional dress; they learned American manners and customs as quickly as possible; and they made heroic attempts to learn English without the benefit of formal schooling—all so that they could "fit in" to their new homeland. Until recently, most people who immigrated to the new country were very willing to acculturate (i.e., to alter their own cultural practices in an attempt to become more like the new culture). The end result was a blending or melting pot of cultures.

However, since the early 1970s, the practice of intentional acculturation by immigrating cultures seems to have fallen by the wayside. Many individuals who migrate to the United States from other countries now cling tenaciously to their traditional cultural practices and languages, thus producing a phenomenon that is called multiculturalism. Rather than blending smoothly into the bigger pot as former immigrants had done, the modern immigrants maintain their own unique flavors and textures, much like the ingredients in a large tossed salad. As an ever-growing phenomenon, multiculturalism is something that health-care providers need to be aware of; they must learn ways of adapting their health practices to allow for these differences.

There are drawbacks and benefits in both approaches. In the era of the "melting pot," individuals who attempted to retain their native beliefs, customs, and languages were often ridiculed, scorned, and generally made to feel that they were outsiders to the mainstream culture. However, when they did become homogenized into the American culture, learned the language of the dominant society, and made an effort to be seen as belonging, they were more likely to be accepted as equals and quickly advanced up the socioeconomic ladder.

The current "salad bowl" trend in society has the advantage of allowing individuals in the dominant culture to gain an appreciation of other cultures for their unique contributions to society. The drawback of the salad bowl is that it tends to create pockets of culturally different individuals who live in, but only have minimal interaction with, mainstream American society. Because they do not speak the language or refuse to accept the customs of the dominant culture, it may be more difficult for them to advance their socioeconomic status.

The salad bowl process has also given rise to cultural relativism among some groups. Cultural relativism occurs when members of a strong cultural group understand their culture and group members only from their own viewpoint rather than from that of the larger culture. They do not try to understand its unique characteristics, values, and beliefs.

Some cultural groups manage to blend the melting pot and the salad bowl together through a rather complex process that is sometimes called heritage consistency. Outwardly, they may become acculturated to the point where they wear business suits, speak passable English, eat fast foods, and go to movies. However, when they are at home, or with groups from their traditional culture, they speak their native language, wear their traditional clothes, eat ethnically correct meals, and generally follow their native customs. This approach to acculturation has the advantages of allowing them to fit in and advance in the larger culture while retaining many of the elements of their traditional culture that provide a sense of stability to their lives. It does, however, create in some individuals a type of cultural confusion that may lead to increased tension and anxiety.

SOCIETAL FACTORS AND ETHNIC POPULATION TRENDS IN THE UNITED STATES

Rapid population growth in ethnic groups has been the trend in the United States for many years. The last comprehensive national census was conducted in 1990 and is the source for the most recent statistics listed in Box 13.1. The U.S. Bureau of Census projects that by the year 2000 between 25% and 33% of the U.S. population will be composed of minority groups and that by the year 2080 the white population will actually be a minority group with only 48.9% of the total population of the United States.

Contributing to the rapid growth in minority populations is the increasing number of immigrants coming to the United States. Between 1970 and 1985, the number of legal immigrants each year increased from

13.1 Ethnic Population Trends in the United States

GROUP	1980	1990	INCREASE
Caucasian	188,372,000	199,668,000	6%
African-American	26,495,000	29,986,000	13.2%
Hispanic	14,609,000	22,354,000	53%
Native-American	1,420,000	1,959,000	37.9%

Data from the U.S. Bureau of Census, 1992.

500,000 to more than 6 million. Currently the largest numbers of immigrants are from Asia, Mexico, and Central and South America. Fewer immigrants have come from Africa and Europe than in previous years.

However, the percentage of minority nurses does not reflect the national population trends. Despite efforts on the part of the National League for Nursing (NLN), American Association of Colleges of Nursing (AACN), and other organizations concerned with nursing education, minority nurses still constitute only 10% of the RNs practicing in the United States. The latest reported statistics by the NLN actually show a decrease in the number of minority students enrolled in basic nursing programs, from 15.8% in 1991 to 15.4% in 1994. In a perfect world, the number and percentage of RNs from the various minority groups would perfectly mirror society as a whole to better meet the needs of a culturally diverse country.

Despite the relatively low number of minority nurses, nurses from one culture should be able to give culturally competent care to individuals from any other culture. Being on the front lines of health care, nursing is the one profession that is continually bombarded with cultural changes that result from ethnic shifts in population. Nurses now recognize that they can no longer use traditional ethnocentric models to guide their practice and protocols. Nurses are beginning to promote an understanding of individuals from other cultures and improve the overall quality of health care.

The Medicare and Medicaid laws that evolved out of the social programs of the 1960s have increased the number of culturally diverse clients with whom nurses come in contact. Historically, many minority groups tend to be among the poorest segments of the population. Before the Medicare and Medicaid legislation that expanded government funded health care to cover all welfare recipients, ethnic minorities were unable to afford health care and were seen only in the health-care setting when severely ill. Ethnic minorities are now covered by these laws and, by their increasing numbers in all levels and areas of health care, have prompted nurses to become more sensitive to the transcultural aspects of health care.

Because it is on the front lines of health care, nursing is the one profession that is continually confronted with cultural changes that result from ethnic shifts in population.

Since the 1970s, transcultural nursing has become an important subject in most nursing programs. However, nursing education has taken only the first unsteady steps on the path to seeking a true integration of cultural competence into daily practice. As technologic and transportation advances bring more and more people from different cultures closer together, there will be an increased demand for nurses who can practice effectively in a culturally diverse society. Many challenges still lie ahead.

DEVELOPING CULTURAL AWARENESS

Developing a cultural awareness is the first step in becoming a culturally competent nurse. One of the main challenges for nurses who practice in a culturally diverse environment is to understand the client's perspective of what is happening in the health-care setting. From a cultural viewpoint, it may be very different from what the nurse believes is occurring.

A nurse develops cultural awareness only when he or she is able to recognize and value all aspects of a client's culture, including their beliefs, customs, responses, methods of expression, language, and social structure. However, merely learning about another person's culture does not guarantee that the nurse will have cultural awareness. Nurses must first understand their own cultural background and explore the origins of their own prejudiced and biased views of others. Several tools have been developed in recent years to measure a person's cultural awareness. Box 13.2 contains a synthesis of several cultural assessment tools. Answer the questions honestly, then check how you rate in terms of cultural awareness. Keep in mind that there is always some degree of inaccuracy in all self-assessment tools and that the validity and reliability of tools vary widely. The specific score is not as important as gaining an insight into and understanding of what factors are important in developing cultural awareness. Cultural awareness begins with an understanding of one's own cultural health-care beliefs and cultural values.

To those unfamiliar with a particular culture's health-care beliefs, many of the health-care practices may appear meaningless, strange, or even dangerous. Beliefs about health care are based in part on knowledge and are often related to religious beliefs. For example, if a particular society has no knowledge of bacteria as a cause of infection, then the use of antibiotics may seem to them useless in achieving a cure for the disease. On the other hand, if a society believes that illness is caused by evil spirits entering the body from curses by witches or medicine men, then practices such as incantations, use of ritualistic objects like bones, feathers, or incense, and even blood-letting and purgatives to "re-

lease" the spirit from the body is a very logical approach to achieving a cure.

The basic belief system of cultures are highly complex and involved and are often maintained as very closely guarded secrets. For example, among some Native-American groups, there is a strong belief that twin births are attributed to witchcraft. Until recent years, it was believed that one of the twin infants had to die so that the other infant might live. These beliefs and practices are usually kept as closely guarded secrets among the group's members, and there may even be some type of sanction or punishment for members who reveal the belief.

Many cultural beliefs develop over time from a trial-and-error process that has both benefits and drawbacks. For instance, several Native-American tribes that live in the Western desert have developed the practice of keeping infants in cradleboards until they begin walking. This practice, from a safety viewpoint, protects the crawling infant from injury and bites from creatures that are commonly found in the desert, such as scorpions, rattlesnakes, and poisonous insects or lizards. However, the practice tends to delay the leg muscle development of the child and increases the incidence of hip dysplasia due to the child's position in the cradleboard.

Some cultural beliefs have a primary purpose of explaining unusual or unpredictable events. For example, many traditional Vietnamese-Americans believe that mental illness results from some action that offended one or more of the gods. They also believe that a family member who is mentally ill brings disgrace upon the family, and thus knowledge of the illness must be kept secret, especially from strangers. As a

> 66 99 *If a society believes that illness is caused by evil spirits entering the body from curses by witches or medicine men, then practices such as incantations, use of ritualistic objects like bones, feathers, or incense, and even blood-letting and purgatives to "release" the spirit from the body is a logical approach to achieving a cure.*

13.2 Cultural Awareness Assessment Tool

Directions: Circle the number that best reflects your honest response to the statement. When you are finished, add up the total number of points and compare them to the Cultural Awareness Scale below.

STATEMENT	ALWAYS	SOMETIMES	NEVER
I feel comfortable when discussing alternative lifestyles with clients.	3	2	1
I support the use of traditional cultural healing practices for hospitalized clients.	3	2	1
I know the limits of my communication skills with clients from different cultures.	3	2	1
Outside the work setting, I make an effort to be involved with people from different cultures.	3	2	1
When assessing clients, I recognize the biologic variations of different ethnic groups.	3	2	1
I accept that there is a strong relationship between culture and health.	3	2	1
I consider the race, gender, and age of my clients when administering medications.	3	2	1
When caring for clients from different cultures, I consider the specific diseases common among their group.	3	2	1
I openly acknowledge my own prejudices and biases when working with clients from different cultures.	3	2	1
I seek out and attend in-service classes that deal with cultural and ethnic diversity.	3	2	1
I remain calm when my health-care values or beliefs clash with those of a client.	3	2	1
I practice culturally competent nursing when dealing with all clients, not only those from different ethnic groups.	3	2	1
When assessing clients initially, I consider their geographic origins, religious affiliation, and occupation as important elements of the care plan.	3	2	1
I have a high level of knowledge about the beliefs and customs of at least two different cultures.	3	2	1
I use a standardized cultural assessment tool when performing admission assessments on clients from different cultures.	3	2	1
I take into consideration the policies of my institution that serve as barriers for the effective provision of culturally competent care.	3	2	1
I recognize the cultural differences between the members of the same culture.	3	2	1

Cultural Awareness Scale
    40 to 51 points = High degree of cultural awareness
    30 to 39 points = Average degree of cultural awareness
    17 to 29 points = Low degree of cultural awareness

result, traditional shamans or priest/doctors are sought to attempt to appease the offended deity through rituals and prayers. Only with great reluctance will a traditional Vietnamese-American family seek therapy or medication for a mental illness.

There are several sources for the development of cultural values, including religious beliefs, worldview and philosophy, and group customs. The values that underlie any particular culture serve as powerful forces that affect all aspects of a person's life, ranging from individual actions and decision making to health-care behaviors and life-goal setting. Values, which are discussed in Chapter 6, are the ideals or concepts that give meaning to an individual's life. They are deeply ingrained, and most individuals will strongly resist any attempt to change their value structure.

Cultural values are neither right nor wrong; they exist in a culture from a long-term process of development that can often be traced back to a need for group survival. However, when judged from the perspective of other cultures, they may seem strange or even harmful. Because it makes nurses feel secure and even superior, there is a tendency to transfer to clients health-care expectations based on the nurse's own cultural framework. However, this approach often leads the nurse to failure when trying to change health-care behaviors.

It is important to recognize that one of the primary functions of nurses is to change clients' values, particularly values about health care. It is not an easy task. The first step, always, is to recognize that the nurse comes from a particular culture that has its own set of health-care values. Like all values, these have developed over time and are dependent on the nurse's education, upbringing, religious beliefs, and cultural background.

The next step is to identify the culture of the client and recognize specific health-care practices that are both similar and different

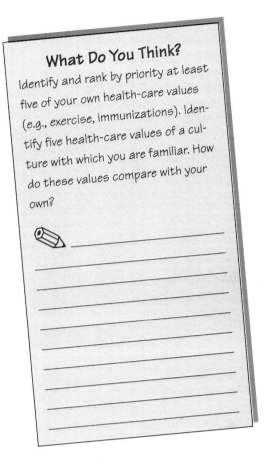

What Do You Think?

Identify and rank by priority at least five of your own health-care values (e.g., exercise, immunizations). Identify five health-care values of a culture with which you are familiar. How do these values compare with your own?

from those of the nurse. The nurse must then make a decision about whether it is desirable or possible to change the client's values, and if the end result is worth the effort.

For example, many cultures have strong values concerning pregnancy and the birth of children. In traditional Middle-Eastern families, the birth process is valued as an event strictly involving women, and the father is usually not present to either witness or assist in the delivery. However, midwives and obstetric nurses from the current American culture place a high value on the father's participation in the birth event as a way of promoting stronger family ties and starting the bonding process as soon as possible. The nurse who takes care of a Middle-Eastern family must decide whether or not to try to convince the father to stay in the delivery room during the delivery. In any event, the ultimate outcome remains relatively unchanged. Even without the father in the delivery room, the child is delivered safely, and only the bonding process with the father is delayed.

Some African cultures have discovered over time that a woman who delivers a small infant will have a much easier time during labor and delivery. Small infants usually have fewer traumatic birth defects or stillbirths and a higher maternal survival rate. In some traditional central African homeland settings where there is little skilled health care available, the value of having small infants helps in the survival of the group. The custom of feeding pregnant women only a corn-mush cereal throughout their pregnancies ensures small babies at birth. In the United States, where good prenatal nutrition is highly valued, this traditional practice is seen as dangerous to both the mother and the infant. Poor prenatal nutrition has been related to developmental delays, mental retardation, and skeletal deformities in infants as well as maternal malnutrition that can lead to infectious diseases and inability to breast-feed. In this situation, the benefits of a change in such practices of traditional African-American women would be rewarded by healthier babies and mothers.

OBTAINING AN ACCURATE CULTURAL ASSESSMENT

Obtaining thorough and accurate cultural assessments of clients from different backgrounds can be time consuming and difficult. However, the only way that nurses can avoid imposing their cultural values and practices on others and develop plans of care based on knowledge about others' beliefs and customs is to make a concerted effort to obtain this information. Several different cultural assessment tools for clients have been developed—some short and directed, others lengthy and complicated. However, all these tools attempt to gather information about clients' beliefs, customs, values, and social group influences, particularly with regard to health-care issues. One of the most thorough cultural assessments developed to date is based on Purnell's Model of Cultural Competence (Box 13.3). Although this tool is lengthy, it is easy to see that once it is completed, the nurse would have an accurate and complete understanding of the client's culture. It would also be a worthwhile undertaking for nurses to complete an assessment of their own culture.

In reality, most busy nurses would not have the time to complete this type of assessment on every client from a different

What Do You Think?

Using Purnell's cultural assessment tool, assess your own cultural background. In what areas of your own culture are you lacking knowledge?

13.3 The 12 Domains of Cultural Assessment—
Purnell's Model for Cultural Competence

I. OVERVIEW, INHABITED LOCALI-
TIES, AND TOPOGRAPHY
Overview
1. Identify the part of the world from
which this cultural or ethnic group
originates and describe the climate
and topography of the country.

Heritage and Residence
2. Identify where this group predominantly resides and include approximate numbers.

*Reasons for Migration and Associ-
ated Economic Factors*
3. Identify major factors that motivated this group to emigrate.
4. Explore economic or political factors that have influenced this
group's acculturation and professional development in America.

Educational Status and Occupation
5. Assess the educational attainment
and value placed on education by
this ethnic group.
6. Identify occupations that individuals in this group predominantly
seek on immigration.

II. COMMUNICATIONS
Dominant Language and Dialects
1. Identify the dominant language of
this group.
2. Identify dialects that may interfere with communications.
3. Explore contextual speech patterns of this group. What is the
usual volume and tone of speech?

Cultural Communication Patterns
4. Explore the willingness of individuals to share thoughts, feelings,
and ideas.

5. Explore the practice and meaning of touch in their society,
within the family, between
friends, with strangers, with
members of the same sex, with
members of the opposite sex,
and with health-care providers.
6. Identify personal spatial and distancing characteristics when
communicating on a one-to-one
basis. Explore how distancing
changes with friends versus
strangers.
7. Explore the use of eye contact
within this group. Does avoidance
of eye contact have special
meanings? How does eye contact vary among family, friends,
and strangers? Does eye contact
change among socioeconomic
groups?
8. Explore the meaning of various
facial expressions. Do specific facial expressions have special
meanings? Do persons tend to
smile a lot? How are emotions
displayed or not displayed in facial expressions?
9. Are there acceptable ways of
standing and greeting outsiders?

Temporal Relationships
10. Explore temporal relationships in
this group. Are individuals primarily past, present, or future-
oriented? How do individuals see
the context of past, present, and
future?
11. Identify how differences in the interpretation of social time versus
clock time are perceived.

BOX

13.3 The 12 Domains of Cultural Assessment—
Purnell's Model for Cultural Competence *(continued)*

12. Explore how time factors are interpreted by this group. Are individuals expected to be punctual in terms of jobs, appointments, and social engagements?

Format for Names
13. Explore the format for a person's name.
14. How does one expect to be greeted by strangers and health-care practitioners?

III. FAMILY ROLES AND ORGANIZATION

Head of Household and Gender Roles
1. Identify the perceived head of the household. How does this change during different developmental aspects of life?
2. Describe gender-related roles of men and women in the family system.

Prescriptive, Restrictive, and Taboo Behaviors
3. Identify prescriptive, restrictive, and taboo behaviors for children.
4. Identify prescriptive, restrictive, and taboo behaviors for adolescents.

Family Roles and Priorities
5. Describe family goals and priorities emphasized by this culture.
6. Explore developmental tasks in this group.
7. Explore the status and role of the aged in the family.
8. Explore the roles and importance of extended family members.

9. Describe how one gains social status in this cultural system. Is there a caste system?

Alternative Lifestyles
10. Describe how alternative lifestyles and nontraditional families such as single parents, blended families, communal families, same-sex families, and so forth are viewed by this society.

IV. WORKFORCE ISSUES

Culture in the Workplace
1. Identify specific workforce issues affected by immigration, e.g., education.
2. Describe specific multicultural considerations when working with this culturally diverse individual or group in the workforce.
3. Explore factors influencing patterns of acculturation in this cultural group.
4. Explore native health-care practices and their influence in the workforce.

Issues Related to Autonomy
5. Identify cultural issues related to professional autonomy, superior or subordinate control, religious issues, and gender in the workforce.
6. Identify language barriers with concrete interpretations of the language.

V. BIOCULTURAL ECOLOGY
Skin Color and Biologic Variations
1. Identify the skin color and physical variations for this group.
2. Explore any special problems or concerns the skin color

13.3 The 12 Domains of Cultural Assessment—
Purnell's Model for Cultural Competence *(continued)*

may pose for health-care practitioners.

3. Identify biologic variations to body habitus or structure.

Diseases and Health Conditions

4. Identify specific risk factors for individuals related to the topography or climate.

5. Identify any hereditary or genetic diseases or conditions that are common with this group.

6. Identify any endemic diseases specific to this cultural or ethnic group.

7. Identify any diseases or health conditions for which this group has increased susceptibility.

Variations in Drug Metabolism

8. Identify specific variations in drug metabolism, interactions, and side effects.

VI. HIGH-RISK BEHAVIORS
High-Risk Behaviors

1. Identify specific high-risk behaviors common among this group.

2. Explore behaviors related to the use of alcohol, tobacco, and recreational drugs and other substances among this group.

Health-Care Practices

3. Identify the typical health-seeking behaviors of this group.

4. Assess the level of physical activity in their lifestyles.

5. Assess the use of safety measures such as seat belts and helmets.

VII. NUTRITION
Meaning of Food

1. Explore the meaning of food to this group.

Common Foods and Food Rituals

2. Identify foods, preparation practices, and major ingredients commonly used by this group.

3. Identify specific food rituals.

Dietary Practices for Health Promotion

4. Identify dietary practices used to promote health or to treat illness in this cultural group.

Nutritional Deficiencies and Food Limitations

5. Identify enzyme deficiencies or food intolerance commonly experienced by this group.

6. Identify large-scale or significant nutritional deficiencies experienced by this group.

7. Identify native food limitations in America that may cause special health difficulties.

VIII. PREGNANCY AND CHILDBEARING PRACTICES
Fertility Practices and Views Toward Pregnancy

1. Explore cultural views and practices related to fertility control.

2. Identify cultural practices and views toward pregnancy.

Prescriptive, Restrictive, and Taboo Practices in the Childbearing Family

3. Identify prescriptive, restrictive, and taboo practices related to pregnancy such as foods, exercises, intercourse, and avoidance of weather-related conditions.

4. Identify prescriptive, restrictive, and taboo practices related to the birthing process, such as reac-

tions during labor, presence of men, position for delivery, preferred types of health-care practitioners, or place of delivery.

5. Identify prescriptive, restrictive, and taboo practices related to the postpartum period such as bathing, cord care, exercise, foods, and the role of men.

IX. DEATH RITUALS

Death Rituals and Expectations

1. Identify culturally specific death rituals and expectations.
2. Explain the purpose of death rituals and mourning practices.
3. What are specific burial practices, such as cremation?

Responses to Death and Grief

4. Identify cultural expectations of responses to death and grief.
5. Explore the meaning of death, dying, and the afterlife.

X. SPIRITUALITY

Religious Practices and Use of Prayer

1. Identify the influence of the dominant religion of this group on health-care practices.
2. Explore the use of prayer, meditation, and other activities or symbols that help individuals reach fulfillment.

Meaning of Life and Individual Sources of Strength

3. Explore what gives meaning to life for individuals.
4. Identify the individual's sources of strength.

Spiritual Beliefs and Health-Care Practices

5. Explore the relationship between spiritual beliefs and health-care practices.

XI. HEALTH-CARE PRACTICES

Health-Seeking Beliefs and Behaviors

1. Identify predominant beliefs that influence health-care practices.
2. Describe the influences of health promotion and prevention practices.

Responsibility for Health Care

3. Describe the focus of acute care practice (curative or fatalistic).
4. Explore who assumes responsibility for health care in this culture.
5. Describe the role of health insurance in this culture.
6. Explore behaviors associated with the use of over-the-counter medications.

Folklore Practices

7. Explore combinations of magicoreligious beliefs, folklore, and traditional beliefs that influence health-care behaviors.

Barriers to Health Care

8. Identify barriers to health care such as language, economics, and geography for this group.

Cultural Responses to Health and Illness

9. Explore cultural beliefs and responses to pain that influence

interventions. Does pain have a special meaning?

10. Describe beliefs and views about mental illness in this culture.

11. Differentiate between the perceptions of mentally and physically handicapped in this culture.

12. Describe cultural beliefs and practices related to chronicity and rehabilitation.

13. Identify cultural perceptions of the sick role in this group.

Blood Transfusions and Organ Donation

14. Describe the acceptance of blood transfusions, organ donations, and organ transplantation among this group.

XII. HEALTH-CARE PRACTITIONERS
Traditional Versus Biomedical Care

1. Explore the roles of traditional, folklore, and magicoreligious practitioners and their influence on health practitioners.

2. Describe the acceptance of health-care practitioners in providing care to each gender. Does the age of the practitioner make a difference?

Status of Health-Care Providers

3. Explore perceptions of health-care practitioners with this group.

4. Identify the status of health-care providers in this society.

5. Describe how different health-care practitioners view each other.

Reprinted with permission from Purnell, LD, and Paulanka, BJ: Transcultural Health Care. FA Davis, Philadelphia, 1998.

---

culture. However, the following key questions can serve as a starting point for a cultural assessment:

- Why do you think you are ill? What was the cause of the illness?
- What was going on at the time the illness started?
- How does the illness affect your body and health?
- Do you consider this to be a serious illness?
- If you were at home, what type of treatments or medications would you use? How would these treatments help?
- What type of treatment do you expect from the health-care system?

- How has your illness affected your ability to live normally?
- If you do not get better, what do you think will happen?

A gradual approach to cultural assessment may be more productive. As discussed earlier, clients from different cultures may often feel uncomfortable with revealing detailed information about cultural beliefs, values, and practices to strangers. By first asking some general questions, which demonstrate to the client that the nurse is interested in that person as an individual and that the nurse really does care about his or her health, an atmosphere of trust can develop. Frequently, only after a warm and

dardized American growth chart because of their genetically smaller stature). Changes in skin color may also affect the interpretation of assessment findings (e.g., with regard to an assessment of cyanosis in people with a light versus a dark complexion). In order to determine whether the client's skin color is normal or abnormal, the nurse must know what constitutes the normal color for a particular ethnic group. In assessing for cyanosis, the nurse may need to examine the client's oral mucosa and may also need to measure capillary refill times to determine whether the client has cyanosis.

The ultimate goal of cultural assessment, as with all assessments, is to provide the best care possible for the client. A fundamental belief that nurses hold to strongly is that all clients have a right to self-determination, including the customs, practices, and values that emanate from their culture. By considering both the cultural and ethnic variables of each client, nurses will avoid practice that is ethnocentric and conducted strictly from the nurse's cultural viewpoint.

PROVIDING CULTURALLY COMPETENT CARE

Cultural competence has become a buzzword for the twenty-first century. The term has several divergent definitions with little consensus among cultural experts. However, cultural competence as it relates to nursing can be regarded as the provision of effective care for clients who belong to diverse cultures, based on the nurse's knowledge and understanding of the values, customs, beliefs, and practices of the culture. Provision of culturally competent care requires the development of certain interpersonal skills that allow nurses to work with individuals and groups in the community. The primary skills required for cultural competence include communication, understanding, and sensitivity. Although the

trusting environment has been established will a client be willing to reveal the more hidden aspects of his or her culture to the nurse.

Physical assessments made on individuals from other cultures require a certain level of cultural awareness and competence on the part of the nurse. Although the assessment techniques used for different individuals may be identical, the nurse needs to possess knowledge of the basic biologic and physical variations among ethnic groups. The interpretation of assessment findings may be affected by ethnic variations in anatomic structure or characteristics (e.g., children from some Asian cultures may fall below the normal growth level on a stan-

basic types of cultural skills are similar, their application within and between cultural groups may differ greatly. The development of cultural competence is not a one-time skill to check off on a skills checklist; rather, it is an ongoing process that continues throughout the nurse's career.

TRANSCULTURAL COMMUNICATION

The ability to communicate is the foundation on which culturally competent care is built. The most obvious barrier to culturally competent care for the non-English-speaking client is the lack of a common language. Communication is a highly complex process that requires both verbal and nonverbal communication. Nonverbal communication includes (but is not limited to) body language, facial expressions, eye contact, personal space, touch and body contact, formality of names, and time awareness (Box 13.4).

Other factors that affect communication are loudness of voice, tone, and acceptable greetings. Often clients communicate differently with family and friends than they do with health-care personnel. Nurses should also be aware that in some cultures (e.g., those with a strong caste system, which involves a class structure) communication between those in the upper and lower classes in that society may be affected. For example, different cultures may hold the role of women or of health-care personnel in more or less esteem.

Nurses must be cautious when interpreting the nonverbal responses from some cultural groups. Some cultures respond to all questions with the reply "yes," a nod, or a smile. This response, in the American culture, usually indicates understanding and compliance. However, particularly in Asian cultures, nodding and smiling are really signs of respect for the nurse's position or an attempt to avoid confrontation.

The classic example of this process occurred when an English-speaking nurse gave a non-English-speaking Asian client preoperative instructions about how to prepare an abdominal surgical site. She thought that she had shown the client how the bottle of povidone-iodine, a powerful skin disinfectant, was to be used in scrubbing the area. The client smiled and nodded throughout the instruction. When asked whether he had any questions, he did not respond. The nurse took the silence to mean that he had no questions. When the nurse left the room, the client promptly drank the whole bottle of povidone-iodine. Fortunately, the error was discovered immediately, and no long-term complications occurred from the accident. Nurses who work with non-English-speaking clients need to develop other ways to measure how much a client understands rather than depending only on a verbal response. Return demonstrations provide more accurate information and better validation of the client's level of understanding in the absence of a common spoken language.

The use of silence by some cultural groups has led to misunderstandings in communication in the health-care setting.

> " " *The use of silence by some cultural groups has led to misunderstandings in communication in the health-care setting.*

For example, Asian-Americans consider silence to be a sign of respect, particularly for elders, whereas Arab-Americans and the English use silence to gain privacy. Among many people in Europe (e.g., the French, Russians, and Spanish), silence often indicates agreement.

Variations in communication style also account for misunderstandings and miscommunications. Factors such as loudness, intonation, rhythm, and speed of speech all

13.4 Guidelines for Communicating with Non-English-Speaking Clients

1. Use interpreters rather than translators. Translators just restate the words from one language to another. An interpreter decodes the words and provides the meaning behind the message.
2. Use dialect-specific interpreters whenever possible.
3. Use interpreters trained in the health-care field.
4. Give the interpreter time alone with the client.
5. Provide time for translation and interpretation.
6. Be aware that interpreters may affect the reporting of symptoms, insert their own ideas, or omit information.
7. Avoid the use of relatives who may distort information or not be objective.
8. Avoid using children as interpreters, especially with sensitive topics.
9. Use same-age and same-gender interpreters whenever possible. However, clients from cultures who have a high regard for the elderly may prefer an older aged interpreter.
10. Maintain eye contact with both the client and the interpreter to elicit feedback and read nonverbal clues.
11. Remember that clients can usually understand more than they express; thus, they need time to think in their own language. They are alert to the health-care provider's body language, and they may forget some or all of their English in times of stress.
12. Speak slowly without exaggerated mouthing, allow time for translation, use active rather than passive tense, wait for feedback, and restate the message. Do not rush; do not speak loudly. Use a reference book with common phrases such as *Roget's International Thesaurus* or *Taber's Cyclopedic Medical Dictionary*.
13. Use as many words as possible in the client's language and nonverbal communication when unable to understand the language.
14. If an interpreter is unavailable, the use of a translator may be acceptable. The difficulty with translation is omission of parts of the message, distortion of the message, including transmission of information not given by the speaker, and messages not being fully understood.
15. *Note:* Social class differences between the interpreter and the client may result in the interpreter's not reporting information that he or she perceives as superstitious or unimportant.

Reprinted with permission from Purnell, LD, and Paulanka, BJ: Transcultural Health Care. FA Davis, Philadelphia, 1998, pp 16–17.

are important in communication. Among certain cultural groups, American nurses' have a reputation for speaking at a rapid rate and for using medical jargon. Some nurses also have a reputation for their tendency to increase the volume of their voices when communicating with clients who do not speak English, as if talking louder will increase understanding. On the other hand, groups such as Native-Americans and Asian-Americans speak more softly and may be difficult to hear even when the nurse is standing at the bedside. These groups may misinterpret the louder, more forceful voice tone of the American nurse as an indication of anger. Arab-American groups are often noted for their dramatic communication styles. Nurses may misinterpret this behavior as hostility, when in reality they are merely trying to demonstrate a point using an emotional communication style. Nurses need to analyze their own speech patterns and consciously modify their tone and pace when working with different cultural groups to prevent misunderstandings.

Nurses also need to recognize that certain groups are much less willing to disclose private matters or personal feelings than others. In general, clients from American or European origins tend to be less secretive about almost all issues, because the practice of sharing has been encouraged from an early age. However, many Asian cultures, particularly the Japanese, are highly reluctant to discuss personal topics with either family or health-care providers. Other groups, such as Mexican-Americans, will discuss personal issues openly with friends and family members but are reluctant to do so with health-care providers who they do not know well. However, even within these groups there are wide variations. American women probably constitute one of the most open groups when it comes to expressing personal feelings, whereas American men tend to have much more difficulty with this type of communication.

Nurses presume that all clients should trust them instantaneously just because they are nurses and should answer even the most personal questions immediately. As discussed earlier, it may be much more productive to start the communication process with small talk and general, nonthreatening questions to establish an atmosphere of trust. Often the use of open-ended questions and statements will allow the client to express beliefs and opinions that would be difficult to discover through closed-end questions that the client can an-swer with a simple "yes" or "no." As the level of trust increases, the client will be more likely to reveal important information in the more sensitive areas of the assessment. In addition, sensitivity to the nonverbal aspects of the communication process will allow nurses to use behaviors that increase trust and avoid gestures, facial expressions, or eye contact that may rely a message of superiority, hostility, anger, or disapproval.

The inappropriate touching of clients from different cultures is a leading cause of miscommunication. American nurses are taught early on in their first nursing classes, usually physical assessment or basic skill courses, that it is necessary to "lay on hands" in order to provide good care. Students who are reluctant to palpate the femoral pulses of their laboratory partner or remove a client's shirt to auscultate anterior heart and breath sounds may receive a failing grade for the course.

However, touching in other cultures conveys a number of alternative meanings, ranging from power, anger, and sexual arousal to affirmation, empathy, and cordiality. For example, it is generally not acceptable for men and women to touch in many Arab cultures, except in the privacy of the home and in the context of marriage. American female nurses who palpate pulses, listen to breath sounds, or palpate for tactile fremitus when assessing men from an Arab culture may be communicating a message that they never intended. Some groups, such as Mexican-Americans or Italian-Americans who frequently touch and hug family members and friends, are much less receptive to touching by strangers during health-care examinations, particularly if the health-care provider is of the opposite sex. In these situations, it would be extremely important for the nurse

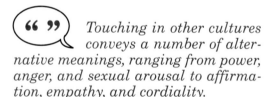

Touching in other cultures conveys a number of alternative meanings, ranging from power, anger, and sexual arousal to affirmation, empathy, and cordiality.

to explain what he or she is going to do and why it is important before the particular physical contact occurs. The nurse should also avoid any unnecessary contact, such as palpation of femoral pulses when the client has pneumonia.

Closely related to the issue of touch is the concept of personal space. Personal space is a zone that individuals maintain around themselves in most casual social situations. When a person's personal space is violated, it often creates a generalized feeling of discomfort or threat, which causes the person to move away from the offending individual. Nurses routinely violate clients' personal space when performing physical assessments or providing basic care.

The actual distance required to maintain a comfortable personal space varies widely from one culture to another. People who belong to the European, Canadian, or American cultures usually require between 18 and 22 inches of distance for a comfortable personal space when communicating with strangers or casual acquaintances. In contrast, individuals from the Jewish, Arab, Turkish, and Middle-Eastern cultures may require as little as 3 to 5 inches of personal space when talking with another person and often interpret physical closeness as a sign of acceptance. In addition, they prefer to stand face to face and maintain eye contact when they are talking. It is easy to understand why misinterpretations in communication might arise. A client from a Middle-Eastern culture might judge an American nurse to be cold and aloof, although she is merely maintaining a comfortable personal space from the client. Likewise, an American nurse may feel physically threatened by the close communication style of a Turkish-American client and find himself or herself continually backing away from the client in an attempt to re-establish his or her personal space.

> **" "** *The actual distance required to maintain a comfortable personal space varies widely from one culture to another.*

Similarly, eye contact communicates different messages to different cultures. Among American and many European cultures, making periodic eye contact during conversations indicates that the person is attentive to the communication as well as acting as a means of measuring the person's sincerity. Common sayings such as, "Look me in the eye and say that," or admonitions for public speakers to "make eye contact" with the audience emphasize the underlying positive value these cultures place on eye contact. Lack of eye contact may be interpreted as inattention, insincerity, or disregard.

In contrast, some Native-American cultures believe that the eyes are the windows of the soul and that direct eye contact by another may be interpreted as an attempt to "steal the soul" from the body. Between Native-American men, direct eye contact is a sign of challenge and aggression and may precipitate a violent, physical confrontation. Among some South-American cultures, sustained eye contact is a sign of disrespect, whereas in other cultural groups, particularly Mexican-Americans, eye contact with a child is believed to convey the *mal de ojo,* or evil eye. Many childhood and adult illnesses among these cultures are attributed to the effects of the evil eye, and practices such as tying red cloths or strings around the children's wrists are used to ward off the illnesses. Eye contact, a routine part of America culture, has diverse and powerful meanings to clients from other cultures.

The complexity and importance of communication should never be underestimated when working with clients from diverse cultures. Merely speaking a language does not encompass the entirety of communication. Awareness of the meanings of gestures, body positions, facial expressions, and eye movements is essential in culturally competent communications.

OTHER ELEMENTS OF TRANSCULTURAL NURSING PRACTICE

There are several other elements to be considered for effective transcultural nursing, including passive obedience, cultural synergy, building on similarities, and conflict resolution. The term *passive obedience* refers to a type of behavior that develops when clients from a different culture believe that the nurse is an authority figure or expert in health-care matters. Although many cultures may display this type of behavior to some extent, it is most commonly seen among Asian-American groups. These cultures try to cope with the uncertainty of their health status and the threat of an authority figure by becoming passively obedient. Rather than asking questions that they think will reveal their lack of knowledge or confusion about some health-care issue or that they believe may challenge the authority of the nurse, they become passively obedient and compliant.

It is inevitable that conflicts will arise from time to time when caring for clients of different cultures. It is important to recognize that the origins of many conflicts reside within the individual. Nurses may label clients from other cultures as noncompliant, when in reality the nurse has an incomplete understanding of the client's culture or unrealistic expectations for behavior.

Other common reasons for noncompliance among culturally diverse clients include the lack of external symptoms of disease, incon-

venient or painful treatments, and lack of external support from family members or close friends. As discussed earlier, the nurse first needs to ask the client what traditional treatments are used in dealing with this disease. In some cases, where the traditional treatments are similar to the ones used by the health-care facility, the nurse may be able to demonstrate to the client that they are really very similar. In other cases, the treatments may be very different. However, if the traditional treatment does not disrupt the facility's treatment plan or threaten the client's health, they can be used simultaneously with the standard medical treatments. Nurses who work in the Native-American health-care system and hospitals have become accustomed to finding bone fragments, feathers, and leather medicine pouches in the beds of their clients.

Nurses who work actively to develop cultural synergy tend to be more successful in the delivery of competent transcultural care. *Cultural synergy* is a term that implies that health-care providers make a commitment not only to learn about other cultures but also to immerse themselves in those cultures. Nurses achieve cultural synergy when they begin to selectively include values, customs, and beliefs of other cultures into their own worldviews. The first step in cultural synergy is the desire to know everything there is about another culture and to purposely establish relationships with individuals from other cultures.

Closely related to cultural synergy is the recognition that cultures are really very much alike in many aspects. It would seem that most books and publications written about cultural diversity present only the diversity of cultures and not the similarities. Although recognition of cultural differences is

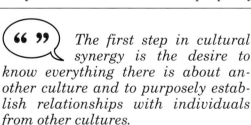
" " *The first step in cultural synergy is the desire to know everything there is about another culture and to purposely establish relationships with individuals from other cultures.*

important, it should be just one step toward the ultimate realization that there are more similarities than differences among cultures. Many colleges offer courses in comparative religions that identify the many similarities of the fundamental beliefs that underlie the major religions. However, many college courses on cultural diversity have not evolved past the point of identifying cultural differences. Perhaps this is due in part to the "salad bowl" approach to cultural communication that exists in current society. It would almost appear that a new approach to acculturation, based on similarities between cultures rather than on the differences, needs to be developed.

INFORMATION SOURCES FOR TRANSCULTURAL NURSING

The recent explosion of interest in cultural diversity and transcultural nursing has led to a proliferation of literature on the topic. The origins of the current transcultural movement can be traced back to 1974, when a transcultural conference on communication and culture was held at the University of Hawaii School of Nursing. Following the success of this conference, a series of transcultural conferences were planned over the next year to bring together nurses, sociologists, anthropologists, and other social scientists to discuss issues that would eventually form the basis for transcultural nursing. Not long after this conference, the Transcultural Nursing Society was organized. It was incorporated in 1981 and began publishing its semiannual official journal, *Journal of Transcultural Nursing,* in 1989. It is now being published four times a year. In 1976, the American Nurses Association (ANA) recommended that multicultural content be included in nursing curricula. Since then, the ANA has organized the Council on Intercul-

tural Nursing, which publishes the *Intercultural Nursing Newsletter.*

During the last decade, a few universities and colleges have begun offering graduate degrees in transcultural, cross-cultural, and international nursing. Graduates are now able to become certified transcultural nurses (CTNs) by completing oral and written examinations offered by the Transcultural Nursing Society. Nurses do not need to be from minority groups to obtain the CTN.

Society has not remained stagnant during this period of development and organization. Growing numbers of immigrants, changing governmental regulations, and grassroots movements all have contributed to the pressure placed on nursing to recognize and effectively care for clients from different cultures.

Site Seeing

Aboriginal Nurses Asociation of Canada
http://www.anac.on.ca/
Contact: mail to:info@anac.on.ca

ACHNE (Community Health)
mail to:listserv@unccvm.uncc.edu
Subscribe ACHNE-L Firstname Lastname

Alternative Medicine Home Page
http://www.pitt.edu/~cbw/altm.html
Contact: Charles B. Wessel
mail to:cbw@med.pitt.edu

American Holistic Nurses' Association
http://www.ahna.org/
Contact: mail to:webmaster@ahna.org

DiversityRx
http://www.diversityrx.org/HTML/DIVRX.htm

GLOBALRN (Culture)
mail to:LISTSERV@ITSSRV1.UCSF.EDU>LIST SERV@ITSSRV1.UCSF.EDU/P>
Subscribe GLOBALRN Firstname Lastname

Conclusion

The major changes in U.S. demographics that have occurred in the 1980s and 1990s require nurses to provide culturally sensitive care. Based on the fundamental belief of professional nursing that all individuals are to be cared for with respect and dignity regardless of culture, beliefs, or disease process, nurses must actively seek multicultural education. However, nurses need to keep in mind that cultural assessments and decisions about care are relative to the nurse's personal experiences, beliefs, and culture. There is a natural tendency to stereotype individuals from other cultures unconsciously on the basis of one's internal value system. There is also a tendency to batch all individuals from one culture into a single group, when in reality, there may be wide variations within the group.

It is a well-accepted belief that nurses who value cultural diversity will deliver higher quality care. Nurses who have a high level of cultural knowledge and sensitivity maximize their nursing interventions when they become co-participants and client advocates for individuals who might otherwise be lost in an impersonal health-care system. Only when nurses can understand the client's perspective, develop an open style of communication, become receptive to learning from clients of other cultures, and accept and work with the ambiguities inherent in the care of multicultural clients will they become truly culturally competent health-care providers.

Critical Thinking Exercises

Consider the following case study:

In 1990, Jose Bisigan, aged 87 years, and his wife Carmen, aged 85, sold their small restaurant and immigrated to Los Angeles from a small town in the Visayan region of the Philippines. They came to join their first-born daughter, nurse Felicia, aged 54, her husband, and their three children aged 10 to 18. Mr. Bisigan speaks limited English and is in a poststroke rehabilitation unit. Since the stroke, he has had mild aphasia, mild confusion, and bladder and bowel continence problems. His hypertension and long-standing diabetes are controlled with medication and diet. His wife, daughter, and grandchildren have been supportive of him during this first hospitalization experience. Mr. Bisigan's family has cooperated with the health team, often agreeing with minimal resistance to the prescribed treatment management. The rehabilitation team recommended subacute rehabilitation treatment as part of the discharge plan.

As a businessman and the elder in the family household, Mr. Bisigan is looked to for counsel by the immediate and extended family. Mr. Bisigan's status, however, has caused friction between Felicia and her husband, Nestor, an American-born Filipino who works as a machinist. Nestor has accused Felicia of giving excessive attention to her mother and father. Felicia's worries about her parents' health have made Nestor very resentful. He increased his already daily "outings with the boys." Felicia maintains a full-time position in acute care and a part-time night shift position in a nursing home.

Mr. Bisigan's discharge is pending, and a decision must be made before Medicare coverage runs out. Felicia has to consider the possible choices available to her father and the family circumstances and expectations. Mrs. Bisigan, who is being treated for hypertension, has always deferred decisions to her husband and is looking to Felicia to make the decisions. Because of her work schedule, the absence of a responsible person at home, her mother's health problems, and intergenerational friction, Felicia considers nursing home placement. She is, however, reluctant to broach the subject with her father, who expects to be cared for at home. Mrs. Bisigan disagrees with putting her husband in a nursing home and is adamant that she will care for her husband at home.

Felicia delayed talking to her father until the rehabilitation team requested a meeting. At the meeting, Felicia indicated that she could not bring herself to present her plan to put her father in a nursing home because of her mother's objection and her own fear that her father will feel rejected. Feeling very much alone in resolving the issue about nursing home placement, she requested the team to act as intermediary for her and her family.

✔ Identify cultural family values that contribute to the conflicts experienced by each family member.

Name _____

Course _____

Instructor _____

Date _____

Critical Thinking Exercises

✔ Identify a culturally competent approach that the team can use when discussing nursing home placement with the Bisigans.

✔ How might the rehabilitation program be presented to Mrs. Bisigan and still allow her to maintain her spousal role?

✔ Discuss at least three communication issues in the family that are culture-bound and suggest possible interventions.

✔ Identify psychocultural assessments that should be done by the rehabilitation team to have a greater understanding of the dynamics specific to this family.

✔ Identify health promotion counseling that might be discussed with the Bisigans' grandchildren.

✔ Identify and explain major sources of stress for each member of this household.

Reprinted with permission from Purnell, LD, and Paulanka, BJ: Transcultural Health Care. FA Davis, Philadelphia, 1998, pp 269–270.

BIBLIOGRAPHY

American Nurses Association: Cultural Diversity in the Nursing Curriculum: A Guide for Implementation. ANA, Kansas City, Mo., 1986.

American Nurses Association: Nursing's Social Policy Statement. ANA, Washington, DC, 1995.

Banks, JA, and Banks, CM: Multicultural Education: Issues and Perspectives. Allyn and Bacon, London, 1997.

Canuso, R: Co-family sleeping: Strange bedfellows or culturally acceptable behavior? Cultural Diversity 3:109–111, 1996.

Chrisman, N, and Schultz, D: Transforming health care through cultural competence training. In Dienemann, J (ed): Cultural Diversity in Nursing: Issues, Strategies and Outcomes. American Academy of Nursing, New York, 1998.

Clinton, J: Cultural diversity and health care in America. Journal of Cultural Diversity 3(1):4–8, 1996.

Cultural diversity in nursing. J Nurs Educ (special issue) 32(5), 1998.

Darks, G: Why don't more African Americans go into nursing? American Nurse 30(5):5, 1998.

Fitzsimons, VA, and Kelly, ML: The culture of learning. NLN Press, New York, Pub number 14-26, 1999.

Ketter, J: Workforce conflicts subject of multi-cultural workshops. American Nurse 27:3, 1995.

Leninger, M: Transcultural nursing: Concepts, theories, and practices. Wiley, New York, 1978.

Lester, N: Cultural competence: A nursing dialogue. Am J Nurs 98(9):36–43, 1998.

Purnell, LD, and Paulanka, BJ: Transcultural Health Care. FA Davis, Philadelphia, 1998.

Sandhaus, S: Migrant health: A harvest of poverty. Am J Nurs 98(9):52–65, 1998.

Smith, P, and Weinman, M: Cultural implications for public health policy for pregnant Hispanic adolescents. Health Values 19(1):3–9, 1995.

Stacqualursi, F, et al: Assessing and implementing diabetes patient education programs for American Indian communities. Diabetes Educator 19(1):31–34, 1993.

Stewart, M: Health care community faces the year 2000. American Nurse 29(6):24, 1997.

Tolley, M: Experiencing the neighborhood: The parish as a clinical site. Oklahoma Nurse 43(1):31, 1998.

Wenger, AFZ: Cultural context, health and health care decision making. J Transcultural Nurs 7(1):3–14, 1996.

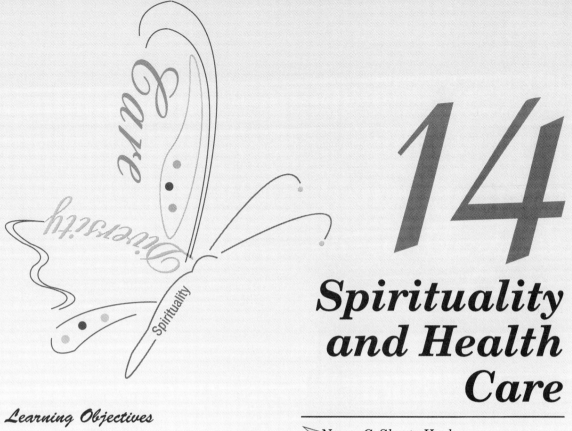

14

Spirituality and Health Care

➤ *Nancy C. Sharts-Hopko*

Learning Objectives

After completing this chapter, the reader will be able to:

1. Develop a working definition of spirituality.
2. Distinguish spirituality from religion.
3. Describe what is meant by the nursing diagnosis Spiritual Distress.
4. Describe research that supports the health benefit of spiritual practices.
5. Describe the relationship between spirituality and one alternative healing modality used within nursing.

The emotional demands of working with people who are experiencing a crisis stimulate many health professionals to examine spiritual issues for themselves. Their interest may be sparked by the diverse spiritual practices that they witness in the course of their work or from a growing body of biomedical research that is showing that spiritual practices bring tangible benefits to health and well-being.

Spirituality refers to people's living with consciousness of a reality beyond that which is knowable through the five senses. This awareness of a transcendent reality may be experienced in terms of a divine creator, or it may be experienced in relation to the wonder of all creation or to fundamental values such as love, truth, or beauty. Health professionals have shown increased interest in spirituality during the 1990s.

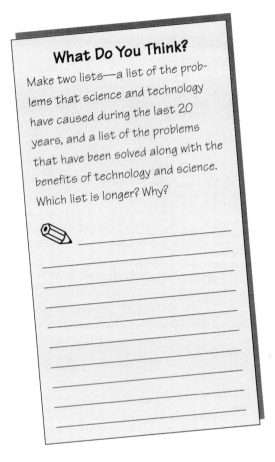

What Do You Think?

Make two lists—a list of the problems that science and technology have caused during the last 20 years, and a list of the problems that have been solved along with the benefits of technology and science. Which list is longer? Why?

It is universally true that the human life cycle is marked by a rhythm of transitions: birth, the entry of a child into society, puberty, sexual awakening, entry into adulthood, marriage, parenthood, illness, loss, old age, and death. In all cultures there are other rhythms that people honor, such as the solar and lunar cycles, the agricultural cycle, and the reproductive cycles. These cycles constitute the rhythm of human life. All people recognize the importance of each of these transitions and in some way have ritualized them through their religions. People learn from their own cultural groups how to behave during each transition, and each cultural group has conceptualized an understanding of these human experiences; however, their importance is universal.

Nurses primarily have contact with clients in the health-care setting within the context of these transitions. Developmental crisis theory holds that these transitions are times of anxiety and vulnerability for families. Therefore, nurses are required to treat people who are going through these transitions with great tenderness and care. It is a sacred trust for nurses to be allowed into a family system in transition. During these transitions, clients and families may seek spiritual support or they may feel spiritual abandonment. Ideally, nurses can help people identify and find the spiritual support that they require.

Over a long period of time, from the enlightenment of the seventeenth century to the dawn of the twenty-first century, political leaders and educated people in Western cultures came to believe that all the answers to human suffering could be found in science and technology. For example, early in the twentieth century, antibiotics were thought of as "magic bullets" that cured diseases and reduced suffering. People were eager to take part in research studies to solve their health-care problems. It was in this context that the nursing profession embraced the Western scientific method as the measure for defining itself. Nurses believed, and some still do believe, that rigorous research involving testing of hypotheses would provide the theoretical base for the practice of professional nursing.

More recently, however, the horrors of modern warfare, the harnessing of nuclear power, space exploration, and the mapping of the human genome are among new capabilities that have given urgency to reconsideration of the question: "What does it mean to be fully human in the universe as it is now understood?" It is evident that science and technology cannot offer the solutions to all human problems; in fact, they have contributed to many of them.

Science, electronic communications, and the great social experiments of the last two centuries are among the influences directing humans to a consciousness of the individual's connectedness to the whole of creation and all peoples. One of the ways in which both consumers of health care and health professionals are responding to this realization is by reintegrating spirituality and spiritual modes of healing into health and illness practices. Another response is the growing inclination to examine and adopt the spiritual wisdom of traditions other than one's own.

A feature of postmodernism is the realization that the concept of truth is a relative one, allowing for an appreciation of diverse perspectives on what is true. Science, including nursing science since the mid-1980s, has expanded its ways of discerning truth, leaving behind traditional hypotheticodeductive, quantitative research.[1] The emergence of **phenomenology** within the discipline of philosophy is one major influence that has led to an appreciation for qualitative methods of discovery within nursing. As a philosophical approach to understanding truth, phenomenology parallels and is closely related to existentialism, advocating the view that consciousness determines reality and truth in space and time. In the health-care setting, a phenomenologic approach appreciates the belief that the client's observations may be more objective than those of the nurse, because they are attached to the client's past experiences and knowledge, which includes rich descriptions of the person's experiences of life transitions. In nursing, intuition has emerged as a phenomenon worthy of further investigation.[2] This change in viewpoint has coincided with increased interest in complementary and alternative therapies and with the importance of spirituality in healing and wellness.

THE NATURE OF SPIRITUALITY

Spirituality is a broad and somewhat nebulous concept that has to do with people's search for answers to questions and issues, such as those listed in Box 14.1. Coles,[3] a Harvard University professor of psychiatry, identified similar concerns among children of various cultural backgrounds in his research on the development of spirituality.

A rich heritage of spiritual practices, including systematic reflection for growth toward wholeness, is found in all the major religions of the world.[4] The roots of the great traditions, including each religion's prayer practices, can be traced to the shift in human consciousness that occurred around 500 B.C. During this period many great teachers and spiritual leaders emerged, including Confucius; Lao-Tze; Siddhartha Gautama, who became the Buddha; Zoroaster; the Greek philosophers Socrates, Plato, and Aristotle; and the Hebrew prophets Amos, Hosea, and Isaiah.[5] St. Augustine, a Roman Catholic bishop who lived in North Africa during the fifth century, is credited with first identifying the relationships among contemplation,

14.1 Questions That are Spiritual in Nature

Why are we here?

How do we fit into the cosmos?

What power or intelligence created and orders the universe?

What is the nature and meaning of divine or mystical experiences?

How are we to make meaning of suffering?

How are we to behave toward other people?

How are we to deal with our own shortcomings and failures?

What happens to us when we die, and where were we before we were born?

action, and wisdom within the Christian tradition.[6,7] For Augustine, the contemplative life was properly focused on discernment of truth and was open to all people. However, Augustine equated truth, ultimately, with God.

Goddard[8] defined spirituality as integrative energy, capable of producing internal human harmony or holism. Other authors refer to spirituality as a sense of coherence.[9] Spirituality also entails a sense of transcendent reality, which draws strength from inner resources, living fully for the present, and having a sense of inner knowing.[10,11] Solitude, compassion, and empathy are important components of spirituality for many individuals.[12,13]

The concept of hope is central to spirituality. Spirituality may be regarded as the driving force that pervades all aspects of and gives meaning to an individual's life. It creates a set of beliefs and values that influence the way that people conduct their lives. Spiritual activity involves introspection, reflection, and a sense of connectedness to others or to the universe. For many people, this connectedness focuses ultimately on a Supreme Being who is sometimes called God.

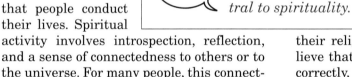

The concept of hope is central to spirituality.

Traditionally, the term *spirituality* has been defined as a sense of meaning in life or associated with a sense of an inner spirit. However, it is difficult to identify what such a spirit is like and how it can be observed. In addition, spirituality can be defined from both religious and secular perspectives. A person with spiritual needs does not necessarily need to participate in religious rituals and practices.

The Religious Perspective

From the religious perspective, Oldnall[14] defines spirituality as encompassing the ideology of the *imago dei* (image of God), or soul, that exists in everyone. The soul makes the person a thinking, feeling, moral, creative being able to relate meaningfully to a Supreme Being and to others. This being or force may be called God, the divine creator and sustainer of the universe, the divine mystery, or other names that convey a profound sense of transcendence and awe. A religious perspective often entails a set of beliefs that help explain the meaning of life, suffering, health, and illness. These beliefs can be crucial to a believer's well-being.

Spirituality is often mistakenly understood to mean just religious practice; however, it should be considered in the broader sense of the term.[15] Religion can be an approach to spirituality, and spirituality is often a component of religion, but the two concepts are different. It is quite possible for the members of a specific religion to be quite limited in their spirituality. Most people have known individuals who dutifully follow the rules of their religious tradition. They strongly believe that if they have adhered to the rules correctly, God will reward them with blessings such as health, success, affluence, social status, and power. For these individuals, adverse events like disease, death of a loved one, or loss of investments can be devastating, because they are perceived as a failure in religious practice or punishments from God. On the other hand, there are many deeply spiritual persons who do not belong to any organized religion but who may be profoundly reflective about the meaning of their life and experiences.

Huston Smith, a scholar of comparative religions at the University of California at Berkeley, has published books and coproduced several public television series with the intent of helping diverse nonacademic audiences appreciate religious traditions other than their own. For Smith,[4] all the world's religions seek to answer the same questions: "Why are we here?", "What does it all mean?", and "What, if anything, are we supposed to be doing with our lives?" Smith proposes that all religions taken together are like a stained glass window that refracts the light in different colors and offers reflections of different shapes. Each of the world's religions is different because it has evolved to respond to unique histories and different cultural developments.

Definitions of religion usually identify a specific system of values and beliefs and a framework for ethical behavior that the members must follow.[8] Religion can be thought of as a social construct that reflects its cultural context and specific philosophical influences. A religion evolves within a specific cultural group, situated in history, and attempts to discern what the group believes are God's commandments as the group has come to understand them.[16,17] Religion, as an institutionally based, organized system of beliefs, represents only one specific means of spiritual expression.[15] Participation in a specific religion generally entails formal education for membership, an initiation ceremony, participation in worship gatherings, adherence to a set of rules of behavior, the participation in prescribed rituals, a particular mode of prayer, and the study of that group's sacred texts. Religious groups vary widely in their tolerance of intragroup diversity of beliefs and behaviors as well as their respect for the belief systems of others. In addition, within a specific religious group there may be a wide range of understanding of what their practices represent.

Occasionally, health-care professionals may encounter individuals whose spiritual practices are highly questionable or discomforting to witness (e.g., worshippers of Satan or those who seek to invoke harm to others through their prayers and rituals).

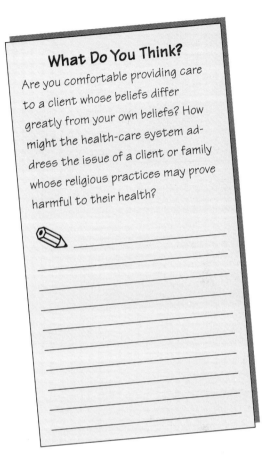

What Do You Think?

Are you comfortable providing care to a client whose beliefs differ greatly from your own beliefs? How might the health-care system address the issue of a client or family whose religious practices may prove harmful to their health?

The Secular Perspective

A secular perspective of spirituality, according to Oldnall,[14] encompasses a set of positive values, such as love, honesty, or truth, chosen by the individual that ultimately become that person's supreme focus of life and organizing framework. These values have the capacity to motivate the individual toward fulfillment of personal needs, goals, and aspirations, leading ultimately to self-actualization.

Manifestation of Spirituality

Both the religious and secular perspectives can exist at the same time in the totality of a person's life. A person's spirituality may

What Do You Think?

How would you define your spirituality—is it religious or secular? Is one form better than the other? Why?

mystical (communal) stage, with its "unseen order of things."

A TRADITION OF SPIRITUALITY IN NURSING

Modern nursing has a rich legacy of the appreciation of spirituality in health and illness. Florence Nightingale's views of nursing practice were based on a spiritual philosophy that she set forth in *Suggestions for Thought*. She was the daughter of Unitarian and Anglican parents,[19] and among her ancestors were famous dissenters against the Church of England. The skepticism fostered by her Unitarian upbringing may have influenced her to question and critique established religious doctrine. Her search for religious truth caused her to become familiar with the writings of Christian mystics (e.g., St. Francis of Assisi, St. John of the Cross) and also with various Eastern mystical writings, including the *Bhagavad-Gita*.

For Nightingale, spirituality involved a sense of a divine intelligence who creates and sustains the cosmos as well as an awareness of her own inner connection with this higher reality.[20] The universe, for Nightingale, was the embodiment of a transcendent God. She came to believe that all aspects of creation are interconnected and share the same inner divinity. She believed that all humans have the capacity to realize and perceive this divinity. Nightingale's God can be described as perfection or as the "essence of benevolence."

Nightingale saw no conflict between science and mysticism. To her, the laws of nature and science were merely "the thoughts of God." Spirituality, for Nightingale, entailed the development of courage, compassion, inner peace, creative insight, and other "God-like" qualities. Based on this belief, Nightingale's convictions commanded her to lifelong service in the care of the sick and helpless. Nightingale endorsed the tra-

be nourished by the ability to give and receive touch, caring, love, and trust. Spirituality may also entail an appreciation of physical experiences such as listening to music, enjoying art or literature, eating delicious food, laughing, venting emotional tension, or participating in sexual expression. Peck[18] has proposed a series of four developmental stages for human spirituality: stage 1, the chaotic (antisocial) stage, with its superficial belier system; stage 2, the formal (institutional) stage, with its adherence to the law; stage 3, the skeptic (individual) stage, with its emphasis on rationality, materialism, and humaneness; and stage 4, the

dition of contemplative prayer, or attunement to the inner presence of God. All phenomena, Nightingale believed, are manifestations of God. A spiritual life entails wise stewardship of all the earth's resources, including human beings. Physical healing was seen by Nightingale as a natural process regulated by natural laws, and as she stated in her *Notes on Nursing,* "What nursing has to do . . . is to put the patient in the best condition for nature to act upon him."[21]

As nursing sought to establish itself as a profession with a legitimate knowledge base, the concern with human spirituality was downplayed and even consciously ignored until the early 1980s. Typically, Oldnall[14] assigns the spiritual domain to the art rather than to the science of nursing, because of its seemingly subjective nature mistakenly equated with aesthetics and intuition. Attention to the spiritual domain in providing holistic care depends on the beliefs and values of both the nurse and the client.

Spirituality and Religion in Nursing Theory

Oldnall[14] analyzed 26 nursing theories and major conceptual frameworks that were developed from the 1960s to the 1980s for content dealing with the spiritual domain. The analysis revealed that, although 14 of them recognized the spiritual domain of health somewhere in their assumptions, only two theories mentioned it directly by name. Rogers' Science of Unitary Human Beings is an example of a profoundly spiritual view of humanity that does not directly name the concept of spirituality. Rogers' framework suggests that there are unbounded human energy fields in interaction with the environmental energy field. Rogers' spiritual definitions can apply as well to the concept of the soul (discussed later). Martha Rogers, who grew up in Tennessee amidst fundamentalist Christians, was loathe to be interpreted in that light; moreover, she had to establish her credibility at New York University during the 1950s, before nursing was accepted as a scientific discipline.

Among the 26 theories analyzed, Neuman,[22] in the later development of her theory, and Watson[23,24] were the only ones who clearly acknowledged the impact of spirituality in the development of their theories. But Watson alone defined and explained the spiritual terminology she used to discuss the spiritual aspect of holistic health.

Watson[23,24] specifically identifies the awareness of the clients' and families' spiritual and religious beliefs as a responsibility of a nurse. She advocates that nurses should appreciate and respect the spiritual meaning in a person's life, no matter how unusual that person's belief system may be. Watson states that nurses have an obligation to identify religious and spiritual influences in their clients' lives at home and to help clients meet their religious requirements in inpatient settings. For example, nurses can facilitate clients' use of measures such as the lighting of candles (real or electric), put flowers and personal objects in the room, ensure privacy, and play music to promote increased comfort and relieve anguish.

Spiritual Crisis

Since 1978, the North American Nursing Diagnosis Association (NANDA) has recognized the nursing diagnosis of spiritual distress.[25] It has most recently been defined as "disruption in the life principle that pervades a person's entire being and integrates and transcends one's biological and psychosocial nature." Defining characteristics of spiritual distress include concerns with the meaning of life and death, anger toward God, concerns about the meaning of suffering, concerns about the person's relationship to God, questions about the meaning of life, the inability to participate in preferred religious practices, seeking spiritual help, concerns about the ethics of prescribed medical regimens, black humor, expressing displaced anger toward clergy, sleep disturbances, and altered mood or behavior. Spiritual distress may occur in relation to separation from religious or cultural supports, challenges to beliefs and values, or intense suffering.

Nurses should be aware that some individuals have been seriously harmed by their religious communities. Examples of harm might include being shunned or excommunicated, being told that they are evil, being forced into a rigidly controlled lifestyle by a cult, or being physically or sexually assaulted by members of the religious community. For these people, illness may be seen as punishment for some sinful action, and they may perceive any offer of spiritual support from the religious community as profoundly threatening. They may believe that God has abandoned them or that the idea of God is foolish or even destructive. Given the rapid turnover of clients in most health systems, there may be little that the nurse can do other than to acknowledge their spiritual pain and accept them, with the assurance that "I am here for you now." If there is more time for contact, the nurse may be able to refer a client or family to appropriate support groups or clergy.

At times clients make health-care decisions that conflict with the beliefs of their religious communities. These often produce high levels of spiritual distress that may affect both the mental and physical well-being of the client. Consider the following case study:

> 66 99 *Spiritual distress may occur in relation to separation from religious or cultural supports, challenges to beliefs and values, or intense suffering.*

When I was a nursing student in the early 1970s, I cared for a woman who was undergoing a therapeutic abortion because of several medical complications of her pregnancy. She had her first child before RhoGAM was available, and she, an Rh-negative mother, had borne an Rh-positive baby. She had only one kidney, and her physicians were concerned that the immunologic complication of carrying a second Rh-positive baby would jeopardize that kidney's function. The decision was difficult for the woman and her husband to make, but they believed the first priority was to care for and raise their 7-year-old son. She needed to protect her kidney so that she could live and participate fully in the child's upbringing.

The night before I cared for this woman, her clergyman came to the hospital and told her that she would go to hell for her decision. Being a devout church member, the woman was extremely distressed the next day. The primary nurse assigned to this woman recognized the spiritual distress caused by the clergyman and requested that a hospital chaplain spend time with her. The chaplain talked and prayed with the woman for several hours. These actions brought great comfort to the woman, who proceeded with the abortion.

Clients often make choices that are difficult for nurses to accept. For instance, based on religious beliefs, clients may refuse commonplace treatments, such as blood transfusions, medications, and even minor surgeries. End-of-life decisions are often based on family members' spiritual beliefs and can be controversial among the health-care personnel who are involved in the decision.

In some acute care settings, regular group sessions are conducted with staff nurses by a chaplain or psychiatrist to assist them in understanding and accepting controversial client decisions.

The Human Energy System and the Soul

Most religious traditions include a concept called "the soul." Religious traditions usually offer explanations of what the soul is, how and when human beings acquire a soul, and what happens to the soul after death. But soul need not be a religious concept. Thomas Moore, a psychotherapist who has written extensively about spiritual development, describes the soul "not as a thing, but a quality or a dimension of experiencing life and ourselves. It has to do with depth, value, relatedness, heart, and personal substance . . . [not necessarily] an object of religious belief or . . . something to do with immortality."[26] Yet Moore observes that the soul must be nurtured, and religious practices can provide that nurturance. For Moore, spirituality is the effort a person makes to identify the soul's world view, values, and sense of relatedness to the whole of the person and of creation. The work of the soul is the quest for understanding or insight about major life questions.

Some people may depict the soul as an image of the person that extends several feet beyond the physical self, or the soul is characterized by color and energetic movement. The soul enters the body at some point during gestation and leaves the body at approximately the moment of death. Reincarnation, or the return of a soul for many earthly lifetimes, is a concept encountered in many religious frameworks, including certain mystical traditions within Judaism and Christianity, although not all denominations ascribe to it.[27] The reason for the soul's return to earthly life is to learn, to develop, and to be purified. Some traditions express this process in terms of earning an improved position in the spiritual world to become closer to God after the final judgment.

The soul would seem to be an exquisitely precise and vast center for communication. Souls have the capacity to communicate with one another, with all living things, and with the divine source of all energy. Their capacity is not limited by the laws of physical matter.[28,29] Some alternative modalities of healing rely on energy movement through the soul. Examples of therapies that capitalize on knowledge of the soul and the movement of a divinely generated en-

Site Seeing

Agency for Health Care Policy and Research (AHCPR)
http://www.ahcpr.gov/ info@ahcpr.gov

American Holistic Nurses' Association
http://ahna.org

Community Health Information Resources
http://chmis.org/
Contact: mail to: baguilar@eskimo.com

Healthtouch Online
http://www.healthtouch.com/

HealthWWWeb
http://www.healthwwweb.com/healthwwweb.html
Contact: mail to: Webmaster@HealthWWWeb.com

National Health Information Center (NHIC)
http://nhic-nt.health.org/
Contact: mail to: NHICinfo@health.org

Office of Alternative Medicine
http://altmed.od.nih.gov/oam

Resources for Nurses and Families
http://pegasus.cc.ucf.edu/~wink/home.html
Contact: Diane Wink, RN
mail to: wink@pegasus.cc.ucf.edu

ergy, life force, or grace (*chi* in Chinese, *ki* in Japanese, or *prana* in Indian traditions) include therapeutic touch, Reiki, and shiatsu. Energy can move in many directions. When a person needs it, energy can be drawn from the divine source of energy into the person; excess energy can be moved from one person to another; and the flow of energy throughout the person's energy field can be balanced to achieve a state of health. Some alternative healing practices that use colors, herbs, aromas, and crystals can be regarded as consistent with a paradigm of repatterning the human energy field or altering the flow of energy throughout the person's body. The circulation of divine energy may be thought of as coming from God and circulating through all living things, the earth, and all the celestial bodies, thus interconnecting all creation.

> **" "** *Some individuals seem to be more aware of the nonphysical or spiritual realms than others.*

Religious traditions of India and other Eastern cultures teach that the human energy system contains seven energy centers, or chakras. These might be considered as the primary openings in the human energy system through which energy flows. Each center has or controls a unique type of energy and spirituality that it allows to enter or leave the body. The root chakra is located at the base of the torso, or the perineum, and its energy has to do with the material world. The crown chakra, the highest level of energy at the top of the head, relates to spirituality.[29]

Examining the religious art of many cultures, over many centuries, artists depict these areas of their subjects' bodies in similar ways. For instance, holy people are depicted with vivid, large, or colorful hearts, and their heads are surrounded by halos. At the very least, the chakras represent a paradigm for ordering the archetypal issues of human life.

Some individuals seem to be more aware of the nonphysical or spiritual realms than others. Many people have had a precognition or déjà vu experience during their lives. However, nurses may have more opportunities to glimpse a different reality than lay people. Nurses have been involved in research on the near-death experience for more than 20 years. Across religious and cultural traditions, and throughout history, a common near-death experience has been documented, but it has been only since the early 1980s that it has gained credence among Western health professionals. Many clients describe the experience of near death as a sensation of floating in the air while visualizing their body lying below on a hospital bed, at the scene of an accident, or where the near death occurred. They often watch healthcare personnel who are working to resuscitate the body. The person then experiences being drawn into a tunnel, perhaps accompanied by other forms or spiritual beings, and moving toward a bright light that emanates great energy or love. They also describe a communication with the light-being, generally identified as God, about whether they are to remain there or return to the earthly body. Obviously, in cases of near death, the decision is made to return. Individuals who have experienced near death often report that they have developed a great inner peace, they no longer fear death, and that their lives have been transformed by what they have experienced.

Nurses who spend much of their time working with clients who are near death, like hospice nurses, are most likely to have witnessed the experience of deathbed visions and gained a glimpse of a different realm of reality. Dying clients who are having a deathbed vision are often aware of multiple realities—the tangible here and

Spiritual Care
Nancy C. Sharts-Hopko

My mother died two weeks after she had a stroke during coronary by-pass surgery. My brother and I implemented her DNR (do not resuscitate) orders the Wednesday before she died on a Monday. During those days of terminal care, although she never had the same nurse two days in a row, we felt well cared for in a spiritual sense.

Some of the things that the staff did included making sure they made us aware that we were not restricted to visiting hours; staying with Mom when we left the room to get something to eat or go to the bathroom; offering to share their food and drinks with us; making sure that we had access to pastoral care— the hospital's or Mom's own; making sure that we had pillows, blankets, and even the other bed in Mom's room for our own use; allowing us as much privacy as we needed; coming in to talk with us; sharing their own stories of the loss of family members; explaining to us where in the physiologic process of dying she was; talking with Mom when they came into the room, both personally and in terms of explaining what they were going to do; handling Mom with great gentleness and respect; allowing us as much time alone with Mom after she died as we wanted; and after she died, calling the undertaker, and explaining clearly what steps we then had to take.

now that family members and caretakers can observe, and "the other side," where they see loved ones who have previously died and are waiting for their arrival. The following personal experience is a good example of this phenomenon:

At the time my maternal grandmother died in 1990 at the age of 98, she had been unable to communicate for many years as a result of a series of strokes. However, one afternoon in the nursing home, where she spent the last 14 years of her life, she rang for a nurse and asked for a glass of water. When the nurse returned 15 minutes later with the water, grandmother said, "Never mind—Frank is here for me." And within a few minutes she was dead. Frank, my grandfather, had died in 1937.

Some medical researchers attribute near death and deathbed experiences to progressive hypoxia in specific brain centers.[30] However, others give the experiences a spiritual interpretation. Could it be that Frank had, indeed, come to meet his wife of many years past? There is a vast amount of literature on angels and spiritual guides emphasizing that people need not feel alone or frightened by future situations or crises. Angels and other spiritual guides are available to comfort them just for the asking.[31]

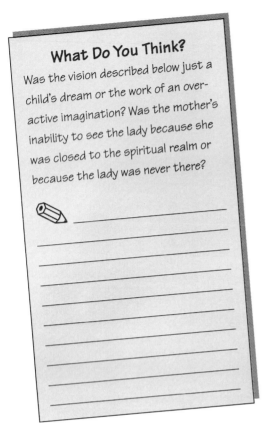

What Do You Think?

Was the vision described below just a child's dream or the work of an over-active imagination? Was the mother's inability to see the lady because she was closed to the spiritual realm or because the lady was never there?

their souls and can apply that knowledge and ability to the physical world, producing changes that science has difficulty explaining and some call miracles. For example, the current-day Hindu holy man in India Sai Baba generates ash that has brought miraculous healing to some people who have touched it. Also, many healing miracles were documented by physicians and scientists during the lifetime of the Italian Franciscan priest Padre Pio before his death in 1968. The common message of mystics from around the world is that people are to live lives of love and compassion for all. The extraordinary love and compassion that most marks the early life of the Dalai Lama, a Buddhist holy man, is depicted in the recent films "Seven Years in Tibet" and "Kundun."

SPIRITUAL PRACTICES IN HEALTH AND ILLNESS

Jung, the Swiss psychoanalytic pioneer of the early twentieth century, was the first to directly propose that all human mental and even physical illnesses are the result of maladjustment between the physical and the spiritual being.[32] Although his father was a Protestant clergyman, Jung was a professed agnostic for most of his life. However, by the end of his life, Jung came to believe in the existence of God.[18] But even before his conversion experience, Jung recognized that the truths contained within the world's religions and in ancient mythology convey knowledge about basic human nature. These truths are embedded in the human biologic being and manifest themselves in the unconscious mind.[33] Modern storyteller-healers, such as the poet Robert Bly,[34] credit Jung with explaining why ancient religious and secular stories survive over the centuries. These stories survive because they continue to resonate at the core of human nature.

Some authorities believe that children are more open to communication from the spiritual world than adults because they have not yet been contaminated with the laws of natural science that are generally accepted by Western society.[31] For example, a young child related the following experience: When she was about 7 years old, she awoke in the middle of the night to find a beautiful lady in a gown of glowing white watching her. She had the experience at least one other time, but her mother, whom she called into the room at the time, was unable to see the lady.

Mystics are believed to be people who have a different relationship to time, space, matter, and energy than most of the population.[29] It seems that they are able to understand the real nature and full capability of

During the last several decades, there has been growing realization that spiritual practices have an important role to play in modern health care. Benson, a Harvard professor of psychiatry, published a ground-breaking book, *The Relaxation Response* in 1975.[35] After reviewing numerous controlled studies of physiologic responses to transcendental meditation and other meditative techniques, Benson outlined a strategy of meditation for use by the general public. In 1975, Benson asserted that this practice required no spiritual underpinnings at all, and meditation on any word, even "potato," would be beneficial. However, 20 years later, Benson[36] was emphatically convinced of the health benefit of spiritual connectedness. He now teaches meditation on a spiritually meaningful word. Following this trend, in the mid-1990s the Harvard University Medical School initiated its conferences on Spirituality and Healing in Medicine.

Two phenomena that have unfolded since the mid-1970s support the trend toward spirituality in health care. First, in the tumultuous managed care environment now characterizing the health industry, clients and consumers increasingly feel that their health needs are not being addressed. More than one-third of American adults are seeking alternative solutions to health and illness problems from various nonmainstream sources, including spiritual practices.[15,37] The second phenomenon is the growth of a body of well-designed and controlled research specifically examining relationships between spiritual practices and health outcomes of both clients and providers of care.[38–40]

In one study, 393 clients admitted to the coronary care unit at San Francisco General Hospital were randomly and blindly assigned to one of two groups.[38] In the first group, 192 clients were assigned anonymously to prayer groups throughout the San Francisco Bay area. The remaining 201

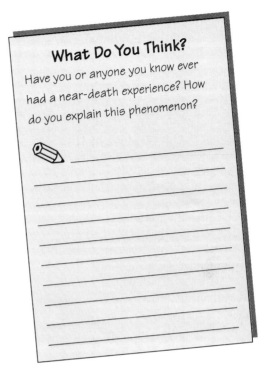

What Do You Think?

Have you or anyone you know ever had a near-death experience? How do you explain this phenomenon?

clients were assigned to a control group where no prayer was involved. Although some of the control group may have been prayed for by their own friends and family, the experimental group received from their assigned prayer groups regular and specific intercessory prayer that requested God's intervention for healing. In all other ways the two groups were similar. The group who received regular intercessory prayer had fewer episodes of cardiac arrest, congestive heart failure, and pneumonia, and they required less ventilatory assistance and fewer antibiotics and diuretics than the control group, who received no prayer interventions.

One of the more dramatic studies was conducted using a sample of 232 open heart surgery clients at Dartmouth-Hitchcock Medical Center. Those clients who indicated that they had social support were one-third as likely to die as those who did not. Those who indicated that they had religious faith were one-third as likely to die as those who

14.2 American Holistic Nurses' Association

The American Holistic Nurses' Association was founded in 1980 by a group of nurses dedicated to bringing the concepts of holism to every arena of nursing practice. They define holism as wellness, that state of harmony between body, mind, emotions, and spirit in an ever-changing environment.

AHNA offers certification in holistic nursing and has endorsed programs in Amma Therapy, Interactive Imagery, and Healing Touch.

Visit the AHNA web site at: http://ahna.org.

14.3 Parish (Congregational) Nursing

Parish (congregational) Nursing is a movement of the last decade in which churches, synagogues, mosques, and other faith communities designate nurses to serve their membership. Parish nursing is viewed as a healing ministry, and parish nurses are attuned to spiritual issues raised by health transitions, as well as the healing nature of spiritual practice. They may function to assist people to remain in their own homes, they may connect them with other health services for which they are eligible, they may provide needed health teaching and support, and at times their role is to simply be present with them.

The Lutheran General Health System established the International Parish Nurse Resource Center in 1986, in Park Ridge, Illinois. They can be contacted at 1-800-556-5368, or on the World Wide Web at www.advocatehealth.com/sites/pnursctr.html.

did not. And those who had both social support and religious faith were one-ninth as likely to die as those who had neither.[41]

In another study, 203 family practice clients were interviewed regarding their views on the relationship between religion and health. They were very positive about their family practice physicians' involvement in spiritual issues; more than one-third of the group wanted their family practice providers to discuss religious issues related to their health with them more frequently, and half of the group wanted their physicians to pray with them. However, two-thirds of the group reported that their family practice physician had never discussed religious beliefs with them.[42]

Family practice physicians have, since the late 1980s, become more open to exploring the spiritual domain of health with their clients. In a 1989 study of 160 family practice physicians, most acknowledged the beneficial relationships among religious practice and both mental and physical health. Many

thought that they should discuss these matters with their clients, and two-thirds of the physicians thought that prayer with their clients was appropriate at times. Yet only one-third of the group had prayed with clients. Praying with clients was more prevalent among younger physicians.[43] When a 1996 Yankelovich survey re-examined this issue among board-certified physicians in family medicine, 79% of that group agreed that prayer can actually effect healing—a substantial increase from previous surveys. There are a number of organizations and agencies that encourage the incorporation of spiritual practices into health care (Boxes 14.2 to 14.5).

Prayer

According to a recent *Newsweek* survey, most Americans pray. Thoughts in general, and prayers in particular, should be regarded as powerful forces, and people need to learn how to direct and use them for positive ends. Individuals with a spiritual orientation have known for a long time that positive thoughts and affirmations influence events for the better, whereas negative thoughts and curses can bring about adversity. Thoughts and prayers should be viewed as exchanges of energy with creation. Prayer is sometimes defined as "communicating with God," or speaking with some type of divine entity.[18] It is believed that all prayers are "heard" because they reverberate in the open system of the spiritual realm.

Dossey, a physician who spent many years studying the impact of prayer on health, observes that some prayers may "backfire" because human wisdom is limited and it is impossible to know all the complexities of a given situation nor what the long-term outcomes may be.[44] Merely praying that a loved one may live does not address quality of life issues. Although the loved one may still be alive, he or she may be in great pain or exist in a vegetative state requiring complete and expensive care. As a physician, Dossey recommends prayers of protection from the ill will or the mistaken, if well-intentioned, assistance of others. Examples of protective prayer include the Lord's Prayer, the Prayer for Peace attributed to St. Francis, and the ancient Irish Prayer of St. Patrick's Breastplate. Rather than seeking a specific outcome to a problem, protective prayers ask for a protective shield of light and love in the time of need or simply that God's will be done.

Once a person believes that prayer can be an effective force in altering the world, he or she must then decide on what type of prayer is most effective. There are many and varying opinions about praying and types of prayer. Dossey and Peck recommend a few simple principles. First, Dossey recommends praying with humility. Truly spiritual people are often characterized by hu-

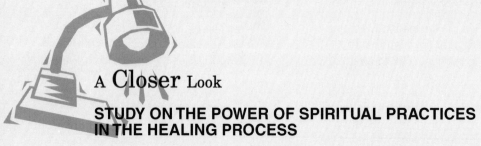

A Closer Look

STUDY ON THE POWER OF SPIRITUAL PRACTICES IN THE HEALING PROCESS

The John Templeton Foundation supports research that brings together science and religion, and medicine and religion in particular.

In December 1997, Beth Israel Deaconess Medical Center and Harvard Medical School released the results of a study that found that 94% of health maintenance organization (HMO) executives believe that personal prayer, meditation, or other spiritual practices aid medical treatment and accelerate the healing process.

In addition, 74% of HMO professionals believe that spiritual practices can reduce health-care costs. Two-thirds of the 300 executives indicated that they are interested in seeing evidence of the clinical effectiveness of spiritual practices for healing and wellness.

Visit the John Templeton Foundation website at www.templeton.org.

---

mility.[18] Prayers that express love and support or that seek forgiveness of self and others are powerful messages to their recipients. Consider the following case as an example of this principle:

A man in the renal intensive care unit (ICU) at a large medical center many years ago was being cared for by a graduate nurse. He had experienced renal failure of unknown etiology. At that time, because of the primitive nature of dialysis and the very limited facilities, if a person did not regain renal function within 30 days, a committee would determine whether treatment should be continued or stopped. If it was stopped, obviously the person would die. Because this man was in his 60s and had seemingly already lived most of his life, he was not considered a priority case for dialysis. He owned a thriving hardware store in a small town in Indiana where he was also the mayor. He was not known to be particularly religious, but after several weeks in the ICU, he began to ask that the Bible be read to him by the night shift nurses before he went to sleep. He also began to pray for the first time in many years. One night he talked with the graduate nurse about his realization that he had lived his life focused primarily on his work, rather than on the people he loved—his wife and his children. In his work he was a success, but in his relationships, he saw failure. He explained to the nurse that he told God that night that if he were allowed to recover, he would change the way that he lived his life. Near the end of the 30-day trial period, for no reason that the doctors could determine, he began to produce urine. Eventually, he recovered full urinary function and was able to leave the ICU to go home. This man's prayers of repentance and for forgiveness seemed to have been answered.

Another interpretation for what was experienced by the man with renal failure is that disease, illness, or injury brings a message or a lesson to persons experiencing them that change their lives in some manner.[45] This interpretation is based on the belief that all elements of creation are embued with consciousness, and that pathogenesis, illness, or disease is but one manifestation of this consciousness. Contemplative, or meditative, prayer is a means by which people can become more sensitive to their internal environment so they can learn what the illness has to teach.

A belief in a universal consciousness is sometimes considered to be the underlying process causing psychosomatic illnesses. It is possible that healing and cure may be produced by therapeutic interventions at a subconscious level, even without the person's recognition or understanding of the message. Like the man with renal failure, however, the person may still need the illness and its message to become open to the healing process. When the person opens up to the message of the illness and understands why it happened, that message can then be absorbed into the whole of the person's life so that the illness is free to leave on its own. Although the recovery may seem to be most mysterious, in reality it is a result of a well-sequenced process.

Meditation and Healing

After 20 years of studying the relaxation response and prayer in relation to many ill-

 It is possible that healing and cure may be produced by therapeutic interventions at a subconscious level, even without the person's recognition or understanding of the message.

nesses, Herbert Benson, like all true scientists, sought to understand the phenomenon that he had observed and measured. He regarded the ability of people to participate in their own healing through prayer or meditation as the use of a source of healing power that he named "remembered wellness,"[36] sometimes called by others "the placebo effect." Benson believed that all people have the capacity to "remember" the calm and confidence associated with emotional and physical health and happiness. Benson saw the benefit of remembered wellness as a source of energy to be tapped into and used for healing, not something to regard suspiciously. However, the effectiveness of remembered wellness depends on the individual's belief system.

Benson also observed that everyone involved in providing health care is in a position to make use of this energy as part of the healing process. One thing that health-care providers can do to promote healing is to speak positively of treatments and medications being used. For example, positive reinforcement occurs when the nurse refers to the clients' medication as the "drug your doctor prescribed to help your heart" or the food tray as "nutrition to help your body fight your infection." Benson notes that remembered wellness depends on three components: belief and expectation of the client, belief and expectation of the caregiver, and belief and expectation generated by a caring relationship between the client and the caregiver. A warm and trusting relationship seems to enhance the effectiveness of the care that is provided.

In contrast, Benson describes the "nocebo effect" as the fulfillment of an expectation of harm. It is also an effect that health professionals can cause. Examples of the nocebo ef-

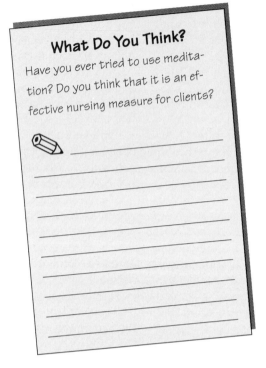

What Do You Think?

Have you ever tried to use meditation? Do you think that it is an effective nursing measure for clients?

fect include advising clients that a medicine will probably make them sick, telling them that chemotherapy will drain their energy and cause their hair to fall out, or informing them that a certain percentage of people die from a given procedure. Such warnings, Benson has documented in a significant percentage of cases, can actually bring about the warned against complications.

The relaxation response, which Benson has studied and taught widely, entails 20 minutes, twice each day, of quiet meditation on a word or image that is spiritually meaningful to the person. When an intrusive thought enters the person's consciousness, the person should lightly dismiss it, as if gently blowing a feather away, and return to the meditation word or image. Over the years of teaching this practice, Benson has demonstrated dramatic results through double-blind controlled studies of people who use the relaxation response. Over time, these individuals have demonstrated lowered blood pressure, decreased incidents of

dysmenorrhea, reduction in chronic pain, and improvement in a number of illnesses.

Siegel, a general and pediatric surgeon and professor at the Yale University School of Medicine, has also successfully used relaxation, meditation, visualization, and hypnosis with hundreds of seriously ill clients, including many with cancer. Meditation as described by Siegel is a technique of listening. However, listening is not a passive process. Rather, it is a way of focusing the mind in a state of relaxed awareness to pay attention to deeper thoughts and feelings, to the products of the unconscious mind, to the peace of pure consciousness, and to deeper spiritual awareness.[46] Some teachers of meditation suggest that the person select a spiritually symbolic word (e.g., God, love, beauty, peace, Mary, Jesus) on which to focus, whereas others suggest watching a candle flame. Still others teach practitioners to focus on their breathing. All these methods are intended to bring the person to a deeply restful state that frees the mind from its usual chatter. This is the experience of being centered. People may experience spiritual insights, but more often they experience a gradual enhancement of well-being.

Visualization is the practice of meditating with an image of a desired outcome or the process of attaining it. It is preferable that the image be selected by the person rather than someone else. For example, a person with a tumor might visualize miniature miners mining the unhealthy tissue and carting it away. Hypnosis is a process of suggesting an image of a desired reality to someone. Both of these techniques have been demonstrated to stimulate the immune system. Siegel has also observed that some seriously ill people believe that they deserve their illness as a punishment for something they did in the past. Helping them forgive themselves often brings about dramatic improvements in their conditions. Releasing fear and hate has a similar effect.

This process reflects back to Nightingale's belief that nurses need to help clients get out of the way of their own healing.

It might seem logical to conclude that clients who do not recover from illness, or who die, have failed to help themselves or did not adequately use their spiritual powers. However, that is not the case. Spiritual modes of healing do not always lead to cure. Spiritual healing takes a much broader view and includes enhanced comfort and an inner peace with disability or death.

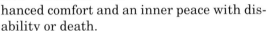

> **❝ ❞** *The practitioner of TT first centers and then assesses the state of the recipient's energy field, noting energy levels and movement around the chakras.*

Therapeutic Touch

Therapeutic touch (TT) is an active alternative healing modality that involves redirecting the human energy system. During the last 25 years, Krieger, who was a professor of nursing at New York University, along with Kuntz have retrieved TT from ancient traditions, studied it, and refined it. They also discovered that TT was consistent with the Science of Unitary Human Beings developed by Martha Rogers. The Science of Unitary Human Beings defines persons as energy fields in interaction with the larger environmental energy field. The energy fields are characterized by patterns of waves. One way of altering the wave patterns of the human energy field is to use TT to move energy into and through it in deliberate ways. According to Krieger, the practitioner of TT acts with the intent of relaxing the recipient, reducing pain and discomfort, and accelerating healing when appropriate.[47] Krieger's earliest controlled study[48] of the effects of TT showed that the hemoglobin levels of a group of clients who received TT increased significantly more than the levels in a control group who did not receive TT.

The TT practitioner should approach the client with compassion and the intent to heal, and the recipient of care ideally approaches the healing encounter with receptivity and openness to change. The practitioner of TT first centers and then assesses the state of the recipient's energy field, noting energy levels and movement around the chakras. Cues may be determined through physical sensations in the practitioner's hands, direct visualization, inner awareness, or other intuitive modes of insight.[49] After assessing the recipient, the TT practitioner, working from the center of the client's energy field to the periphery, directs energy from the environment into the client's field as needed, stimulates energy flow through the client's field, clears congested areas in the energy field, dampens excess energetic activity, and synchronizes the rhythmic waves of the energy flow depending on the client's needs. The practitioner is not diverting his or her own energy into the client because it would be detrimental to the practitioner. Rather, the TT practitioner redirects the client's energy field or directs energy from the environment outside the client.

NURSING PRACTICE AND SPIRITUAL WELLNESS

Although the nursing profession is deeply rooted in religious traditions, modern nursing has spent considerable energy attempting to distance itself from this aspect of its history. Nursing as vocation has given way to nursing as profession. The current healthcare system has required nurses to shift their identity from vocation to profession in order to achieve appropriate value in a system that is increasingly economically oriented.

Yet nursing is much more than the mere secular enterprise the modern world perceives it to be. Perhaps it is time that nurses re-evaluate the work they do and consider it a vocation, that is, a life calling in the spiritual sense of that word. The world's religions consistently allude to the symbolic and deep meaning of the work that nurses do. Nursing practice has the capacity to be richly imaginative and to speak to the soul on many levels. Nursing practice can be carried out mindfully and artistically, or it can be done routinely and unconsciously, like any other job. When nursing is practiced with deep consciousness and purpose, it nurtures the nurse as well as the client.

Some experts perceive that nursing is directly connected to the nurse's fantasy life, family myths, ideals, and traditions. The profession of nursing may be one way that nurses sort out their major life issues. Although the choice of nursing as a career may seem to have been serendipitous, in the spiritual context, it is reasonable to question whether anything really happens by accident. Moore[26] speaks of work as opus, or those undertakings that are central to the soul's lifetime work of self-definition and self-identification. As nurses practice nursing, they craft themselves.

As with most professions, at times it may become difficult, even impossible perhaps, to feel good about the work that is being done. Negative attitudes about work are detrimental to a person's self-development and tend to cause people to become overly invested in the surface trappings of work, such as money, power, and success. The phenomenon of burnout among nurses has been identified and studied for many years (see Chapter 10). Burnout can be viewed from a spiritual perspective, in which the well runs dry, energy fields become imbalanced, or the person experiences a prolonged "dark night of the soul," or even a finding that the nurse's life work is devoid of meaning.

People working in the helping professions, whose work is rooted in compassion and concern for others, are prone to depression and burnout.[26] A concerted effort at spiritual development, or the nourishment of the soul, is essential to nurses' overall mental and physical well-being. Consider the following personal exchange:

A nursing faculty colleague who is a psychotherapist recently confided in me that her burnout is caused precisely because she strives to live as Jesus would live in the same circumstances. I reminded her that Jesus also rested, partied enthusiastically with friends, and went on 40-day retreats when he needed to do so. I suggested to her that in her attempt to "live like Jesus," she might also consider caring for herself the way Jesus cared for himself.

In the attempt to maintain an internal state of balance, the first thing that nurses need to do is to take time to feed their spirit. Daily prayer or meditation is an important source of both insight and energy. Belonging to a group or community that actively pursues spiritual growth is also a powerful source of spiritual nourishment. Many individuals find that their spirit is nourished within the setting of a formal religion, although not necessarily the one in which they were reared. It is not uncommon for people to seek a faith community in midlife or later life, perhaps after being away from one for many years. The experience of trying vari-

> **❝ ❞** *Although the choice of nursing as a career may seem to have been serendipitous, in the spiritual context, it is reasonable to question whether anything really happens by accident.*

ous religions and modes of worship is, all by itself, a broadening, nurturing experience.

Periodic retreat from the hustle and bustle of modern living can be highly restorative of the spirit. A retreat may be for a few hours, a half-day, a weekend, a week, or longer. For some people, keeping a journal regularly is a retreat-like experience. For others, it may be a stroll through a beautiful park, a few hours watching waves on a beach, or a trip to the woods. Retreat is most effective when time is consistently set aside for introspection and reflection rather than for tasks.

A sense of sacredness can infuse everyday life with meaning and zest if nurses would only open themselves to it. It is a part of normal human activity to celebrate seasonal and family holidays with specific rituals, music, decorations, group gatherings, and foods. These types of activities honor life cycles that are greater than the individual and nurture important relationships that serve as a **support system.**

Many people have routines for their weekends or days off that allow time for self-restoration. These special activities may include a large country breakfast while listening to favorite music; baking cookies, bread, or a pie; sitting for an extended period of time in a favorite easy chair; or even playing a physically demanding sport like basketball. Many people have favorite coffee mugs or dishes or special objects in their homes that are not only beautiful but may remind them of loved ones, wonderful trips, religious experiences, or other events that nourish them each time they view the object. One of the most spiritual aspects of a person's life is the enjoyment of beauty. It costs little or nothing to plant or cut flowers or listen to music. It is in these moments that a person's creativity and insight are most evident.

The hectic modern world continually urges people to enhance their capacity for dealing with multiple concerns at the same

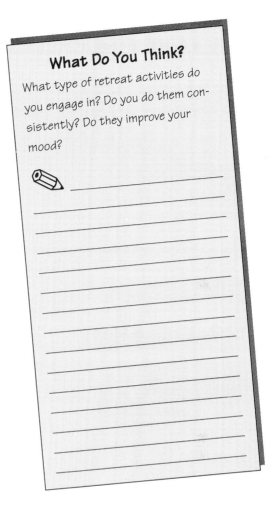

What Do You Think?

What type of retreat activities do you engage in? Do you do them consistently? Do they improve your mood?

time. Some people even define success by looking at how many balls they can juggle simultaneously. *Multitasking* is the new buzzword for the health-care environment of the twenty-first century. Nurses must be able to talk on the telephone, send faxes and e-mail, surf the net, and use a word processor for entering client data at the same time that they are developing care plans, evaluating clients, answering call lights, supervising unlicensed assistive personnel, and providing physicians with information. Although this is highly productive, the more nurses multitask, the more disconnected they become from themselves. Multitasking can be thought of as the antithesis of spiritual nurturance. Spirituality is about personal wholeness, whereas multitasking is about fragmentation. Only when nurses begin to slow down and start centering their energy fields will they have the capacity to be fully present and be able to attend with complete consciousness to their loved ones, colleagues, and clients and focus completely on the present moment.

Conclusion

Spiritual development is not merely a task to be accomplished and checked off like an item on a checklist for personal improvement. Rather, spirituality is a way of life that involves a profound respect for self and for others and true living of the Golden Rule. Once individuals realize their self-goodness and the goodness of all creation, they have no choice but to live a spiritual life. Their ability to see their lives as abundantly blessed begets more goodness. Over time, they will feel more sustained, and the change will be recognized by the people for whom they are providing care. Spiritual development is a synergistic process. Some people may wonder whether there is a personal cost to spiritual development. Spiritual development does not cost the person anything, but it requires a shifting of priorities. What is regarded as abundant living may shift from a material focus to a focus on health, love, beauty, and a joy in life. It is never too late to begin to live in this way—but neither is it ever too soon.

Name _____

Course _____

Instructor _____

Date _____

Critical Thinking Exercises

Mrs. Jan Steiner, 73 years old, has outlived two husbands. Ted, her second husband, died 20 years ago. Reared in the Roman Catholic faith, Mrs. Steiner converted to Judaism when she married Ted. Her two daughters by her first husband were also reared in the Roman Catholic tradition, one of whom, Kathy, continues to practice her religion. The other daughter, Judith, is Unitarian.

Mrs. Steiner experienced a stroke 2 years ago that left her moderately disabled. At that time she moved into a long-term care facility. Still, she was able to read and to enjoy visits with friends and family. But a second stroke 3 months ago left her incontinent and aphasic.

Mrs. Steiner has just had a major heart attack. Although bypass surgery could extend her life, she has never articulated any end-of-life desires. Her daughters are in conflict over how Mrs. Steiner's medical management should proceed. Kathy strongly believes that as long as Mrs. Steiner is alive, life should be actively supported. It would be morally wrong to do less than that. Judith, on the other hand, believes that what had been the "life" of Mrs. Steiner is essentially over and it is a waste of resources to merely delay the inevitable. The nursing staff, as they attempt to facilitate communication between the family and the medical staff, feel caught in the middle.

✔ What are your own spiritual beliefs about the proper approach to Mrs. Steiner's medical management?

✔ Analyze the positions of Kathy and Judith from both their ethical and spiritual context.

✔ What resources are likely to be available in the hospital or the community to help the daughters come to a decision?

Bypass surgery is not performed, and Mrs. Steiner returns to her long-term care facility. Her overall condition continues to deteriorate, and within 3 months she is very near death. She seems to have little awareness of her surroundings and she does not consistently recognize or respond to her daughters.

✔ Knowing the religious divergence within Mrs. Steiner's family, how might the nursing staff facilitate their preparation for the death of their mother and her funeral?

✔ What would happen within Mrs. Steiner's circle of family and friends if any "side"—Catholic, Jewish, or Unitarian—"won" in planning her end-of-life care?

✔ Have you seen blending of religious traditions in rituals such a marriage or burial? What are the advantages and disadvantages of such an approach?

✔ What might be the outcomes of handling their mother's death in a strictly secular or nonsectarian way and allowing all relatives and friends to mourn privately in accordance with their own spiritual traditions?

References

1. Belenky, M, et al: Women's Ways of Knowing. Basic Books, New York, 1986.
2. Benner, PE: From Novice to Expert: Excellence and Power in Clinical Nursing Practice. Addison Wesley Longman, Reading, Mass., 1984.
3. Coles, R: The Spiritual Life of Children. Houghton Mifflin, Boston, 1990.
4. Smith, H: The Illustrated World's Religions: A Guide to Our Wisdom Traditions. HarperCollins, New York, 1994.
5. Greeley, DL: Christians and the global experience of prayer. In Eigo, FA (ed): Prayer: The Global Experience. Villanova University Press, Villanova, Pa., 1997.
6. Butler, C: Western Mysticism: The Teaching of SS Augustine, Gregory and Bernard on Contemplation and the Contemplative Life, ed 2. Constable, London, 1926.
7. Hadot, P: Philosophy as a Way of Life: Spiritual Exercises from Socrates to Foucault. (Davidson, A, ed; Chase, A, trans). Blackwell, Boston, 1995.
8. Goddard, NC: "Spirituality as integrative energy": A philosophical analysis as requisite precursor to holistic nursing practice. J Adv Nurs 22:808–815, 1995.
9. Post-White, J, et al: Hope, spirituality, sense of coherence, and quality of life in patients with cancer. Oncol Nurs Forum 23(10): 1571–1579, 1996.
10. Burkhardt, M, and Nagai-Jacobson, M: Reawakening spirit in clinical practice. Journal of Holistic Nursing 12(1):9–21, 1994.
11. Howden, JW: Development and psychometric characteristics of the Spirituality Assessment Scale. Unpublished dissertation, Texas Women's University. Abstract accessed on Medline, 1992.
12. Learn, CD: Crafting the quilt: A phenomenology of older women's experience of spirituality. Unpublished dissertation. University of Colorado Health Sciences Center. Denver, CO, 1993.
13. Long, A: Nursing: A spiritual perspective. Nursing Ethics: An International Journal for Health Care Professionals 4(6):496–510, 1997.
14. Oldnall, A: A critical analysis of nursing: Meeting the spiritual needs of patients. J Adv Nurs 23:138–144, 1996.
15. Eisenberg, D, et al: Religion and spirituality defined according to current use in nursing literature. J Prof Nurs 8(1):41–47, 1992.
16. Frank, G, et al: Jewish spirituality through actions in time: Daily occupations of young Orthodox Jewish couples in Los Angeles. Am J Occup Ther 51(3):199–206, 1997.
17. Sevensky, RL: Religion and illness: An outline of their relationship. South Med J 74(6):745–750, 1981.
18. Peck, MS: The Road Less Traveled and Beyond. Touchstone, New York, 1997.
19. Widerquist, JG: The spirituality of Florence Nightingale. Nurs Res 41(1):49–55, 1992.
20. Macrae, J: Nightingale's spiritual philosophy and its significance for modern nursing. Image J Nurs Sch 27(1):8–10, 1995.
21. Nightingale, F: Notes on Nursing. Dover, New York, 1969. (Originally published, 1860)
22. Neuman, B: The Neuman Systems Model: Application, Nursing Education and Practice. Appleton Century Crofts, Norwalk, Conn., 1989.
23. Watson, J: Nursing: The Philosophy and Science of Caring. Colorado Associated University Press, Boulder, Colo., 1985.
24. Watson, J: Nursing: Human Science and Human Theory of Care. Theory of Nursing. National League for Nursing, New York, 1988.
25. North American Nursing Diagnosis Association: Nursing Diagnosis: Definitions and Classification, 1997–1998. NANDA, Philadelphia, 1998.
26. Moore, T: Care of the Soul. HarperCollins, New York, 1992.
27. Cooper, D: God is a Verb: Kabbalah and the Practice of Mystical Judaism. Putnam, East Rutherford, N.J., 1997.
28. Kunz, D (ed): Spiritual Healing. Quest Books, Wheaton, Ill., 1995.
29. Myss, C: Anatomy of the Spirit. Harmony Books, New York, 1996.
30. Houran, J, and Lange, R: Hallucinations that comfort: Contextual mediation of deathbed visions. Perceptual Motor Skills 84(3), pt 2):1491–1504, 1997.
31. Burnham, S: A Book of Angels. Ballantine, New York, 1990.
32. Bendit, LJ: The spirit in health and disease. In Kunz, D (ed): Spiritual Healing. Quest Books, Wheaton, Ill., 1995, pp 92–100.
33. Jung, CG: Man and His Symbols. Dell, New York, 1962.
34. Bly, R: Iron John. Addison-Wesley, Reading, Mass., 1990.
35. Benson, H: The Relaxation Response. William Morrow, New York, 1975.

36. Benson, H: Timeless Healing. Fireside, New York, 1997.
37. Spiegelblatt, L, et al: The use of alternative medicine by children. Pediatrics 94(6): 811–814, 1994.
38. Byrd, RC: Positive therapeutic effects of intercessory prayer in a coronary care unit population. South Med J 81(7):826–829, 1988.
39. Kass, J, et al: Health outcomes and a new index of spiritual experience. Journal for the Scientific Study of Religion 30:203–211, 1991.
40. Tsai, SL: Effects of relaxation training, comforting imagery and meditation on the stress levels of Chinese nurses working in modern hospitals in Taiwan. Issues in Mental Health Nursing 14(1):51–66, 1993.
41. Oxman, T, Freeman, D, and Manheimer, ED: Lack of social participation or religious strength and comfort as risk factors for death after cardiac surgery in the elderly. Psychosom Med 57:5–15, 1995.
42. King, D, and Bushwick, B: Beliefs and attitudes of hospital inpatients about faith healing and prayer. Journal of Family Practice 39(4):349–352, 1994.
43. Koenig, H, L, Bearon, and Dayringer, R: Physician perspectives on the role of religion in the physician-older patient relationship. J Fam Pract 28(4):441–448, 1989.
44. Dossey, L: Be Careful What You Pray For . . . You Just Might Get It. HarperSanFrancisco, New York, 1997.
45. Progoff, I: Finding the message of illness. In Kunz, D (ed): Spiritual Healing. Quest Books, Wheaton, Ill., 1995, pp 197–209.
46. Siegel, BS: Love, Medicine and Miracles. Harper & Row, New York, 1986.
47. Krieger, D: Accepting Your Power to Heal. Bear, Santa Fe, N.M., 1995.
48. Krieger, D: Therapeutic touch: The imprimatur of nursing. Am J Nurs 79:784–787, 1979.
49. Macrae, J: Therapeutic Touch: A Practical Guide. Alfred A. Knopf, New York, 1996.

BIBLIOGRAPHY

Calkins, D, and Delbanco, T: Unconventional medicine in the United States: Prevalence, costs, and patterns of use. N Engl J Med 328:246–252, 1993.

Donahue, MP: Nursing the Finest Art: An Illustrated History, ed 2. Mosby, St. Louis, 1996.

Lelis-Grice, D: Loving, human touch helps family cope with loss. AACN News 15(9):4–6, 1998.

Loscalzo, F: The essence of nursing is touching another soul. AACN News 15(10):3, 1998.

Troussman, S: The human connection: Nurses and their patients. American Nurse 30(5):1–8, 1998.

Wilson, J: Healing and curing. Oklahoma Nurse 43(1):4–5, 1998.

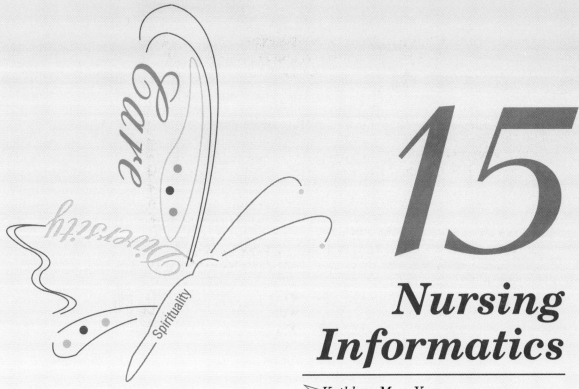

15

Nursing Informatics

➤*Kathleen Mary Young*

Learning Objectives

After completing this chapter, the reader will be able to:

1. Discuss the impact of the information revolution on society in general and on health care specifically.
2. Define nursing informatics.
3. Explain the importance of nursing informatics to nursing practice.
4. Analyze the availability of resources and references in the practice site.
5. Evaluate the importance of human factors engineering on equipment design.
6. Compare the electronic health record to the paper record system.
7. Analyze the ethical issues concerning data ownership.

A worldwide information revolution is exploding the systems of modern culture. Although no one can predict the full effect of the current information revolution, it is easy to see the changes that it creates in our daily lives. The information revolution changes both the way that teachers teach and the way that learners learn. Teaching in the public school, and even in colleges, now demands fast-moving, entertaining lessons that capture the student's attention, because the classroom teachers must compete with television and the computer games with which this generation has been raised. School children and college students no longer read whole books. Technology has accustomed them to 30-second "sound bites" of information. Libraries are evolving from repositories of hardbound volumes and journals to providers of Internet access to on-line journals and books.

TECHNOLOGY AND COMMUNICATION

The information revolution has changed both the form and the format of communication. Before the advent of the telephone, people communicated through the written word. Letter writing was an art. Before television and the computer were invented, people gathered together in neighborhoods and developed a sense of community. Today the whole world is the community, and every corner can be reached from a home computer. Senior citizens in Blacksburg, Virginia, use their computers not only to chat but also to organize get-togethers. "It's like wandering into the town center to meet friends and to check the bulletin board," says Dennis Gentry, a retired Army officer. "Only you can do it in pajamas anytime you want."[1]

The award of the Nobel Prize in economics in 1996 illustrates the increasing role of information in today's society. Two microeconomic theorists won the prize for explaining how the lack of information helps to shape modern business decisions. The theorists study an area of economics called asymmetric information. According to an Associated Press report in the fall of 1996, "asymmetric information refers to when both sides do not have the same facts. The buyer of a house or a used car, for example, is unlikely to have all the information that the seller has. Without the same facts, the seller has an advantage over the buyer, who must spend additional time and money to learn more." The fact that the person with more information has an advantage seems like common sense, but a grasp of the impact of asymmetric information will lead to a better understanding of day-to-day economic activity.

Not only does technology change the way in which people communicate and work, but it also creates a new decision-making process that affects all aspects of industry and commerce. Informed decisions produce better outcomes. Competition has become a driving force in the pricing and marketing of health care. Payment methods that promote competition are encouraged by Medicare and Medicaid **prospective payment systems** (**PPSs**), health maintenance organizations (HMOs), **preferred provider organizations** (**PPOs**), and managed care. To offer a competitive and quality organization, information must be available to make decisions. More information is available to decision makers with information technology.

The application of the increased information available through technology to decision making in health care gives technologically driven organizations a competitive edge. A leadership survey conducted by _Hospitals and Health Networks_[2] reveals that the addition of information technology is either number one or number two among the high-priority goals listed by hospitals, managed care organizations, and group practices. To stay competitive in national and international health care, the health-care delivery system, and specifically nursing, must open itself to new information and ideas.

The health-care information revolution is progressing at the speed of light. Computers will be involved in almost every area of client care; the assessment of the quality of care; and the enhancement of decision-making, management, planning, and medical research.[3]

DEFINITION OF INFORMATICS

Two definitions of informatics are used in the health-care field. The term *medical informatics* was coined in the mid-1970s. Borrowed from the French expression *informatique medicale,* it described "those collected informational technologies which concern themselves with the client care, medical, decision-making process."[4] Mandil[5] uses the term *health informatics,* which is defined as the use of information technology with information management concepts and methods to support the delivery of health care. Mandil's definition encompasses medical, nursing, dental, and pharmacy informatics as well as all other health-care disciplines. The definition for health informatics focuses attention on the recipient of care rather than on the discipline of the caregiver.

The nursing community, however, is developing a discipline of informatics that is specific to the delivery of nursing care and is based on the science of nursing. Nursing has distinct and discrete information needs. The "data, information and knowledge of nursing are symbolic representations of phenomena of peculiar interest to nursing. The structure of this nursing information is substantively different from that of other disciplines. These information structures pose discipline-specific problems for the management and processing of nursing information."[6]

In 1989, Graves and Corcoran suggested a model for nursing informatics. In this model, nursing informatics is identified as "a combination of computer science, information science, and nursing science designed to assist in the management and processing of nursing data, information and knowledge to support the practice of nursing and the delivery of nursing care."[6]

Computer science refers primarily to the configuration and architecture of the computer system. Information science refers to the computer software, including how data or tasks are processed, how problems are solved, and where products are produced. Nursing science refers to the practice of nursing.[7] Turley[8] added a fourth element, cognitive science, to the model for nursing informatics. He defined cognitive science as an interdisciplinary field that results from the convergence of psychology, linguistics, computer science, philosophy, and neuroscience. It is concerned with perception, thinking, understanding, and remembering. Turley's model unites information science, computer science, and cognitive science into a framework of nursing science.

Data, Information, and Knowledge

When Graves and Corcoran developed their classic definition of nursing informatics, they defined *data* as raw and unstructured facts. The numbers 102 and 104 are raw data. By

> " " To stay competitive in national and international health care, the health-care delivery system, and specifically nursing, must open itself to new information and ideas.

themselves, these numbers have little meaning because they lack interpretation.

Information consists of data that have been given form and have been interpreted. If the number 102 is given additional data so that it becomes a 102-degree oral temperature of a 25-year-old man taken at 9 A.M., it becomes information that has meaning.

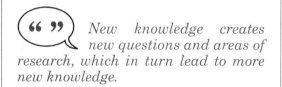
New knowledge creates new questions and areas of research, which in turn lead to more new knowledge.

Knowledge takes the process one step further, because it is a synthesis of data and information. Combining the information that an oral temperature of 102 degrees is higher than normal for a 25-year-old man with an understanding of human physiology and pharmacology provides the practitioner with the knowledge that enables him or her to make a decision concerning a course of treatment. This process is the basis for critical thinking and decision making and can also be used in research to create new knowledge.

The Graves and Corcoran model of "data to information to knowledge" is linear, but the process of synthesizing data into information to create knowledge is actually circular. New knowledge creates new questions and areas of research, which in turn lead to more new knowledge. To answer the research questions, new data are required that must be processed into information to create more knowledge. The goal of this process is to provide the most accurate and current information so that nurses can make informed decisions in their daily practice.

Areas of Focus in Informatics

Turley[8] suggests that the specialty of nursing informatics has evolved through three levels of special interest: technology, concepts of nursing theory, and function.

Early in the evolution, definitions of nursing informatics focused strictly on the use of technology. For example, in 1985 Hannah[9] defined nursing informatics as "any use of information technology by nurses in relation to the care of patients or the educational preparation of individuals to practice in the discipline is considered nursing informatics." Similarly, Saba and McCormick[7] continued to define nursing informatics in terms of technology: The use of technology and/or a computer system to store, process, display, retrieve, and communicate timely data and information in and across health care facilities that:

Administer nursing services and resources

Manage the delivery of patient and nursing care

Link research resources and findings to nursing practice

Apply educational resources to nursing education.

A further evolution in the focus of nursing informatics is seen in those experts who advocate the underlying concepts of nursing theory. They argue that without a well-articulated theoretical basis to guide the gathering of data, nursing will soon be overwhelmed with meaningless data and information. They point out the need for definitions, a standardized nursing language, and criteria for organization of the data.

Those who focus on the concept of function in nursing informatics take the process one step further. They focus on how the management and processing of information help nurses enter, organize, or retrieve information. They stress the usability of the applications to achieve specific purposes. Whereas technology and concept are important in forming the foundation of informatics, the nurse's ability to use the system and make it function is the real test of the system's effectiveness.

In reality, nursing informatics includes all three of these areas of focus. However, the field of informatics has become so large that it is difficult for any one person to be an expert in all three areas.

Broader Definition

From the earlier definitions given by Hannah and Saba, a broader definition has evolved, and nursing informatics is now recognized as a nursing specialty for which one can receive certification. The Catalog of the American Nurses Credentialing Center (ANCC)[10] states that the nursing informatics practice "encompasses the full range of activities that focus on the methods and technologies of information handling in nursing. It includes the development, support, and evaluation of applications, tools, processes, and structures that assist the practice of nurses with the management of data in direct care of clients."

In the broadest sense, nursing informatics is the management and processing of information to support decision making in nursing practice. It encompasses all information needs related to the practice of nursing. Strictly speaking, information systems do not have to be electronic; however, electronic systems greatly increase accessibility to and accuracy of the information.

Nursing informatics supports all areas of nursing, including practice, education, administration, and research. It facilitates and guides the management of data.

IMPORTANCE OF NURSING INFORMATICS

Informatics is no longer just an elective subject. In today's competitive and rapidly changing health-care delivery system, informatics is an essential. The importance of the role of informatics is apparent in the need for the articulation of nursing practice.

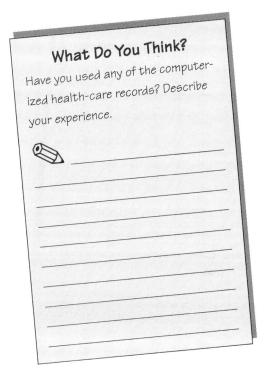

What Do You Think?

Have you used any of the computerized health-care records? Describe your experience.

Articulation is an important way for nursing to demonstrate its accountability and credibility so that nursing can remain an essential element of the health-care system.

Articulation

Historically, the nursing profession has had difficulty in locating relevant nursing information quickly, because there was no universally agreed upon nomenclature and taxonomy for either nursing clinical information or management data. This lack of access to information has presented several seemingly insurmountable challenges for nurse executives, including being able to identify what the nursing staff actually does, determining the impact nurses have on outcomes, and establishing appropriate reimbursement for nursing activities.[11]

For example, how does a nurse interpret the term *weak grasp* when it is seen in the

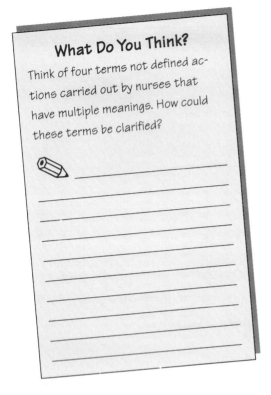

chart of a client? The meaning of weak grasp differs widely depending on the client. If the client is a premature infant with a weak grasp, the term has an entirely different meaning than if it is applied to a 25-year-old professional football player with a head injury or even a 60-year-old client with a stroke. Imagine the difficulty that a researcher will have when he or she is investigating the phenomenon of weak grasp because of the lack of a standardized definition among the nursing community. Because of the need to standardize nursing language to name and communicate what nurses do, nursing classification schemes, taxonomies, or vocabularies have come to the forefront with the evolution of nursing informatics.

The American Nurses Association Database Steering Committee was formed in 1991 to develop a common nursing language called the Unified Nursing Language System (UNLS). UNLS maps concepts and identifies common terms from different vocabularies and acknowledges them as synonyms of the same concept. Table 15.1 lists the criteria used to recognize a nursing classification system.

Four classification systems are recognized as meeting the criteria for classification schemes: North American Nursing Diagnosis Association (NANDA), Omaha Classification System (OCS), Home Healthcare Classification (HHC), and Nursing Interventions Classification (NIC).

NANDA is a classification system for nursing diagnosis. The list began in 1973 with 37 nursing diagnoses. The association meets biannually and updates the list. In 1996, the list included more than 100 nursing diagnoses.

The Omaha system originated as the Problem Classification Scheme at the Visiting Nurse Association of Omaha, Nebraska. The Omaha system is a taxonomy designed to document interdisciplinary practice in a community setting.

The Home Healthcare Classification (HHC) originated from a study funded by the federal government "to develop a method to assess and classify home health Medicare clients to predict resource requirements and measure outcomes of

Table 15.1	Criteria for Selection of Classification Schemes

Be clinically useful for making diagnostic, intervention, and outcome decisions.

Be stated in clear and unambiguous terms, with terms defined precisely.

Demonstrate evidence of testing for reliability.

Have been validated as useful for clinical purposes.

Be accompanied by documentation of a systematic methodology for development.

Be accompanied by evidence of process for periodic review and provision for adding, revising, and deleting terms.

Provide a unique identifier or code for each term.

care."[12] The HHCC assesses, documents, codes, and classifies home health nursing diagnoses, their expected outcomes, nursing interventions, and types of nursing intervention actions according to their components of care.

The Nursing Interventions Classification (NIC) developed at the University of Iowa classifies both nurse- and physician-initiated interventions. NIC is designed for use in all settings and with clients of all ages.

Nursing Outcome Classification (NOC) is in the process of development at the University of Iowa. It will classify nursing-sensitive client outcomes. When complete, the NOC is expected to contain client outcomes, indicators, and measurement activities at five to six levels of abstraction. The accumulation of such detailed information about the effectiveness or lack of effectiveness of nursing interventions and the linkages among nursing diagnoses, interventions, and outcomes will add to nursing knowledge and allow nurses to identify areas of practice that need improvement.[13]

Standardization of the data in a client's record is the first step toward unifying information. The second step has been the development of criteria to determine the necessary elements that must be included in every client record or encounter. The Nursing Minimum Data Set (NMDS) developed in 1985 and accepted by the American Nurses Association in 1990 is a list of the data elements necessary in any computerized client record system or national database. The NMDS is considered to be the umbrella for other nursing process schemes. The purpose of the NMDS is to (1) describe the nursing care of clients and their families in various settings, both institutional and noninstitutional; (2) establish comparability of nursing data across clinical populations, settings, geographic areas, and time; (3) demonstrate or project trends regarding nursing care provided and allocation of nursing resources to clients according to their health problems or nursing diagnoses; (4) stimulate nursing research through linkages of detailed data existing in nursing information systems and in other health-care information systems; and (5) provide data about nursing care to influence health policy and decision making.[14] The NMDS has 16 elements divided into three main categories: nursing care (e.g., nursing diagnosis, intervention, outcome, and degree of nursing care), client demographics (e.g., the client's personal identification, date of birth, sex), and service elements (e.g., the unique service agency number, the admission and discharge dates, client's condition, and expected payer).

Accountability

Intuitively, the nursing profession has long known that the increased use of nurses improves the quality of care and also client outcomes, while decreasing the cost of health care. However, nurses traditionally have not been very good at documenting their worth and effectiveness. According to the Congressional Office of Technology Assessment,[15] better use of nurse practitioners could result in savings for clients, employers, and society owing to the cost-effectiveness of both their training and their services. Nurses affect client outcomes positively and contribute measurably to the goals of a competitive health-care delivery system.

In order to measure effectiveness with accurate information about client care and outcomes, nurses must use standardized language in both practice and documentation. The ability to measure the resources

> **❝ ❞** *Intuitively, the nursing profession has long known that the increased use of nurses improves the quality of care and also client outcomes, while decreasing the cost of health care.*

used and the client outcome achieved will help distinguish one health-care provider from another. As nursing practice becomes more efficient and can demonstrate improved client outcomes, both the quality of care will increase and health-care organizations will become more financially stable.

Credibility

The credibility of the nursing profession rests on the state of its documentation. Nurses must be able to measure their effectiveness with accurate information about both the care given and the client outcomes achieved. Nursing professionals must have control over the process of care as well as the information and assessments of the quality of care. Improvements in quality do not occur in isolation. Quality improvements result from a continual process of assessing care and measuring outcomes that produce improvements in treatments, changes in care procedures, and an increased number of support services.[16]

A standardized language will facilitate the nursing profession's ability to delineate the cost and benefits of nursing care from the costs and benefits of other health-care providers. If the nursing profession cannot articulate and measure the unique contributions that nurses make to the client's health and well-being, then the profession will continue to have difficulty justifying its higher costs over less educated and less qualified health-care providers.

ACCESS TO INFORMATION

An information explosion continues to restructure the world of health-care journals and textbooks. The amount of health-care information contained in scientific journals has grown to a point where no single individual is able to read all of the material. In 1994, 34,000 references from 4000 journals were added each month to the National Library of Medicine Medline database from among the more than 100,000 scientific journals published.[17] Coping with the volume of biomedical and nursing literature is an enormous task. With just a nightly perusal of the latest journals, even the most conscientious practitioners will have difficulty in keeping up with all the current research and new developments in their specialty field.

Although a great amount of new information is available, it would seem that only a small portion is actually transferred into the minds and practice of many health-care professionals. The traditional paradigm that seems to guide the decision-making process for many nurses is to (1) refer back to the knowledge learned in school, (2) confer with a colleague, (3) look up the problem in any textbook/reference book available in the work setting, and (4) use previous experiences and "gut" instincts. Although this

What Do You Think?

What do you remember from the last professional nursing journal that you read? Have you used any of the information in your nursing practice?

process is useful and has some merit, it is questionable whether it is adequate for the delivery of high-quality care.

Consider a new paradigm for decision making that may be more appropriate for the information age. This process includes (1) accessing current literature concerning the latest diagnostic techniques and treatment modalities, (2) conferring with a knowledgeable colleague, and (3) evaluating the effectiveness of previous experiences. Research shows that nursing interventions based on research produce better client outcomes.[18] This process is called evidence-based practice.

Ironically, even though evidence-based practice produces higher quality care, the health-care culture has been slow to implement its use. With increasing client care responsibilities, nurses rarely have time to go to the library to research solutions to client care problems. Furthermore, nurses are not rewarded for taking the initiative to do so. However, leaving the practice site in order to access relevant information is no longer necessary in the information age. Literature searching can be available at the point of care using automated systems.

Royle described a Canadian study where literature searching via a personal computer was available on the nursing unit. Nurses had access to six databases, the Health Science Library's on-line catalog, user manuals, search aids, textbooks, and reference books on medical-surgical and oncology nursing. The study extended over a 6-month period, and the nurses received 6 hours of training in the use of the system. Even after the training sessions, the nurses found that they still had difficulty finding time to use the system. However, with practice, they became more familiar with information that was available. They also claimed that "having access to literature about clinical issues gave them confidence in dealing with clients and other health professionals and allowed them to contribute

BOX

15.1 Principles for Access to Library and Information Services

1. All nurses should have access to a free library service funded by their employer that contains appropriate literature and multimedia resources.
2. Library services should have flexible opening hours and be staffed by qualified librarians.
3. Nurses should have equal rights, similar to those of other healthcare professionals, to paid study time to update their practice.
4. Every nurse should have access to training on the Internet and appropriate databases.
5. Every nurse should be educated in electronic systems and services to support evidence-based practice.

Source: Urquhart, C, Davis, R: The impact of information. Nursing Standard 12(8), 23–31, 1997.

more fully to the multidisciplinary health care team"[19] (Box 15.1).

Nurses must continue to demand access to and time for information searches that promote improved client care. The creation of workplaces in which nurses can easily access client information, including research information, is essential to high-quality nursing practice.

HUMAN FACTORS THAT AFFECT INFORMATICS

The human factors that influence informatics include knowledge about human abilities, limitations, and characteristics that are relevant to the design of tools, machines, systems, and jobs. "Human factors," "human engineering," "usability engineering," and "ergonomics" are often used interchangeably. The study of human factors examines how to make the interaction of people and equipment safe, comfortable, and effective. Cognitive science, one of the components of informatics discussed earlier, forms part of the foundation for the study of human factors. Cognitive science includes the human acts of perception, thinking, understanding, and remembering. In order to manage and process information, especially with an automated system, the individual must be able to understand and remember a great deal of data. The more logically that this information is arranged, the easier it is to use the system.

Every day in their client care, nurses use complex machinery, including many types of monitors, ventilators, intravenous (IV) pumps, feeding pumps, suction devices, electronic beds and scales, lift equipment, and assistive devices. The directions for use of many of these machines are not self-evident and may be highly complicated. Although hospital equipment producers are becoming better at incorporating the human factor in the design and use of this complicated equipment, it would seem that consulting with practicing nurses or "field testing" equipment in the workplace prior to its mass production would make it more user friendly.

Similarly, new computer systems present many learning difficulties for health-care providers. Many computer systems are not user friendly. Computer systems designers are notorious for supplying computers with numerous advanced but obscure functions, but these systems often lack the ability to make daily tasks easier to accomplish. Millions of dollars have been wasted on computer systems that are not used or are underused because the user needs were not assessed before the systems were designed.

Individuals encountering complicated computer systems for the first time commonly feel that they are stupid, incompetent or too old to learn because they cannot quickly master the use of the new technology. However, the fault often lies not with the individual but rather with the design of the technology. Nurses, through their education and philosophical orientation, are generally more in tune with the human factor than equipment designers, particularly as it relates to client care. Nurses can use their human factor orientation in the process of evaluating new technology before it is purchased. Also, nurses may be able to make suggestions to medical equipment producers to help improve the equipment after it has been used for some time.

Poor user design is responsible for thousands of health-care "accidents" each year. Complex medical devices are often used under extremely stressful conditions in which the user's cognitive abilities are not as fo-

What Do You Think?

What equipment have you used recently that made you feel stupid or inadequate? Could the equipment have been improved to make it more usable?

_____

_____

_____

_____

_____

_____

_____

_____

cused as they might be in a less stressful situation. Often the users are not considered during the design phase, because the designers believe that they know what is needed. The inevitable result of poor design in all types of equipment, ranging from paper laboratory forms to life-support devices, is an increased error rate. Cognitive science studies have shown that the average person's memory can retain only six to eight pieces of information at the same time. A well-designed system will take these elements into account (Box 15.2).

In a Harvard Medical Practice Study[20] 30,121 client records were randomly selected from 51 New York hospitals. Adverse events were documented in 3.7% of the hospitalizations. Of the adverse events 27% were determined to be preventable. Of the preventable events, 10% to 20% were related to the system or to devices. The authors suggest that the use of computerization and system analysis (human factors) would reduce the number of incidents. Most agree, however, that computers can just as easily contribute to errors as help reduce them.

Training employees how to use a system is a common methodology for reducing error. Although training is important, by itself, it may not be adequate. According to McDonald,[21] error frequency was not well correlated with level of training, but a computer-based reminder system helped clinicians reduce errors significantly. Even with more training, errors returned to the previous level when the computerized reminder system was removed.

When automated and computer systems are properly designed using human factors engineering techniques, they can be a valuable part of the monitoring and prevention of error in clinical practice. As nursing professionals, it is important to understand that human performance is not perfect and cannot be perfected through education and training. Professionals must look for well-designed systems that can reduce and even eliminate errors.

ELECTRONIC HEALTH RECORD

A health record serves multiple purposes. It is used to document client care and provides communication among health-care team members. It is a financial and a legal record. It is used for research and continuous quality improvement (CQI). Although the health record can take many forms, the most common forms are either paper or electronic. Both forms have advantages and disadvantages (Table 15.2).

Electronic health records (EHRs) have many advantages. They are accessible from remote sites to multiple care providers at the same time. They can provide reminders about completing information or carrying through with protocols as well as providing warnings about incompatibilities of medications or variances from normal standards. Redundancy is reduced with the

---

BOX 15.2 Elements of a Good Technology Design

1. Can be operated intuitively with minimal reliance on complicated manuals.
2. Easy-to-read displays that are logically arranged.
3. Easy to use and reach controls.
4. Positive and safe electrical and mechanical connections.
5. Alarms that sound only when there is a real problem so that they are not turned off because of annoyance.
6. Long-life reliability with few malfunctions.
7. Easy and quick to repair and maintain.

Table 15.2	Advantages and Disadvantages of the Paper Record

Advantages

- People know how to use it.
- It is fast for current practice.
- It is portable.
- It is nonbreakable.
- It accepts multiple data types, such as graphs, photographs, drawings, and text.
- Legal issues and costs are understood.

Disadvantages

- It can be lost.
- It is often illegible and incomplete.
- It has no remote access.
- It can be accessed by only one person at a time.
- It is often disorganized.
- Information is duplicated.
- It is hard to store.
- It is difficult to research, and CQI is laborious.
- Same client has separate records at each facility (physician office, hospital, home care).
- Records are shared only through hard copy.

EHR. Rather than every health-care worker asking a client for his or her past health history, allergies, and current medications, the information is captured once and then transmitted to every record requiring the information. EHRs require less storage space, are more difficult to lose, and are much easier to research. Improved communication, increased completeness of documentation, and reduction in error are the most important advantages of the EHR.

However, EHRs have some obvious disadvantages. There is a high front-end cost in buying and converting from a paper to an electronic system. Employees may have problems adapting to the new system because of the large learning curve involved in converting from a paper system to an electronic system. EHR systems are nonportable but are breakable. Decisions must be made about who can enter data into the system and when the entries should be made. Many legal and ethical issues involving privacy and also access to information still remain to be resolved.

The ideal EHR will be a lifelong continuous record of all the care that the client has received rather than the episodic, piecemeal data that it now provides. This one record will reflect an individual's current health status and lifetime medical history. It will be unique to the person and not to the institution. This record will reside in multiple data sites and will accept multiple data types (e.g., graphs, pictures, x-rays, text) and be accessible worldwide.

The information on the EHR does not physically reside in one place. When viewed from a computer workstation, the EHR only appears to be in one place. In reality, the individual records are retrieved from many information systems, such as laboratory, radiology, document imaging, anatomic pathology, anesthesiology, bedside, accounting, and others.

With proper authorization, this record could be accessed from anywhere in the world, at any time. Many people around the world could look at the same record at the same time. If an individual became critically ill abroad, this would be a valuable tool to facilitate the diagnosis and treatment.

Many barriers must be overcome before the ideal EHR can be fully implemented. The issues of maintaining confidentiality and security must be solved. The high cost of starting up the system is still a barrier. Bob Boysen, Chief Information Officer of Iowa Health System, believes the universal ID or a unique client identifier could become the biggest bombshell to hit health-care informatics this century.[22] Many organizations use either their own client numbering system or social security numbers to identify individual records. Neither of these systems is adequate for the global access of the future. Fingerprinting, iris and retinal imaging, face prints, and voice prints all are identification methods under investigation for use as the universal ID.

Information can be entered through a bedside system, a point-of-care system, or a unit system. A bedside system, as the name implies, is a computer terminal installed in each client's room or next to each bed. A point-of-care system has a broader meaning and includes not only the bedside but also many other points of care in the health-care environment and community, including locations such as the laboratory, radiology department, outpatient clinics, and even the home for home-health-care providers. Many facilities currently have a unit system that can be accessed at only one terminal in the client care area (e.g., the nurses' station).

Taking a paper record and typing it into a computer does not, in itself, constitute a modern electronic record. Automating the paper record in its present form only automates inefficient practices based on outdated requirements. Modern systems go beyond merely computerizing current paper records. These new systems gain control over the generation of information and develop new techniques for using it creatively. One of the most important characteristics of a bedside or point-of-care system is that client information can be input directly from the terminal rather than keeping notes or charting from memory at the end of the shift. Documentation at the time of care is an important change in workflow for most health-care workers who are accustomed to documenting at the end of a shift in a workroom with other professionals.

The re-engineering and streamlining of departmental workflow is accomplished by the automatic and continual routing of electronic documents and medical images from one person or department to another throughout the shift. With this system, traditional manual tasks are now automated, thus increasing the efficiency of management decisions and improving the distribution and evaluation of complex client records and electronic documents by autho-

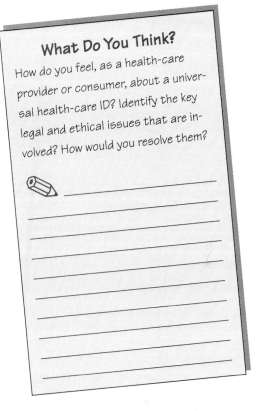

rized staff. It is this radical redesign of the old manual processes that provides the real return on investment for implementing the electronic health record.

ETHICS, SECURITY, AND CONFIDENTIALITY

Most people assume that all doctor-client communications are confidential. However, "confidentiality is now becoming a commodity to be traded in exchange for health care," experts warned at the eighth annual Conference on Computers, Freedom and Privacy.[23]

Examples of violation of client confidentiality abound. In 1996, a convicted child rapist working as a technician in a Boston hospital rifled through 1000 computerized records looking for potential victims. He was caught when the father of a 9-year-old girl used caller ID to trace the call back to

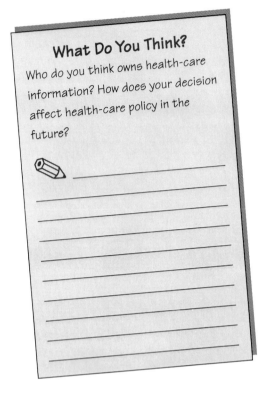

What Do You Think?

Who do you think owns health-care information? How does your decision affect health-care policy in the future?

curred—can they claim some ownership to the information, particularly if it is stored there? Or do all these groups and individuals own a part of the information?

Those who argue on the "individual rights" end of the ethical spectrum believe that each individual should have total and exclusive control over the information concerning his or her health and the care rendered. Those on the utilitarian or "social good" end of the ethical spectrum believe that society as a whole benefits from shared information about disease occurrence and treatment. Therefore, the information should be available to all interested parties. As with most ethical dilemmas, a single definitive answer has not been proposed regarding who owns the data.

However, public policy debates concerning the collection of health-care information for use as aggregate databases to underpin health-care planning are increasing. Many consumers are concerned about the status of future physician-client relationships. Driving the development of data collection policy is the public's fears about the damages that may result from excessive and uncontrolled health-care information disclosures through automated information systems.[25]

When clients enter the health-care system, they are generally asked to sign consents so that other organizations can obtain information about their health status and the care that they received (particularly insurance companies so that bills can be paid). They are usually unaware that this information can be supplied to many other organizations or institutions. For example, reports to the trauma registry are made about injuries resulting from accidents. The tumor registry collects information about benign and malignant tumors, and infectious disease reports are made to the Public Health Department. In the future, sharing of health-care information will be used to support the development of payment systems, examine access to care, identify cost

the hospital. A banker on Maryland's State Health Commission pulled up a list of cancer clients from the state's records, crosschecked it against the names of his bank's customers, and revoked the loans of those clients diagnosed with cancer. At least a third of all Fortune 500 companies regularly review health information before making hiring decisions. More than 200 subjects in a case study published in the *Science and Engineering Ethics* reported that they had been discriminated against as a result of genetic testing.[24]

One of the key ethical questions is "Who owns the client's health-care data?" Does the individual's health-care information belong exclusively to him or her? Does it belong to the organization (e.g., insurance company, PPO) that paid for the care? Or should the information belong to the physician who directed and ordered the care? What about the facility in which the care oc-

differences of treatment modalities, research disease trends and epidemiologic implications, and expand consumer information. Policies guiding the collection, development, and use of these data must be created around the core issues of confidentiality and security.

Even today, there is an expanded use of client information that would have been unacceptable only a few years ago. Some current, commonly accepted uses for client records include quality assurance, institutional licensing and accreditation, biomedical research, third-party reimbursement, credentialing, litigation, regional and national databases, court-ordered release of information, and managed care comparisons. Although automated information systems did not cause these information uses, automation does make acquiring this information much easier. Unauthorized sharing of health-care information is generally unethical but is not always illegal. The code of ethics for most health-care professionals prohibits the unauthorized or unnecessary access to client information. In addition, most health-care institutions have policies prohibiting unauthorized access to confidential information. Although individuals can lose their jobs because of unauthorized access or sharing of client information, it is not illegal to do so.

Unauthorized access or sharing of information is not a new problem. It is just as easy to gain unauthorized access to a manual paper record as it is to the automated electronic record. The professional codes of ethics that stress client confidentiality have always been the primary protector of client information. Access to the paper record is available to anyone who picks up the chart. In some ways, the automated electronic record provides greater privacy to an individual. Access to the automated record is generally restricted to employees who have been issued a password. Also, most organizations have periodic **audits** that can track each person who has accessed a record, and some systems can even detect unauthorized access at the time of entry into the system.

Threats to the security of information can be either accidental or intentional and affect both paper and electronic systems. Accidental threats involve naturally occurring events such as floods, fires, earthquakes, electrical surges, and power outages. The paper record has little security against many natural events. Typically, paper records are secured in a locked file cabinet or medical records room. Although current safety regulations require fire detection and suppression systems in these areas, even small fires can destroy a large number of paper records very quickly. There is little that can be done to protect paper records against major flooding. Once the charts are destroyed, they cannot be reproduced.

Facilities with automated systems usually have well-developed natural disaster plans built into the system design. These plans include the automatic production and storage of a back-up tape of the data at a protected location some distance from the health-care facility. The frequency of data back-up varies with the organization's requirements.

 Facilities with automated systems usually have well-developed natural disaster plans built into the system design.

Most systems automatically save all the data in the system every 24 hours, although this time interval can be shortened or increased to meet the facility's needs. Although these measures provide a high degree of protection from major natural events such as floods and fires, power surges and outages create problems for electronic systems that leave paper systems unaffected. Anyone who works at all with computerized equipment recognizes the major disruptions in service and work that occurs when the

Nursing Informatics Expands Professional Nursing

How are your computer skills? Can you access and surf the Internet with ease? What was your last Power Point Presentation? How do you see yourself using informatics in your professional practice? In the near future, employers of both nurse educators and staff nurses may very well be asking these questions during employment interviews.

In the educational setting, *informatics* is a term that is used to describe on-line distance learning through computer technology. Although the ability to use computer technology for educational purposes has been widely available since the late 1980s, the development, acceptance, and use of multimedia Internet presentations in the classroom are still in early developmental stages. Community colleges are the pioneers in attempting to use multimedia and electronic networking on a widespread basis. However, there are still relatively few actual courses that are offered by the Internet for student and working nurses as revealed by on-line searches.

With an ever-shrinking pool of students, colleges have identified a need for finding alternative means of presenting traditional classroom courses, particularly in rural areas where students must drive considerable distances to attend classes. Use of on-line informatics helps free students from rigidly scheduled classes in specific locations. However, the search for and development of safe, reliable, and high-quality alternative educational methods is ongoing.

Currently, the primary methods of delivering informatics is through long-distance learning (LDL) and the Internet. These methods have been used on a limited basis for several years and are generally considered reliable. Classes conducted through LDL and the Internet are generally presented in a traditional format, except that the students are located at any number of sites distant from the originating source of the presentation. Students are able to both hear and see the professor, and the professor is able to hear and see the students. Responses and contributions from students are instantaneous.

Electronic bulletin board (EBB) is another technology that is being developed for class work, although it is not as widely available as LDL and the Internet. Unlike the instructor-centered LDL and Internet, EBB has the advantage of being learner-centered. Ideally, in the EBB classroom, the student who may be somewhat shy has an opportunity to contribute to the class without being placed under the spotlight when speaking. With EBB, students have time to consider and prepare their answers and comments before placing them on-line. It is hoped that their responses will be more thorough and detailed than those contributed in the LDL and Internet environment.

As EBB develops and becomes more widely accepted, it is anticipated that it will provide the adult learner with an educational environment that is convenient and primarily oriented to their individual learning needs. Discussion on EBB overcomes the factors of distance and time that often prevent students from sharing and interacting in a traditional setting.

Any of these modes of informatics (LDL, Internet, and EBB) also benefit students by developing their skills in the use of computer technology. Computer technology in the hospital setting is commonplace, and a facility with computers is viewed by employers as a necessary skill in today's health-care system. At some point in the near future, all nurses will be required to be able to use the computer as a tool in health care, much as they now use intravenous pumps, electronic thermometers, and the telephone.

Sources: Beaman, ML: Nursing Informatics Partnership Workshop. MAINlines 18(4):8, 1997; Mills, A: Nursing Informatics Workshop—St. Louis University. MAINlines 18(4):9, 1997; Adelman, DS: Teaching nursing on-line: One community college's experience. MAINlines 18(4):12–14, 1997; and Ruchala, P: On-line nurse practitioner education at St. Louis University. MAINlines 18(4):15, 1997.

"system goes down." Again, some safeguards can be built into the system so that not all the most recent information is lost when the power goes out. Power surges can be controlled with surge protection devices.

Intentional threats to the security of information involve the actions of an individual or individuals who wish to damage, destroy, or alter the records. In most cases, it is difficult to protect paper records from intentional tampering. It is a rather simple task for a determined individual to gain access to paper records and either erase, add to, or rewrite sections of the chart. These changes are often very difficult to detect. In addition, a person could simply remove the chart and destroy it so that there would be no record left at all.

Although automated electronic records are vulnerable to several different intentional threats, they are, over all, more secure than the paper record. All current automated systems have computer virus-checking programs that protect the automated record from the introduction of both intentional and accidental computer viruses into

the system that will destroy information. Once data have been entered into the automated system, the data are difficult to alter. Modern automated systems are now designed with the "write once, read many" (WORM) programs. If a legitimate change in the electronic record needs to be made, it must be added as an addendum. Any changes made in the electronic record are logged by the time and the person who made them and can always be tracked to the point of origin. Although it is true that a determined and gifted hacker can still obtain access to almost any electronic database, electronic security systems are becoming more and more difficult to breach.

USES OF THE INTERNET

For nursing professionals, the Internet has become a valuable resource for communicating with colleagues and professional organizations, researching clinical information, and educating consumers about health resources and information. Because of the lack of standardization and regulation, it is important that the nurse evaluate each site for accuracy of information, authority, objectivity, currency or timeliness, and coverage.[26]

Most professional organizations maintain a Web site containing information about the organization. Many include policy statements and lists of publications. **Continuing education units (CEUs)** can be obtained via the World Wide Web to help nurses remain current and retain licensure. *The Nursing Forum* (http://forums.msn.com/nursing), for example, is a site that lists nursing education courses, nursing position vacancies, nursing conferences, and other pertinent information. The news groups provide professional information and access to experts in specific areas of interest.

Disease-specific Web sites publish clinical information for both the consumer and the professional. OncoLink is an example of a resource for information about cancer. Often the most recent information about a disease is found on the Internet. Publishing is quicker and easier on the WWW than in a peer-reviewed journal. Web-based support groups disseminate information on both technical and consumer levels. Protocols and policies are shared through Web sites and news groups.

Today, consumers are more knowledgeable about health care through use of the Internet. Clients are better informed than they were in the past, because they now have easy access to a wide range of health-care information. Preventive and wellness services are available electronically through articles, chat groups, and health risk assessment surveys posted on consumer Web sites. Kaiser Permanente has started an ambitious on-line pilot project that offers members various services, including 30,000 pages of disease-specific information; participation in discussion groups; and the ability to ask questions of a nurse, pharmacist, or specialist. In the future, members will be able to schedule themselves for nonurgent appointments at various clinics, order prescription refills or over-the-counter medications from an "on-line drug store," and send e-mail messages directly to their physicians.[27]

Healthfinder is a consumer health and human services information Web site cre-

---

Site Seeing

AMIA Nursing Informatics Working Group
http://www.gl.umbc.edu/~abbott/nurseinfo.html
Contact: Patricia A. Abbott
mail to:abbott@gl.umbc.edu

Community Health Information Resources
http://chmis.org
Contact: baguilar@eskimo.com

Computers in Nursing Interactive
http://www.cini.com
Contact: Leslie H. Nicoll
lnicoll@maine.maine.edu

Healthcare Informatics Standards
http://www.mcis.duke.edu/standards/guide.htm
Contact: Al Stone
mail to:stone001@mc.duke.edu

Idea Nurse (Informatics)
http://ideanurse.com/
Contact: Peter Ramme
mail to:peter@silcom.com

Medical Informatics at McGill University
http://mystic.biomed.mcgill.ca/
Contact: Zs Bencsath-Makkai
zsuzsi@biomed.mcgill.ca

Northern California Nursing Informatics Association (NCNIA)
http://www.dnai.com/~mmoore/ncia.html
Contact: mmoore@dnai.com

NRSING-L
listserv@library.unmed.edu
Subscribe NRSING-L Firstname Lastname

On-Line Journal of Nursing Informatics
http://milkman.cac.psu.edu/~dxm12/OJNI.html
Contact: Dee McGonigle, PhD, RNC, FACCE
mail to:dxm12@psu.edu

ated and maintained by the federal government. The site links the user with on-line government publications, clearinghouses, databases, web sites, support and self-help groups, as well as the government agencies and not-for-profit organizations that produce reliable information for the public. The goal of this information source is to help consumers make better choices about their health and human services needs for both themselves and their families.

TELEHEALTH

For more than 30 years, clinicians, health services researchers, and others have been investigating the use of advanced telecommunications and information technologies to improve health care. Physicians examine and treat clients from distant sites with video cameras, thus saving money by exchanging office visits for on-line appointments. Telehealth is becoming more common in emergency rooms across the United States. The University of Pittsburgh offers neurological consults to physicians at seven linked hospitals. In Baltimore, providers are taking telehealth to the streets, using cellular telephone lines to transmit live video and client data back to home base.[28] With expenditures for home health services expected to double within the next 5 years, health maintenance organizations (HMOs) and home health agencies are investing in telemedicine and information technologies to control costs and meet increased service demands.[29]

The terms *telehealth* and *telemedicine* are often used interchangeably. As defined here, telehealth is the use of electronic information and communications technologies to provide and support health care when distance separates the physician and the client. Telehealth includes a wide range of services and technologies, ranging from the "plain old telephone service" (POTS) to highly sophisticated digitized cameras,

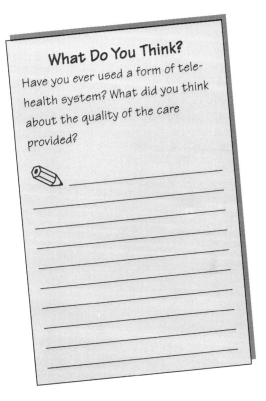

What Do You Think?

Have you ever used a form of telehealth system? What did you think about the quality of the care provided?

telemetry, and voice systems. Telemedicine is just one of the services provided by the overall telehealth system that primarily involves consultation with a physician.

Some uses of telehealth, such as emergency calls to 911, are so common that they are often overlooked when considering telehealth systems. Other applications such as telesurgery involve exotic technologies and procedures that are still in the experimental stage.

Historically, consumer concerns about access to health care have been the driving force behind the development of many clinical telehealth systems. Early applications focused on remote populations scattered across mountainous areas, islands, open plains, and arctic regions where medical specialists, and sometimes even primary care practitioners, were not available. Many telehealth projects from the 1960s through the early 1980s failed because they were expensive, awkward to use, and often not guided by the strategic plans of the facilities using them.

Renewed interest in telehealth has been spurred by managed-care initiatives seeking to reduce health-care costs while maintaining or increasing the quality and access to care. Overall costs have decreased for many of the information and communications technologies used by telehealth systems. In addition, the ever-developing National Information Infrastructure is making these technologies more accessible and user friendly. Currently, Medicare, Medicaid, or third-party insurance does not reimburse interactive telemedicine consults. However, provisions included in future federal budgets that mandate Medicare reimbursement for telehealth services in remote areas will be initiated in 1999. Because Medicare and other payers do reimburse for radiology consultations, teleradiology (the transmission of x-ray via Internet) is a frequently used service of the telehealth system.

Telehealth offers many advantages affecting the cost of and access to the health-care system of the future. The telehealth system allows access to centralized specialists who can support primary care providers in outlying areas. Outlying areas can be either rural or urban areas that lack access to the full range of health-care services. Outlying clinics staffed only with nurse practitioners or physician assistants have immediate access to physician referrals through the telehealth system. University medical centers can offer specialist consulting services to primary care physicians at distant locations, thus reducing unnecessary travel and increased cost to clients. Here is an actual example of how the telehealth system functions in an emergency situation:

In 1996 a 72-year-old man with a collapsed lung walked into the emergency room (ER) in a small town in North Dakota. The general practitioner who usually saw routine emergency cases immediately called the trauma II medical center in Bismark and arranged a teleconsult with an ER physician and a thoracic surgeon. The man would die without a thoracotomy. Following the surgeon's instructions, the physician was able to insert the chest tubes needed to safely transport the client by helicopter to Bismark.[28]

Telehealth services often save lives and prevent permanent disability, especially when time is a factor in treatment. For example, health-care providers know that if thrombolytic medications are given within 3 hours after the onset of symptoms of a stroke, the likelihood of death or permanent disability is reduced by 50%. Using telehealth technology, neurology specialists can evaluate a client's condition while he or she is still in the ambulance en route to the hospital, thus saving valuable time in making the decision about using lifesaving medications. The ER is prepared to administer the medications as soon as the client enters the department rather than having to wait several hours for all the routine evaluations and consults to be completed.

In the future, home care may benefit the most from telehealth. By investing in telehealth technologies, home-care providers should be able to balance cost reductions with increased quality of care. Clients can be monitored at home using a combination of telephone calls, home visits, video visits, and in-home monitoring via the telehealth system. In-home monitoring devices for conditions ranging from congestive heart failure and diabetes to cancer and cardiac conditions can send information from the client's

> 66 99 *The telehealth system allows access to centralized specialists who can support primary care providers in outlying areas.*

home to a central base for assessment by professionals. A Kaiser Permanente study in California demonstrated that when instant access from home to health-care professional was provided by telehealth systems, it reduced the cost of care by one-third while increasing its quality. Furthermore, the study showed that client anxiety levels were reduced, as noted in the agency's client satisfaction surveys.[28]

Future challenges remain for telehealth applications. Many of the older technical systems are poorly designed and do not meet the needs of the user's environment. As discussed earlier, human factor design and user assessments must be carefully considered when developing any new technologies. Although the overall costs of electronic systems continue to gradually decrease, initial expenditures are still a barrier to implementation, especially in smaller facilities. Lack of Medicare, Medicaid, and **third-party payment** for telehealth systems also limits their development and use. Several legal issues still need to be resolved, including health-care provider licensure when consults are given across state lines and the liability incurred by providers who examine a client by television rather than in a face-to-face, hands-on encounter. Federal and state policies protecting privacy and confidentiality need to be developed with specific provisions for telehealth systems.

The telehealth system also affects nursing practice. Nurses are the primary users of telephone triage systems that rely on computerized decision-making trees to suggest appropriate actions when given a set of client symptoms. Nurses who practice in rural and underserved urban areas will have more autonomy and provide higher quality care when linked electronically with the support services of a large medical center. The use of remote monitoring devices provides nurses with immediate information about changes in their clients' conditions, improves outcomes, reduces complications, and lowers the number of re-admissions to the hospital.

The same types of technology used for telehealth can be used for distance and **nontraditional education** applications. Widespread use of continuing education is achieved through distance technology. Courses are video-conferenced with two-way interaction. Continuing education credits can be earned through courses on the Internet. Even college credits can be earned via Internet access. Grand rounds are conducted at multiple sites with video conferencing equipment and in-services are beamed to multiple locations.

Conclusion

The information revolution affects every aspect of health care, not only in the United States but also throughout the world. The advent of advanced communications technology and its increased availability worldwide promotes ties between people and nations, bridging the gap between isolated rural communities and major metropolitan areas. The nursing profession needs to be actively involved in developing clinical information systems and the electronic health record, establishing care standards, safeguarding client privacy, using the Internet, and researching better ways of improving access and the quality of care through technology. The nursing profession is transformed, enhanced, and enriched as nurses become active participants in the information revolution.

Critical Thinking Exercises

✔ Debate the ethical issues of personal privacy and the greater social good in relation to availability of health-care information.

✔ Discuss how the design of equipment increases or decreases error rate.

✔ Discuss uses of telehealth for patient teaching and monitoring of home health clients.

✔ Write a vision paper describing your view of technology in health care in the year 2030.

✔ List all the pieces of data you had to give at your last visit to the doctor or hospital.

✔ Was all of the information necessary to provide your care?

✔ Who needed the information?

✔ How was the information recorded or transmitted?

References

1. Swerdlow, JL: Information revolution. National Geographic, October 1995, pp 5–11.
2. American Hospital Publishing: The 1997 Hospitals & Health Networks Leadership Survey, 5 August, 1997. Hospitals and Health Networks [on-line serial]. Available January 15, 1998 at http://www.amhpi.com/hhn/doc16188.htm.
3. van Bemmel, JH, and Musen, MA (eds): Handbook of Medical Informatics. Springer-Verlag, Heidelberg, 1998.
4. Greenburg, AB: Medical informatics: Science or science fiction. Unpublished material, 1975.
5. Mandil, S: Health informatics: New solutions to old challenges. World-Health 2–5, August–September, 1989.
6. Graves, J, and Corcoran, S: The study of nursing informatics. Image: Journal of Nursing Scholarship 21:227–231, 1989.
7. Saba, VK, and McCormick, KA: Essentials of Computers for Nurses, ed 2. McGraw-Hill, New York, 1995, p 226.
8. Turley, Toward a model for nursing informatics. Image: Journal of Nursing Scholarship 28(4): 309–313, 1996.
9. Hannah K: Current trends in nursing informatics: Implications for curriculum planning. In Hannah, K, Guillemin, E, and Conklin, D (eds): Nursing Uses of Computer and Information Science: Proceedings of the IFIP-IMIA International Symposium on Nursing Uses of Computers and Information Science. Calgary, Alberta, Canada, 1–3 May 1985. Elsevier Science Publishers BV, Amsterdam, 1985.
10. American Nurses Credentialing Center Catalog. Washington, DC: American Nurses Publishing, 1994.
11. Simpson, RL: Information is power. Nurs Admin 20(3):86–89, 1996.
12. Bowles, KH, and Naylor, MD: Nursing intervention classification systems. Image J Nurs Sch 28(4):303–307, 1996.
13. Maas, ML, Johnson, M, and Moorhead, S: Classifying nursing sensitive patient outcomes. Image J Nurs Sch 28(4):295–301, 1996.
14. Prophet, CM: Nursing interventions classifications. In Grobe, SJ, and Pluyter-Wenting, ESP (eds): Nursing Informatics: An International Overview for Nursing in a Technological Era. Elsevier, New York, 1994, pp 692–696.
15. Congressional Office of Technology Assessment, 1988.
16. Casey, A: Nursing, midwifery and health visiting teams project. In Grobe, SJ, and Pluyter-Wenting, ESP (eds): Nursing Informatics: An International Overview for Nursing in a Technological Era. Elsevier, Amsterdam, 1994, pp 639–642.
17. Elliott, S: Information overload and medical progress: When is enough too much? Minimally Invasive Surgical Nursing 8(1):23–27, 1994.
18. Bostrum, J, and Suter, W: Research utilization: Making the link to practice. Journal of Nursing Staff Development 9(1):28–34, 1993.
19. Blythe, J, et al: Linking the professional literature to nursing practice: Challenges and opportunities. American Association of Occupational Health Nursing 43(6):342–345, 1995.
20. Brennan, TA, et al: Incidence of adverse events and negligence in hospitalized patients. Results of the Harvard Medical Practice Study I. N Engl J Med 324:370–376, 1991.
21. McDonald, CJ: Protocol-based computer reminders, the quality of care and the non-perfectability of man. N Engl J Med 295:1351–1355, 1976.
22. Childs, B: A quick look forward. Healthcare Informatics 87–88, January 1994.
23. Miller, L, and Weise, E: Database sharing eroding medical confidentiality. USA Today, 23 February 1998, p. 10D.
24. Quittner, J: Invasion of privacy. Time, 25 August 1997, pp 29–35.
25. Mills, ME: Data privacy and confidentiality in the public arena. In Proceedings of the AMIA Annual Fall Symposium on the Emergence of Internetable Health Care. Systems That Really Work. Nashville, Tenn., 25–29 October 1997. Hanley & Belfus, National Commission on Nursing Implementation Project, 1997.
26. Alexander, J, and Tate, M: The web as a research tool: Evaluation techniques. Available July 1996 at URL, http://www.science. widener.edu/~withers/alaslides/pptfirst. htm.
27. Schneider, P: Patient informatics is growing. Healthcare Informatics 14, August 1997.
28. Davies, P: Delivering emergency care—In a heart beat. Telemedicine and Telehealth Networks 28–32, October 1997.
29. Kincade, K: Growing home-care business benefits from telemedicine tlc. Telemedicine and Telehealth Networks 23–27, October 1997.

BIBLIOGRAPHY

Adelman, DS: Teaching nursing on-line: One community college's experience. MAINlines 18(4):12–14, 1997.

American Nurses Association: The Scope of Practice for Nursing Informatics. American Nurses Association, Washington, DC, 1994.

Beaman, ML: Nursing informatics partnership workshop. MAINlines 18(4):8, 1997.

Brown, JS, and Dugid, P: Universities in the digital age. Change 28(4):11–19, 1996.

DeBack, V, Murphy, M, and Waite, R: The Nation's Nurses: A Credible Profession Doing an Incredible Job [Brochure]. W.K. Kellogg Foundation, Milwaukee, WI, 1988.

Mills, A: Nursing Informatics Workshop—St. Louis University. MAINlines 18(4):9, 1997.

Nicoll, LH: Nurses' Guide to the Internet, ed 2. Lippincott, Philadelphia, 1998.

Ruchala, P: On-Line nurse practitioner education at St. Louis University. MAINlines 18(4)0:15, 1997.

Werley, HH, and Lang, NM (eds): Identification of the Nursing Minimum Data Set. Springer, New York, 1988.

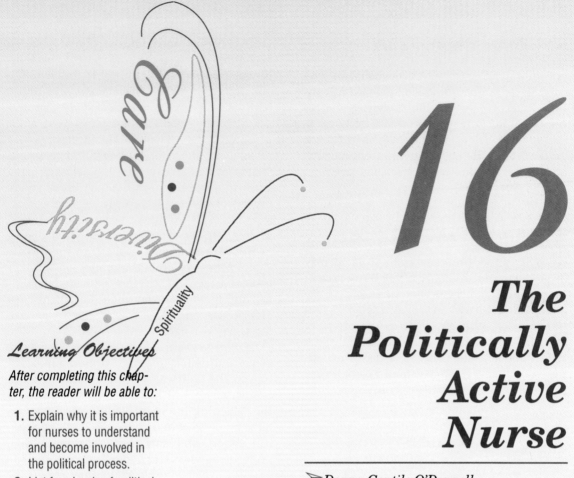

16

The Politically Active Nurse

➤ *Donna Gentile O'Donnell*

The word *politics* conjures up various images—some positive and some negative. There are images of great statesmanship, like the inaugural speech of John F. Kennedy exhorting the nation, "Ask not what your country can do for you, but what you can do for your country." Or images of more ignoble moments, like the conviction of former Vice-President Spiro Agnew, the national tragedy of Watergate, the resignation of Richard Nixon, and the impeachment proceedings against Bill Clinton, or the numerous negative campaign commercials vilifying a political opponent. Politics touches peoples lives at all levels, crossing national boundaries, affecting individual states, and permeating local governments.

Almost everyone has something to say about politics, ranging from political candidates, academicians, and members of the press to regular citizens. People define politics in many ways. One of the most cynical definitions of politics is offered by Ambrose Brice in *The Devil's Dictionary,* describing it as "a strife of interests masquerading as a contest of principles. The conduct of public affairs for private advantage." Other, more widely accepted definitions include "the art or science of government," "the art or science concerned with guiding or influencing government policy," or "the total complex of relations between men in society."[1]

GOVERNMENT AND POLITICS

Keep in mind that *government* is a very broad term that refers to almost any type of hierarchical structure that functions to organize and direct an organization. From this context, the governance structure of any health-care facility can be considered a type of government that has its own politics. At this level, nurses should have a considerable amount of political influence.

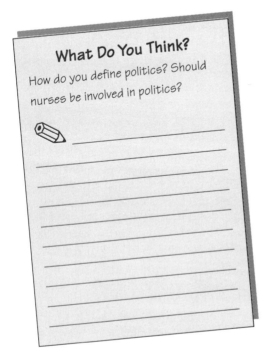

What Do You Think?

How do you define politics? Should nurses be involved in politics?

Historically, most nurses have avoided becoming engaged in government, perhaps because they share definitions similar to the one presented by Mr. Brice. However, nurses, both as individual citizens and as a professional group, need to recognize that their personal lives and professional practice are affected by the political world. Some recent trends in health care, particularly managed care and cost containment, have made nurses increasingly susceptible to the "bottom line." In addition, because of politics, nurses are confronting major changes in health care on a daily basis. They have experienced the erosion of the profession through their replacement with less educated personnel and have seen the quality of client care deteriorate. Nurses, if they decide to act, are not powerless against such trends.

As a large group of voters, nurses have the power, influence, and skill to take an active role in the political process. Senator Daniel Inouye of Hawaii has referred to nurses as the "sleeping giant in health care." Nurses have much to gain by using the tools of political action, and now more than ever their professional survival depends on it.

There are attainable, deliberate actions individual nurses can take that can create a powerful, political force. However, before nurses can realize their full potential, a basic knowledge and understanding of the political system is necessary. Henry Adams stated long ago that "Knowledge of human nature is the beginning and end of a political education." If he is correct, it is logical to conclude that nurses, who are among the most astute observers of human nature, are in many ways ideally suited to the art and science of politics. The goal of this chapter is to provide a foundation for understanding the political basics by using a "nuts and bolts" approach and to motivate nurses to become active in the political world. Politics is examined both within the profession of nursing and within society at large. In addition, this chapter discusses the forces that drive politics and the three concepts it comprises—partisanship, self-interest, and ideology.

WHY SHOULD NURSES BE INVOLVED?

A widely accepted definition of politics is the process of influencing public policy, including all forms and levels of governmental regulations. The effects of politics are pervasive and related to almost every aspect of life. On a personal level, politics influence where children go to school, the quality of food eaten, the water that flows from your kitchen tap, what medications are prescribed, and the speed limit on roadways. On a professional level, politics influences where nurses work, what they do and how they do it, the ability to organize professionally, and even the nurse's professional status through licensure and certification. The effects of politics on a person's life would seem to have no limits.

Nurses experience the effects of governmental regulations both directly and indirectly. Examples of directly experienced government regulations include some recent reforms that many states have initiated. Some state delegations have considered nurse-patient ratios. All states now have granted advanced practice nurses prescriptive privileges, although the regulations governing their implementation vary widely from state to state. Earlier attempts at national health-care reform have resulted in massive restructuring of the health-care system that led to dramatic decreases in the number of nurses employed in acute care hospitals. These reforms, initiated to forestall proposed legislation, continue to influence health care even today. Many nurses respond to these changes with sad acceptance and believe that they are beyond their control.

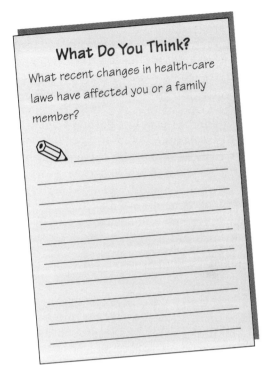

What Do You Think?

What recent changes in health-care laws have affected you or a family member?

DEFINITIONS OF POLITICS, POLITICAL ACTION, AND RELATED CONCEPTS

As a dynamic process, politics plays a key role in all forms and levels of government, including federal, state, and local. It can be seen as the complex interaction between the public policy and various public and constituent interests. Politics is directly and indirectly influenced by the self-interest of political officials, both elected and appointed. The mass media also have both a direct and indirect impact on the political process through numerous political commentators, political commercials, and investigations into the backgrounds of selected political figures.

Political action is a set of activities, methods, tactics, and behaviors that affect or have the potential to affect governmental and legislative processes and outcomes.[2] Examples of political action include grass-roots efforts to change policies, the activities of lobbyists to change elected officials' opinions or votes, the give and take of political compromise within legislative bodies, and even the power of veto by the chief executive of a governmental structure. Government is often thought of as a series of processes used to maintain society. As both an element of and result of politics, government is also influenced by the forces that drive politics and the three concepts that constitute it: (1) partisanship, (2) self-interest, and (3) ideology.

 Self-interest is almost always the most important factor in politics.

Partisanship refers to membership in a political party. Because of the limited nature of this chapter, it focuses on Democrats, Republicans, and to a lesser extent, Independents.

Self-interest is almost always the most important factor in politics. It dictates the kind of issues that legislators become involved in and present to their constituencies as the key issues. For instance, a congressman who resides in a district that has a Catholic majority who support a pro-life position will almost always be a pro-life congressman. The legislative structure in the United States was designed so that elected officials represent the people in their districts rather than having the whole population of the United States trying to make policy decisions. If a candidate does not represent the beliefs of the district, it is unlikely that he or she will succeed in that district.

In the larger world of electoral politics, the principle of self-interest often means that an elected official will not make legislative or political decisions that could lead to professional damage, namely loss of an election. Occasionally, there are exceptions to this rule. There have been a few cases in which elected officials were so ideologically committed to an issue that they defied conventional wisdom and made decisions that went against their self-interest. Generally, in order to be effective in politics, a person needs to understand and accept the self-interests of his or her constituents and use these self-interests as the driving force in their political decision making.

Ideology is a broad concept that embodies beliefs and principles of an individual or group. Conservatives, liberals, populists, libertarians, and radicals represent five examples of ideologies.

Conservatives. Traditional conservatives support less governmental regulation and involvement in everyday life, fewer taxes, and smaller social programs. The general characterization of the conservative belief system is "less government equals better government." Applied to the current range of issues, conservatives tend to be anti-abortion, anti–gun control, anti–socialized health care, and pro-choice on education.

Liberals. Traditional liberals believe that government has a moral responsibility to do good for society and that government intervention is necessary for the greater good of the citizens. This ideology, traditionally, translates into larger government structures, increased taxes, and larger spending for a wide range of social programs. Liberals are traditionally pro-choice, pro-gun control, pro–governmental regulated health care, and anti-choice on education.

Populists. Populists are probably the most dominant political force in America at a grassroots level. Although populists in general do not like paying high taxes, ideologically they may represent a variety of positions on any particular issue. For instance, one group of populists may be anti-abortion, whereas another may be pro-choice. The common bond among all populists is that they have a sense of being burdened by a large, oppressive governmental structure. "The middle class is under siege" is a major theme that has resonated throughout several recent presidential campaigns.

Libertarians. Libertarianism is both a political party and an ideology. As a political partisan group, they represent an electoral fringe element. Ideologically, Libertarians differ from populists because they do not have the underlying middle-class anger that often drives the populists to take political action. Although they do believe in fiscal conservatism and dislike paying high taxes, Libertarians tend to be "laid back" in their approach to politics. Typically, they avoid ideological battles because they do not want to be burdened with decisions about choice on gun control, health care, schools, or abortion.

Radicals. Radicals exist at either end of the ideological spectrum in both of the major parties. It is important to recognize that although most voters tend toward the middle of the political spectrum between conservatism and liberalism, radicals attempt to force their parties to the extreme ends of the spectrum. For instance, Republicans are challenged by the radical right, which consists of the anti–big government and pro-life forces that make conspicuous demands on the party. To counteract the rhetoric of the radicals, the Republican party will try to find candidates who are ideologically near the middle of the spectrum because they know that most Republican voters have opinions near the middle of the spectrum.

UNDERSTANDING THE PLAYING FIELD

Structure

The three branches of the government are the executive, judiciary, and legislative branches. These branches exist simultaneously at the federal, state, and local government levels. At the federal level, the executive branch consists of the President, Vice-President, Cabinet, and various executive administrative bodies. The executive of a state is the governor. Boards and commissions can also be construed as part of the executive branch because they are appointees of the chief executive. Locally, in county government, one or more county commissioners function as executives.

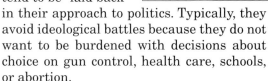

The judiciary branch of government should not be discounted as unimportant to nurses.

Larger cities usually have a mayor. Smaller cities and townships sometimes also elect mayors.

The judiciary branch is the court system. It is important to note that there is a distinction between state court and federal court; however, appeals and supreme courts are found at both levels. At the state level, there are supreme courts, appeals courts, and the lower courts. At the federal level, there is the Supreme Court, federal courts of appeal, and district or circuit courts. Additionally, many cities and counties have a local court system.

The judiciary branch of government should not be discounted as unimportant to nurses. Over the years, several important issues have been decided by courts that have an effect on the practice of nursing. These include the Supreme Court's decision regarding the right of nurses to organize into collective bargaining units (see Chapter 11 for more discussion), the requirement of health-care providers to report potentially violent patients to the police, the obligation for nurses to refuse to carry out physician orders they deem dangerous, and criteria for when nurses can withdraw life support measures. New test cases that are continually being brought before the Supreme Court have the potential to dramatically change the way that nurses are perceived and what they are permitted to do in the workplace.

At the federal level, the legislative branch of government consists of the House of Representatives and the Senate. Each state also has a legislative branch of government, and, except for Nebraska, all states have a bicameral legislature with both a House of Representatives and a Senate. The primary function of the legislative branch of government is the formation of policy by the making of laws.

> 66 99 *In most cases, the majority party has the capacity to pass almost any bill they support over the objections of the minority.*

Key Players in the Formation of Policy (Agenda) and the Legislative Process

Members of the legislative branch of government have a wide range of ability and influence. It is important to remember that legislators are human, and they respond to the same forces that all people respond to, including interpersonal dynamics, peer pressure, and both internal and external factors.

The majority leader in the House is the person who generally supervises and directs the activities on the House floor. Some consider it to be the most powerful job in politics. The majority leader has control over the legislative calendar, which ultimately determines when many of the House session activities take place and even when bills are introduced for consideration. The majority leader is also the central figure in crafting the budget, which is the single most important activity the legislature performs on an annual basis.

The majority whip is responsible for collecting votes when legislators may be leaning toward voting against their party. At the same time the majority leader is supporting a bill, the whip is negotiating on the House floor for the votes necessary to successfully pass the bill. The whip is responsible for collecting support and votes for various issues both during the legislative session and when they are in recess.

The minority leader represents the party that does not have a numerical majority in the House and helps organize support against bills introduced by the majority leader. The minority leader presents an alternative point of view. There is an expression in the legislature: "The majority will have their way, and the minority will have their say." In most cases, the majority party has the capacity to pass almost any bill they support over the objections of the minority. The minority leader usually only has the capacity to speak against it. However, there are some issues that legislators will almost never vote against—"mom," "pop," and the "little guy." When these issues are included in a bill, most legislators will support it even if they must vote against their party.

The conference committee attempts to reconcile differences in bills from the House and the Senate. The rules governing the structure, composition, and function of the conference committee vary from state to state. Generally, they consist of an equal number of appointed members from both the House and the Senate. Often a specified combination of votes, such as two votes from the house and two votes from the senate, are necessary to approve a compromise bill and move it out of committee.

Caucuses are formed when the legislature divides into groups comprising of people with mutual interests. These groups operate as a unit, trading on their capacity to bring a block of votes for or against an issue or bill, rather than an individual vote. Examples are the Black Caucus, the Women's Caucus, the Hispanic Caucus, and the Business Community Caucus. Although caucuses may be bipartisan, many are partisan in nature. For example, the largest caucus groups are the Democratic Caucus and the Republican Caucus. Each caucus develops its own internal governance structure and version of leadership, including a speaker who leads the caucus and speaks for the group. After a group member achieves a leadership role, he or she must try to balance the wishes of the group against his or her own political survival in the caucus and the political pressures exerted by the larger world.

The media and the voters are external forces that influence policy makers. The media has become a tangible power in government, often driving and shaping public opinion that eventually evolves into a legislative agenda. Although they claim to be objective, in reality the major news organizations decide what is and what is not news. The public often perceives media personalities as the people who know, write, and speak about the important public issues and matters of substance. One study performed at a large research university investigated how the media reported political campaigns for the years 1975-1995. The study compared the actual number of words recorded in writing or spoken on television by the candidates with the number of words spoken or written by the media about the candidate, which acted as a filter, translator, or commentator for the public. The

results showed that the media consistently outcommunicated the candidates at all levels.

Before media campaigns became the norm and millions of dollars were spent on television and radio advertising, the printed news media used to publish what the candidate said and often printed whole speeches. This approach allowed the public to read the speeches and make up their minds about which issues the candidate supported. Today, the trend is to give a 30-second sound bite of a speech, then have 10 minutes of political analysis by some well-known commentator who tells the public what the candidate is saying. Some of the printed media have adopted a similar approach to political issues. In newspapers, it is not unusual to see a lengthy editorial comment positioned right next to a statement made by a candidate. All elected offi-

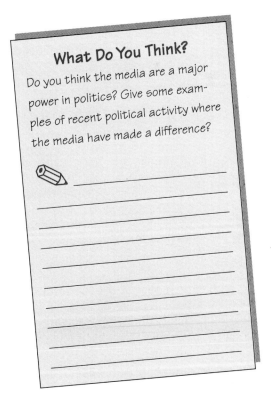

What Do You Think?

Do you think the media are a major power in politics? Give some examples of recent political activity where the media have made a difference?

cials have a great respect for the power of the media to influence public opinion. Those who are good elected officials learn to use this to their advantage.

Legislators, while recognizing and using the power of the media, have also become wary of it. They know that although they can use the media to proclaim their message, the media also pose a risk to their political survival, depending on the vulnerability of their position. Some legislators have a false sense of invulnerability because of the nature of their constituency base; for example, a legislator may have a large population of senior citizens in his district who have supported him for many years. The legislator publicly supports senior citizen issues and believes that the senior citizen support will always be there. However, during an election campaign, a political opponent's investigation uncovers information that the legislator actually voted against several bills that would have increased senior citizens' benefits. In addition, the opponent discovered that the legislator was having an affair with his married secretary. The opponent leaks this information to the media, which immediately put it on television and report it in the newspapers. If the story develops "legs," meaning it takes on a life of its own and continues to grow even without further information from the opponent, it will be on television news programs and in the newspapers every day. The major networks will do investigative reporting on the issues, and eventually the talk show and television tabloid programs will become interested and begin interviewing people who know or have heard about more "dirty little secrets" about the legislator. At this point, the legislator who is the subject of that story is in political jeopardy. There is little

> **" "** *There is little that a politician fears more than being the subject of a negative story that develops "legs."*

that a politician fears more than being the subject of a negative story that develops legs.

THE POLITICAL PROCESS
Who Introduces Legislation?

Laws serve to maintain order in a complicated society and regulate the interactions of its citizens. As society becomes more complex, more laws are needed to ensure the survival and smooth functioning of the population. For example, although computers and electronic communications have increased the quantity of information individuals can process and the speed at which it is transmitted, they have also added to the complexity of the world. Just a few years ago, there were no laws that dealt with "hacking," computer fraud, or computer theft of bank funds. Today, there is an ever-growing body of law that deals with computers, and whole sections of police agencies have been dedicated to enforcing these laws, such as the Federal Bureau of Investigation's Computer Crime Unit. However, where do ideas for laws and policies come from? And how do these ideas become laws?

Any elected official, including governors, mayors, county commissioners, and city council members, can propose a program or initiative that requires passage by the legislature (i.e., a bill). The elected official will go to the legislative leadership in the parties and ask them either to submit the bill or to help move the bill through the legislative process.

Lobbyists, constituency groups, and advocates are a major source of proposed legislation. They represent various interests ranging from public interest groups to corporate lobbyists. Lobbyists frequently craft legislation and then pass it to a friendly legislator. Consumer groups are often visible at the legislature through demonstrations and lobbying.

Constituency groups can best be described by example, such as the American Association of Retired Persons (AARP). These groups are made up of individuals interested in advancing an agenda that promotes a range of issues based on self-interests. Advocates, in contrast, can be described as groups who have a single issue or point of view that they are trying to advance, such as housing or abortion rights.

Legislation is also generated from governmental agencies. When agencies are seeking fee increases, or another type of policy reform, they can introduce legislation. For example, the recent policy reforms in the Internal Revenue Service (IRS) were a type of agency-initiated legislation. Frequently the employees of the agency will draft the legislation and then direct it toward a supportive legislator.

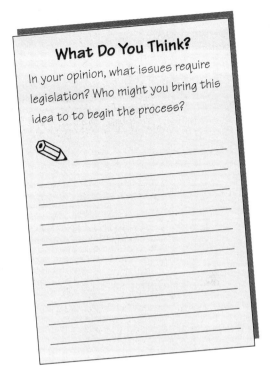

What Do You Think?

In your opinion, what issues require legislation? Who might you bring this idea to to begin the process?

What Issues Drive the Development of Legislation?

Funding. Because almost all government agencies depend on legislative funding to sustain their operations, they become actively engaged, overtly or covertly, in seeking the passage of a budget that will sustain their survival.

Public Demand. Legislators are very careful to listen to the demand of their voters and avoid voting against an issue to which the public is emotionally attached. A classic example of this process was seen in New Jersey, where a child was sexually molested and murdered by a known convicted sex offender who unknowingly moved into the child's neighborhood. The tragedy prompted a public outcry: How could this happen? Something needs to be done! Ultimately, the outcry produced the now famous Megan's Law, which requires public disclosure of a known sexual offender's residence.

Programmatic Issues. These issues recur periodically and require legislative attention. Requests for increases in television cable rates constitute an example of a programmatic issue. The cable industry will be very interested in the outcome of legislation that may affect what they can charge for their services. Both cable and consumer group lobbyists actively seek the ear of key legislators at these times.

Constituent-Specific Issues. Groups of voters may have specific interests that can lead to an introduction of a bill. For example, in legislative districts where a large population of senior citizens resides, the escalating cost of prescriptions may be an important issue. Legislation specific to that constituency will be introduced at a greater rate than in areas with fewer senior citizens in their populations.

What is the Process of Introducing Bills?

Any legislator can introduce a bill from any source. Additional legislators can sign on as the bill's cosponsors. A bill is considered to be strong if it has strong sponsorship, including a number of powerful cosponsors, a high degree of bipartisanship, and the interest of powerful individuals, both political and nonpolitical. After the bill is introduced, it is taken to the chief clerk who assigns it a number that permits it to be tracked throughout the process.

After the bill is assigned a number, it is referred to a committee. The House and Senate leaders make the decision on which committee considers the bill. This decision, greatly influenced by politics, is critical to the survival and ultimate passage of a bill. It is no coincidence that most bills die in committee. Invariably, the leadership discusses their expectation for the bill with the committee chairs, and if the leadership wants a bill to fail, it is referred to a committee where it will never be voted on or passed on to the House.

At the federal level, bills are referred to full committee and, generally, because of the enormous number of bills being introduced, to a subcommittee. It is within the committee structures that most of the work of Congress takes place. Committee action is perhaps the most important phase of the Congressional process, for this is where the most intensive consideration is given to proposed measures and where people are provided with an opportunity to be heard. The subcommittee studies the issue carefully,

holds hearings, and reports the bill back to the full committee with recommendations. There are numerous standing committees in the House and Senate. In addition, there are several select committees and several standing joint committees. Each committee has jurisdiction over certain subjects, and often has two or more subcommittees. In the U.S. Congress, the committees with greatest jurisdiction over health matters and their subcommittees are:

1. **House Ways and Means Committee:** Social Security and Medicare (healthcare subcommittees)
2. **House Commerce Committee:** Health legislation including Medicaid (Subcommittee on Health and the Environment)
3. **Senate Finance Committee:** Medicare and Medicaid (health subcommittees)
4. **Senate Labor and Human Resources Committee:** Health legislation in general; it also works cooperatively with the Senate Finance Committee in considering issues involving Medicare and Medicaid
5. **House and Senate Appropriations Committee:** Authorizes all money necessary to implement action proposed in a bill (Subcommittees for Labor, Education, and Health and Human Services)

As a result of full committee hearings, several things may happen to a bill. It may be:

- Reported out of committee favorably and be scheduled for debate by the full House or Senate
- Reported out favorably, but with amendments
- Reported out unfavorably
- Killed outright

For example, a bill reforming the way that judges are elected ideally would go to the judiciary committee; however, there is no legal requirement that the speaker or the Senate Pro Tem President send the bill to any particular committee. For political reasons, the speaker may refer the bill to the committee on intergovernmental affairs, where it will languish and die.

In order for a bill to survive, the bill sponsor must have the knowledge and the political standing to move the bill out of committee. If sponsors are truly committed, they will trade on their political capital. *Political capital* is a term that generally refers to some type of favor or action that a politician can exchange for something he or she wants. It is an extremely important element in the legislative process and consists of, but is not limited to, votes, amendments to bills, appointments, and support from constituency groups. Political capital often consists of an "If you vote for my bill, I'll vote for your bill" type of exchange.

After a bill has been reported out of a House committee (with the exception of Ways and Means or Appropriations Committees), it goes to the Rules Committee, which schedules bills and determines how much time will be spent on debate and whether or not amendments will be allowed. In the Senate, bills go on the Senate calendar, after which the majority leadership determines when a bill will be debated. After a bill is debated, possibly amended, and passed by one chamber, it is sent to the other chamber, where it goes through the same procedure. If the bill passes both the House and the Senate without any changes, it is sent to the President for his signature.

If the House and Senate pass different versions of a bill, however, the two bills are sent to a Conference Committee, which consists of members appointed by both the House and the Senate. This committee seeks to resolve differences between the two bills; if the differences cannot be resolved,

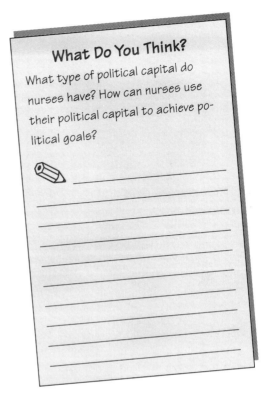

What Do You Think?

What type of political capital do nurses have? How can nurses use their political capital to achieve political goals?

the bill dies in committee. After the Conference Committee reaches agreement on a bill, it goes back to the House and Senate for passage. At this juncture, the bill must be voted up or down, because no further amendments are accepted.

If the bill is approved in both houses, it then goes to the chief executive. At the federal level the President, or at the state level, the Governor, who then make determinations about bills. Governors can do one of two things: sign the bill into law or actively veto the bill. At the federal level, the President has the same options, with the addition of the pocket veto. Pocket vetoes, found only at the federal level, occur when the President rather than actively vetoing a bill, simply does not sign it so that it does not become law. If vetoed, it is sent back to the House and Senate. In order to override

Know the Structure to Play the Game

One of the keys to creating power is understanding the organizational structure of the government. The Constitution of the United States establishes three separate branches of the federal government: legislative, judicial, and executive. The Constitution also ascribes certain auxillary powers to the individual states. It is the role of the state governments to serve its citizens within these parameters and to delegate discrete areas of activity to local governments.

Beneath the federal level of government in the United States, there exist state governments and five layers of local government identified by the US census bureau: county, municipal, township, school district, and special district governments (which include various utility, construction, and facility authorities). The qualifications for the classification of these local government structures are generally determined by the parent state governments. State governments are governed by their individual state constitutions and in turn delineate responsibility for the local governments.

It is important for nurses to understand that there are three levels in each governmental sector: federal, state, and local. These distinctions are important and are the most common source of confusion for nurses.

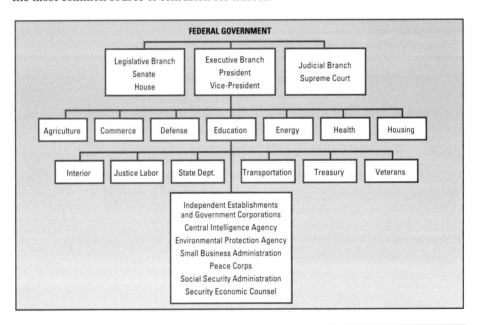

➤ Figure 16-1

The organizational structure of the government.

the veto, a two-thirds vote by both chambers is required.

Clearly, the passage of a law can be a long and difficult process. This is often quite frustrating for "action-oriented" nurses who are used to seeing immediate outcomes, forming plans, and making things happen quickly.

All bills that are passed need a fiscal note attached to them. Therefore, the appropriation committee is operationally very power-

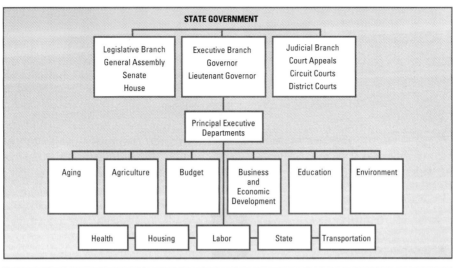

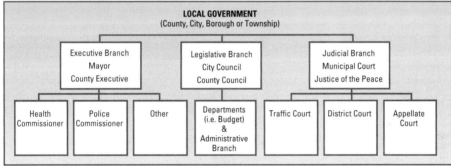

> Figure 16-1 (continued)

ful. A piece of legislation that is passed without a fiscal note attached will never become a reality. Over the years, many pieces of legislation have been passed by the legislature, but have been starved to death financially.

Major regulatory change occurs in laws in the form of housekeeping bills. Legislators can use this tactic to move a piece of legislation through the process, especially when the bill is more significant than the leadership acknowledges it to be. Although regulatory reform and change may seem tedious, they are important to the legislative process

and have the capacity to do enormous public good or harm.

Executive Orders

Executive orders provide the Chief Executive, the Governor, or the President with a means for moving an agenda item forward. Executive orders are in many cases a convenient way to formulate policy with minimal involvement from the legislature. They also allow the executive to make a statement about an issue that can be entered on the public record. The legislature can leave executive orders uncontested or challenge them, by characterizing them as beyond the scope of the executive branch. This may involve turning to the third branch of government, the judiciary.

Regulatory Agencies

Regulatory agencies are also arenas where policies are made and amended. For instance, the role of the Intergovernmental Regulatory Reform Commission (IRC) is to examine regulatory issues across the state.

HOW TO BE POLITICALLY ACTIVE

Why Organize or Be Politically Active?

The first step in becoming politically active is to identify the specific goals that nurses, as a group, want to accomplish. Nurses recognize many important issues in today's health-care system, including the increasing acuity of hospitalized clients who require higher levels of care and more complex level of support than ever before, increasing responsibilities for nurses in supervision of rising numbers of unlicensed health-care personnel, loss of control of the work environment through managed-care organizations, and ever-shortening hospitalizations resulting in clients being sent home "quicker and sicker." Any one of these issues can become a focal point at which nurses aim their considerable political power.

For example, most nurses are concerned that registered nurses who have traditionally been at clients' bedsides are being replaced by individuals who are less prepared and less able to deal with high-acuity clients. Nurses believe that when they are replaced in large numbers by unlicensed assistive personnel including nursing assistants, as well as with personnel who provide specific services, like monitor technicians who sit in front of cardiac monitors, the quality of client care decreases. Nurses know that these technicians are many times taking on responsibilities for which they have had little training. Rarely are there established national standards for these assistive personnel that require them to demonstrate their ability to provide a specific level of care or that even protect the public safety.

Nurses are usually employees at will and can be fired for any reason. Whistle blower protection is generally not available to protect nurses who wish to speak out against unsafe staffing levels or employment practices. Nurses are, at times, torn between their obligations to maintain high standards of safe, ethical care and their obligations to their families. Although nurses often feel powerless against a giant monolithic health-care bureaucracy, in reality they have the potential to be a potent political force. Nationally, with 2.2 million nurses licensed to practice, the nursing profession constitutes the largest single body of health-care providers in the country.

Nurses in all health-care settings are saying "somebody's got to do something about this situation." The reality of the situation is that the "somebody" is nurses. Once nurses identify exactly what it is that needs to be accomplished and understand what is possible within the political framework, then they can use their considerable political power to make changes that will benefit both the clients and the profession.

> 66 99 *Nurses believe that when they are replaced in large numbers by unlicensed assistive personnel, the quality of patient care decreases.*

The Need for Organization at the State Level

Donna Gentile O'Donnell

Why do nurses need to organize at the state level?

There is a debate that is just starting in nursing about the political activity the ANA is involved in at the federal level.

The ANA over the last several years has successfully raised money through telemarketing in every state in the country. Many nurses do not realize that the ANA Political Action Committee (PAC) is now the second largest federal versus state published action (PAC) in Washington. In the last election cycle they raised $1.2 million that was spent on political activities exclusively at the federal level. However, it is important to realize that many of the political battles that nurses have to fight are at the state level.

There is an ongoing discussion between the federal and state governments about what constitutes a legitimate course of action for the federal government and what constitutes a legitimate course of action for the state government, particularly with respect to the current trends. The tenth amendment to the Constitution essentially says that any powers that are not expressly articulated to be part of the federal government mandate go to the states. This amendment underlies the current debate about Medicaid and Medicare and whether or not the states should be responsible for its administration.

The concept of unfunded mandates has come to the forefront in the past few years as a result of the states' rights push. There is an ongoing discussion among the National Governors' Association demanding that the federal government give more latitude to the way that governors are permitted to govern their states. They are saying: "Don't give us mandates. Give us the opportunity to set our own standards, to set our own regulatory actions, and to set our own legislative and governmental agenda." The nation is moving toward greater state control governmentally. It would be great if nurses could organize and just concentrate on issues at the federal level in Washington, but because most of nursing's issues are at the state level, this strategy is probably not going to work.

For nursing organizations to be effective, there has to be organized political action among nurses and by nurses in every state in this country. Those states that are not active and organized politically are going to be in trouble, and the nurses in them will fare badly. Nurses need to be conscious of the fact that the trend is toward states becoming more active politically and determiners of their own fate in government. Consequently, nurses need to organize politically at the state level.

Another thing to keep in mind is that nurses' licensure, as well as the certification and regulation of hospitals, is a function of the state. Again, it does not make sense to concentrate all of nursing's resources at the national level. Of course there are some issues and programs, particularly with respect to funding, in which federal action is necessary. But most of the issues that nurses are going to be dealing with occur at the state level, and that is where attention needs to be focused. The reality of the situation is that the states have the capacity to define and regulate objective standards for both nurses and hospitals. The mandate for nursing is to define how those standards are established and then develop an achievable agenda for political action by nurses at the state level.

Rules for Radicals

Saul Alinksky, in *Rules for Radicals,* hypothesizes that human beings are divided into three groups: "the have's, the have nots, and the have a little and want mores." Nursing typically falls in the last group.

One problem nurses in this group encounter is the ongoing conflict between the status quo and progress. They want to obtain more power and control, gain more benefits, earn more money, and have more respect as professionals. However, the strong desire to advance is counterbalanced by fear of jeopardizing their current jobs and their professional standing. Their motivation to be something more, to do something new, or to believe in something bigger is held back and pulled in another direction by their fear of change. The result of this internal tug-of-war is an attitude of inertia and ambivalence that has prevented nurses from organizing politically and effectively using their numerical power.

Despite the inertia and ambivalence problems of individuals in the "have a little and want more" category, some of the most notable revolutionaries in history have come from this group, including Thomas Jefferson, Napoleon Bonaparte, Martin Luther King, Jr., and Vladimir Lenin. Each of these individuals came from the working middle class with a belief that it could be made better. Nurses can use their actions as examples of what individuals can accomplish to raise their own motivation levels to a point where it overwhelms the inertia of the status quo.

A fourth group of people, who seem to evolve from the inertia found among the "have a little, want more" group are the "do nothings." These individuals can be heard saying things like, "I agree with what you are saying, I just don't agree with your means," "I'm not going to get involved in this," or "I'm too busy to belong to the organization." The "do nothings" tend to watch the activities of others, and if their efforts are successful, then they will join in as a beneficiary because they feel they have supported the effort from an ideological standpoint. However, they avoid any active involvement in politics. Edward Burke recognized the danger in the do nothings. He said, "The only thing that is necessary for the triumph of evil, is for good men (and women) to do nothing."

What Can One Nurse Do?

It is important to remember that politics is a free market enterprise open to anyone who is willing to become involved and play the game. Success in the political arena is contingent on three elements: (1) knowledge and understanding of the process; (2) the ability to offer something of value to the political figure; and (3) the capacity to identify what will be necessary to accomplish the objective. Anyone who is interested in becoming politically active must recognize that all candidates and elected officials need three things: resources to run their political operation (money and volunteers), votes, and a means to shape public opinion.

Sufficient resources are essential to running a political campaign. The first and most necessary resource is always money. Would-be candidates soon discover that a lack of money to fund a campaign will inevitably lead to political failure. An unfunded candidate cannot travel, send mailings, produce radio and television commercials, post signs, or organize a telephone bank. Voters often fail to realize that political candidates are only as available as finances permit. Frequently, good candidates lose because they fail to garner the financial resources necessary to run an effective campaign. Nurses can gain a candidate's support for issues by donating to his or her campaign chest.

A second important resource in an election campaign is volunteers. Volunteers work in campaigns by manning telephone banks, making literature drops, placing signs, and conducting voter registration drives. Usually political candidates are very glad to have the free help for their campaigns. Although nurses may not be able to make large monetary contributions to a candidate's campaign, they can always volunteer some time. Working closely with a candidate on a volunteer basis allows individuals to discuss important issues on a personal basis and helps candidates win who support issues important to nurses.

Obviously, votes are essential to any candidate. If a candidate does not have votes,

> ## What Do You Think?
> Have you ever helped a political candidate you supported in any way? How?
>
> ✏ _____
> _____
> _____
> _____
> _____
> _____
> _____
> _____
> _____
> _____

he or she will not be elected. One of the most significant activities nurses can become involved in is to join and support a political party. The chosen party should reflect the nurse's value system and fundamental beliefs. Keep in mind that there is never a perfect fit with any political party. Almost everyone who belongs to a political party will disagree at some point with some element of the party, usually with the extremist views. However, differing opinions and beliefs should not serve as a barrier to membership in a political party. The only way to change a view or opinion is by active participation from within the party. The ultimate political power is the vote. Nurses need to be registered to vote and then actually go to the polls on election day to cast their ballots for the candidates who support legislation that empowers nurses and recognizes the needs for beneficial health-care reform.

Candidates need endorsements from their constituents so that they can build their support base. They generally consider endorsements from nurses as one of the most valuable assets to their campaign. By carefully selecting candidates who support legislation favorable to nursing and health care, endorsements can give nurses the capacity to shape public opinion. The periodic polls conducted by national news magazines asking readers to rank various professions on how much they were trusted have consistently shown that the public views nurses very highly, in the same category as police officers and teachers.

Nurses should use endorsements by choosing candidates in campaigns that have an impact on important issues. Often the campaigns for governor fall into this category, because governors, as chief executives, have a great deal of political power and can appoint people to a number of boards, committees, and positions. Nurses need to recognize that the members of the board of nursing in their state, as well as other important appointed positions in the health departments and other regulatory agencies, may be appointed by the governor and that this board has the final decision in the way that nurses practice. When nurses establish a working political relationship with the chief executive of the state, the governor is more likely to look favorably on those who have sustained him or her, supported him or her financially, and given him or her endorsements during the political campaign. They will be the people that he or she is going to appoint to a board position.

Targeting endorsements will prevent nurses from making blind political decisions. Candidates should be assessed first on their willingness to be supportive to issues that nurses are interested in and then on their capacity to win the election.

In 1992, Chalich and Smith[3] offered a model for individual political development that encourages grassroots involvement in local issues. As a nurse activist herself, Chalich contends that whereas some involvement in partisan politics may be desirable, grassroots efforts may be more fulfilling and should certainly not be discounted. This model is an activity-oriented ladder, including activities at four distinct levels:

- Rung 1—Civic involvement: Children's sports, parent-teacher association (PTA), neighborhood improvement group
- Rung 2—Advocacy: Writing letters to public officials and newspapers and making organized visits to officials on local issues
- Rung 3—Organizing: Independent organizing on local issues, incorporation of single-issue citizens' groups, and networking with similarly situated citizens' groups
- Rung 4—Long-term power wielding: Campaigning for oneself or another, local government planning, and agenda setting

Nurses usually shudder at the thought of running for political office. They tend to perceive political campaigns as something that is underhanded and tawdry and just do not want to be involved. However, it is not impossible for nurses to achieve high status in public office. Several nurses hold elected office in state and local government level, including Barbara Hafer, RN, State Treasurer of Pennsylvania, and Marilyn Goldwater,

> **" "** *By carefully selecting candidates who support legislation favorable to nursing and health care, endorsements can give nurses the capacity to shape public opinion.*

RN, who serves in the Maryland State Senate and has been a delegate to the national convention.

One way that nurses can direct their political activities is to develop a political relationship with a legislator or a political operative who can mentor and guide the nurse in finding a route through the political maze. As discussed earlier, the principle of self-interest is one of the most critical elements in politics, and in order to establish a relationship with a political figure, nurses must demonstrate that the issues they support have value to both themselves and to the politician.

> 66 99 *One way that nurses can direct their political activities is to develop a political relationship with a legislator or a political operative who can mentor and guide the nurse in finding a route through the political maze.*

There are several ways that a nurse can make decisions on who to support when becoming involved in the political process. A first step is to begin identifying the issues particular legislators are interested in and will vote for. Opinion editorial pieces in the editorial section of newspapers can provide a sense of the issues of concern to legislators. It is a good idea to begin with local legislators and candidates, like the state representative, state senator, or the council person serving the neighborhood. Call their offices and find out when and where they are scheduled to speak, then go and listen to the speech to get a sense of who they are and what issues they support. Their speeches and the way that they answer questions will reveal their ideology and partisanship. Also, during question and answer periods, ask elected officials what they think about issues important to you.

Another way to become familiar with prominent political figures is by attending some of the many partisan events that occur during an election season. A good way to visualize the local political landscape is by observing who is talking to whom at the event. Nurses can make their own assessments of political candidates based on observations of the candidates in action, calling their offices for information, reading published literature, or talking to people who know the candidate. Beginning the process may seem difficult, but once a decision is made to become politically active, you'll become more confident.

Know the Issues

For nurses to be successful in the political process, they must know and understand the issues. At times an issue may be readily apparent in the nurses' community, for example, an increased number of homeless people. Other issues are easily identified by reading newspapers. Issues are generally presented in the editorial section; most newspapers also have a political watch section, which reports the results of any significant votes at the state and federal levels.

The ANA newspaper, *American Nurse,* is an excellent source of information on issues of concern to the profession. In addition, the American Journal of Nursing *Newsline* feature and Nursing and Health Care's *Washington Focus* serve as excellent, easily readable sources of information in journals. *Capitol Update,* the ANA legislative newsletter for nurses, reports on the activities of its nurse lobbyists and on significant issues in the Congress and regulatory agencies. This publication requires a subscription but is available in most nursing schools and hospital libraries.

State nurses' associations and many specialty nursing groups also publish newsletters or legislative bulletins. Many of these are free to members but may be sent only when requested. When one is a member of a nursing organization, Action Alerts may also be sent to inform members of vital issues and the action needed by nurses.

Tactics

Tactics, essential tools for those who desire to be politically active, are the conscious and deliberate acts that people use to live and deal with each other and the world around them. In a political sense, tactics usually means using whatever resources are available to achieve a desired goal. Hannibal, one of the great tacticians in political history, said, "We will either find a way or we will make a way." Nurses, with their long history of accomplishing much with few resources, are natural tacticians. As nurses learn how to organize themselves for political purposes, they can use their well-developed tactical skills to achieve important political goals. Listed below are some easy-to-use tactics for political action.

Use the Resources That Have the Most Power (Money, Endorsements, Votes). For example, there are approximately 270,000 licensed nurses in Pennsylvania. By enlisting 25% of those nurses and collecting minimal dues, a powerful political force can be organized. If 25% of 270,000 nurses contribute $75 to a political action committee per year, approximately $5 million in annual revenue will be produced. In most states, $5 million would almost guarantee a win in any election.

Engage in Bipartisan Tactics. Both Republican and Democratic nurses need to be politically active to achieve unified goals.

> " " *In politics, getting the facts and laying the groundwork are analogous to developing a nursing care plan.*

Political action across the spectrum of issues and across partisan lines is necessary to achieve the goal of bipartisanship. Nurses should understand that only by supporting candidates who favor nursing and its agenda, whether they are Democrat or Republican, can the profession make changes that will advance the agenda of the discipline. The most important thing, always, is the issue being addressed and not the personality or party of the candidate.

Sometimes communications with legislators take the form of lobbying. Lobbying may be defined as attempting to persuade someone (usually a legislator or legislative aide) of the significance of one's cause or as an attempt to influence legislation. Lobbying methods include letter writing; face-to-face communication or telephone calls; mailgrams, telegrams, or e-mail; letters to the editor; and providing testimony (verbal or written).

In order to lobby effectively, one should be both persuasive and able to negotiate. Lobbying is truly an art of communication, an area in which nurses can become skilled. Before beginning any lobbying effort, it is vital to gather all pertinent facts. In politics, getting the facts and laying the groundwork are analogous to developing a nursing care plan. Before visiting or writing a legislator, gather facts, delineate a problem or concern you wish to discuss, and develop a plan to articulate your concerns. Determine a method for evaluating your effectiveness.

If the plan is to visit the legislator's office, an appointment should be set up in advance. Most often the meeting may actually be with the legislative aide, particularly at the federal level. This should not be discouraging because this is the individual who is often responsible for assisting in the development of position statements and

16.1 Alinski's Rules for Tactics (with O'Donnell's Comments)

- Power is not only what you have but what the enemy thinks you have.

  This is widely used in political organizing. Fund raising reports are a classic example. Candidates will work very hard to get their financial commitments before filing their candidacy, to inform people of their ammunition.

- Never go outside the experience of your own people.

  This is the fundamental mistake that has been made in some efforts to organize nurses. The American Nurses Association and the state associations too often reflect an elite group not connected to the real world. Their leadership tends not to be nurses from the bedside or intimately connected with front-line nursing. Their issues, although legitimate, are not the experience of the nurses entrenched in patient care issues.

- Wherever possible, go outside the experience of your enemy. Pick your battlefields.

  During a press conference around the March on Washington in 1996, nurses talked about their experiences that were foreign territory to the press. They presented a compelling picture. Most of the press were not accustomed to listening to nurses talk about high-tech procedures and gained a new level of respect for what nurses do. To the extent to which you can impress people with your knowledge and go outside their experience, it forces them to compete.

- Make them live up to their own book of rules.

  An example of this rule happened many years ago. Bob O'Donnell, former speaker of the Pennsylvania House, tells a story about when he was first breaking into the political world. There was a party machine that was not interested in supporting the common interests of the neighborhoods. Undaunted, he learned the rules for which the next ward leader and committee person election would be held. Ward leaders and committee people are the smallest unit of the partisan political system. Usually committee people are responsible for districts. The districts add up to the ward. The ward leader oversees the committee people who manage those districts and register people to vote. Standing within the system is necessary in order to be successful in a political system. The way to do that in the ward structure is to either be ward leader or to have significant influence over the ward leader. Over a period of several years, O'Donnell assisted his allies in obtaining committee people positions. When there was an election for the ward leader, the committee people elected O'Donnell to the position of ward leader. The party machinery refused to seat the ward leader. O'Donnell used their own rule book to bring the issue to federal court and forced them to seat the new ward leader. He beat them at their own game.

- Ridicule is man's and woman's most potent weapon.

  This is also known as the Dan Quayle phenomenon. Dan Quayle has been repeatedly characterized as a

BOX

16.1 Alinski's Rules for Tactics *(continued)*

political buffoon. Dan Quayle is not as unintelligent as people assume him to be. Unfortunately for him, Vice-President Quayle did some uninformed things while he happened to be standing in front of a magnifying glass with the national press behind it. More recently, Bill Clinton became the focus of many a political joke because of his involvement with Monica Lewinski. His Republican enemies seized on the incident to the point where they made it an issue of impeachment.

- A good tactic is one that your people enjoy.

    The 1996 March on Washington is a wonderful example. Laura Gasparis Vonfrolio did a wonderful job of tapping into the anger disseminated all over the country. Nurses enjoyed the national forum that permitted a massive demonstration for their voices to finally be heard.

- A tactic that drags on too long, becomes a drag; use the concepts of reward and momentum.

    This is the most dangerous element for nurses attempting political organizing. The process is difficult and takes time to reach a successful conclusion. Nurses can become discouraged by the slow pace of the change process in the political arena. Rather than only focusing on long-range goals, it is important to concentrate on smaller objectives as, for instance, achieving a significant role in a city council race.

- Keep the pressure on. Become the constant by which all other variables are defined.

Currently, the American Nurses Association (ANA) defines issues and concepts at the national level. The ANA has raised money in every state and has translated that money into a political power base in Washington. When a senator or congressman who has been a beneficiary of the ANA's largess takes a position, it is with the ANA in mind. Nurses need to become the standard by which all related variables are measured in their states. State legislators need to consider nurses' opinions the same way they do now with the teachers' association.

- The threat is usually more terrifying than the thing itself. Threat is multiplied by the unknown and the imagination of someone under attack.

    This principle can be used very effectively over time. Imagine if someone opposed pro-nursing legislation and nurses threatened to demonstrate. The public image of thousands of nurses donning their uniforms would be a very powerful image for legislators to contend with.

- The major premise for tactics is the development of operations that will maintain a constant pressure on the opposition. The pressure must be sustainable over time.

    This is the concept of what/then. In a tactical plan, you have to be able to look beyond and determine what happens after you reach the end of this tactic.

- Pick the target. Freeze it. Personalize it. Polarize it. And use a focused and strategic attack.

Essentially, nurses need to be focused in their political activities. For example, imagine that nurses have considerable support from various legislative groups for objective standards and want to pass a law. A solid bill has been drafted. But a Democrat or Republican will not introduce your bill. The strategy is to target the one person who is slowing it down, whether it is the speaker, the senate pro tem president, or majority leader. Pick the target. Freeze it. Go after it with a vengeance. Personalize the attack and look at their constituencies. If they have a large senior citizen constituency, proclaim to the media that the prevention of the passage of your legislation is putting senior citizens in your legislative district in danger. The legislator will have to respond. Remember the one cardinal tenet of legislative action, never hurt "mom," "pop," or the "little guy." That is a focused and strategic attack.

offering committee amendments for the legislator.

To ensure that legislators listen to your concerns, it is important not only to be well prepared but to show that others support your position. When one person speaks, legislators may listen, but when many people voice the same concern, legislators are much more likely to pay attention.

Benefit Through Collaboration. Nurses can increase their political power by making alliances with other powerful constituency groups who support similar issues, such as the American Association of Retired Persons (AARP). The AARP is very interested in health-care issues, particularly managed care, national health insurance, and the decreased quality of care from the increased use of nonlicensed personnel. Nurses who are organized into collective bargaining units can use the alliance with powerful unions. Unions are traditionally concerned with issues such as working conditions, including staffing patterns in hospitals, wages, job security, and benefits. Nurses are concerned about the same issues.

Alinsky provides useful pointers regarding tactics that nurses can use. Box 16.1 summarizes and gives examples for Alinsky's rules for tactics.

How to Organize

"Know thyne enemy" is one of the most fundamental rules that tacticians must follow, whether it is in war or politics. Napoleon was successful as a tactician and general because before he fought any battle, he walked the battlefield. He knew what the terrain was like, and he knew where the rocks and crevices were. He knew what to anticipate when he arrived on the battlefield. Nurses who want to be successful in a political battle must first learn the hills and valleys and rocks and crevices of the primary political battlefield, their own state demographics.

Important demographics for organizing nurses at the state level:

- *Total population of the state.* The total population of the state provides a demographic overview of the political arena.
- *Total number of registered voters.*

- *Total number of registered voters by political party.*
- *Total number of likely voters in any given election cycle.* To determine this number, the difference between an on-year election cycle and off-year election cycle should be understood. An on-year election cycle occurs when there is a major race in the state, usually during a presidential or gubernatorial race. An off-year cycle is when a major race is not being run. There may be city council races or even a state representative or senate race, but the majority of the population do not consider these major races, and fewer people tend to vote. Also, lower levels of political activity are seen in an off-year election cycle.
- *Total number of registered nurses.* The total number of registered nurses in a state can be obtained from the state board of nursing. Comparing the number of actual voters with the number of registered nurses in a state provides an indication of the potential power of an RN voting block. For example, if there are 800,000 people who regularly vote in a state and there are a total of 300,000 nurses in the state who are organized into a voting block about a particular issue, then that group of nurses represents a significant percentage of voters, and candidates running for statewide office will be interested in having nurses' support. Nurses must be encouraged to register and vote to increase the power of the block.

Comparing numbers helps define the political landscape of a state.

Important Characteristics of an Organizer

Many of the characteristics of an organizer listed in Box 16.2 are the same characteristics that are required of nurses on a daily basis in the practice of their profession. Although these characteristics may have varying degrees of value for the organizer, the one critical element a political organizer has to have is the capacity to communicate. Although nurses usually have a well-developed ability to communicate at the bedside, they may lack the confidence to communicate in the larger public and political arenas. Nurses need to recognize that the communication skills that they use on a daily basis, when explaining complicated medical jargon to clients, are the same skills they can use in translating health-care issues into a language that the public and elected officials can understand. One way to gain the public's interest and elected officials' support is to personalize health-care issues by stressing the fact that nurses are the professionals who provide the bulk of direct care for their mothers, fathers, brothers, and children. Communication of issues that touch people personally is usually the most effective method.

BOX 16.2 Characteristics of an Organizer

Curiosity
Motivation
Reverence
Realism
Flair for the dramatic
Sense of humor
Charisma
Self-confidence
Communication skills
Clear vision of the future
Capacity to change
Persistence
Ability to organize
Imagination

AFTER ORGANIZATION— WHAT THEN?

Drafting Legislation and Creating Change

The critical questions must be asked. The first question always must be, "Who is the decision maker?" For example, if there is an issue that needs to be resolved in the state board of nursing, the first step is to identify who makes the decisions at the board. Although the board members make decisions, it is important to remember that the people who sit on the board are appointed. Who appoints them and what is the basis of those appointments? If they are political appointees, they usually have some sort of political benefactor or a political relationship with someone in power. By understanding these types of relationships, it becomes easier to determine their ideological and parti-

san positions on many issues. For example, if a nursing board is newly appointed by a recently elected Republican governor, it is probably safe to assume that most of the board members are Republicans who agree with the governor on many key issues.

The second question to address is: "How accessible is the appointee's benefactor?" Sometimes board members are appointed by the legislative leadership and not the governor. It is important to discover who appointed the board and whether or not individual voters have access to them. Generally, the access by individual voters to the power figures who make these types of appointments is very limited. Organized groups, like the American Nurses Association, provide the best avenue of access at the federal level. Other questions that need to be answered include:

- How successful have nurses been in the past in achieving specific goals?
- What positions do nurses hold in government?
- What does the state board look like politically?
- Which legislators have supported nursing issues in the past?
- Which legislators traditionally oppose nursing and health-care issues?

Because of the failure to ask and answer these questions, numerous pieces of pronursing legislation that have been introduced have died in committee or lacked sponsors to move the bill through the process. Nurses in those states where nurses are in tune with the political issues and powers have more success moving bills through the legislative process so that they become law than in states where nurses are apathetic about the political process.

Even if a bill favorable for nurses or health care does not pass the first time, the fact that it was brought to a vote is important for several reasons. First, it has

16.3 A Political Nurse's Bedtime Story

Once upon a time in a far-off place many years in the future, there exists a world where nurses have real political power. In every state, there is an organized and successful political nursing organization. A small group of committee nurses organized and ultimately phone-banked their way across the state. Committed nursing students telerecruited 50,000 nurses, at $75 a piece, for a total of $3.75 million in annual revenue minus operating expenses. Bipartisan contributions were made to political candidates who met the following criteria:

These candidates have gone on the record endorsing a pro-nursing, pro-–health care agenda in a pre-endorsement questionnaire that they were asked to complete. They actually completed it and mailed it in, and they even called to make sure it was received, because nurses' support is now important to them.

The selected candidates now have a reasonable chance of election or re-election, particularly when supported by nurses at the level they are requesting. If one calls requesting a $50,000 contribution, with $3.75 million in the bank, $50,000 is not a hard check to write.

They have demonstrated their interest in the profession by developing a real relationship with the American Nurses Association. This relationship goes far beyond the traditional political greeting cards to the point where, when a call is placed to their political headquarters, the candidate—and not a volunteer staff person—actually speaks with the nurse. This relationship is evidenced by other events. For example, several nurses have been appointed to influential committees, boards, commissions, and other influen-

tial positions in state government. In addition to having access to the newly elected governor, nurses have played substantial roles in the election or re-election of two dozen legislative seats.

All the political players know the nursing organization and the power it represents. They say, "You should call the nurses. They'll give you a contribution. But you'd better support their issue." Members from both sides of the aisle and both chambers are available to sponsor and lobby legislation the nursing organization has drafted. Nurses hire their own experts to testify at the committee hearings and to put nursing legislation together and guide it through the process. Nurses know that if they play "political hardball" and remain cohesive on an issue, they can control a block of votes that is so substantial that legislators will quake in their shoes with the knowledge that nurses will vote against them. But, nurses hardly ever have to do that, because the threat that the nurses will be against an elected official is enough to make even the most seasoned elected official cower.

Because of nursing's influence, the governor has established an independent regulatory commission that reviews the practices of hospitals, including nurse-patient ratios and independent standards of care. A senior nursing organization member chairs the health-care regulatory commission. The legislature has passed legislation giving specific protection to nurses who are whistle blowers; thus, if a nurse reports an institution for delivering unsafe patient care, he or she will not risk termination of his or her employment. The prime sponsor of the protective leg-

BOX

16.3 A Political Nurse's Bedtime Story *(continued)*

islation was a nurse who was recently elected to the state legislature. In addition, several nurses were appointed to various high-ranking posts in state government. Other members are now high-ranking aides to legislative leaders on both sides of the aisle. There are more jobs for nurses everywhere. Unlicensed personnel are moved into appropriate roles. Nurses are respected in the health provider community, and that respect translates into salaries commensurate with experience and lifestyles that reflect that new standing.

Is this a dream? It is now, but it doesn't have to be. Consider it as a vision of what can be. But, this vision will have to be realized by recognition among our colleagues that this is a battle worth fighting and worth winning.

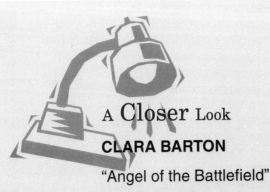

A Closer Look

CLARA BARTON

"Angel of the Battlefield"

Clara Barton was a woman who broke barriers of all kinds. She began her career in nursing on the battlefield of the Civil War. While other famous nurses like Florence Nightingale and Dorothea Dix served in theaters of war, Clara was literally on the battlefield. The sleeves of her dress bore testament with the hole of a bullet that narrowly missed her.

In between her battlefield service, she traveled to Washington to lobby the Congress for better care for soldiers and more support for their families. She was really one of the first "nurse lobbyists." She may have been the only woman to testify before Congress and the Committee on the Reconstruction and one of the few private citizens to receive appropriated federal dollars for her work. She earned widespread respect for her work on and off the battlefield, which gave her the standing and resources she needed to found the Red Cross. As a true political operative and lobbyist, she cultivated and sustained long-term relationships among men of power and prestige in Washington, DC.

From Oakes, S: Woman of Valor: Clara Barton and the Civil War. The Free Press, New York, 1994.

brought an issue to the attention of the whole legislature that they may otherwise have dismissed as unimportant. Second, the legislative process brings to light the proponents and opponents of the issue and allows nurses to specifically target those legislators who voted against the bill. One of two approaches can be used at this point. Nurses can either communicate with the legislators to explain why the bill is important in hopes of changing their minds, or they can organize as a voting block and attempt to vote the opposing legislators out of office. Third, after a bill has gone through the process the first time, it becomes much easier to identify the obstacles and sticking points in the language of the bill. Before the bill is re-introduced in a later session of the legislature, it can be modified and amended to eliminate those parts that may have caused ideological problems for specific legislators.

Other Factors That Have Potential Political Powers for Nurses

Historically, very few nurses have either sought or been elected to governmental positions. However, it is important to realize that not all nurses who hold elected positions are allies for nursing. Unless elected nurses identify themselves as nurses and support the profession, they may not be willing to support nursing issues politically. For example, a nurse currently elected to Congress from a Southern state refused to speak to the nurses who participated in the March on Washington Nurses. Although she is a nurse and has had a number of articles published in nursing journals in the past, she refused to support the nurses who marched. Elected officials must always be judged by what they do and what they deliver, and not by what they say, or look like, or think, or what people think they think (Box 16.3).

Conclusion

There is nothing magical about nurses becoming involved in politics. It is a matter of hard work and use of the critical thinking skills nurses already possess. It is clear that nurses can and do make a difference in the political arena. Nurses must ask how and where they can make a difference and how they can become involved in the process. Not every nurse may choose to run for political office, but each nurse can and should make a contribution. Betts[4] believes that nursing's interest in public policy and politics is "the prescription for the power so necessary to our future." Carpe diem!

Critical Thinking Exercises

How Do Politics Affect You and Your Family?

Why should nurses be involved in politics? Does it really make a difference who is elected and who makes the laws? Take a minute to go through the questions below and check the items that you think may be affected by politics.

Between the time you wake up and the time you leave the house several things usually happen to you. Do you think any of the following subjects are affected by politics?

✔ The water with which you wash your face and brush your teeth.

✔ The electricity that lights the room.

✔ The price and quality of food you have for breakfast.

✔ The safety of the products you buy.

As the average person's life span grows longer and the retirement age is lowered, these later years become more meaningful. Are any of the following decisions affected by our political systems?

✔ The age at which you can retire.

✔ The income that you get during retirement.

✔ The quality and cost of health care.

✔ The life expectancy of each of us.

We value our leisure time and the chance to get away from it all. Are any of the following areas affected by politics?

✔ The parks and lakes where vacationers fish and swim.

✔ The air that you breathe.

✔ The radio and television programs that entertain you.

References

1. Webster's New Collegiate Dictionary, 1997.
2. O'Donnell, 1996.
3. Chalich, T, and Smith, L: Nursing at the grassroots. Nurs Health Care 13:242–244, 1992.
4. Betts: Nursing's agenda for health care reform policy, politics and power through professional leadership. Hospital Administration Quarterly 20(3):8, 1996.

BIBLIOGRAPHY

AACN/PAC List, Nurse State Legislators. Washington DC, January 1998.

Abdellah, FG: Nursing's Role in the future: A Case for Health Policy Decision Making. A Case For Monograph Series. Sigma Theta Tau International Center Nursing Press, Indianapolis, Ind., 1991.

Aburdene, P, and Naisbitt, J: Megatrends for Women: From Liberation to Leadership. Fawcett Columbine, New York, 1993.

American Nurses Association: Nursing Facts. American Nurses Publishing, Washington, DC, 1994.

Bagwell, MM: The politics of nursing. In Schoolcraft, V (ed): Nursing in the Community. John Wiley, New York, 1984.

Curtis, B, and Lumpkin, B: Political action committees. In Mason, D, Talbott, S, and Leavitt, J (eds): Policy and Politics for Nurses. WB Saunders, Philadelphia, pp 562–576.

DeKieffer, D: The Citizens Guide to Lobbying Congress, Chicage Review Press, 1997.

Duskin, M: Who voted and why, Washington DC. National Voter 46(2):5, 1997.

Goldwater, M, and Lloyd Zusy, MJ: Prescription for Nurses: Effective Political Action. CV Mosby, St. Louis, 1990.

Helms, LB, Anderson, MA, and Hanson, K: Doin' politics: Linking policy and politics in nursing. Nurs Admin Q 20(3):32–41, 1996.

Hoffman, S: Nurses must unify to bring change for patients and profession. American Nurse 29(6):5–7, 1997.

Hopey, D: Close-up. The Pittsburgh Post-Gazette, 17 July 1994, pp 3, 11.

Kelly, L: Dimensions of Professional Nursing. Pergamon Press, New York, 1991.

Majewski, J: Local government. In Mason, D, Talbott, S, and Leavitt, J (eds): Policy and Politics for Nurses. WB Saunders, Philadelphia, 1993, pp 421–432.

Mason, D, Talbott, S, and Leavitt, J (eds): Policy and Politics for Nurses: Action and Change in the Workplace, Government, Organi-zations, and Community. WB Saunders, Philadelphia, 1993.

Munro, N: Public policy: A new paradigm grows from grass roots. Crit Care Nurse 18(5):76–85, 1998.

N-STAT (Nurses Strategic Action Team): Program Report: Victory in Key Committee. American Nurses Association, Washington, DC, 1994.

O'Donnell, D.G.: Political Action in Nursing, OTM Enterprises, (videoseries), 1995.

Sharp, N: All politics is local: And other rules. Nurs Man 25:22–25, 1994.

Siebber, JR, et al: Missing in action: Nurses in the media. Am J Nurs 98(12):55–56, 1998.

Trossman, S: Stepping onto the stage: RNs take on the role of political player. American Nurse 29(6):1–18, 1997.

Uhlman, M: Medical market in transition. Philadelphia Inquirer, 24 July, 1994, pp A1, A6.

Winter, K: Educating nurses in political process: A growing need. Cont Educ Nurs 22:143–146, 1991.

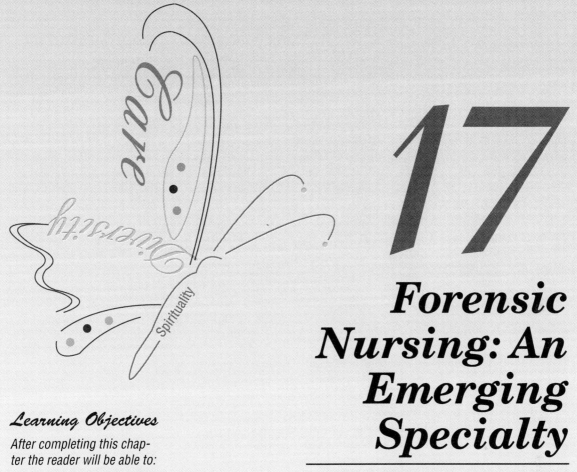

17

Forensic Nursing: An Emerging Specialty

➤ *Anita G. Hufft and Cindy Peternelj-Taylor*

Forensic nursing is an evolving specialty that has emerged as a dynamic and influential factor in the health care of individuals and communities. As society becomes more concerned about violence and its impact on daily life, it becomes more likely that the health-care system will interface with the criminal justice system. With their orientation to holistic and comprehensive client care, their keen clinical skills, and an ability to collaborate with others, forensic nurses are ideally situated to provide quality care to both victims and perpetrators of crime. Trends in nursing education and nursing practice indicate that increased specialization and differentiation of practice will dominate career opportunities.

Learning Objectives

After completing this chapter the reader will be able to:

1. Define forensic nursing.
2. Discuss specialties in forensic nursing practice.
3. Describe settings in which forensic nurses practice.
4. Describe the populations for whom forensic nurses provide care.
5. Identify resources for education and practice in forensic nursing.

DEFINITION OF FORENSIC NURSING

Forensic nursing is still in its early stages of development. The American definition of this specialty is somewhat different from the definition found in the British literature. In order to provide for the broadest interpretation, a working definition of forensic nursing that bridges these two perspectives is presented.

Forensic nursing, which was first introduced in the United States as a term in 1991 by Lynch,[1,2] was identified within the scope of four distinct nursing roles:

1. Clinical forensic nursing
2. **Sexual assault nurse examiner**
3. Forensic psychiatric nursing
4. Correctional/institutional nurse

Burrow[3] offers a more succinct definition of forensic nursing as it is commonly understood in Great Britain. Based on an understanding of forensic psychiatry, Burrow refers to forensic nursing as nursing management of any client behavior that "links psychiatric symptomatology and offending behavior." A related, but distinct definition of the forensic nurse was proposed by Scales and associates: "One who practices in a facility or program where the primary mission is the evaluation or treatment of mentally ill offenders."[4]

The American Nurses Association (ANA) recognized forensic nursing as a specialty in 1995 and further defined forensic nursing as the "application of forensic science combined with the biopsychosocial education of the registered nurse, in the scientific investigation, evidence collection and preservation, analysis, prevention and treatment of trauma, and/or death related to medical-legal issues."[5]

Although there are different classifications of nursing specialties within forensic nursing in the United States and abroad, the clarification of the role is dependent not only on what the nurse does (role expectations) but also on where the nurse works (role setting). The British approach emphasizes nursing relationships with perpetrators of crime, whereas the American approach emphasizes nursing relationships with the victims of crimes.

For the purposes of this discussion, forensic nursing is defined as a nursing specialty practice that integrates nursing science and forensic science to apply the nursing process to the health and well-being of individual clients, their families, and communities to help bridge the gap between the health-care system and the criminal justice system. This definition builds on the paradigm presented by Lynch,[1] which emphasizes the "expanded role of the nurse in meeting the needs of victims and perpetrators of violent crime through enhanced quality of care and preventive services. Implementation of these roles occurs in many settings" (Box 17.1).

BOX 17.1 Settings for Forensic Nursing Practice

Individuals practice forensic nursing in many settings, both in and out of formal institutions such as hospitals and correctional facilities. They work with both victims and perpetrators of crime and may focus their practice in various ways, including:

- Physical injury and violence
- Mental illness
- Dysfunctional family systems
- Community health promotion and accident prevention
- Policy making

Such a wide variety of clinical applications make forensic nursing an exciting opportunity for both new and experienced nurses.

In order to make nurses visible and recognized for their contributions, any definition of forensic nursing should emphasize the uniqueness of nursing and clearly promote the idea that nurses do something different than other health-care providers or other members of a forensic team. The widest scope of practice within the forensic nursing specialty should be considered when defining forensic nursing. This consideration allows for the broadest possible application of forensic nursing knowledge in many settings and with as many populations as possible.

FORENSIC NURSING KNOWLEDGE

Nursing practice traditionally has been referred to as an art and a science. The knowledge that guides nursing actions is grounded in humanities, biology, physical sciences, and everyday experience. Nurses use knowledge from all of these areas to understand human systems and the environments in which they practice.

Nursing science explains the relationships between the domain concepts of nursing: human systems, environment, and health. Lynch and Burgess[6] report that the scientific knowledge base of forensic nursing is derived from forensic science, criminal justice, police science, and legal studies. Forensic nursing uses forensic science as the context for nursing, incorporating knowledge of defining people and groups, understanding forensic communities and forensic environments, and identifying nursing therapeutics that differentiate forensic practice from other kinds of nursing. For example, people can be categorized as either victims or perpetrators of crime. Knowledge of theories that explain the behavior of victims and criminals is important information for the nurse (Box 17.2). Environments in which forensic nursing can be applied include **secured settings,** such as locked hospital units, jails, or correctional institutions. Environments also include se-

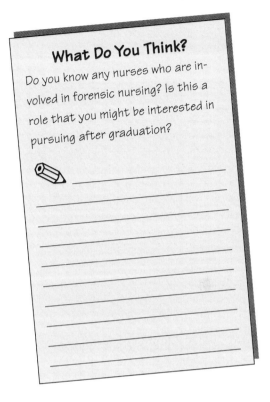

What Do You Think?

Do you know any nurses who are involved in forensic nursing? Is this a role that you might be interested in pursuing after graduation?

cured or special settings such as a medical examiner's office, a crime scene, or a shelter for women. Still other nurses may practice forensic nursing in emergency rooms or schools, adapting their nursing interventions to assess potential for violence or self-harm. The way in which nurses dispose of a contaminated dressing, how they touch a client, and how they set goals with a client can all be affected by whether or not the client is a victim of a crime or violence or an initiator of crime or violence. These are a few examples of how forensic nursing is different from other types of nursing and how knowledge of forensic nursing concepts can be valuable for any nurse. Forensic science is relevant to contemporary nursing, ensuring that clinicians are prepared to identify and report victims of crime, collect and preserve forensic evidence, evaluate issues of competence, and protect the rights and health of victims and perpetrators of crime.[1]

BOX

17.2 Application of Nursing Theory

Based on the Roy Adaptation Model, an approach to identifying characteristics specific to the prison environment that affect the health care of women prisoners has been proposed.[26] A conceptual framework for understanding women's health issues in correctional settings includes the assessment of contextual stimuli and also factors in the background experiences and conditions that support the individual inmate's response to the prison experience and current health-care needs.

A profile of women offenders reveals common characteristics that include chaotic lifestyle prior to incarceration, significant drug or alcohol abuse, lack of control over their lives, previous contact with the criminal justice system, inconsistent and exploitative relationships, and marginalized roles in society. What may be more significant is the generally poor attitude toward the health-care system that most inmates have. The health assessment of the female offender, therefore, would be focused on adaptations that accompany the response to these types of stressors, looking for history of coping with these types of problems and creating opportunities for developing a relationship in a generally mistrusting environment.

Source: Roy C: Introduction to Nursing: An Adaptation Model, ed 2. Englewood Cliffs,

CONCEPTS RELEVANT TO FORENSIC NURSING

Professional nursing practice is based, in part, on the use of theoretical knowledge and concepts in making decisions about client care. There are essential concepts that must be understood by nurses working in forensic settings and in forensic roles. The concepts of victimization, violence, manipulation, custody, and human rights serve to clarify the nursing profession's understanding of the client and his or her environment, to better guide the selection of therapeutic interventions and to give meaning to nursing interactions with the client.

Victimization

In the 1970s, when the victim movement began, its primary goals were to help victims recover from the emotional trauma and physical injuries resulting from crime. Another goal included prevention of secondary victimization by ensuring that the criminal justice, health, and social services systems treat victims with dignity, respect, and compassion. Although significant advances in the care of victims has taken place in the past since then, the belief that violence and victimization are caused only by criminals has proved to limit strategies for prevention of secondary victimization from the system.[7] The current trend is to treat violence as a major criminal justice and health problem. Public health concepts have been used to provide a health-oriented model for understanding victims, treating victims, and preventing victimization.[7] This approach focuses on public education, controlling the spread of violence (and the victim self-concept), and early detection of victimization.

Treatment of victims of violence and violence itself as a health issue, in addition to a criminal justice issue, opens the door to more health-care intervention. Early intervention and treatment by the health-care system, combined with criminal justice efforts, have the potential to decrease the experience of victimization. Recognizing the significance of this issue, Friedman[7] offers an example of the victim's rights (Box 17.3).

Violence

As a major example of antisocial behavior, violence is a concept integral to the understanding of forensic nursing. Family violence (including abuse of children, spouses, and the elderly) represents a long-standing concern of health-care professionals. The American Medical Association (AMA) has linked violence in the family with the escalation of violence in the world at large.[8] Nurses use their knowledge of violence in the application of specific skills and interventions such as (1) increased awareness of family violence as a public health problem, (2) recognition of the risk factors and symptoms of abuse and neglect, (3) use of therapeutic communication techniques to ask questions nonjudgmentally, and (4) treatment and referral of clients for shelter and services when needed. The AMA has published guidelines for the diagnosis and treatment of abuse and neglect. Basic nursing diagnosis and care planning books contain chapters devoted to interventions with clients who are victims of abuse. Forensic nurses need to keep abreast of current research, which includes studies of the development of individual violent behavior, the effect of testosterone on aggression on children, the father's role in child/adolescent development and delinquency, effects of neighborhood characteristics on drug use and sales, peer social networks, and the relationship of child care arrangements to delinquency.[9]

Manipulation

Manipulation is not necessarily a maladaptive or antisocial behavior. Its value is dependent on the context in which it occurs for its meaning. Negative use of manipulation is a common characteristic of victims and perpetrators of crime, who often resort to maladaptive behaviors in order to have their needs met.[10] For example, an inmate

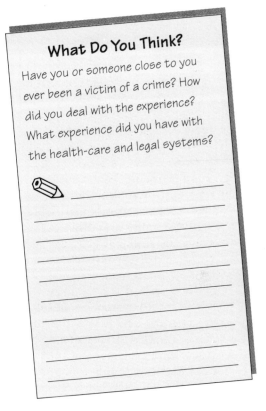

What Do You Think?

Have you or someone close to you ever been a victim of a crime? How did you deal with the experience? What experience did you have with the health-care and legal systems?

may tell prison authorities secrets or privately inform them of everyday illnesses to get special favors, such as release from work detail.

The following are characteristics of destructive or antisocial manipulation:

1. It is the primary method used to have needs fulfilled.
2. The needs and feelings of others are disregarded.
3. People are treated as objects and dehumanized in order to fulfill the needs of the manipulator.[11]

Often associated with manipulation are maladaptive behavior patterns involving impulsiveness, aggression, and detachment. These behaviors are characteristics that define actions and relationships among perpetrators and victims. Forensic nursing applications focus on the assessment of these characteris-

A Closer Look

THE SILENT EPIDEMIC OF SEXUAL ASSAULT

Although sexual assault has received increasing publicity in recent months, it still remains the most common, unreported crime in the United States. The American Medical Association (AMA) estimates that one woman or child is sexually assaulted every 45 seconds, for a total of more than 700,000 sexual assaults per year. Of this group of victims, 61% are females younger than the age of 18; only 5% are male. Studies have also shown that 75% of the perpetrators of sexual assault are friends, acquaintances, intimate partners, or family of the victims.

Large numbers of sexual assaults remain unreported because of social attitudes and biases that make the victims seem responsible for the crimes. Victims are afraid to step forward to report the crimes or seek help from health-care providers because they fear ridicule and blame. In cases that go to court it is often "her word against his," and defense lawyers routinely bring in the past sexual behavior of the victim to make it seem as though "she was asking for it."

Concerned groups of health-care providers, such as the AMA, American Nurses Association (ANA), and several psychiatric groups have begun publication and distribution of literature concerning sexual assault. Many of the pamphlets and brochures encourage the victims to talk to health-care providers about their experiences. Psychiatric providers often can trace a client's depression and/or suicide attempts back to episodes of sexual assault during childhood. Materials have also been distributed to physicians and nurse practitioners to provide general information about the symptoms of sexual assault, its incidence, and about types of questions to ask suspected victims. Some studies suggest that victims of sexual assault are more comfortable talking about it with health-care providers than clergy or police.

The hope of the health-care community is to break the code of silence that surrounds sexual assault by educating both victims and care providers. All health-care providers, no matter what the setting, are likely to come into contact with victims of sexual assault sometime during their careers. It is essential that the health-care practitioner recognize the symptoms and take appropriate action to help the victim express himself or herself without guilt or fear.

Source: Sexual assault called "silent violent epidemic." Washington Post, 7 November 1995, p 2.

BOX 17.3 Crime Victim's Bill of Rights

The right to be treated with fairness and with respect for the victim's dignity and privacy.

The right to be reasonably protected from the accused offender.

The right to be notified of court proceedings.

The right to be present at all public court proceedings related to the offense, unless the court determines that testimony by the victim would be materially affected if the victim hears other testimony at trial.

The right to confer with an attorney for the government in the case.

The right to restitution.

The right to information about the conviction, sentencing, imprisonment, and release of the offender.

From Friedman, LN: Adapting the health care model to prevent victimization. National Institute of Justice Journal 228:16–19, 1994.

What Do You Think?

Should prisoners have the same human rights as everyone else? Make a list in two columns of the rights that you think they should have or not have. Which list is longer? Why?

tics and the assignment of meaning within the framework of criminal activity in which they occur.

Custody

Confinement of individuals who are accused of breaking the law or convicted of a crime involves sanctions that are unique, and these, in turn, influence nursing. Goffman[12] refers to these settings as "total institutions" and identifies them in terms of their control over all aspects of an individual's life and daily routine, as is seen in the regimentation of scheduled activities and sequencing of events, the relinquishment of individual identity among those in custody, and the fact that the primary concern of all procedures and policies centers on what is best for the institution rather than the individual inmate. Lloyd[13] observes that these characteristics are common to mental hospitals, prisons, and forensic psychiatric facilities.

Providing health care in an environment where health-care delivery is not the primary goal leads to many complex challenges for the forensic nurse. The priorities of the correctional system are built on confinement and security. As a result, nurses in this setting commonly face basic value conflicts, because the principles of security are often at odds with the principle of treatment. For example, if a prison has sick call only at 6:00 A.M., and an inmate becomes ill at 2:00 P.M., the inmate must wait until the following morning to obtain treatment. Unless the sickness is life threatening, prison officials do not want to risk a lapse in security by altering the normal routine. Forensic nurses working with incarcerated perpetrators often struggle to find the balance between the security limitations of the institution and the health-care needs of the prison population. This contradiction, known as "custody and caring," can be immobilizing to nurses, who frequently find themselves caught between the proverbial "rock and a hard place."[14] In other words, no matter how therapeutic a specific health-care program a nurse develops, a correctional institution will consistently sacrifice individual health needs to institutional needs.

Human Rights

The basic human rights that are taken for granted in most nursing environments become an important issue of nurse advocacy in forensic nursing. There is little debate in the general health-care settings over the individual's right to self-determination, protection from discomfort and harm, maintenance of dignity, fair treatment, and respect for privacy. However, when viewed against the backdrop of the criminal justice system, these rights become controversial and complex issues. Take, for example, the case of the rape victim who wants to remain anonymous. She may fear the shame and retaliation if her identity is made public. The district attorney believes that public exposure of such cases will help destigmatize rape, encourage other women to testify, and increase the successful conviction of rapists, ultimately leading to a decrease of violence in society. When seen within a forensic context, the right of the individual rape victim to privacy comes into conflict with the right of society to be free from harm. Also, the issue of long-term best interests of the victim must be taken into consideration. Although public exposure of the rape victim may lead to immediate distress and possibly to further victimization, it may also increase the likelihood of successful resolution of the trauma through public dialogue and psychological processing of the event. The duty to do good for the client (beneficence) comes into conflict with the duty to protect from harm and to advocate for the patient's right to self-determination.

FORENSIC NURSING SPECIALTIES

Clinical Forensic Nursing Specialty

Clinical forensic nursing is the management of crime victims from trauma to trial. Nurses working in clinical forensics collect evidence through assessment of living victims, survivors of traumatic injury, or those whose death is pronounced in the clinical environment.[2] Clinical forensic nursing involves making judgments related to client treatment associated with court-related issues.[15] The clinical forensic nurse assesses victims of child and elder abuse and domestic violence. Forensic nurses are asked to differentiate between conditions that simulate accidental injury and those that are purposefully in-

 An essential skill required by the forensic nurse is the ability to assess patterned injury by identifying marks such as defense wounds, grab marks, and fingernail marks.

flicted. An essential skill required by the forensic nurse is the ability to assess patterned injury by identifying marks such as defense wounds, grab marks, and fingernail marks. Clinical forensic nurses focus on observation of the communication and interaction patterns of suspected abuse victims and perpetrators. Many nurses come to forensic nursing from acute care settings of emergency room nursing, critical care nursing, and perioperative nursing.

In the coroner's office, death notification entails stabilization of the family situation and grief support, skills that are basic to nursing practice. Expert skills in physical assessment, clinical history taking and interviewing, and use of technology have helped advance this nursing role.

Because of their awareness of the effects of violence in society and their ability to assess situations in which potential for violence exists, clinical forensic nurses are often called upon for consultation. By identifying risk factors and cues for violence in health-care and workplace settings, these nurses can assist in the development of strategies, policies, and protocols to manage risk and reduce violence and injury. They will also assist in the debriefing or resolution of violent events in a workplace or community.

The sexual assault nurse examiner (SANE) is a registered nurse who has received specialized training to provide care to the sexual assault victim.[16] The SANE performs physical and psychosocial examination and collection of physical evidence, therapeutic interactions to minimize the trauma and initiate healing, coordination of referral and collaboration with community-based agencies involved in the

rehabilitation of victims, and the judicial processing of sexual assault. The first programs training SANEs were developed in the United States in the late 1970s. It is expected that national certification will be mandated in the near future.

Forensic Psychiatric Nursing Specialty

Forensic psychiatric nurses integrate psychiatric/mental health nursing philosophy and practice with knowledge of the criminal justice system and assessment of the sociocultural influences on the individual client, the family, and the community to provide comprehensive psychiatric and mental health nursing.[17] Forensic psychiatric nurses work with mentally ill offenders and with victims of crime. They help victims cope with their emotional wounds and assist in the assessment and care of perpetrators.[4] They focus on identification and change of behaviors linking criminal offenses or reactions to them. These nurses assist perpetrators and victims of crime in dealing with the courts and other aspects of the criminal justice system, minimizing further victimization and promoting functional abilities.

 Forensic psychiatric nurses integrate psychiatric/mental health nursing philosophy and practice with knowledge of the criminal justice system and assessment of the sociocultural influences on the individual client, the family, and the community.

Functional applications of forensic psychiatric nursing include assessment of inmates for mental and physical fitness, criminal responsibility, disposition, and early release. Forensic psychiatric nurses also provide mental health treatment for convicted offenders and those who are not found criminally responsible. In the criminal justice system, forensic psychiatric

Issues

Forensic Nurses Help Rape Victims

A program started in Tulsa, Oklahoma, in 1994 has been copied and implemented across the nation. Designed originally to provide more compassionate care for rape victims, the program has also secured more convictions for prosecutors in sexual assault cases.

The sexual assault nurse examiner (SANE) program was started as an experimental effort coordinated by the Tulsa Police Department with local health-care providers and trauma centers. An initial grant of $100,000 from the Ford Foundation, plus smaller grants from public and private sources, allowed for the education of registered nurses to perform the forensic examination of rape victims. The special examination uses a 16-step procedure that includes the collection of saliva, semen, and hair samples. Prior to the SANE program, it was not unusual for victims to wait 6 to 8 hours for an examination by an emergency room (ER) physician. During the long wait, the victim could not eat, drink, change clothes, or take a shower to avoid destroying useful evidence. Some victims decided to walk out rather than endure the wait and emotionally traumatic procedures.

Under the guidelines of the SANE program, the victim is met at the ER door by the nurse examiner. Victims are quickly counseled, examined, and treated in special treatment areas that provide a maximum amount of privacy. A special waiting room is set aside for police and family members. The examination by the SANE is generally completed in less than 2 hours. During the first 3 years of the program, SANEs performed more than 700 examinations of rape and sexual assault victims.

In addition to achieving its primary goal of providing more compassionate and timely care for the victims, the SANE program has provided a bonus of increased convictions for rape and sexual assault crimes. The streamlined process helps in the gathering and maintenance of key evidence as well as providing better witnesses. The quality of the evidence gathered by the SANEs is on a par with the evidence gathered at other crime sites by trained forensic police technicians. Rape and sexual assault victims are more inclined to testify if they feel that they are not being victimized a second time during the examination at the hospital.

Source: Program to help rape victims also helps win more sexual-assault cases. New York Times, 30 December 1994, section B6, p 3.

nurses deal with destructive, aggressive, and socially unacceptable behavior. These nurses provide interventions that encourage individuals to exercise self-control, foster individual change in behavior, and, in the process, protect other members of society and property.

There has been an increase in the involvement of forensic psychiatric nurses (especially those prepared for advanced practice) in the assessment and treatment of forensic psychiatric clients. These practitioners are involved in the development and refining of clinical roles in forensic psychiatric nursing and are in a position to promote intervention strategies that increase the likelihood of rehabilitation and reintegration of the forensic client into society.

Correctional/Institutional Nursing Specialty

Correctional/institutional nurses work in secure settings, providing treatment, rehabilitation, and health promotion to clients who have been charged with or convicted of crimes. Settings include jails, state and federal prisons, and halfway houses. Laben and Blum[18] observe that before the 1960s, nurses in general gave little thought to working in the correctional system, even though jails and correctional facilities have always been a part of the community at large. There is a growing awareness of the potential for the correctional population as a target of successful health interventions. Some nurses have created private practices or consultation services in which they identify the health needs and arrange for the care of people detained in custody.[19] This service is provided separate from acute care, which is located in a secured hospital or infirmary section of the institution. Such services are just emerging as health-care alternatives and will serve as the model from

which community-based care, aimed at decreasing recidivism among those incarcerated, will develop. To guide professional nursing practice, the ANA first published Standards for Nursing Practice in Correctional Facilities in 1985; these standards were revised and updated in 1995.[20] In addition to the specialties of forensic nursing noted earlier, nurses are continuing to develop roles based on the integration of forensic knowledge into nursing practice (Box 17.4).

Nurses in General Practice

In addition to nurses in specialty practice, nurses in general practice find forensic nursing knowledge of growing importance. Forensic applications in the acute care setting emphasize the use of forensic knowledge and awareness of criminal justice implications for the assessment, documentation of care, and reporting of information to police or other law enforcement agencies. Nurses who work in emergency rooms and

17.4 **Subspecialties of Clinical Practice Identified by the International Association of Forensic Nurses**

Forensic nurse educators/consultants

Nurse coroners

Death investigators

Legal nurse consultants

Nurse attorneys

Clinical nurse specialists and those specializing in trauma

Transplant and critical care nurses

Forensic pediatric nurses

Forensic gerontology nurses

in critical care units are often in positions to preserve evidence of what might be a criminal offense. Victims of automobile accidents or apparent accidental overdoses are not always what they appear to be. Knowledge of what to look for and how to collect evidence, in addition to knowing whom to call and when, can be valuable in finding out what really happened in such cases. Clients often come into acute care settings with what is first thought to be an injury that is the result of an accident. However, preservation of evidence such as stomach contents, clothing residue, or marks on the skin surface can provide a very different picture—one of injury caused by a self-inflicted wound or violence perpetrated by another person.

CLINICAL APPLICATIONS

Hatmaker[16] reports on the advantages of using a sexual assault nurse examiner to care for victims of rape. Sexual assault victims are usually seen in a busy emergency room, and they are often not on the top of the triage list, where traditionally, life-threatening cases are taken first. The wait for the rape victim can be agonizing. The

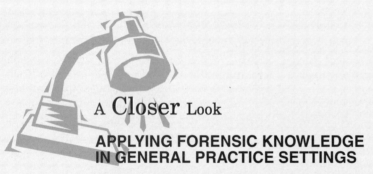

A **Closer** Look

APPLYING FORENSIC KNOWLEDGE IN GENERAL PRACTICE SETTINGS

The following case emphasizes the importance of applying forensic skills to preserve evidence. A nurse working in an emergency room cares for a client who eventually succumbs to cardiac arrest. Circumstances surrounding the death are confusing and troublesome to the nurse.[27] The sisters of the deceased seemed unusually angry with the husband, who had refused to bring the sisters in to see the deceased the day before. An empty prescription bottle of medication, the contents of which were found in lethal doses at autopsy, was filled only a couple of days before. Stomach contents, which showed the medication, had been discarded at autopsy and were no longer available for analysis. At first the nurse was uncertain of her responsibility, of what all the circumstances meant, or whether they meant anything at all. By the time she reported the situation to the police, there was not enough evidence to conclude whether the death was an accident, an assisted suicide, or an outright murder. If the medical examiner could have examined the gastric contents, he would have known how many pills had been ingested at once; however, the evidence was gone. No legal action was ever pursued. All that remained were accusations from the family and the nurse's feeling of frustration.

victim has a long time to think about the rape, fear the worst, and worry about the pain and humiliation from the physical examination. The victim may feel alone and abandoned at a very stressful time in her life. Nurses are trained to listen, observe, support, and take care of the client. When the SANE intervenes, a multidisciplinary approach is used. The police officer is responsible for interviewing the victim about the sexual attack, whereas the nurse focuses on the forensic examination, collection of evidence with the use of a rape kit, and noting the presence of any injuries with written and photographic documentation.

Comprehensive nursing care includes an evaluation of immediate trauma as well as a referral to a rape crisis center, individual therapist, follow-up medical care, or other community health resources. In one case, the SANE noticed the presence of a dry, shiny substance on the victim's cheek. She sent a swab of the substance to the crime laboratory along with clothes and other body tissue evidence. None of the other evidence linked the victim to a perpetrator. However, the cheek swab did establish a DNA link to the accused rapist and was an important factor in the conviction of the assailant. Hatmaker goes on to state that benefits of a community-based SANE team approach to sexual assault includes state-of-the-art evidence collection, compassionate care of victims, increased confidence among police and district attorneys that evidence collected is credible, and an increased likelihood that the process will yield convictions in court.[16]

ENVIRONMENTS FOR PRACTICE

The practice of forensic nursing can take place in several settings. The clinical foren-

sic nurse may work in organizational settings under the control of local or state government, usually the coroner's office or the medical examiner's office. Similar to the emergence of nurse practitioners in the 1960s, the development of the role of nurse medical examiner appears to be related to the shortage of forensic pathologists. Nurses are adept at mastering the clinical skills required to assist in the investigation of death and violence. It is estimated that the need for forensic pathologists will increase from the current 350 to 400 to 800 to 1000 in the near future (Corrie, M, MD, personal communication, November 3, 1996).

Clinical Forensic Nursing Settings

Clinical forensic nurses work in the laboratory, in the examination office, in the autopsy room, and in the field at crime scenes. Roles include field investigation, autopsy assistant, family liaison, and custodian of evidence. When investigating a death scene, the clinical forensic nurse interviews witnesses, takes charge of the body, examines the body, photographs the body, secures physical evidence, arranges body transport, and gathers records. When working with living victims, the tasks are similar but focus on injury assessment and the collection of evidence.

> **" "** *Clinical forensic nurses work in the laboratory, in the examination office, in the autopsy room, and in the field at crime scenes.*

The coroner is usually in charge of death investigation. Nurses working in this capacity initiate or assist with death investigation under selected circumstances of homicide, violence, suicide, and suspicious circumstances that would indicate a violation of criminal law (e.g., the presence of illegal drugs, body found in water, fire, explosion) (Evans, E, personal communication, September 22, 1997).

Correctional Care Settings

Custody settings include jails, state and federal prisons, halfway houses, and other settings in which the individual who is accused of a crime or sentenced for a crime is held in confinement. In some states, private companies have been given contracts to manage either the entire secure setting or the health-care delivery system used by that setting. Prior to the 1970s, there was little in the way of systematic or planned health care for inmates of secured settings. Since the 1970s, the criminal justice system and the health-care system have worked both independently and in collaboration to develop systems of health care for those in custody. Whatever the custody setting, the nurse is responsible for identifying and performing a role that is consistent with professional standards and state law in which he or she is licensed. Many health-care facilities in secure settings choose to be accredited, subjecting themselves to scrutiny of an outside agency that verifies the quality of the health care delivered in that setting. Most certified correctional health care facilities in the United States affiliate with the National Commission on Correctional Health Care.

"Few issues, aside from overcrowding, cause correctional administrators more concern than providing health services for inmates."[21] Limited resources constitute a persistent concern for health-care delivery in any setting. In correctional settings, the problem is compounded by political influences, legal issues, ethical concerns, inmates with special needs, and emphasis on security. Nurses working in correctional settings must always frame their care planning within the limitations of the requirements of the institution and the characteristics of those for whom they provide care.

Prison and jail inmates are overwhelmingly from an impoverished environment and disproportionately represent minority groups.[22,23] In the prison setting, many per-

BOX 17.5 The Skill Set of the Correctional Nurse

The skill set of the correctional nurse includes strategies to break barriers to nurse-client relationships, including mistrust, low self-esteem, chaotic and chronically unhealthy lifestyles, and poor communication abilities that characterize many inmates. Issues such as ethical standards, confidentiality, and informed consent have unique dimensions when considered within the correctional setting. Essential knowledge for the correctional nurse includes:

1. Understanding of the history of health care in corrections
2. Legal issues surrounding the provision of care in prisons
3. Ethical principles, including inmate participation in biomedical research
4. The organizational structure of prison health services
5. Staffing concerns related to custody rules and regulations
6. Inmates with special health needs, such as chronic illness and communicable diseases.

Elements of the aforementioned content areas, along with an overview of a model health-care program that meets accreditation standards, should be part of any orientation program for new nurses working in correctional settings.

sonal rights are lost, and individuals in confinement are subject to health care that is controlled by the confining agents, whether that is the local, state, or federal government. Inmates do not vote; they essentially have no power and few special interest groups to champion their welfare. In the prison setting, physical touch is discouraged; access to medication and comfort measures is limited; movement is restricted; and even talking is prevented at certain times. Inmates usually harbor strong negative attitudes and deep resentment toward authority figures or anyone identified with the correctional system, including nurses. In order to provide quality nursing care in correctional settings, nurses must excel in both clinical skills and interpersonal competencies (Box 17.5)

EDUCATION FOR FORENSIC NURSING

Nursing education for forensic nursing is developing rapidly in many areas. It is the responsibility of nursing educators to ensure the inclusion of forensic content in basic nursing curricula by teaching the basic skills for routine assessment, identification, treatment, and referral of victims of child, elder, and spouse abuse.[24] Currently, there are growing numbers of schools of nursing that integrate forensic nursing into existing nursing courses, such as family nursing courses, comprehensive health and physical assessment courses, community health courses, and critical care or trauma courses. Elective nursing courses and programs of graduate nursing education in forensic nursing are slowly emerging. There is also an increase in the clinical placement of undergraduate and graduate students in forensic settings. These placements are found in research courses, nursing of adult courses, nurse practitioner courses, and psychosocial nursing courses.

Some hospitals and other health-care institutions are beginning to offer continuing education programs that integrate forensic science and nursing practice. Current programs include a wide range of academic offerings, such as the Utah Crime Scene

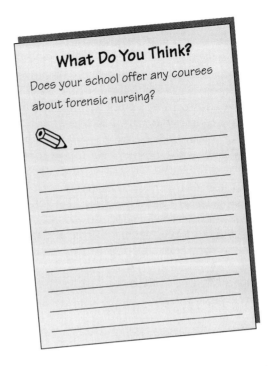

What Do You Think?

Does your school offer any courses about forensic nursing?

Academy, the American Association of Legal Nurse Consultants' education program, and the College of Nursing, University of Massachusetts–Boston forensic nursing course. The Mercy College in New York incorporates prison sites into an RN program, as does the Indiana University Southeast baccalaureate program. The University of Virginia offers a forensic nursing major at the graduate level. Forensic nursing education has even come to the Internet via a comprehensive program of offerings from Mount Royal College, Alberta, Canada. Two courses of a seven-course series have already been developed and are currently available. Specific information about these and other educational opportunities are found in the Site-Seeing Box.

In general, most programs screen and carefully select students for experiences in a forensic setting. Students must understand the logistical and behavioral restrictions that are inherent in forensic settings, whether they are in a correctional institution or a medical examiner's office (Box 17.6).

The International Forensic Nurses Association (IAFN) is a professional association of registered nurses working in the medicolegal nursing area whose purpose is to develop, promote, and disseminate information about the science of forensic nursing.
IAFN National Office, c/o Slack, Incorporated, 6900 Grove Road, Thorofare, New Jersey 08086
Phone: (609) 848-8356
Fax: (609) 848-4274
E-mail: iafn@slackinc.com

American Forensic Nurses Association (AFN) An organization with headquarters in Palm Springs, California. Specifically established to meet the needs of law enforcement agencies in the collection of forensic evidence. Offers distance education courses via the World Wide Web.
http://www.amrn.com.aboutus.htm

CLFORNSG (Forensics)
mail to:listserv@ulkyvm.louisville.edu
Subscribe CLFORNSG Firstname Lastname

Fitchburgh State College, Fitchburgh, Massachusetts, offers a master's degree in forensic nursing. Call (508) 665-3181 or contact http://www.fsc.edu/forensic.htm

Forensic Health Studies are offered over the Internet through Mount Royal College, Alberta, Canada. Contact Arlene Kent-Wilkinson at the Center for Health Studies, Mount Royal College, 4825 Richard Road, SW, Calgary, Alberta, Canada T3E 6K6
Call toll free: 1-888-240-7201
E-mail: srunquist@mtroyal.ab.ca

The Legal Nurse Consultant Resource Directory was developed to provide nurses with a general understanding of legal nurse consulting and a list of resources for further investigation. American Association of Legal Nurse Consultants, 4700 W. Lake Ave., Glenview, Illinois 60025-1485.
Phone: (847) 375-4713
Fax: (847) 375-4777
http://www.aalnc.org/consulting.htm

National Alliance of Certified Legal Nurse Consultants Medical Legal Consulting Institute, Inc.
P.O. Box 2476, Bolsover, Suite 632, Houston, Texas 77005
Phone: (713) 349-9182
Fax: (713) 349-0616
http://www.legalnurse.com

Rutgers University College of Nursing offers Correctional Health Certificate courses.
http://nursing.rutgers.edu/nursing/ce/bcorrect.htm

Sexual Assault Nurse Examiner Program
http://www.state.ky.us/agencies/gov/sane.htm

The University of Colorado, Colorado Springs, offers forensic nursing education programs, including graduate education as a forensic clinical nurse specialist. Call UCCS at (719) 262-4424, or access website at Iafn@slackinc.com for multiple programs.

The Utah Crime Scene Academy provides on-site training each spring and fall. Classes are held at the Utah Peach Officer Standards and Training Academy. Write for application: Mr. Kevin M. Patrick, Utah Crime Laboratory, 4501 South 2700 West, Salt Lake City, Utah 84119.
http://www.ps.ex. state.ut.us/cl/CSA.htm

CHARACTERISTICS OF THE FORENSIC NURSE

As with any other nursing specialty, forensic nursing is not for everyone. Who should be a forensic nurse? The same characteristics that predict a successful student learning experience in forensic settings (see Box 17.6) also apply to the practitioner. Social maturity, adaptability, analytical skills, and an optimistic disposition are critical to career management in any stressful setting. The nurse working in forensic settings should feel comfortable working in settings that demand adherence to strict protocols and many rules. At the same time, the suc-

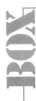

17.6 Preferred Characteristics for Students in a Forensic Setting

Characteristics that promote optimal student experiences in forensic settings:

1. *Social maturity*—Skills interacting with diverse and unfamiliar groups of individuals
2. *Objectivity*—The ability to think critically, process information analytically, and be nonjudgmental
3. *Adaptability*—Constructive responsiveness to changing environmental demands
4. *Sense of humor*—Maintenance of idealism and optimism by not taking things personally and striving to see the positive aspects of situations

cessful nurse will apply nursing knowledge to decisions about client care. Nurses who choose clinical forensic roles often have an acute care or emergency care background and enjoy working in situations that demand technological as well as organizational expertise and interpersonal skills.

Nurses working in custody or correctional settings need well-developed psychosocial assessment skills and must acquire a nonjudgmental attitude toward offenders. Studies have demonstrated that nurses who think of the criminal as someone who deserves respect and professional care, who believe in the ability of offenders to be rehabilitated, and who see their roles as caregivers will experience increased work satisfaction, increased work productivity, and increased job longevity. Nurses who dislike working with offenders, see the role of prisons primarily as punishment, and consider their primary role as exerting control over offenders have low levels of job satisfaction with poor productivity and frequent job turnover.

Role conflict has been recognized as a major threat to job satisfaction and a source of stress for nurses working in forensic settings. An active involvement in professional organizations, combined with a well-defined program of career development that decreases isolation and places a strong emphasis on research-based clinical knowledge, reinforces the self-concept and the coping skills of the nurse in forensic practice. Networking with other forensic nurses can diminish the feelings of isolation that forensic nurses sometimes experience and can contribute further to the ongoing professional development of the forensic nurse.[14,18]

Many opportunities are available for nurses to take an active role in forensic nursing. The practice of forensic nursing intersects with various professional and governmental groups that are traditionally viewed as being outside the domain of nursing, including forensic pathologists, law enforcement agents, and defense attorneys.[5] However, Standing Bear[25] cautions nurses to adhere to the skills and practices that are unique to the nursing profession whenever they interface with the allied fields. Nurses need to cooperate with other disciplines but not be absorbed by them. Territoriality among health professionals can and does exist. As members of the nursing profession, forensic nurses must remain faithful to the principles of professional nursing.

Equipped with strategies to support independent and accountable nursing judgments, and with sensitivity to the roles and needs of others in the work setting, the forensic nurse is ideally situated in a position of power and influence in the criminal justice system. The ability to control aspects of the work environment and to achieve positive outcomes with clients results in increased job satisfaction and constructive, satisfying work relationships.

Conclusion

Forensic nursing is a developing nursing role that consists of two major practice specialties: clinical forensic nursing and correctional nursing. Clinical forensic nursing focuses on the application of forensic science to nursing interventions with victims of crime. Correctional nursing specialty practice involves the evaluation and treatment of those in custody. Forensic nursing takes place in various settings, including, but not limited to, medical examiner and coroner's offices, prisons and jails, and psychiatric facilities. Opportunities for nursing education in forensic nursing and for affiliations in professional organizations dedicated to forensic nursing are essential components of the growth of this role. Rewards for this area of practice include autonomous professional practice, challenges to expand repertoire of nursing skills to nontraditional settings, high demand for skills, diversity of clients and settings, and opportunities to work with peers in other disciplines.

Challenges often faced by the nurse in forensic practice include highly stressful work environments, threats to security and risk of physical violence, and risk of a confusing role with that of medical specialists, security officers, or other professionals. An exciting aspect of forensic nursing practice is involvement in a dynamic nursing specialty as it evolves within many settings. The opportunity to contribute to the increasing body of knowledge known as forensic nursing science provides the potential to make nursing for the twenty-first century relevant and responsive to the needs of society.

Critical Thinking Exercises

Application of Human Rights

What information do you need to make a decision? The reader is encouraged to explore applications of human rights from the point of view of the victim and the perpetrator of the crime. Think about how the issue of human rights would be defined and protected in the following examples. What is the nurse's role?

✔ A married father of two, an upstanding member of the community, is accused of child molestation and is admitted to the unit for psychiatric evaluation and submission of tissue samples.

✔ A female inmate becomes pregnant in prison and does not want anyone to know who the father is.

✔ A young man has a history of substance abuse and mental illness. He refuses medication to control psychotic behavior and is confined in a forensic psychiatric facility because of the claim that he is incompetent to stand trial for car theft.

✔ A mother of an infant is being interviewed in a suspected child abuse case. She admits that she was sexually and physically abused as a child and throughout her marriage. The priority is to establish her role in the current charges involving injury of her 3-month-old infant.

If You Were the Nurse on Duty, What Would You Do?

Below are scenarios that exemplify typical situations for the nurse in general practice. Identify your probable response. Critically analyze each situation in terms of what you know and do not know. What types of facts or skills are not part of your current knowledge base?

You are working on a maternity unit when a woman who is an inmate from a correctional institution is admitted in an advanced stage of labor. A correctional officer is in attendance; the woman is shackled at the feet and hands. As she is wheeled to the labor room, you note that the client has had 10 previous pregnancies and four live births.

✔ What factors make the care of this woman different from other pregnant women?

✔ Is she dangerous?

Critical Thinking Exercises

✔ How do you maintain confidentiality with this client?

✔ As an offender in custody, does she surrender any rights?

You work in a hospital setting that is experiencing an increase in violence in the work-place. Perpetrators of street, child, and domestic violence often follow their victims to the hospital setting and continue to pose a significant threat to the whole hospital community. It is important to assess the potential for violence.

✔ How will you contribute to the reduction of risk in the workplace?

✔ Identify risk factors and cues for violence.

✔ How would you implement strategies to assist violence management in the acute care setting?

A halfway house for paroled offenders is due to be constructed in your community. Residents are angry and afraid to have ex-convicts living in their neighborhood. A town meeting is scheduled in which the issue will be discussed. Does nursing have anything to contribute to the discussion?

✔ What do we know about mentally ill offenders, sex offenders, perpetrators of domestic violence, and others?

✔ What is the therapeutic outcome for those mentally ill offenders who have completed rehabilitation programs?

✔ What is the risk to the community?

✔ What stress management strategies are helpful to a community?

You work at a junior high school, providing sex education and health promotion pro-grams for young teenagers. You notice that more and more young people are wearing gang colors and using gang-related language and hand signals.

✔ How does this affect your work?

✔ Does this change your priorities?

✔ Are there referrals or strategies that should be initiated because of the gang affiliations of your students?

Acknowledgments

Special thanks to Arlene Kent-Wilkinson for the preparation of this list of resources.
   Additional thanks to Amber M. Fischer and Michael A. Hufft for their assistance in the research, editing, and general preparation of this chapter.

References

1. Lynch, VA: Forensic aspects of health care: New roles, new responsibilities. J Psychosoc Nurs 31(11):5–6, 1993.
2. Lynch, VA: Clinical forensic nursing: A new perspective in the management of crime victims from trauma to trial. Nurs Clin North Am 7:489–507, 1995.
3. Burrow, S: An outline of the forensic nursing role. British Journal of Nursing 2(18):899–904, 1993.
4. Scales, CJ, Mitchell, JL, and Smith, RD: Survey report on forensic nursing. J Psychosoc Nurs 31(11):39–44, 1993.
5. International Association of Forensic Nurses and the American Nurses Association: Scope and Standards of Forensic Nursing Practice. American Nurses Association, Washington, DC, 1997.
6. Lynch, VA, and Burgess, AW: Forensic nursing. In Burgess, AW (ed): Advanced Practice Psychiatric Nursing. Appleton & Lange, Stamford, Conn., 1998, pp 473–490.
7. Friedman, LN: Adapting the health care model to prevent victimization. National Institute of Justice Journal 228:16–19, 1994.
8. Witwer M: Doctors focus on the threat to health from violence. National Institute of Justice Journal (228):8, 1994.
9. Visher, CA: Understanding the roots of crime. National Institute of Justice Journal (228):9–15, 1994.
10. Hufft, A, and Fawkes, LW: Federal inmates—A psychiatric nursing challenge. Nurs Clin North Am 29(1):35–41, 1994.
11. Fortinash, KM, and Holoday-Worret, PA: Psychiatric Nursing Care Plans, ed 2. CV Mosby, St. Louis, 1995.
12. Goffman, E: Asylums. Doubleday, New York, 1961.
13. Lloyd, C: Forensic Psychiatry for Health Professionals. Chapman & Hall, London, 1995.
14. Peternelj-Taylor, CA, and Johnson, RL: Serving time: Psychiatric mental health nursing in corrections. J Psychosoc Nurs Ment Health Serv 33(8):12–19, 1995.
15. Whyte, L: Forensic nursing: A review of concepts and definitions. Nursing Standard 11(23):46–47, 1997.
16. Hatmaker, D: A SANE approach to sexual assault. Am J Nurs 97(8):80, 1997.
17. Peternelj-Taylor, CA, and Hufft, A: Forensic psychiatric nursing. In Johnson, BS (ed): Psychiatric-Mental Health Nursing: Adaptation and Growth, ed 4. JB Lippincott, Philadelphia, 1997.
18. Laben, JK, and Blum, J: Persons with mental illness in jail. In Worley, NK (ed): Mental Health Nursing in the Community. CV Mosby, St. Louis, 1997, pp 368–384.
19. Evans, A, and McGilvray, L: RN's trial: A forensic nursing service. Australian Journal of Advanced Nursing 14(2):11–15, 1996.
20. American Nurses Association: Scope and Standards of Nursing Practice in Correctional Facilities. American Nurses Association, Washington, DC, 1995.
21. Huggins, MW: Foreword. In Anno, BJ (ed): Prison Health Care: Guidelines for the Management of an Adequate Delivery System. National Commission on Correctional Health Care, Chicago, 1991, p. xv.
22. Anno, BJ: Prison Health Care: Guidelines for the Management of an Adequate Delivery System. National Commission on Correctional Health Care, Chicago, 1991.
23. Shields, KE, and deMoya, D: Correctional nurses' attitudes toward inmates. Journal of Correctional Health Care 4(1):37–59, 1997.
24. Lynch, VA: Forensic nursing in the emergency department: A new role for the 1990's. Critical Care Nurse Quarterly 14(3):69–86, 1991.
25. Standing Bear, SG: Forensic nursing and death investigation: Will the vision be co-opted? J Psychosoc Nurs Ment Health Serv 33(9):59–64, 1995.
26. Peternelj-Taylor, CA: Forbidden love: Sexual exploitation in the forensic milieu. J Psychosoc Nurs Ment Health Serv 36(6):14–23, 41–42, 1998.
27. Cramer, C: Forensic nursing: Unanswered questions. Journal of Emergency Nursing 22(3):236–238, 1996.

BIBLIOGRAPHY

Aiyebusi, A: Clinical view. Nursing Times 94(8):51, 1998.

Carroll, V, and Morin, K: Workplace violence affects one-third of nurses. American Nurse 30(5):15, 1998.

Nawar, M: Workplace violence: One nurse's night of fear. American Nurse 30(5):15, 1998.

Peternelj-Taylor, CA, and Johnson, RL: Custody and caring: Clinical placements of student nurses in a forensic setting. Perspectives in Psychiatr Care 32(4):23–29, 1996.

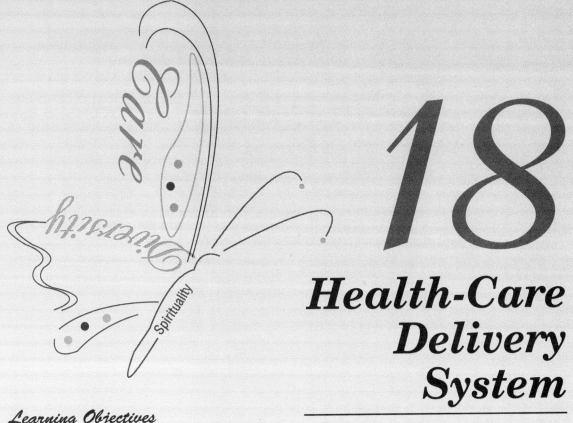

18

Health-Care Delivery System

➤ Deborah L. Finfgeld

Learning Objectives

After completing this chapter, the reader will be able to:

1. Analyze the evolution of the health-care delivery system in the United States.

2. Evaluate the factors that are influencing the evolution of the health-care delivery system.

3. Synthesize the concerns surrounding the uninsured in this country.

4. Analyze industry efforts to manage health-care costs.

5. Evaluate the efforts being made to ensure quality cost-effective health care.

The health-care delivery system in the United States has been evolving since before the Declaration of Independence was signed. Originally, medical remedies and nursing procedures were passed down from one generation to the next and were often combined with superstitious and spiritual rituals. Health care was provided within the home, with women as the primary caretakers. Lay midwives not only assisted women in labor but were also occasionally required to treat clients with acute illnesses.

As formal education for physicians developed, centralized locations for clinical practice were needed. In many cases, physician education constituted the vital force behind the construction of hospitals. Hospitals required nursing staff, thus nursing schools were developed and were modeled closely on the Nightingale model to solve the staffing problems. The Nightingale model was essentially a hospital-based diploma program with some theory presented in the classroom, but most of the education was gained in clinical practice at the bedside.[1]

Early health care involved a minimal knowledge of effective therapies and cures. For this reason, hospitals were initially considered to be places where people went to die. As technology evolved and the growing pharmaceutical industry began to offer life-saving medications, hospitals evolved into acute care facilities where people went to be treated, cared for, and recover. Gradually, acute care of the sick, which is known as **secondary intervention,** was moved from the home to the hospital setting.

Another layer of care developed when technology provided the resources necessary to perform advanced procedures, such as open heart surgery and organ transplants. To meet the demand for these types of interventions, centralized hospitals offering advanced services were developed to draw clients from large geographical areas. These facilities provide what are known as **tertiary interventions.** Unfortunately, as tertiary and acute care facilities became more popular, less attention was devoted to **primary intervention,** which focuses on health promotion, illness prevention, early diagnosis, and treatment of common health problems.

To a great extent, delivery of health care became centralized within hospitals, where professionals were thought to hold the key to well-being through technology. Individual responsibility was minimized, and concerns about cost were diminished because **third-party reimbursers** were responsible for paying a large proportion of the bills. Health care was essentially removed from the hands of consumers, as clients became pawns in an expansive, expensive, and highly technical system.

Consumers, health-care providers, and third-party reimbursers remained relatively satisfied with this system until it became obvious that health-care costs were out of control and millions of Americans had little or no access to care. It also became evident that failure to focus on promoting health and preventing illness was resulting in countless cases of unnecessary suffering and death. To solve these problems, the health-care industry is gradually moving toward a decentralized system in which more and more care is being provided on an outpatient basis; emphasis is being placed on health promotion, illness prevention, and responsible self-care practices; and health-care providers are implementing cost-containment measures. Within today's highly competitive marketplace, health care is being provided in a more coordinated and comprehensive manner along the wellness to illness and acute to chronic continua (Table 18.1).

During the current period of rapid change, provider roles and reimbursement practices are being drastically overhauled. It is important for nurses to understand

Table 18.1	Health Care Delivery System Changes	
FROM	TO
Hospital-based care	Community-based care
Acute care	Illness prevention, health promotion, long-term and rehabilitative care
Incidental fragmented care	Comprehensive, continuous, coordinated care
Patients as passive participants	Patients assuming responsibility for self-care with support of family members
Expensive high-tech care	Cost-effective care provided at an appropriate level
Health-care delivery system	Competitive health-care marketplace monopoly
Service use increases profits	Service use decreases profits

these changes in the health-care delivery system to ensure that their services are fully used and that their ability to function independently and autonomously is protected. In addition, third-party reimbursers must be cognizant of the important role that nurses fulfill and the importance of fair reimbursement practices.

MEMBERS OF THE HEALTH-CARE DELIVERY TEAM

Within the health-care delivery system, large numbers of diagnosticians, technicians, direct care providers, administrators, and support staff are employed. It is estimated that there are more than 300 job titles used to describe health-care workers.[2] Among these are nurses, physicians, physician assistants, social workers, physical therapists, occupational therapists, respiratory therapists, clinical psychologists, and pharmacists. All these individuals provide services that are essential to daily operation of the health-care delivery system in this country.

Of particular importance among this array of health-care workers are various types of nurses: registered nurses, licensed practical (vocational) nurses, nurse practitioners, case managers, and clinical nurse specialists. Each of these individuals requires a different type of educational background, clinical expertise, and, sometimes, professional credentialing. In general, all nurses make valuable contributions within the health-care delivery system. There has been an increased demand for nurses who are educated to deliver care in the community setting and in long-term health-care settings rather than in the hospital. There has also been a need for nurse case managers who are prepared to coordinate care for vulnerable populations requiring costly services over extended periods. Nursing education programs are attempting to meet these

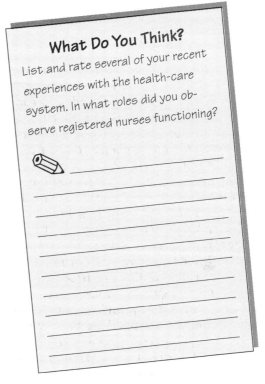

What Do You Think?

List and rate several of your recent experiences with the health-care system. In what roles did you observe registered nurses functioning?

needs by preparing individuals who can practice independently and autonomously, network, collaborate, and coordinate services. These programs also offer more clinical experiences in rehabilitation, nursing home, and community settings.

Registered Nurses, Licensed Practical Nurses, and Unlicensed Assistive Personnel

Registered nurses (RNs) who have been educated at the associate, diploma, or baccalaureate level have traditionally been considered the cornerstone of the current health-care delivery system. In the past, most RNs worked within hospital settings and provided direct client care and nursing administration functions within these facilities. Owing to current trends in health-care funding, there have been fewer hospital admissions, thus decreasing the demand for

RNs in these facilities. However, as health care has moved more to the community setting, there has been an increased need for well-prepared nurses who can function autonomously within the community. Within institutional settings, there still remains a need for licensed practical nurses (LPNs) and unlicensed assistive personnel (UAP) who work under the supervision of an RN. This pattern of care is particularly evident in nursing homes and other long-term care facilities.[3]

Advanced Practice Nurses

For individuals who are unfamiliar with the health-care delivery system, it is sometimes difficult to understand the similarities and differences between nursing titles and roles. This confusion is particularly evident in the case of clinical nurse specialists (CNSs) and nurse practitioners (NPs), who

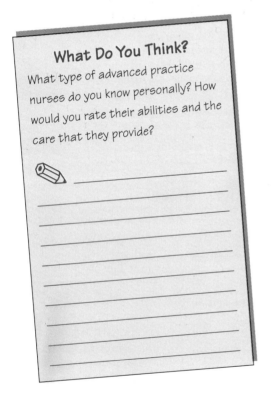

What Do You Think?

What type of advanced practice nurses do you know personally? How would you rate their abilities and the care that they provide?

are sometimes collectively referred to as advanced practice nurses (APNs). In general, NPs are prepared to provide direct client care in primary care settings, focusing on health promotion, illness prevention, early diagnosis, and treatment of common health problems. Their educational preparation varies, but in most cases individuals successfully complete a graduate nurse practitioner program and are certified by the American Nurses Credentialing Center (ANCC) or an appropriate professional nursing organization. Depending on the individual state practice act, NPs have a range of responsibility for diagnosing diseases and prescribing both treatments and medications. Eleven states now grant NPs direct third-party reimbursement for their services without a physician.

Clinical nurse specialists usually practice in secondary or tertiary care settings and focus on care of individuals who are experiencing an acute illness or an exacerbation of a chronic condition. In general, they are prepared at the graduate level and are ANCC certified. CNSs are highly skilled practitioners who are comfortable working in high-tech environments with seriously ill individuals and their families. Because of the nature of their work, they are excellent health-care educators and physician collaborators.

Attempts have been made to combine the roles of the CNS and NP so that the best qualities of both roles are preserved. The goal of this combination is to provide high-quality care to individuals in a wide array of health-care settings who have a wide range of health problems. Advocates of this movement include the National League for Nursing (NLN), American Association of Colleges of Nursing (AACN), and American Nurses Association (ANA). Titling for this new blended role is unconfirmed, and state legislatures may make the final decisions through their licensing laws.[4] As such, titling, educational preparation, and practice privileges will probably vary from one state to another.

Case Managers

One argument for the blended NP/CNS role is the need for case managers who possess the expertise of both levels of preparation.[4] **Case managers** coordinate services for clients with high-risk or long-term health problems who have access to the full continuum of health-care services. Case managers provide services in various settings, such as acute care facilities, rehabilitation centers, and community agencies.

> **" "** *One argument for the blended NP/CNS role is the need for case managers who possess the expertise of both levels of preparation.*

They also work for managed-care companies, insurance companies, and private case management agencies. Their roles vary depending on the circumstances of their employment; however, their overall goal is to coordinate the use of health-care services in the most efficient and cost-effective manner possible. **Case management** is the "glue" that holds health-care services together across practitioners, agencies, funding sources, locations, and time. Titling, educational preparation, and certification of nurse case managers are now available. The ANCC has developed certification eligibility criteria for nurse case managers, and an examination is available. At this time, case managers can be physicians, social workers, registered nurses, and even well-intentioned lay persons with little health-care education.

Other Key Health-Care Team Members

Physicians. Physicians in health care today include four groups and represent many subspecialties. Physicians (MDs) are the most common group of doctors; however, osteopaths (DOs), chiropractors (DCs), and podiatrists (DPMs) also play significant roles in the delivery of health care. Osteopaths are licensed to practice medicine and have the same clinical privileges as MDs. The main difference between MDs and DOs relates to their philosophical underpinnings of their training. Osteopaths have traditionally placed more emphasis than MDs on the importance of the relationship between body movement to overall health. Chiropractors tend to have a more limited scope of practice than MDs or DOs. They are not licensed to prescribe medications or perform surgery. Instead, they focus on the spinal column and its effect on the nervous system. They intervene by making therapeutic adjustments of the vertebrae. Like DCs, DPMs have a limited scope of practice and focus on the diagnosis and treatment of foot problems. They typically use medications, corrective devices, special shoes, and surgery to treat ordinary foot conditions.[2]

Among MDs and DOs, family practitioners are gradually becoming primary care providers for many individuals. From this initial point of service, clients may be referred to higher-priced specialists for conditions requiring expertise in specific body systems. This channeling of clients has come about in large part because of the efforts of managed care companies to limit the high cost of specialists.

For many years, physicians were considered to be at the pinnacle of the health-care delivery system. Physicians wrote orders, and the rest of the health-care delivery system workforce dutifully carried them out. However, as the health-care system has evolved, so has the role and position of physicians. One reason for this change relates to the fact that assessments, diagnoses, interventions, and evaluation of outcomes are no longer exclusively carried out in hospitals or physicians' offices. Instead, community-based services are representing an increasing portion of traditional care so that quality care can truly be provided at every level—primary, secondary, and tertiary. In addition, delivery of health care has become increasingly complex, and no one professional group can realistically maintain singular control over the entire system. Finally, payers are seeking to reimburse qualified individuals who deliver care in the most efficacious and cost-effective way possible. As such, the health-care delivery baton is gradually being passed to other practitioners, such as advanced practice nurses and physician assistants.

Physician Assistants. The evolution of physician assistants (PAs) can be traced to the post–Vietnam War period, when medical corpsmen returned to the United States and wished to pursue further medical education. This group has always been closely aligned with physicians, and unlike nurses, they have no individual licensure, but practice under the licensure of the supervising physician as regulated by the medical practice acts of each state. Their responsibilities include assessment and history taking, delineation of health problems, performance of routine procedures, implementation of individualized treatment plans under a physician's supervision, client education, and counseling. PAs sometimes work for individual physicians but are more commonly employed by hospitals, clinics, and group practices.[5] As in the case of advanced practice nurses, PAs have been well accepted by the public and are perceived to provide valuable and effective health care services.[6]

> 66 99 *As in the case of advanced practice nurses, PAs have been well accepted by the public and are perceived to provide valuable and effective health care services.*

Social Workers. Just as some physician responsibilities have been delegated to PAs and NPs, some responsibilities traditionally within the domain of nursing have been assumed by other health-care personnel. In particular, social workers have become increasingly important as the health-care delivery system has developed into a complex matrix of care providers and payers. These individuals play an important role in providing direct social services to clients in community and hospital settings. Their interventions are directed toward resolving financial, housing, psychosocial, and employment problems. In many cases, social workers also serve in case-management roles to ensure seamless coordination of services. They are frequently involved in discharge planning and assist clients to smoothly transfer from one care environment to another.

Physical Therapists. The high incidence of neurological and musculoskeletal health-care problems has made physical therapists important health-care providers. Physical therapists focus on helping individuals maintain or regain the highest level of function possible despite serious afflictions such as strokes, spinal cord injury, arthritis, or residual effects of traumatic accidents. Preventing physical decline and regaining the abilities to groom, eat, and walk are common therapeutic goals, which are accomplished mainly through individualized range of motion and exercise programs. Therapy occurs in hospitals, clinics, or in the community, where clients may be trained to use assistive devices such as canes, walkers, braces, and wheelchairs.[2]

Occupational Therapists. Occupational therapists focus on enhancing the quality of life of individuals who typically have problems that inhibit activities of daily living, such as strokes and spinal cord injuries. Care may be provided in homes or institutional settings and is directed toward assisting individuals to maintain or regain meaningful roles within and outside the home. Skills needed in work settings or the home are frequently honed to enhance independent functioning and self-confidence.[2]

Respiratory Therapists. Respiratory therapists have become increasingly valuable clinicians in the treatment of lung conditions. These individuals strive to restore normal or as near normal pulmonary functioning as possible by conducting diagnostic tests and administering treatments that have been prescribed by a physician.[2] This role is an excellent example of a position that has largely emerged as a result of technological developments in the treatment of respiratory problems and was once considered a part of the nurse's domain.

Clinical Psychologists. Within the health-care arena, clinical psychologists have traditionally played a role in assisting clients to manage mental health problems. In recent years, psychologists have found it more difficult to secure third-party reimbursement for outpatient services. This lack of reimbursement relates mainly to the fact that the efficacy of psychological counseling, especially of long duration, has not been well established. For this reason, some psychologists who were formerly in private practice have been seeking salaried positions within institutional settings where their focus is largely diagnosis and short-term intervention.

Pharmacists. A mere glance at any pharmacology textbook gives an indication of how numerous, complex, and technically sophisticated medications have become. In addition to their role as distributors of prescribed and over-the-counter medications, pharmacists have increasingly taken on the responsibility of educating clients, monitoring appropriate medication selections, and detecting interactions and untoward responses. These activities take place in community pharmacies as well as institutional settings.[3] Pharmacists are a valuable resource for nurses who are seeking to enhance their knowledge base and safely administer medications.

FACTORS INFLUENCING THE HEALTH-CARE DELIVERY SYSTEM

Demographics

One of the most important demographic trends affecting the health-care delivery system is the aging of Americans. Between now and the year 2050, the number of persons 65 years of age or older is estimated to double. It is projected that by 2050, 1 in 5 Americans will be elderly, and their numbers will reach an estimated 80 million. Of this number, many will eventually become more dependent on the health-care delivery system as a result of chronic health problems.[7]

Although aging Americans comprise a sizable number of persons who will potentially require expensive long-term health care, their community activism and powerful influence at the

> **" "** *Between now and the year 2050, the number of persons 65 years of age or older is estimated to double.*

ballot box may provide them with better access to health care than other less vocal and politically savvy groups. Additional at-risk groups consist of persons residing in urban areas with limited incomes as well as individuals living in remote rural areas where access to care is limited.

Health Problems

Another factor that is influencing the climate of health-care delivery in the United States is the long-term and expensive nature of many health problems. Although significant strides have been made in the treatment of some acute infectious diseases, many challenges still exist in the management of health concerns such as cancer, heart disease, Alzheimer's disease, diabetes, chronic obstructive lung disease, and human immunodeficiency virus (HIV). Additional concerns include environmental and occupational safety, drug abuse, and mother and child health care.

Health-Care Priorities

In light of the health problems being faced in the late twentieth century, the United States Department of Health and Human Services (DHHS) outlined proactive strategies for the year 2000 and beyond in the areas of health promotion, protection, and prevention. Health promotion priorities involved physical fitness, adequate nutrition, reduced use of tobacco and other harmful substances, family planning, preservation of mental health, avoidance of violence and abusive behavior, and community support services. Health-protection areas that were emphasized included reduced numbers of accidents, occupational safety and health, improved oral health, improved environmental quality, and food and drug quality.

In addition, mother and child health, heart disease, stroke, cancer, sexually transmitted diseases, HIV, and other infectious diseases were targeted for new preventive strategies. Finally, emphasis was placed on access to health-care services and the importance of individual, family, employer, community, and government responsibility in improving the profile of the nation's health.[8]

In the mid-1990s, the DHHS reported that 8% of these stated objectives had been reached, and progress was being made toward another 40%. The greatest progress had been made in heart disease, stroke, cancer, and unintentional injuries. However, in 18% of the targeted areas there had actually been a decline in rate of goal achievement. Areas in which there was movement away from the target objectives included diabetes and other chronic conditions, occupational safety and health, physical activity, mental health and mental disorders, and violence and abusive behavior. Finally, the gap between infant mortality among minority and nonminority groups widened, with

What Do You Think?

What are the leading health-care problems you have identified? How might these affect the health-care system of the future?

minorities experiencing an increasing number of infant deaths.[9]

Rising Costs

Rising costs are also affecting health-care delivery in this country. In 1996, health-care spending exceeded $1 trillion, which represents an average of $3759 per individual. Although overwhelming, these figures actually reflect a slowdown in the overall annual increase in spending to 4.4%.[10]

Many factors account for this spending pattern. Among them is the way third-party payers customarily reimbursed health-care services with little attention paid to cost-control measures. Other factors include the high cost of innovative technology, the increased need for long-term care, providers who have not always delivered care in the most cost-conscious manner, care provided to uninsured individuals, and the limited ability and motivation of consumers to compare health-care prices.

> **❝ ❞** *In 1996, health-care spending exceeded $1 trillion, which represents an average of $3759 per individual.*

WHO PAYS FOR HEALTH CARE?

There is no simple answer to the question of who pays for health care. Citizens of the United States have traditionally valued independence, individualism, competition, and private entrepreneurship over government control. They have also felt the need to provide care based on humanitarian concerns and a commitment to reduce suffering. These values have led to the development of one of the most fiscally complex health-care systems in the world. Paying for health care involves all levels of government, private enterprise, and innovative commercial financing structures.

It is important for nurses to be familiar with health-care reimbursement practices for several reasons. First, judgments about whether or not to perform diagnostic tests or to use certain treatment strategies are sometimes based on third-party payer guidelines. Second, decisions relating to how long a client is allowed to stay in a care facility are frequently determined by reimbursement policies. Third, plans of care based purely on financial incentives may raise legal and ethical questions. Fourth, the type of care individuals seek depends to some degree on the health-care benefits they have. For example, it is common for people who lack adequate coverage to seek care in an emergency department rather than using more economical primary care agencies such as community health centers or physicians' offices. As client advocates, nurses must understand reimbursement practices in order to offer clients appropriate advice and to make necessary referrals. Finally, advanced practice nurses need to understand reimbursement practices so that they can confidently negotiate fair salaries for themselves and lobby for appropriate reimbursement legislation.

Private Health-Care Insurance

As of 1998, approximately 70.2% of Americans have some kind of private health insurance.[11] These plans are most commonly offered by employers and are **retrospective payment systems** based on actual care rendered. This type of insurance is often used by the working population and covers more than 34% of hospital costs, 47% of physician services, and 47% of dental services. These policies cover a much smaller proportion of home care (13%) and nursing home expenses (3%).[5] An attractive aspect of most private health insurance is that the consumer can choose any health-care facility or physician and still receive the same insurance benefit. Private health insurance is offered through two primary mechanisms, commercial insurance companies and Blue Cross and Blue Shield.

Blue Cross and Blue Shield. Blue Cross and Blue Shield plans evolved during the Great Depression. Financial hardships among the rich resulted in fewer philanthropic donations, and nonprofit hospitals were forced to seek out new sources of revenue. The Blue Cross plan was sponsored by hospitals, and subscribers received hospital services in exchange for their **premiums,**

hence the term **point-of-service plans.** Physicians became involved when they saw an opportunity to guarantee payment for their services and to deter the government-sponsored national health insurance movement. As a result, Blue Shield coverage became readily available.[12]

From the beginning of the Blue Cross and Blue Shield programs, the physician's role in managing these plans raised questions. Traditionally, Blue Cross was controlled by hospital boards, which consisted mainly of physicians. Likewise, physicians made up a large percentage of the Blue Shield governing bodies. Moreover, physicians on Blue Cross and Blue Shield boards also frequently administered federal Medicare and state Medicaid programs. In short, those receiving payments had the most control over establishing prices. In recent years, sensitivity to this conflict of interest has led to an increased number of community representatives on Blue Cross and Blue Shield boards and in more private insurance companies administering these programs.[12]

Another criticism of Blue Cross and Blue Shield plans is that they have traditionally been oriented toward treating illness, with little emphasis placed on health promotion or illness prevention. Because of their size, Blue Cross and Blue Shield have had a significant impact on health-care legislation, but unfortunately, they have not led the way toward a primary health care focus.[12]

Commercial Insurance Companies. Commercial insurance companies, such as Metropolitan Life, Travelers, and Aetna, gained popularity after World War II when unions began to promote benefit packages in lieu of wage increases. A common feature of these **indemnity insurance** plans is that the client is responsible for a **copayment.** Copayments are charges the client is expected to pay when services are rendered. The insurer then directly reimburses either the consumer or provider for the balance of charges. Traditionally, these companies have avoided introducing cost controls except in cases where there appeared to be excessive use or abuse of services.

Unlike most traditional Blue Cross and Blue Shield companies, commercial insurance companies are **for-profit,** versus **not-for-profit,** and surplus income is paid to shareholders rather than automatically put back into the operating budget of the company.[5] For-profit status raises concerns for some in that loyalties to stockholders may be perceived as more important than providing the highest quality care possible to clients. In spite of this concern, more and more Blue Cross and Blue Shield companies have been moving toward for-profit status in recent years.

Self-insurance Arrangements. In an attempt to reduce costs, approximately 75% of the larger employers in this country are choosing to become self-insured.[13] This means that businesses are taking on the financial risk of offering their own self-funded health-care plans.

Employers perceive that there are several advantages to self-funded plans. First, under the **Employee Retirement Income Security Act** (**ERISA**) of 1974, outside regulators who supervise private insurance plans are eliminated. Second, employer self-funded plans are shielded from state regulations and can act as a tax shelter for the company. As a result of these exclusions, the cost of insuring employees is reduced.

Despite the advantages of self-insured plans, authorities have expressed concern about the lack of regulation and consumer protection. Although employers may fabricate other reasons for not hiring someone, there is the possibility that they may reject potential employees based on existing health problems, although this practice has become much more difficult under the Americans with Disabilities Act. However, the question remains whether the nation's workforce should be determined by these types of criteria.

Government-Funded Health Care

The creation of Blue Cross and Blue Shield in the 1930s only temporarily slowed the movement toward government involvement in health-care financing. By the mid-1960s, it became clear that changes needed to be made to ensure adequate health care for the elderly and the indigent. In 1965, legislation was passed that resulted in the establishment of the Medicare and Medicaid programs.[12] By 1996, these two programs financed $351 billion in health-care services, more than one-third of the nation's total health-care bill. Since 1989, this figure reflects an average annual increase in spending of 9.7%, versus 5.8% in the private sector.[10]

Medicare

Medicare is a federally run program that is financed primarily through employee payroll taxes. In 1996, Medicare paid out $203.1 billion in health-care costs.[10] This program covers any individual who is 65 years of age or older as well as permanently disabled workers of any age and their qualifying dependents. In addition, persons with end-stage renal disease are covered under this plan.

Medicare consists of two parts. Part A of Medicare is free in most instances and covers acute hospital, nursing home, hospice, and home-care services.[5] Part B may be purchased for a monthly premium, and 97% of the individuals participating in Part A are enrolled in the program.[14] Participants are covered for physician services, outpatient hospital care, laboratory tests, durable medical equipment, and certain other selected services. Although Medicare was designed for older Americans, long-term care is not covered, and health promotion and illness prevention benefits are limited. In addition, the cost of outpatient medications is not covered, which can account for a considerable portion of an elderly or disabled person's total monthly income. For this reason, it is estimated that a large majority of middle-income and upper-income individuals purchase private insurance, also known as **Medigap policies,** to cover these expenditures.[15]

Medicare was originally designed so that many services were fully covered. This arrangement did not provide cost-containment incentives, nor was the cost-benefit ratio of services taken into consideration. For example, heroic and costly measures were used to extend life with little consideration given to the quality of that existence, precipitating a financial crisis that peaked in the middle 1980s. Since then, cost-control measures have been implemented.

In 1983, a **prospective payment system** (**PPS**) was implemented in which hospitals are reimbursed based on a fixed rate, with incentives to reduce the length of hospital stays. At the core of this program is a classification system made up of hundreds of **diagnosis-related groups** (**DRGs**). Based on the particular DRG in which a client is placed, hospitals are reimbursed for a predetermined amount. In the event that a client is discharged early or costs are kept under the allotted amount, the hospital keeps the difference. In contrast, if a client's bill exceeds the maximum reimbursable amount, the hospital absorbs the cost.

From the outset, developers of the DRG classification system feared that quality of care might be compromised in favor of cost containment. To prevent misuse of the DRG

prospective payment system, the **Medicare Utilization and Quality Peer Review Organization** (**PRO**) was instituted. The purpose of this group is to ensure quality care and prevent misuse of the system.

Cost shifting has become a common practice since the implementation of the DRG prospective payment system. For example, to make up for lost revenues for clients on the DRG system, clients with other forms of insurance have been charged inflated amounts for health-care services. Reports of paying $7 or more for an aspirin tablet are not uncommon.[16]

Under the DRG prospective payment system, physician reimbursement remained untouched. Physicians continued to be reimbursed based on **customary, prevailing, and reasonable charges.** In other words, what was normally charged by physicians in a given geographic area is what they received for their services. If a physician charged more than the customary, prevailing, and reasonable rate for a service, he or she could bill the client for the remaining amount that Medicare did not pay. Attempts to control physician costs were resisted strongly by the American Medical Association (AMA), and as a result, between 1961 and 1991 the price of physician services increased more than sixfold.[17]

In an attempt to contain physician costs, Congress passed legislation in 1989 to establish (1) a standardized physician reimbursement schedule, (2) limits on **out-of-pocket expenses** for clients, (3) ceilings on the volume of services provided by physicians annually, and (4) federal practice guidelines to identify the most effective and efficient means of managing client care.[14]

In part, because uniform practice guidelines were established, CNSs and NPs argued that in addition to physicians, they too

> Cost shifting has become a common practice since the implementation of the DRG prospective payment system.

should receive direct Medicare reimbursement. Their rationale was that both APNs and physicians perform the same procedures using the same practice guidelines, thus, there should be no barriers to equitable and direct reimbursement for nurses. Thanks to the ardent efforts of many nurse lobbyists, Medicare legislation was passed in 1997 such that nurses now receive unrestricted Medicare reimbursement. In the past, only CNSs and NPs in rural areas could receive direct payments.[18,19]

Medicare is currently in a state of change because of the enormous number of baby boomers who will soon become eligible for Medicare benefits and the diminishing numbers of individuals who will be supporting the program through payroll taxes. It is thought that to sustain the Medicare program in a similar form, national health-care insurance is inevitable.[5] Even though many Americans are opposed to such a trend, Congress appears to be incrementally moving the country in this direction. For example, in an attempt to avoid Medicare fraud and cut costs, Congress passed legislation that severely penalizes physicians for accepting out-of-pocket payments for Medicare-reimbursable services. Physicians who accept such payments are subsequently ineligible to receive Medicare reimbursement for 2 years, a penalty that would seriously affect most practices.

This legislation has caused considerable confusion among the public, who perceives the Medicare program to be financially vulnerable but feels compelled to seek services within the parameters of the system. Individuals who have tried to provide insight into this situation suggest that this legislation is essentially a covert movement toward national health insurance. Other interesting developments that support this notion are

overall growth rates in Medicare spending versus diminishing growth rates of employer-sponsored health insurance premiums[10] and initiatives to lower the Medicare eligibility age from 65 to 55. Although purported to be self-supporting through participant premiums,[20] this latter initiative has the potential to greatly increase costs and force total reform of the Medicare financing mechanism.

Although Medicare has traditionally been a fee-for-service benefit, and individuals have typically been able to freely choose their health-care providers, managed-care initiatives have begun to change these practices. This is an example of a private sector initiative affecting a government program. The full impact of this trend is still unknown; however, it may foretell the emergence of a unique, albeit complex, reimbursement system that blends private and government reimbursement strategies. This trend also compels NPs and CNSs to join a **panel of approved providers** to ensure their reimbursement eligibility under Medicare.

Medicaid

Medicaid is a state-administered entitlement program that is designed to serve the poor. Funds are generated at the federal, state, and local levels; and each state has the freedom to customize its program based on the needs of its residents. Because the financial status of each state is different, Medicaid eligibility and services vary from place to place. States with more money tend to offer better benefit packages or cover more people than states that have limited resources. In fiscal year 1996, Medicaid paid out $147.7 billion for health services and supplies.[10]

 States with more money tend to offer better benefit packages or cover more people than states that have limited resources.

Services that are typically covered include hospitalization, diagnostic tests, physician visits, and rehabilitative and outpatient care. Medicaid often covers long-term nursing home costs after personal funds have been exhausted. States can opt to offer services such as home care, for which they receive federal matching funds. Because Medicaid covers the poor and may reimburse at relatively low levels, some practitioners are reluctant to treat patients covered under this program.

Although Medicaid was originally developed to serve the poor, some states are changing their eligibility requirements. In some areas of the country, individuals who are classified as **medically indigent** qualify for Medicaid benefits. Medically indigent refers to individuals who, if faced with medical expenses, would experience financial hardships. For all practical purposes, however, they are not considered poor. Some analysts have suggested that this is one more way in which health-care financing is surreptitiously moving toward a government-controlled system.

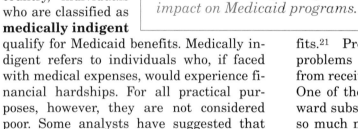

" " *Managed care initiatives are beginning to have an impact on Medicaid programs.*

Managed care initiatives are beginning to have an impact on Medicaid programs, and participants in some states are being asked to select from a panel of approved providers rather than having unlimited freedom to choose a practitioner. Capitated versus fee-for-service payment systems are also being instituted. Unfortunately, direct reimbursement under Medicaid is not guaranteed to qualified nurses; thus, continued lobbying efforts are necessary on a state-by-state basis.

Uninsured

Despite what may appear to be a plethora of reimbursement options, there were an estimated 41.7 million U.S. citizens (15.6%) in 1996 who had no health insurance.[11] It is a common misconception that these individuals receive adequate care through charitable donations. In reality, the insured receive 54% more ambulatory care services and 90% more hospital care than the uninsured.[21]

The uninsured tend to be from minority groups, lack higher education, unemployed or working part-time versus full-time, foreign born, poor, and between 18 and 24 years of age. Employees of small businesses (fewer than 25 individuals) also tend to be less well insured.[11] On the whole, white-collar workers have better health-care benefits than blue-collar workers and workers in service industries. Those in manufacturing still have relatively good benefits.[21] Preexisting or long-term health problems can preclude some individuals from receiving coverage at reasonable rates. One of the reasons that the movement toward substantial health-care reform gained so much momentum during the 1990s was because of the large number of uninsured.

HEALTH-CARE REFORM

In an attempt to meet the health-care needs of individuals in the United States, efforts were made at the federal level in the early 1990s to implement a system under which all American citizens and legal residents would have adequate health insurance coverage. The Clinton administration favored a plan in which the financial responsibility of **universal health-care coverage** would be placed on employers. Many were critical of this strategy because they feared government intervention into private enterprise and escalating costs of products and services. Others were skeptical that employer mandates would cover the cost of universal coverage and predicted that tax increases would be inevitable.[22]

Nurses also took an official position on health-care reform in the early 1990s, and the ANA called for employer-mandated universal coverage. Within this plan, a case-management approach was prescribed in which nurses acted as client advocates to provide and coordinate cost-effective comprehensive care. A care-versus-cure philosophy was part of the plan, combined with health promotion and illness prevention strategies.[23]

Group Practice Arrangements

A precursor to many of the ongoing changes in the health-care delivery system was the development of **group practices.** A group practice usually consists of three or more physicians, or nurse practitioners, who are formally organized to provide medical care. They distribute income according to a prearranged plan and jointly use equipment, records, and personnel.

Group practice arrangements are thought to be advantageous for a number of reasons. First, they preserve the ideal of private entrepreneurship while cutting overhead. Second, they are attractive to providers who prefer to hire professional managers. This arrangement enables practitioners to spend more time caring for clients and less time worrying about the mechanics of running a business. Group practice arrangements are also appealing because they offer providers more time off, better client coverage, and professional camaraderie. Finally, group practices frequently employ an array of specialists, and consumers are offered convenient, centralized, and comprehensive services. Because of these advantages, the number of group practices is continuing to increase.

Most group practices were originally set up such that individuals paid for services at the time care was rendered. As early as the 1890s, however, prepaid service contracts were offered by physicians working within

What Do You Think?

How did you feel about the proposed changes of the Clinton health-care system? How would these changes benefit or hurt health care?

group practices. Under these arrangements, potential clients prepaid a flat yearly fee in return for health-care services. At the time care was actually rendered, there were no additional costs to the client. As such, physicians were ensuring a certain level of income for the practice, but they were also accepting a calculated risk that they would procure enough prospective payments to generate a profit. In retrospect, these creative financing ventures foreshadowed current industry efforts to ensure a profitable health-care industry.[5]

Industry's Efforts to Manage Health-Care Costs: Managed Care

Managed care is a term used to describe health-care services that are administered to enhance their efficient and effective use. The primary purpose of these business ventures is to deliver, finance, buy, and sell quality health-care services as economically as possible. In theory, costs are limited by reducing the number of hospitalizations, decreasing the length of inpatient stays, providing more home care, and offering health promotion and illness prevention services.

One way that managed care is being enacted is through the use of **precertification.** Precertification requires that health-care providers receive preapproval from third-party reimbursers for a plan of care before it is initiated. This practice enables managed care organizations to cut costs by eliminating unnecessary procedures and encouraging practitioners to adhere to efficacious practice guidelines. Precertification approval also assures the client and provider that expenses will be covered. Nurses are frequently responsible for communicating with reimbursers to solicit precertification approval for a treatment plan. Although precertification is in widespread use, disconcerting questions loom regarding potential conflicts of interest. These conflicts include the impact that financial analysts have on making health-care decisions based on cost.

To date, the actual advantages of managed care systems are yet to be fully determined owing to a lack of data that fully reflect actual health-care outcomes and the comprehensive cost of health promotion, illness activities, and home-care services. The total cost of administering a comprehensive managed care system, which services the chronically ill with complex health problems as well as healthy individuals who merely access the system for acute care, is yet to be determined.

Managed-care systems consist of administrators, providers, and the physical facilities in which health care is delivered. Many times hospitals are the focal point of managed care organizations, with ancillary services providing an array of complementary care. These delivery systems are of interest to nurses, particularly advanced practice nurses, because of the autonomous practice opportunities they offer.

Several different administrative structures are characteristic of managed care arrangements. Some of the more common structures include **health maintenance organizations (HMOs), independent practice associations (IPAs), independent practice organizations (IPOs), preferred provider organizations (PPOs),** and **point-of-service (POS) plans** (Table 18.2). It should be noted that these systems are in a state of flux, and efforts are continually being made to refine them. To reduce costs, private insurance companies have had a major role in encouraging their development.

Health Maintenance Organizations. HMOs can be organized according to one of two ways: the staff model and the group model. In the staff model, the employees of the HMO both provide health care services and function as administrative personnel to supervise and manage the organization. With the group model there is a medical group that accepts a contract from an HMO to provide health-care services for its participants. The administrative functions are carried out by individuals from the HMO's own administrative staff. Regardless of their structures, the primary purpose of HMOs is to ensure profits by decreasing referrals to specialists, restricting diagnostic studies, decreasing client hospitalizations, reducing lengths of hospital stays, and using a **capitated payment system.**

In a capitated payment system, participants pay a flat rate, usually through their

> **" "** *Nurses are frequently responsible for communicating with reimbursers to solicit precertification approval for a treatment plan.*

ISSUES IN PRACTICE

Cost Containment in a Managed-Care Environment

Individuals working for managed care companies are sometimes asked to make difficult decisions about whether health-care services should be reimbursed. As former medical director of a health maintenance organization (HMO), Dr. Linda Peeno knows about this situation firsthand. Peeno was asked to precertify payment for a computerized voice box. This expensive equipment was requested for a female patient who was unable to speak as a result of a severe brainstem stroke. In this case, precertification was questioned because of the dubious medical necessity of the appliance. That is, the voice box was not deemed necessary to sustain life, rather, it would merely improve the quality of the person's existence. As such, it did not fall under the HMO's explicit guidelines for approval, and there was no precedent for blanket authorization.

In light of the company's recent financial losses, Dr. Peeno experienced pressure from supervisors, colleagues, and subordinates to deny payment for the voice box. Some HMO employees were so worried about the company's financial status, they expressed concern that they would lose their jobs if Peeno continued to precertify nonessential equipment. There was also concern about the financial toll this particular patient had already taken and would continue to take on the company because of the severe nature of her stroke and lengthy rehabilitation period. In short, high-quality care for this stroke victim meant fewer profits for the HMO, and Peeno felt pressure to deny precertification for the voice box.

In spite of company pressure, Peeno approved the voice box. Not only that, she approved the more expensive type—one with a female versus a male voice. Currently, Dr. Peeno reports that the voice box recipient has resumed work and is leading a productive life. As a result of this and other similar situations in which Peeno made decisions that were frowned upon by her supervisors, however, she resigned from the HMO. She now chairs the ethics committee at the University of Louisville Hospital and consults nationally and internationally on medical ethics.

Source: Brink, S: What is the value of a voice? US News & World Report 124(9):40–43, 46, 1998.

employer, to belong to an HMO for a prescribed period of time. Expenses incurred by the HMO in excess of the capitated rate during the contract period are considered financial losses. Amounts that remain after services have been rendered and costs have been covered are profit. In short, health-care practitioners who function within an HMO have strong incentives to keep costs down and ensure profits. The uniqueness of this system is that health-care providers share in the financial risk. The ideal HMO is one in which there is a large pool of healthy members who require few services

Table 18.2	**Comparison of Indemnity Insurance and Some Managed-Care Options**			
	INDEMNITY INSURANCE	HMO	IPA (HMO)	PPO
Copayment	Yes	Nominal	Nominal	Varies
Fee for service	Yes	No	Yes	Yes
Limited number of providers	No	Yes	Yes	Yes
Out-of-plan provider option	N/A	Emergencies only	Emergencies only	Penalty applies
Utilization guidelines	No	Yes	Yes	Yes

and relatively few unhealthy clients who require more and expensive care.

HMOs appear attractive to clients for two reasons. First, after premiums are paid, care is free or requires only a small copayment if a designated HMO provider is used. Second, cost-containment incentives are in place to keep expenses down. Less attractive aspects of HMOs include a limited number of providers under contract at any one time. Clients must select a practitioner from a list of providers (**provider panel**) that may exclude the client's preferred clinician. If individuals choose to use providers who are not included in their HMO's panel, they must pay for those services themselves. The only exception is in emergency situations, such as when an individual is injured in a car accident away from home.

Independent Practice Associations. A variation of the traditional HMO is the IPA, which is usually organized by physicians. Within this structure, HMOs contract with physicians and hospitals to provide care for their members. Physicians are paid on a **fee-for-service** basis at rates that are usually predetermined and attractive to payers. Fee-for-service means that IPA members are charged for each service at the time care is provided, unlike most HMO plans, in which members pay premiums and are not charged for each service individually. Similar to traditional HMOs, IPAs do not reimburse for payments to nonmember providers. Finally, hospitals and physicians must adhere to **utilization guidelines** to contain costs that limit the number of services they can provide. Independent practice organizations (IPOs) are a variation of IPAs in that a group of providers deals with more than one payer at a time.

What Do You Think?

How do you feel about health-care providers making a profit on the care they provide? Do you belong to an HMO? What is the quality of care you receive?

Preferred Provider Organizations.
PPOs are another type of managed care organization that can be sponsored by providers, insurance companies, or employers. Contracts are established with a limited number of health-care facilities and professionals, and lower than customary rates are usually negotiated. In an attempt to contain costs, providers are required to adhere to PPO utilization guidelines. In return for these concessions, provider services are used by greater numbers of clients.

Within PPO systems, physicians are reimbursed on a fee-for-service basis and members are charged each time care is provided. In addition to the fee-for-service arrangement, some PPO plans require participant copayments in which individuals pay a percentage of the cost of services. The copayment requirement is thought to decrease client use and thus reduce costs.

A critical difference between HMO and PPO plans is that use of the PPO providers is encouraged through preferential rates; however, benefits extend beyond the use of these services. Penalties apply if providers are used outside of the PPO, but their use is not prohibited.

Point-of-service (POS) plans are similar to the PPOs, in that they allow clients to access designated practitioners outside the prescribed panel of providers for an additional fee. This option is provided to ensure comprehensive care. Americans have traditionally valued the freedom to choose their health-care providers, making PPOs and POS options more popular than traditional HMO plans.

Current and Future Managed Care

One of the primary goals of managed care is to reduce costs. Studies suggest that this goal is being achieved in some instances as a result of fewer hospital admissions, shortened lengths of stay, and expanded home care services.[24] In spite of these optimistic findings, hospital expenditures rose 3.4% in 1996 to reach a grand total of $358.5 billion.[10]

Additional expenses that may not have been accounted for in this total include the comprehensive costs of running managed care operations and the actual price of providing care in the home. The problem of determining home-care costs stems from the fact that a standardized and accurate system for pricing, billing, and reimbursement is still in the state of development.[25] Also in development are ways to control the quality of care being provided in community settings, assessment of long-term client outcomes, and measurement of overall client satisfaction. As solutions to these problems emerge, the overall effectiveness of managed care will be more clearly determined and the health-care delivery system will continue to evolve.

For most consumers, as well as many health-care providers, the current health-care delivery system has become a confusing alphabet soup of options, some of which include HMOs, IPAs, IPOs, PPOs, and POS plans. Nurses need to remain informed about health-care delivery options to ensure the best possible practice environments and to promote the most efficacious and cost-effective delivery system for clients. It is also important to be knowledgeable about these issues in order to talk informatively to legislators and make wise decisions at the ballot box.

Issues that still require resolution include the following: Should privatization of the health-care delivery system be continued, with an emphasis on fewer and less

> " " *For most consumers, as well as many health-care providers, the current health-care delivery system has become a confusing alphabet soup of options.*

confusing options? Will increased government-controlled interventions make the health-care system more cohesive and comprehensive? Should the current dual-track system, consisting of government and private sector options, be maintained but with the goal of streamlining the system? Nurses need to become involved in these issues and can play an important part in the transformation process occurring in the health-care system.

CARE DELIVERY MODELS

The organizational structure of a facility reflects how the nursing department participates in the delivery of client care. Various models may be used in the delivery of nursing care. Many health-care facilities are currently in a period of transition from one model to another and may even incorporate several different models at the same time. The nurse must recognize which model is being used as well as its strengths and weaknesses. These models include functional nursing, team nursing, primary care nursing, and modular nursing.

Functional Nursing

Functional nursing (Fig. 18-1) has as its foundation a task-oriented philosophy—each person performs a specific job that is narrowly defined according to the needs on the unit. The medication nurse, for example, focuses on the duties concerned with administering and documenting medications for the assigned group of clients. In this organizational unit, the nurse manager is called the "charge nurse," whose main responsibility is to oversee the various workers. Charge nurses are also appointed for each shift to manage the care during that time. This model relies on ancillary health workers such as nurse aides and orderlies. Some believe this model fragments care too much. Because many people have specific tasks, coordination can be difficult, and the holistic perspective may be lost.

Team Nursing

Team nursing (Fig. 18-2) has a more unified approach to client care, with team members functioning together to achieve client goals.

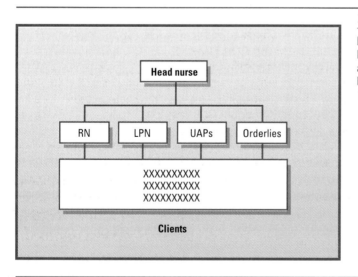

➤ Figure 18-1

Functional nursing. (Adapted from Marquis, BL, and Huston, CJ: Management Decision Making for Nurses. JB Lippincott, Philadelphia, 1994, p 141, with permission.)

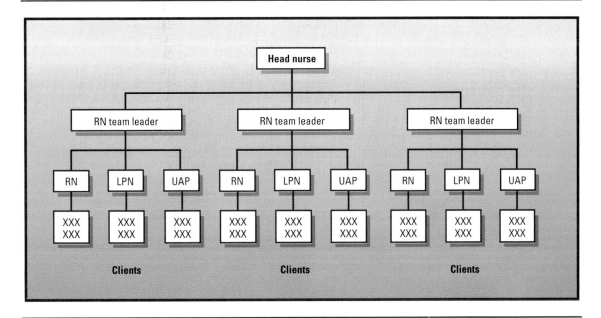

➤ Figure 18-2

Team nursing. (Adapted from Marquis, BL, and Huston, CJ: Management Decision Making for Nurses. JB Lippincott, Philadelphia, 1994, p 142, with permission.)

The team leader functions as the person ultimately responsible for the clients' well-being. More cohesiveness is present among the members of the team than is found in the functional model. Rather than having a narrow task to accomplish, team members focus on team goals under the coordination of the team leader. The team conference provides for effective communication and follow-up between and among team members and is the key to successful team nursing.

Primary Care Nursing

The primary care nursing model (Fig. 18-3) provides nurses the opportunity to focus on the whole person. The primary care nurse provides and is responsible for all of the client's nursing needs. The nurse manager in this model becomes a facilitator for the primary care nurses. Primary care nurses are self-directed and concerned with the consistency of care. The primary care model is similar to the case management model, which has one nurse caring for one client. Many home health agencies use this method of assigning a registered nurse to work with an individual or family for the duration of the services rendered.

Modular Nursing

Modular nursing (Fig. 18-4), also called client-focused care, is one model that was developed in response to professional nursing personnel shortages and to the downsizing of professional nursing staffs. This model is based on a decentralized organizational system that emphasizes close interdisciplinary collaboration. Redesigning the

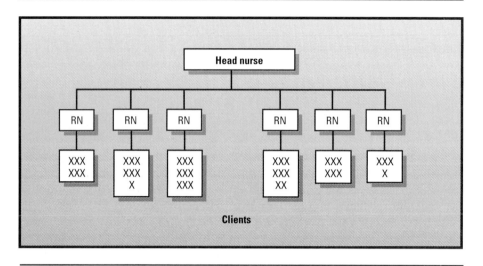

➤ Figure 18-3

Primary nursing. (Adapted from Marquis, BL, and Huston, CJ: Management Decision Making for Nurses. JB Lippincott, Philadelphia, 1994, p 142, with permission.)

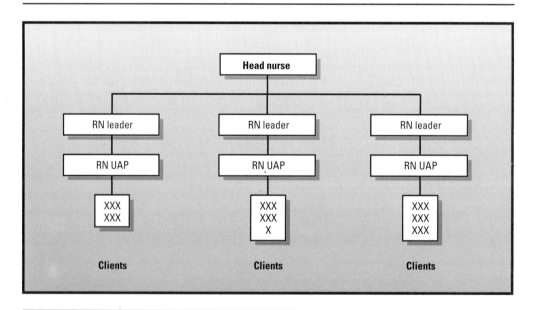

➤ Figure 18-4

Modular nursing. (Adapted from Marquis, BL, and Huston, CJ: Management Decision Making for Nurses. JB Lippincott, Philadelphia, 1994, p 143, with permission.)

method of nursing care delivery takes much planning and input from the various departments involved, such as nursing, respiratory therapy, physical therapy, radiology, laboratory, and dietary.

Important aspects of modular nursing include relying on unlicensed assistive personnel (UAP), also called unit service assistants, for the provision of direct care; grouping clients with similar needs; developing **relative intensity measures** (**RIMs**); and emphasizing team concepts in small groups that remain constant. Cross-training of personnel is another important aspect of modular nursing; for example, using this system, respiratory therapists do not just provide respiratory treatments but also help clients to the bathroom and turn bedridden clients. Nurse managers in this system are responsible for providing explicit job descriptions, maintaining the work group's cohesiveness, carefully monitoring each staff person's abilities, delegating tasks as appropriate, and evaluating the effectiveness of care.

The role of UAP is one area of the client-focused care model that needs more definition, particularly in relation to the registered nurse's accountability and responsibilities in supervising these workers. State boards of nursing across the country are in the process of considering possible changes in nurse practice acts necessitated by the use of UAP.

Benefits of this care delivery model include decreased staffing cost and greater autonomy of cross-trained personnel. The nurse manager must be a strong leader for this model of care delivery to succeed. Consistent collaboration between the nurse manager and physician is of utmost importance in planning client care.[26]

> _Delivering high-quality services is valued above all else, and the ideal goal is that every constituent be completely satisfied with the services provided._

QUALITY ASSURANCE

Continuous Quality Improvement

Quality assurance initiatives have become very important during this turbulent time of change in which efforts are being made to cut costs and, at the same time, maintain high standards of care. In order to ensure high-quality care, the health-care industry borrowed the philosophy of **continuous quality improvement** (**CQI**) from the business world. The **Joint Commission on Accreditation of Healthcare Organizations** (**JCAHO**) was so impressed with its potential to improve health-care delivery, that in 1994 it began requiring hospitals to implement CQI strategies.

CQI, also known as **total quality management** (**TQM**), is based on the belief that the organization with the higher-quality service will capture a greater share of the market than competitors with lower-quality services. Emphasis is placed on not only meeting the expectations of the customer (in this case, the health-care consumer) but exceeding those expectations. Within the CQI philosophy, there are internal customers and external customers. The external customers are clients and their families, whereas internal customers are individuals working within the health-care setting. Delivering high-quality services is valued above all else, and the ideal goal is that every constituent be completely satisfied with the services provided.

CQI requires that the process used to deliver services receive close and constant scrutiny, and everyone is encouraged to generate ideas for improving quality. Although change based on systematically documented evidence is encouraged, standardization of

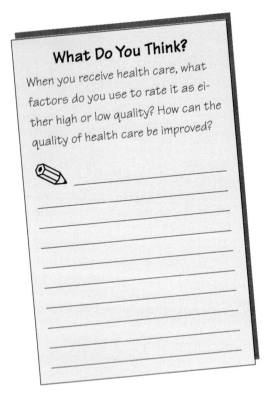

the process is also valued so that efficiency is maximized. CQI is proactively oriented so that the emphasis is placed on anticipating and preventing problems rather than reacting to them after the fact.[27]

Nurses are in an excellent position to implement CQI strategies. On a daily basis, they assess how the health-care delivery system is functioning and the effectiveness of specific treatment approaches. For example, based on evidence that inexpensive saline is as effective as heparin in keeping intermittent intravenous catheters patent, nurses at one hospital implemented a new protocol and saved $70,000 within 1 year.[28]

Case Management Protocols

Another mechanism that has been instituted for monitoring cost-effective quality care has been outcomes based case management protocols, also known as **clinical pathways.** The development of clinical pathways grew out of a need to assess, implement, and monitor cost-effective quality client care in a systematic manner. Clinical pathways were an outgrowth of nursing care plans but had the advantages of streamlining the charting process, encouraging documentation across multidisciplinary team members, and systematically monitoring variances from prescribed plans of care. The ability to identify how client care and progress varied from a predetermined plan enabled more accurate assessment of client care costs and maintenance of quality control measures. Integration of clinical pathways into practical usage has been enhanced by computerization of client records and on-line, bedside documentation.[29]

Integrated Information Systems

Although yet to be fully implemented in today's health-care delivery system, another important element in ensuring quality and providing coordinated care is an information network in which client data are efficiently shared not only from one unit to another but also from one facility to another. By sharing information, all health-care team members can make informed decisions about a client's plan of care based on an understanding of both the client's past health history and current problems. For example, if a client was transferred from an acute to a subacute facility, a full accounting of the person's physical condition and psychosocial status could be made available by on-line computer to physicians, nurses, social workers, and physical therapists at the receiving facility. In addition to promoting higher quality care, a computerized information network has the potential to cut costs by preventing duplication of services and streamlining billing. Before such a system is fully realized, however, issues surrounding unauthorized access to records and client confidentiality need to be resolved.

HEALTH CARE AGENCIES

Outpatient Care

In recent years, several factors have led to greater demand for outpatient services, also known as alternative ambulatory services. First, implementation of the Medicare prospective payment system resulted in shorter hospital stays. Second, private insurers and managed care companies encouraged use of ambulatory versus inpatient services to reduce costs. Third, new technology made procedures that were formerly complicated or dangerous available on an outpatient basis. Finally, consumers demanded less expensive and more user-friendly health-care services.

Some hospitals are embedding themselves within a cluster of outpatient services. Others are establishing satellite clinics in surrounding suburbs and rural communities. Outpatient facilities are also cropping up in retail malls, where families can shop or eat lunch while significant others are receiving health-care services. Services commonly provided in ambulatory care settings include general medical examinations; treatment of injuries; diagnoses of illnesses such as upper respiratory infections, hypertension, and otitis media; and medication therapy.[30]

Nursing Homes and Other Long-term Care Facilities

Today, more senior citizens need long-term care. In addition, individuals of all ages are managing their lives with conditions such as HIV, traumatic head injuries, and other debilitating problems. Such individuals require extended care and rehabilitative ser-

What Do You Think?

List some nontraditional health-care settings that you are familiar with. How is the quality of the care provided? Would you be willing to work in one of these settings after you graduate? Why, or why not?

vices. Hospitals and nursing homes are attempting to meet these demands by developing units to accommodate the long-term needs of these clients.

Some hospitals are beginning to provide care in home-like atmospheres. Large client rooms, comfortable dining areas, and space for activities are important to meet the psychosocial needs of clients who stay for extended periods of time. Emphasis is also being placed on interacting with family members and involving them in the client's care. Because the restorative process may be slow, priority is placed on long-term goals and adjusting to ongoing health concerns.[31]

Nursing homes are another place where long-term health care is being provided. Although clients in these settings experience complex health problems, acute care is usually not necessary. Nursing homes generally provide care for two types of clients. Some individuals are admitted to recuperate after being hospitalized and generally stay fewer than 90 days. They may be recovering from surgery and require assistance until they are able to manage independently. Other clients need care for lengthier periods of time because they are more disabled or do not have significant others who can assist them at home. They may require services ranging from help with activities of daily living to skilled nursing care.

The nursing home industry has experienced considerable growth in recent years, and there are now more beds in these facilities than in acute care hospitals. Traditionally, nursing homes were nonprofit agencies sponsored by organizations such as churches. Today, approximately 75% of all nursing homes are for-profit institutions, and they rely heavily on Medicaid and Medicare reimbursements.[5] Medicare benefits may be limited, and private insurance frequently pays the balance charged.

Assisted Living Centers

Assisted living centers are becoming increasingly appealing to both the public and those in the health-care industry as the need for a comprehensive continuum of cost-effective health-care services grows. Assisted living centers have the advantage of allowing clients to maintain the greatest amount of independence possible, while providing a protective living environment where assistive services are available as needed. Individuals in these centers frequently maintain their own private living quarters; prepare some or all of their own meals; and may transport themselves via their own vehicles to shopping malls, church, and social events.

These centers are increasingly being developed or bought by integrated long-term care companies so that as client acuity levels rise, individuals who require care can be easily integrated into company-owned nursing homes. Likewise, when less acute care is required, clients can be easily transferred back to their assisted living quarters.[32]

Adult Day Care Centers

In an attempt to meet the health-care and psychosocial needs of a growing number of individuals in the community, adult day care centers are becoming more common. These centers provide services primarily for elderly clients who need supportive care for physical problems, organic brain dysfunction, or mobility problems that make them vulnerable to social isolation. Care is available during the day, and clients return to supervised home settings at night. Adult day care services may provide an alternative to more expensive nursing home residency or home-care services.

Comprehensive adult day care centers provide holistic services, including nursing care, rehabilitation therapy, assistance with activities of daily living, transportation, social services, and recreational activities. As such, they employ a wide array of professional staff such as dietitians, art therapists, social workers, physical and occupational therapists, as well as nurses. Some adult day care centers have a more narrow focus, such as those that provide care for individuals with mental health problems. More and more, adult day care centers are becoming vertically integrated into a network of health-care services, which helps to ensure a client referral base for all agencies involved.

In the past, it has been common for adult day care centers to be funded by government agencies, philanthropic organizations, and private payments. Today, these facilities are relying less on government and philanthropic subsidies and are looking more toward traditional third-party payment sources. Currently Medicaid is assuming a large portion of the cost of these services, whereas Medicare has not traditionally reimbursed for such care. Commercial long-term care insurers have been slow to reimburse for adult day care; however, there is increased interest in this option versus more expensive alternatives such as nursing home placement.[33] The general public is also expected to put more pressure on commercial insurers to reimburse for these services because of their growing popularity.

Home Care Agencies

More and more, nurses employed by home care agencies are assuming responsibilities in private residences that public health nurses previously assumed. These nurses may work for hospital-based or local independent agencies, regional-national chains, or private duty registries. In recent years, many independent home care agencies have been vertically integrated into health-care system networks. Home care agencies have benefited from this restructuring because it provides them with a continual source of client referrals. Likewise, parent agencies have benefited by being able to enhance continuity of client care. In the past, home care agencies focused on the provision of long-term care. In recent years, however, this focus has shifted more toward short-term care that can be funded through

Medicare or other payment sources. To supplement home-health-care services, home health aide and homemaker assistance may also be available. Homemakers typically do not help with bathing and grooming but provide services such as housekeeping, meal preparation, and transportation.

Hospice

The philosophy behind hospice care originated in Great Britain and has grown in popularity in this country over the last few decades. Today, hospices are designed to offer compassionate care to terminally ill clients and their family members. Services are provided in homes or institutional settings, usually by nurses and homemakers. Psychological support, respite care for family members, and comfort and pain control measures are common interventions. Preservation of client and family dignity, integrity, and overall well-being is of utmost importance. Medicare provides reimbursement for hospice services if clients meet the guidelines for care.

Community Health Centers

Community health centers provide services primarily for medically underserved and disadvantaged individuals. Based on their philosophical origins, community health centers make a special effort to tailor services to meet local needs, and community members are intimately involved with their operation, development, and governance. These centers are supported by federal funds, and their focus is on health promotion and disease prevention. Some centers offer emergency assistance, home care, mental health counseling, and

> **" "** *More and more, nurses employed by home care agencies are assuming responsibilities in private residences that public health nurses previously assumed.*

rehabilitative support. Diagnostic, laboratory, and pharmaceutical services may also be available.

Community health centers use a team approach, and nurses along with physicians and physicians' assistants are the main care providers. The variety of ambulatory services offered tends to vary as government funding fluctuates. As Medicare and Medicaid funding declines, **sliding-scale fees** are relied on more heavily. Using sliding-scale fee schedules, clients pay differing amounts depending on their incomes. Along with public hospitals, community health centers are being influenced by the capitated payment movement, and some fear that their long-term survival is in jeopardy unless they incorporate with integrated health-care delivery agencies and managed care operations.[34]

School-Based Health Care

Nurses provide a variety of services within local school systems. These services include screenings, health promotion and illness prevention programs, and treatment of minor health-care problems. Emphasis is placed on physical, social, and psychological well-being. Concerns relating to self-esteem, stress, drug abuse, and adolescent pregnancy are frequently addressed by the school nurse. In addition, children and adolescents with long-term health problems often attend school, and it is not uncommon for the nurse to be consulted about such issues as seizure management, colostomy care, or gastric tube feedings.

Students who have health concerns are frequently referred to providers within the community; and an important role of the school nurse is that of community liaison. For this reason, the nurse must be knowledgeable about community resources and adept at getting clients into the system in a timely and efficient manner.

Workplace Health Centers

As a result of rising health-care costs and lost productivity related to health problems, employers are increasingly supporting workplace health promotion, illness prevention, and safety programs. It is estimated that 80% of businesses employing 50 workers or more have some sort of health program.[5] Some programs are mainly educational; others provide health screenings and referrals; and still others offer classes on topics such as stress management, nutrition, exercise, and substance abuse. In industrial settings, health-care services are typically more comprehensive, and preliminary emergency services may be provided in the event of an accident. Nurses usually staff industrial health-care centers; however, company health promotion programs are commonly run by health educators.

Nurse-Run Health Centers

Similar to community health centers, nurse-run health centers tend to focus on health promotion and disease prevention. Historically, they have been service versus profit oriented and remain so today. Nurses who are interested in autonomous practice often work in these settings.

Several types of nurse-run health centers have been identified. Among these are community health and institutional outreach centers. These facilities may be freestanding or sponsored by a larger institution, such as a university or public health agency. Primary care services are generally offered to the medically underserved, and these centers are typically funded by public and private sources. Wellness and health promotion clinics are another type of nurse-run clinic that offer services at work sites, schools, churches, or homeless shelters. Many of these centers are affiliated with schools of nursing, providing health-care services while offering educational experiences for nursing students. A final type of nursing center includes faculty practice, independent practice, and nurse entrepreneurship models. These facilities are owned and operated by nurses and may be solo or multidisciplinary practices. Services are typically reimbursed through fee-for-service, grant monies, and insurance. The ability of nurses in these centers to secure payments through the newly emergent and complex health-care reimbursement network will in large part determine the future financial viability of these types of clinics.[35]

Public Health Departments

Epidemics in the eighteenth and nineteenth centuries forced community leaders to take measures to prevent and control communicable diseases in their communities. Along with this mission came an emphasis on public education and home care. Today, public health departments are administered by state, county, or city governments. The emphasis of public health departments is now on prevention and the management of acute and chronic conditions among the population rather than home care. Foci include prenatal care, children's health, detection and treatment of tuberculosis, control of sexually transmitted diseases, and mental health problems. Although a large percentage of clients seen in these settings are indigent, receive Medicaid, or are Medicare recipients, the services are available to all members of the community.

Parish Nurses

It is estimated that approximately 2000 parish nurses throughout the country are attempting to meet the needs of individuals who are without adequate primary care or who are experiencing escalating health-care costs. Many of these nurses work part-time or are volunteers, and some work in conjunction

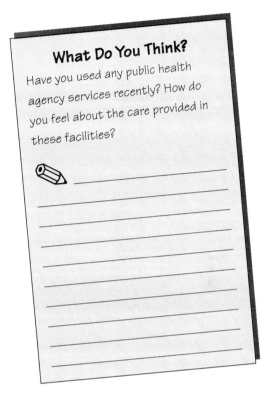

What Do You Think?

Have you used any public health agency services recently? How do you feel about the care provided in these facilities?

with community-based programs. Churches are engaging parish nurses to (1) serve as health educators and counselors, (2) do health assessments and referrals, (3) organize support groups, (4) make visits to parishioners who are sick or elderly, and (5) serve as client advocates or case managers.[36]

Parish nurses are in a unique position to exercise their skills as case managers. As nurses, they possess clinical knowledge and skills, understand the health-care delivery system within their communities, and know many of the key health-care providers. As members of their parish, they are intimately familiar with their communities, understand the cultural climate of their clientele, and are familiar with the services that are available. Moreover, as members of the church community that they serve, they are likely to be familiar with the spiritual, psychosocial, and financial needs of their clients. However, direct reimbursement is not yet available for parish nurses.

Voluntary Health Agencies

Since their inception in 1892, voluntary health agencies have experienced steady growth to the point where they currently number more than 100,000. The first voluntary health agency was the Anti-tuberculosis Society of Philadelphia.[12] Some of the more well known agencies that exist today include the American Cancer Society, The American Heart Association, The National

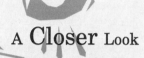

A Closer Look

PARISH NURSE CASE MANAGER

Margaret has been a parish nurse for the past 5 years in a moderate-sized Protestant church. Charlie, an elderly member of the congregation, has congestive heart failure. Up until now, he has managed this condition by himself. Recently, however, his wife of 60 years died, and he experienced an exacerbation of his condition that required hospitalization. During this inpatient stay, his physician suggested nursing home placement, which Charlie strongly opposed. Formerly a farmer, he now lives in a small home in town. His two daughters are supportive; however, they live elsewhere and are unable to offer day-to-day assistance.

Margaret has known Charlie since her childhood and is well acquainted with his home, church, family, and community environment. As the parish nurse case manager, Margaret is recruited to assist in monitoring Charlie's health status as well as organizing social services that will enable him to stay in his home. Margaret has a working relationship with the community's older adult services organization and quickly arranges to have meals delivered to Charlie's home daily. A homemaker is also scheduled to do laundry and clean once a week. Members of the congregation are enlisted to do his weekly shopping and accompany him to church functions. In addition, Margaret arranges for Charlie to participate in a government-subsidized transportation program so that he can attend social and recreational functions at the community senior citizen center. This service also enables him to independently keep regularly scheduled appointments with his physician. Between physician visits, Margaret goes to Charlie's house to do periodic health assessments and monitor his medications. She routinely assesses for signs of side effects and monitors for drug use compliance. As a result of the availability of these services, Charlie has been able to stay in his home, and the inconvenience and expense of nursing home care has been avoided.

A Closer Look

A RURAL NURSING CENTER

The Sinclair School of Nursing at the University of Missouri-Columbia operates a Nursing Center in Moberly, Mo., a rural community in the north-central sector of the state. The Center is located on the campus of Moberly Area Community College and services faculty, staff, students, and their family members. This rural community is approximately 40 miles from the closest comprehensive health-care complex and is generally perceived to be an underserved area.

The mission of the Nursing Center is to provide primary care, which includes health promotion and illness prevention programs and treatment of commonly occurring acute conditions such as colds and influenza. Nurses conduct physical examinations and diagnostic screenings, monitor long-term health problems such as hypertension and diabetes, offer health education programs, and prescribe and administer medications such as antibiotics, contraceptives, and flu vaccines. Weight reduction, smoking cessation, and stress management programs are commonly offered at the Center. Short-term mental health counseling is provided for individuals experiencing psychosocial crises and as adjunctive therapy for persons in the center's weight reduction and smoking cessation programs. Persons with chronic mental health concerns frequent the Center to ask questions and seek intermittent supportive counseling.

The Center is staffed by master's prepared nurse practitioners, clinical nurse specialists prepared at the master's or doctoral level, one RN with an associate's degree, and a secretary. Most of the clinical staff are faculty members at the University of Missouri-Columbia Sinclair School of Nursing, as is the Director of the Center. The Director is a master's prepared clinical nurse specialist with extensive administrative experience. The facility provides a site for faculty practice and student clinical experiences. It also offers a rich source of data for faculty and student research projects.

Currently, the Nursing Center is funded through a federal grant, and client fees are being waived. Steps are being taken, however, to electronically integrate the Nursing Center's billing procedures with a computerized system at the University of Missouri-Columbia Health Science Center. Efforts are also being made to implement a student health fee and to qualify for direct third-party reimbursement. Client billing is anticipated to begin in the near future.

Client response to the Center has been positive, and except for mental health counseling, appointments are unnecessary. Individuals tend to drop by between classes for services. The Center's record keeping was recently computerized; thus, outcomes and cost effectiveness are being monitored in a systematic manner.

Foundation for the March of Dimes, The National Easter Seal Society for Crippled Adults and Children, and the Alliance for the Mentally Ill. These agencies provide many valuable services, some of which include fundraising in support of cutting-edge research and public education. Others, such as the American Cancer Society, which has a strong emphasis on education and research, also help individuals secure special equipment such as hospital beds for the home and wigs for chemotherapy patients. The Alliance for the Mentally Ill is very politically active and organizes support groups for the mentally ill and their families. These groups are not-for-profit organizations, so that all revenue in excess of cost goes toward improving services.

RURAL HEALTH CARE

Delivery of health care in rural areas presents unique challenges. These challenges result from low numbers of physicians, nurses, and allied health-care professionals who are willing to live and practice in re-

---

Site Seeing

Agency for Health Care Policy and Research (AHCPR)
http://www.ahcpr.gov/ info@ahcpr.gov

American Nurses Association
http://www.ana.org/
http://www.nursingworld.org/
Contact: mail to:webfeedback@ana.org

Community Health Information Resources
http://chmis.org/
Contact: mail to:baguilar@eskimo.com

Global Health Network
http://www.pitt.edu/HOME/GHNet/GHNet.html
Contact: Amy Brenen
mail to:brenena@ghnet.org

HCFA: The Medicare and Medicaid Agency
http://www.hcfa.gov/
Contact: mail to:webmaster@hcfa.gov

Healthcare Information Systems Directory
http://www.health-infosys-dir.com/
Contact: mail to:hisd@health-infosys-dir.com

National Health Information Center (NHIC)
http://nhic-nt.health.org/
Contact: mail to:NHICinfo@health.org

National League for Nursing
http://www.nln.org/
Contact: mail to:nlnweb@nln.org

Nightingale
http://nightingale.con.utk.edu/index.htm
Contact: mail to:mackbo@utk.edu

Nurses' Station (Downsizing)
http://www.hci.net/~nursecline
Contact: Joseph A. Cline, RN, BSN
mail to:nursecline@hci.net

Thomas (U.S. Government Legislative Information)
http://thomas.loc.gov/

mote areas; decreased access to advanced medical technology; and the fact that rural hospitals often have more expenses than revenues. In recent years, many rural hospitals have been forced to close or severely curtail their services.

Rural health-care delivery problems are being overcome through integrated delivery networks that provide primary, secondary, and sometimes tertiary care to residents in designated regions. Rural health-care providers are often employees of large multi-layered networks and function under the aegis of a single administrative staff. These systems are composed of physicians, nurse practitioners, nurses, physicians' assistants, and other ancillary health-care personnel who provide local primary health care. To receive secondary and tertiary care within the network, rural residents must frequently travel considerable distances. Although complex and sometimes inconvenient, this layering of services under the same administrative umbrella makes rural health care financially feasible.

Paying for health-care services is another concern for rural residents. Many of these individuals are farmers or employees of small businesses that do not offer health benefits. To overcome this problem, the use of **health insurance purchasing cooperatives** (**HIPCs**) has been proposed. These are large groups of people or employers who band together to buy insurance at reduced costs. HIPCs may be organized by private groups or the government. A typical concern in establishing such groups is estimating the minimum number of individuals necessary to make the organization financially viable. For example, taking into consideration the health status of the population in question, it is important to correctly estimate the minimum number of individuals who will need to pay into the system to cover the resultant costs of those who need services.

Conclusion

The health-care delivery system in this country offers a variety of care facilities, payment plans, and providers. Nurses have traditionally played key roles as direct care providers. As the delivery system changes, however, that role will be expanded and transformed. It is anticipated that nurses will take on additional responsibilities in primary care, case management, and the community. Nurses must understand this system so that they can provide cost-effective quality services and so that they can also help shape the health care delivery system of the future. Nurses must also be aware of risk factors and hazards in places of employment to advocate for the health and safety of the caregiver.

Critical Thinking Exercises

✔ Select three clients you are familiar with who have different health-care needs. Describe these clients' medical histories, current problems, and future health-care needs, then determine which health-care setting and which health-care practitioners would be most appropriate for them. Identify any difficulties that might be encountered during their entry into the health-care system. How can the nurse facilitate the process?

✔ Skilled nursing facilities, subacute care facilities, and assisted living facilities all are forms of long-term or extended health care. Identify five specific problems that nurses working in such facilities encounter. What is the best way to resolve these problems?

✔ Identify cost-cutting measures used at a health-care facility with which you are familiar. Have these measures affected the quality of client care? What other measures to cut costs can be implemented? How have changes within the health-care delivery system altered nursing practice?

✔ Identify four health-care priorities that may be initiated by the year 2000. How are these likely to affect the profession of nursing?

✔ Describe the advantages and disadvantages of various health-care reimbursement plans. Which ones will produce the highest quality care? Which ones are best for the profession of nursing? Are there any payment plans that do both?

✔ Identify those elements in health-care reform that are most necessary. Should nurses support these changes and why?

References

1. Donahue, MP: Nursing the Finest Art: An illustrated history, ed 2. Mosby, St. Louis, 1996.
2. Birchenall, JM, and Streight, ME: Health Occupations: Exploration and Career Planning. CV Mosby, St Louis, 1989.
3. O'Neil, EH: Health Professions Education for the Future: Schools in Service to the Nation. Pew Health Professions Commission, San Francisco, 1993.
4. Busen, NH, and Engleman, SG: The CNS with practitioner preparation: An emerging role in advanced practice nursing. Clinical Nurse Specialist 10:145–150, 1996.
5. Jonas, S: An introduction to the U.S. health care system. Springer, New York, 1998.
6. Williams, SJ: Essentials of Health Services. Delmar, Albany, NY, 1995.
7. United States Census Bureau: Statistical brief: Sixty-five plus in the United States. [On-line] 1997. Available at http://www.census.gov/socdemo/www/agebrief.html.
8. Institute of Medicine: Healthy People 2000: Citizens Chart the Course. National Academy Press, Washington, DC, 1990.
9. Department of Health and Human Services: DHHS releases latest progress report on prevention: Healthy people 2000 review, 1995–96 shows progress in almost half of objectives [On-line] 1997. Available at http://www.cdc.gov/nchswww/releases/96facts/hp2knchs.htm.
10. Health Care Financing Administration: Highlights: National health expenditures, 1996. [On-line] 1998. Available at http://www.hcfa.gov/stats/NHE-OAct/hilites.htm.
11. United States Census Bureau: Health Insurance Coverage: 1996 Highlights. 1998.
12. Hawkins, JW, and Higgins, LP: Nursing and the American Health Care System. Tiresias, New York, 1993.
13. Schultz, EE: Advantages of employer health plans are disappearing. Wall Street Journal, 7 June 1994, pp C1, C15.
14. Lockhart, CA: Physician payment reform: Implications for nursing. In Aiken, L, and Fagin, C (eds): Charting Nursing's Future: Agenda for the 1990s. JB Lippincott, Philadelphia, 1992, pp 448–461.
15. Hall, MA: Making Medical Spending Decisions: The Law, Ethics, and Economics of Rationing Mechanisms. Oxford University, New York, 1997.
16. Wasley, TP: What Has Government Done to Our Health Care? Cato Institute, Washington, DC, 1992.
17. Congressional Budget Office: Trends in Health Spending: An Update. U.S. Government Printing Office, Washington, DC, 1993.
18. Franklin, KR, and Reed, S: Washington watch: ANA lobbies for nursing issues. Am J Nurs 97(7):16, 1997.
19. Reed, S: Washington watch: A successful year on Capitol Hill. Am J Nurs 98(1):17–18, 1998.
20. White House, Office of the Press Secretary: President Clinton announces new proposals to provide Americans ages 55 to 65 improved access to health insurance. [Online] 1998. Available at http://www.pub.whitehouse.gov/uri-res/I2R?urn:pdi://oma.eop.gov.us/1998/1/8/10.text.1.
21. Davis, K, and Rowland, D: Uninsured and underserved: Inequities in health care in the United States. In Lee, PR, and Estes, CL (eds): The Nation's Health. Jones and Bartlett, Boston, 1990, pp 298–308.
22. White House Domestic Policy Council: The President's Health Security Plan: The Clinton Blueprint. Times Books, New York, 1993.
23. American Nurses Association: Nursing's Agenda for Health Care Reform. American Nurses Association, Washington, DC, 1993.
24. Papenhausen, JL: Discovering and achieving client outcomes. In Cohen, EL (ed): Nurse Case Management in the 21st Century. Mosby, St. Louis, 1996, pp 257–268.
25. Gingerich, BS, and Ondeck, DA: Home Health Redesign: A Proactive Approach to Managed Care. Aspen, Gaithersburg, Md., 1996.
26. Sullivan, TJ: Collaboration: A Health Care Imperative. McGraw-Hill Book Co, New York, 1998.
27. Brooks, RH, McGlynn, EA, and Cleary, PD: Quality of health care: Part 2: Measuring quality of care. N Engl J Med 335(13):966–970, 1996.
28. Buterbaugh, L: TQM: The quality-care revolution. Medical World News 33(6):17–21, 1992.
29. Shendell-Falik, N, and Soriano, KB: Outcomes assessment through protocols. In Flarey, DL, and Blancett, SS (eds): Handbook of Nursing Case Management: Health Care Delivery in a World of Managed Care. Aspen, Gaithersburg, Md., 1996, pp 136–169.
30. National Center for Health Statistics: Monitoring health care in America—Spotlight on ambulatory care in the U.S. [On-line] 1997. Available at http://www.cdc.gov/nchswww/releases/97facts/97sheets/mhc0697.htm.

31. Eubanks, P: Outpatient care: A nationwide revolution. Hospitals 64(15):28–35, 1990.
32. Snow, C: One-stop shopping. Modern Healthcare 26(48):32–37, 1996.
33. Handy, J, and Bellome, J: Adult day services: The next frontier. Caring Magazine 15(12):24–26, 28, 30–33, 1996.
34. Schauffler, HH, and Wolin, J: Community health clinics under managed competition: Navigating uncharted waters. Journal of Health Politics, Policy, and Law 21:461–488, 1996.
35. Frenn, M, et al: Symposium on nursing centers: Past, present, and future. J Nurs Educ 35:54–62, 1996.
36. Tolley, M: Experiencing the neighborhood: The parish as a clinical site. Oklahoma Nurse 43(1):31, 1998.

BIBLIOGRAPHY

Brink, S: What is the value of a voice? US News & World Report 124(9):40–43, 46, 1998.

Carroll, V, and Morin, K: Workplace violence affects one-third of nurses. American Nurse 30(5):15, 1998.

de Tornay, R: Critical challenges for nurse educators. J Nurs Educ 35(4):146–147, 1996.

Diamond, K: Primary nurse directs interdisciplinary care for cardiac patient. AACN News 14(11):14–15, 1998.

Health and safety on the job: Nurse protect thyself. American Nurse September/October:1, 12–13, 22, 1997.

Hunt, R: Community-based nursing: Philosophy or setting? Am J Nurs 98(10):44–49, 1998.

Hunt, R, and Zurec, EL: Introduction to Community Based Nursing. Lippincott-Raven, Philadelphia, 1997.

Keepnews, D: Does APRN:MD = UAP:RN? American Nurse 29(4):7–9, 1997.

King, JM, Lakin, JA, and Striepe, J: Coalition building between public health nurses and parish nurses. J Nurs Adm 23:27–31, 1993.

Maffeo, R: Divorcing the UAP: Heresy or solution? American Nurse 30(1):5, 1998.

Malone, B: 'Tis the season: systematic caring for self. American Nurse September/October:2, 1997.

Malone, B: Professionalism: An exercise in stretching. American Nurse 30(3):5, 1998.

Marks, D: Nurse-managed health centers gain recognition for innovation. American Nurse 29(4):10, 1997.

Mohr, WK: Values, ideologies and dilemmas: Professional and occupational contradictions. J Psychosoc Nurs 33(1):29–34, 1995.

Munro, N: Public policy: A new paradigm grows from grass roots. Critical Care Nurse 18(5):76–85, 1998.

Rodgers, B: Is health care a risky business? American Nurse September/October:5, 1997.

Sindul-Rothschild, J, Long-Middleton, E, and Berry, D: 10 Keys to quality care. Am J Nurs 97(11):35–43, 1998.

Slattery, M: Caring for ourselves to care for our patients. American Nurse 30(5):12–13, 1998.

Stewart, M: Managed care law blocks quality care to indigent patients. American Nurse 29(6):12, 1997.

Theisen, BA, and Pelfrey, S: The advantages and risks of being a tax-exempt, nonprofit organization. J Nurs Adm 23:36–41, 1993.

Ubell, E: You can get quality care in an HMO world. Parade Publications, 21 September 1997, pp 10–11.

Whetsell, GW: Total quality management. Topics in Health Care Financing 18(2):12–20, 1997.

GLOSSARY

abandonment Leaving a client without the client's permission; terminating the professional relationship without providing for appropriate continued or follow-up care by another equally qualified professional.

accountability Concept that each individual is responsible for his or her own actions and the consequence of those actions; professional accountability implies a responsibility to perform the activities and duties of the profession according to established standards.

accreditation Approval of a program or institution by a voluntary professional organization to provide specific education or service programs.

act Legislation that has become law.

active euthanasia Acts performed to help end a sick person's life.

acute-severe condition Health problem of sudden onset; a serious illness or condition.

adaptation Process of exchange between a person and the environment to maintain or regain personal integrity; the key principle in the Roy Model of Nursing.

administrative A governmental agency that implements legislation agency.

administrative rule or regulation An operating procedure that describes how a government agency implements the intent of a statute; state boards of nursing implement the nurse practice act.

advanced nursing education Master's or doctoral level education that provides knowledge and skills in areas such as research, education, administration, or clinical specialties.

advanced placement A process by which a student is given credit for a required course through transfer or examination rather than by enrolling in and completing the course.

advanced practice Extended role; increased responsibilities and actions undertaken by an individual because of additional education and experience; nurse practitioners are advanced practice nurses.

advocate One who pleads for a cause or proposal; one who acts on behalf of another.

affidavit Written sworn statement.

affiliation agreement A formal agreement between an educational institution and another agency that agrees to provide clinical areas for student practice.

aggressiveness Harsh behavior that may result in physical or emotional harm to others.

ambulatory care center Type of primary care facility that provides treatment on an outpatient basis.

answer Document filed in the court by the defendant in response to the complaint.

anxiety Uneasiness or apprehension caused by an impending threat or fear of the unknown.

apathy Lack of interest.

appeal Request to a higher court to review a decision in the hopes of changing the ruling of a lower court.

appellant Person who seeks an appeal.

arbitrator Neutral third party who assesses facts independently of the judicial system.

articulation Type of education program that allows easy entry from one level to another; for example, many BSN programs have articulation for nurses with an associate degree.

artificial insemination Insertion of sperm into the uterus with a syringe.

assault Attempt or threat to touch.

assertiveness Ability to express thoughts, feelings, and ideas openly and directly without fear.

assessment Process of collecting information about a client, to help plan care.

associate degree nursing program Type of nursing education program that leads to an associate degree with a major in nursing; usually located in a community or junior college, these programs nominally last 2 years.

audit Close review of records or documents to detect the presence or absence of specific information.

auscultation Assessment technique that requires listening with a stethoscope to various parts of the body to detect sounds produced by organs.

autonomy State of being self-directed or independent; the ability to make decisions about one's future.

autopsy Examination of a body after death to determine the cause of death.

baccalaureate degree nursing program Type of nursing education program that leads to the bachelor's degree with a major in nursing; usually located in a college or university, the length of the program is 4 years.

bargaining agent Organization certified by a governmental agency to represent a group of employees for the purpose of collective bargaining.

baseline data Initial information obtained about a client that establishes the norms for comparison as the client's condition changes.

basic human rights Those considerations society deems reasonably expected for all people; right to self-determination, protection from discomfort and harm, dignity, fair treatment, and privacy.

battery Nonconsensual touching of another person that does not necessarily cause harm or injury.

behaviorism Psychological theory based on the belief that all behavior is learned over time through conditioning.

behavior modification Method to change behavior through rewards for positive behavior.

belief Expectations or judgments based on attitude verified by experiences.

beneficence Ethical principle based on the beliefs that the health-care provider should do no harm, prevent harm, remove existing harm, and promote the good and well-being of the client.

bereavement State of sadness brought on by the loss or death of a significant other.

bill Proposed law that is moving through the legislative process.

bill of rights List of statements that outline the claims and privileges of a particular group, such as the Client's Bill of Rights.

bioethical issues Issues that deal with the health, safety, life, and death of human beings, often arising from advances in medical science and technology.

biofeedback Ability to control autonomic response in the body through conscious effort.

body substance isolation (BSI) Universal precautions; guidelines established by the Centers for Disease Control and Prevention (CDC) and the Occupational Safety and Health Administration (OSHA) to protect health-care professionals and the client from diseases carried in the blood and body fluids, such as HIV and hepatitis B; involves the use of gloves whenever one is in contact with blood or body fluids and the use of masks, gowns, and eye covers if a chance of aerosol contact with fluids exists.

brain death Irreversible destruction of the cerebral cortex and brain stem manifested by absence of all reflexes; absence of brain waves on an electroencephalogram.

breach of contract Failure by one of the parties in a contract to fulfill all the terms of the agreement.

burden of proof Requirement that the plaintiff submit sufficient evidence to prove a defendant's guilt.

burnout syndrome A state of emotional exhaustion that results from the accumulative stress of an individual's life, including work, personal, and family responsibilities.

cadaver donor Clinically or brain-dead individual who previously agreed to allow organs to be taken for transplantation.

capitated payment system System of reimbursement in which a flat fee is paid for health-care services for a prescribed period of time. Expenses incurred in excess of this fee are provider losses.

capricious Unpredictable; arbitrary.

career ladder Articulation of educational programs that permit advancement from a lower level to a higher level without loss of credit or repetition of coursework.

career mobility Opportunity for individuals in one occupational area to move to another without restrictions.

case management Health-care delivery in which a client advocate/health-care coordinator helps the client through the hospitalization to obtain the most appropriate care.

case manager Health-care provider who coordinates cost-effective quality care for individuals who are generally at high risk and require long-term complex services.

certification Official recognition of a degree of education and skills in a profession by a national specialty organization; recognition that an institution has met standards that allow it to deliver certain services.

challenge examination Examination that assesses levels of knowledge or skill to grant credit for previous learning and experience; passing a challenge examination gives the individual credit for a course not actually taken.

chart Legal document that contains all the pertinent information about a client who is in a hospital or clinic; usually includes medical and nursing history, medical and nursing diagnosis, laboratory test results, notes about the client's progress, physician's orders, and personal data.

charting Process of recording (written or computer-generated) specific information about the client in the chart or medical record.

civil law Law concerned with the violation of the rights of one individual by another; it includes contract law, treaty law, tax law, and tort law.

client More modern term for patient; an individual seeking or receiving health-related services.

client goal Statement about a desired change, outcome, or activity that a client should achieve by a specific time.

clinical education Hands-on part of a nursing program that allows the student to practice skills on actual clients under the supervision of a nursing instructor.

clinical forensic nurse Professional nurse who specializes in management of crime victims from trauma to trial through collection of evidence, assessment of victims or making judgements related to client treatment associated with court-related issues.

clinical ladder Type of performance evaluation and career advancement in which nursing positions for direct client care have two or more progressive levels of required skill leading to advancement in salary and responsibility; it allows nurses to remain in direct client care while making career advancements rather than having to move into administration.

clinical pathways Case-management protocols used to enhance quality care, encourage cost-effectiveness, and promote efficiency.

closed system System that does not exchange energy, matter, or information with the environment or with other systems.

code of ethics Written values of a profession that act as guidelines for professional behavior.

collective bargaining Negotiations for wages, hours, benefits, and working conditions for a group of employees.

collective bargaining unit Group of employees, recognized as representatives of the majority, with the right to bargain collectively with their employer and to reach an agreement on the terms of a contract.

committee Group of legislators, in the House or Senate, assigned to analyze bills on a particular subject.

common law Law based on past judicial judgments made in similar cases.

comparable worth Method for determining employees' salaries within an organization so that the same salary is paid for all jobs that have equivalent educational requirements, responsibilities, and complexity regardless of external market factors.

competencies Behaviors, skills, attitudes, and knowledge that an individual or professional has or is expected to have.

competency-based education Courses or programs based on anticipated student outcomes.

complaint Legal document filed by a plaintiff to initiate a lawsuit, claiming that the plaintiff's legal rights have been violated.

compliance Voluntary following of a prescribed plan of care or treatment regimen.

computer technology Use of highly advanced technologic equipment to store, process, and access a vast amount of information.

concept Abstract idea or image.

conceptual framework Concept, theory, or basic idea around which an educational program is organized and developed.

conceptual model Group of concepts, ideas, or theories that are interrelated but in which the relationship is not clearly defined.

confidentiality Right of the client to expect the communication with a professional to remain unshared with any other person unless a medical reason exists or unless the safety of the public is threatened.

consensus General agreement between two or more individuals or groups regarding beliefs or positions on an issue or finding.

consent Voluntary permission given by a competent person.

consortium Two or more agencies that share sponsorship of a program or an institution.

constitutional law Law contained within a federal or state constitution.

continuing care Nursing care generally provided in geriatric day care centers or in the homes of elderly clients.

continuing education Formal education programs and informal learning experiences that maintain and increase the nurse's knowledge and skills in specific areas.

continuing education unit (CEU) Specific unit of credit earned by participating in an approved continuing education program.

continuous quality improvement (CQI) A type of total quality management whose primary goal is the improvement of the quality of health care.

contract Legally binding agreement between two or more parties.

contractual obligation Duty to perform a service identified by a contract.

copayment Percentage of the cost of a medical expense that is not covered by insurance and must be paid by the client.

core curriculum Curriculum design that enables a student to leave a career program at various levels, with a career attained and with the option to continue at another higher level or career; it is organized around a central or core body of knowledge common to the profession.

coroner Elected public official, usually a physician, who investigates deaths from unnatural causes, including homicide, violence, suicide, and other suspicious circumstances.

correctional nurse Registered nurse who specializes in the health care of those in custody in secure settings such as jails or prisons.

credentialing Process whereby individuals, programs, or institutions are designated as having met minimal standards for the safety and welfare of the public.

crime Violation of criminal law.

criminal action Process by which a person charged with a crime is accused, tried, and punished.

criminal law Law concerned with violation of criminal statutes or laws.

criterion-referenced examination Test that compares an individual's knowledge with predetermined standard rather than to the performance of others who take the same test.

critical thinking The intellectual process of rationally examining ideas, inferences, assumptions, principles, arguments, conclusions, issues, statements, beliefs and actions for which all the relevant information may not be available. This process involves the ability to use the five types of reasoning (scientific, deductive, inductive, informal, practical) in application of the nursing process, decision making, and resolution of ambiguous issues.

curriculum Group of courses that prepare an individual for a specific degree or profession.

customary, prevailing, and reasonable charges The typical rate in a specific locale that payers traditionally reimburse physicians.

damages Money awarded to a plaintiff by a court in a lawsuit that covers the actual costs incurred by the plaintiff.

database Information collected by a computer program on a specific topic in a specified format.

defamation of character Communication of information that is false or detrimental to a person's reputation.

defendant Person accused of criminal or civil wrongdoing. A party to a lawsuit against whom the complaint is served.

delegation Assignment of specific duties by one individual to another individual.

deontology An ethical system based on the principle that the right action is guided by a set of unchanging rules.

dependent practitioner Provider of care who delivers health care under the supervision of another health-care practitioner; for example, a physician assistant is supervised by a physician, or an LPN is supervised by an RN.

deposition Sworn statement by a witness that is made outside the courtroom; sworn depositions may be admitted as evidence in court when the individual is unable to be present.

diagnosis Statement that describes or identifies a client problem and is based on a thorough assessment.

diagnosis-related groups (DRGs) Prospective payment method used by the U.S. government and many insurance companies that pay a flat fee for treatment of a person with a particular diagnosis.

differentiated practice Organizational process of defining nursing roles based on education, experience, and training.

dilemma Predicament in which a choice must be made between two or more equally balanced alternatives; it often occurs when attempting to make ethical decisions.

directed services Health-care activities that require contact between a health-care professional and a client.

discharge planning Assessment of anticipated client needs after discharge from the hospital and development of a plan to meet those needs before the client is discharged.

disease Illness; a functional disturbance resulting from an individual organism's inability to adapt to certain stressors; an abnormal physiologic state caused by microorganisms, cancer, or other conditions.

distributive justice Ethical principle based on the belief that the right action is determined by that which will provide an outcome equal for all persons and will also benefit the least fortunate.

due process Right to have specific procedures or processes followed before the deprivation of life, liberty, or property; the guarantee of privileges under the Fifth and Fourteenth Amendments to the U.S. Constitution.

duty Obligation to act created by a statute, contract, or voluntary agreement.

emerging health occupations Health care occupations that are not yet officially recognized by government or professional organizations.

employee Individual hired for pay by another.

Employee Retirement Income Security Act (ERISA) Federal law that grants incentives to employers to offer self-funded health insurance plans to their employees.

employer Individual or organization that hires other individuals for pay to carry out specific duties during certain hours of employment.

empowerment Process in which the individual assumes more autonomy and responsibility for his or her actions.

endorsement Reciprocity; a state's acceptance of a license issued by another state.

end product Output of a system not reusable as input.

energy Capacity to do work.

entry into practice Minimal educational requirements to obtain a license for a profession.

environment Internal and external physical and social boundaries of humans; all those things that are outside a system.

essentials for accreditation The minimal standards that a program must meet to be accredited.

ethical dilemma An ethical situation that requires an individual to make a choice between two equally unfavorable alternatives.

ethical system System of moral judgments based on the beliefs and values of a profession.

ethics Principles or standards of conduct that govern an individual or group.

ethnic group Individuals who share similar physical characteristics, religion, language, or customs.

euthanasia Mercy killing; the act or practice of killing, for reasons of mercy, individuals who have little or no chance of recovery by withholding or discontinuing life support or by administering a lethal agent.

evaluation Fifth step in the nursing process used to determine whether goals set for a client have been attained.

evaluation criteria Outcome criteria; desired behaviors or standards.

expanded role Extended role; increased responsibilities and actions undertaken by an individual because of additional education and experience.

expert witness Individual with knowledge beyond the ordinary person because of special education or training who testifies during a trial.

external degree Academic degree granted when all the requirements have been met by the student; a type of outcomes-based education in which credit is given when the individual demonstrates a certain level of knowledge and skill, regardless of how or when these skills are attained; challenge examinations are often used.

false imprisonment Intentional tort committed by illegally confining or restricting a client against his or her will.

family Two or more related individuals living together.

Federal Tort Claims Act Statute that allows the government to be sued for negligence of its employees in the performance of their duties; many states have similar laws.

feedback Reentry of output into a system as input that helps maintain the internal balance of the system.

fee for service Payment is expected each time a service is rendered. Includes physician office visits, diagnostic procedures (laboratory tests, x-rays) and minor surgical procedures.

fellowship Scholarship or grant that provides money to individuals who are highly qualified or highly intelligent.

felony Serious crime that may be punished by a fine of more than $1000, more than 1 year in jail or prison, death, or a combination thereof.

fidelity The obligation of an individual to be faithful to commitments made to self and others.

for profit Health care agencies in which profits can be used to raise capital to pay stock holders dividends on their investments. Also called proprietary agencies.

foreign graduate nurse Individual graduated from a school of nursing outside the United States. This individual is required to pass the U.S. NCLEX-RN CAT to become a registered nurse in the United States.

forensic nurse A registered nurse who specializes in the integration of forensic science and nursing science to apply the nursing process to individual clients, their families, and the community, bridging the gap between the health-care system and the criminal justice system.

forensic psychiatric nurse A registered nurse who specializes in application of psychosocial nursing knowledge linking offending behavior to client characteristics; nurse specializing in forensic psychological evaluation and care of offender populations with mental disorder.

forensic science Body of empirical knowledge used for legal investigation and evidence-based judgment in police or criminal cases.

fraud Deliberate deception in provision of goods or services; lying.

functional nursing Nursing care in which each nurse provides a different aspect of care; nurses are assigned a set of specific tasks to perform for all clients, such as passing medications.

general systems theory Set of interrelated concepts, definitions, and propositions that describes a system.

genetics Scientific study of heredity and related variations.

gerontology Study of the process of aging and of the effects of aging on individuals.

goal Desired outcome.

Good Samaritan Act Law that protects health-care providers from being charged with contributory negligence when they provide emergency care to persons in need of immediate treatment.

grievance Complaint or dispute about the terms or conditions of employment.

group practice Three or more physicians or nurse practitioners in business together to provide health care.

health Complete physical, mental, and social well-being; a relative state along a continuum ranging from severe illness to ideal state of being; the ability to adapt to illness and to reach the highest level of functioning.

health-care consumer Client or patient; an individual who uses health care service or products.

health-care team Group of individuals of different levels of education who work together to provide help to clients.

health insurance purchasing cooperative (HIPCs) Large groups of people or employers who band together to buy insurance at reduced costs. HIPCs may be organized by private groups or the government.

health maintenance organization (HMO) Prototype of the managed health-care system; method of payment for a full range of primary, secondary, and tertiary health-care services; members pay a fixed annual fee

for services and a small deductible when care is actually given.

health policy Goals and directions that guide activities to safeguard and promote the health of citizens.

health practitioner Individual, usually licensed, who provides health-care services to individuals with health-care needs.

health promotion Interventions and behaviors that increase and maintain the level of well-being of persons, families, groups, communities, and society.

health systems agency (HSA) Local voluntary organization of providers and consumers that plans for the health-care services of its geographic region.

hearsay Evidence not based on personal knowledge of the witness and usually not allowed in courts.

holistic Treatment of the total individual, including physical, psychological, sociologic, and spiritual elements, with emphasis on the interrelatedness of parts and wholes.

home health care Health care services provided in the client's home.

hospice care Alternative way of providing care to terminally ill clients in which palliative care is used; the major goals of hospice care are control of pain, provision of emotional support, promotion of social interaction, and preparation for death; family support measures and anticipatory grieving counseling are also used if appropriate.

hospital privileges Authority granted by a hospital, usually through its medical board, for a health-care practitioner to admit and supervise the treatment of clients within that hospital.

hypothesis Prediction or proposition related to a problem, usually found in research.

ideal role image A projection of society's expectations for nurses that clearly delineates the obligations and responsibilities, as well as the rights and privileges those in the role can lay claim to. Is often unrealistic.

illness Disease; a functional disturbance resulting from an individual organism's inability to adapt to certain stressors; an abnormal physiologic state caused by microorganisms, cancer, or other conditions.

indemnity insurance Health insurance in which the contractual agreement is between the consumer and the insurance company. Providers are not involved in these arrangements, and rates are not pre-established.

intentional tort A willful act that violates another person's rights or property and may or may not cause physical injury.

implementation Fourth step in the nursing process, in which the plan of care is carried out.

incidence Number of occurrences of a specific condition or event.

incident report Document that describes an accident or error involving a client or family member that may or may not have resulted in injury; the purpose of the incident report is to track incidents and to make changes in the situations that caused them; the incident report is not part of the chart.

incompetency Inability of an individual to manage personal affairs because of mental or physical conditions; the inability of a professional to carry out professional activities at the expected level of functioning because of lack of knowledge or skill or because of drug or alcohol abuse.

indemnity insurance policy Method of payment for health-care services; policy holders pay fixed periodic payments for insurance and are compensated, in whole or in part, for their health-care expenses, usually through payment to the provider.

independent nurse practitioner Nurse who has a private practice in one of the expanded roles of nursing.

independent practice association (IPA) Type of HMO usually organized by physicians that requires fee-for-service payment.

independent practice organization (IPO) Type of IPA in which a group of providers deals with more than one insurer at a time.

independent practitioner Health-care provider who delivers health care independently with or without supervision by another health-care practitioner.

indirect services Health-care actions that do not require direct client contact but that still facilitate care, such as the supply and distribution department of a hospital.

informed consent Permission granted by a person based on full knowledge of the risks and benefits of participation in a procedure or surgery for which the consent has been given.

injunction Court order specifying actions that must or must not be taken.

input Matter, energy, or information entering a system from the environment.

inquest Formal inquiry about the course or manner of death.

institutional licensure Authority for an individual health-care provider to practice that is granted by the individual's employing institution; the institution determines the educational preparation, training, and functions of each category of provider it employs; no longer legally permitted, UAPs act under a form of de facto institutional licensure.

interrogatories Written questions directed to a party in a lawsuit by the opposing side as part of the discovery process.

intervention Nursing action taken to meet specific client goals.

invasion of privacy A type of quasi-intentional tort that involves (1) an act that intrudes into the seclusion of the client; (2) intrusion that is objectionable to a reasonable person; (3) an act that intrudes into private facts or published as facts or pictures of a private nature; and (4) public disclosure of private information.

Joint Commission on Accreditation of Healthcare Organizations (JCAHO) Organization that performs accreditation reviews for health-care agencies.

judgment Decision of the court regarding a case.

jurisdiction Authority of a court to hear and decide lawsuits.

justice Fairness; giving people their due.

Kardex Portable card file that contains important client information and a care plan.

law Formal statement of a society's beliefs about interactions among and between its citizens; a formal rule enforced by society.

legal complaint Document filed by a plaintiff against a defendant claiming infringement of the plaintiff's legal rights.

legal obligations Obligations that have become formal statements of law and are enforceable under the law.

legal rights (welfare rights) Rights that are based on a legal entitlement to some good or benefits and are enforceable under the legal system with punishment for violations.

legislator Elected member of either the House of Representatives or the Senate.

legislature Body of elected individuals invested with constitutional power to make, alter, or repeal laws.

liable Obligated or held accountable by law.

libel Written defamation of character.

license Permission to practice granted to an individual by the state after he or she has met the requirements for that particular position; licensing protects the safety of the public.

licensed practical nurse (LPN) Licensed vocational nurse; technical nurse licensed by any state, after completing a practical nursing program, to provide technical bedside care to clients.

licensing board Government agency that implements the statutes of a particular profession in accordance with the Professions Practice Act.

licensure Process by which an agency or government grants an individual permission to practice; it establishes a minimal level of competency for practice.

licensure by endorsement Method of obtaining a license to practice by having a state acknowledge the individual's existing comparable license in another state.

licensure by examination Method of obtaining a license to practice by successfully passing a state board examination.

living will Signed legal document in which individuals make known their wishes about the care they are to receive if they should become incompetent at a future date; it usually specifies what types of treatments are permitted and what types are to be withheld.

lobbyist Person who attempts to influence political decisions as an official representative of an organization, group, or institution.

locality rule standard of care Legal process that holds an individual nurse accountable to both what is an acceptable standard within his or her local community and to national standards as developed by nurses throughout the nation through ANA, national practice groups, and health-care agencies.

malfeasance Performance of an illegal act.

malpractice Negligent acts by a licensed professional based on either omission of an expected action or commission of an inappropriate action resulting in damages to another party; not doing what a reasonable and prudent professional of the same rank would have done in the same situation.

managed care System of organized health-care delivery systems linked by provider networks; health maintenance organizations are the primary example of managed care.

mandatory licensure Law that requires all who practice a particular profession to have and to maintain a license in that profession.

manslaughter Killing of an individual without premeditated intent; different degrees of manslaughter exist, and most are felonies.

mediation A legal process that allows each party to present their case to a mediator, who is an independent third party trained in dispute resolution.

medical examiner Coroner; a physician who investigates deaths that appear to be from other than natural causes.

Medicaid State health-care insurance program, supported in part by federal funds, for health-care services for certain groups unable to pay for their own health care; amount and type of coverage vary from state to state.

medically indigent Individuals who cannot personally pay for health-care services without incurring financial hardship.

Medicare A federally run program that is financed primarily through employee payroll taxes and covers any individual who is 65 years of age or older as well as blind and disabled individuals of any age.

Medicare Utilization and Quality Peer Review Organization (PRO) Organization that reviews the quality and cost of Medicare services.

Medigap policies Health insurance policies that are purchased to cover expenses not paid by Medicare.

midwife Individual experienced in assisting women during labor and delivery; they may be lay midwives, who have no official education, or certified nurse midwives, who are RNs in an expanded role, having received additional education and passed a national certification examination.

misdemeanor Less serious crime than felony punishable by a fine of less than $1000 or a jail term of less than 1 year.

model A hypothetical representation of something that exists in reality. The purpose of a model is to attempt to explain a complex reality in a systematic and organized manner.

morality Concept of right and wrong.

moral obligations Obligations based on moral or ethical principles but are *not* enforceable under the law.

morals Fundamental standards of right and wrong that an individual learns and internalizes during the early stages of childhood development, based primarily on religious beliefs and societal norms.

mores Values and customs of a society.

mortality Property or capacity to die; death.

motivation Internal drive that causes individuals to seek achievement of higher goals; desire.

multicompetency technician Allied health care provider who has skills in two or more areas of practice through the process of cross-training.

multiskilled practitioner Health-care professional who has skills in more than one area of health care, such as an RN who has training in physical therapy.

national health insurance Proposed system of payment for health-care services whereby the government pays for the costs of the health care.

negative entropy Tendency toward increased order in a system.

negligence Failure to perform at an expected level of functioning or the performance of an inappropriate function resulting in damages to another party; not doing what a reasonable and prudent person would do in a similar situation.

no code order Do not resuscitate (DNR) order; an order by a physician to withhold cardiopulmonary resuscitation and other resuscitative efforts from a client.

nonfeasance Failure to perform a legally required duty.

nonmaleficence Ethical principle that requires the professional to do no harm to the client.

nontraditional education Methods of education that do not follow the traditional lecture and clinical practice methods of learning; may include computer-simulated learning, self-education techniques, or other creative methods.

normative ethics Questions and dilemmas requiring a choice of actions where there is a conflict of rights or obligations between the nurse and the client, the nurse and the client's family, or the nurse and the physician.

norm-referenced examination Examination scored by comparison with standards established on the performance of all others who took the same examination during a specific time; the NLN achievement examinations are norm referenced.

not-for-profit (nonprofit) agencies Agencies in which all profits must be used in the operation of the organization.

nurse clinician Registered nurse with advanced skills in a particular area of nursing practice; if certified by a professional organization, a nurse clinician may also be a nurse practitioner, but more often this designation refers to nurses in advanced practice roles such as nurse specialists.

nurse practice act Part of state law that establishes the scope of practice for professional nurses, as well as educational levels and standards, professional conduct, and reasons for revocation of licensure.

nurse practitioner Nurse specialist with advanced education in a primary care specialty, such as community health, pediatrics, or mental health, who is prepared independently to manage health promotion and maintenance and illness prevention of a specific group of clients.

nurse specialist (clinical nurse specialist) Nurse who is an expert in providing care focused on a specialized field drawn from the range of general practice, such as cardiac nurse specialist.

nurse theorist Nurse who analyzes and attempts to describe what the profession of nursing is and what nurses do through nursing models or nursing theories.

nursing assessment Systematic collection and recording of client data, both objective and subjective, from primary and secondary sources using the nursing history, physical examination, and laboratory data, for example.

nursing diagnosis Statements of a client's actual or potential health-care problems or deficits.

nursing order Statement of a nursing action selected by a nurse to achieve a client's goal; may be stated as either the nurse's or the client's expected behavior.

nursing process Systematic, comprehensive decision-making process used by nurses to identify and treat actual and potential health problems.

nursing research Formal study of problems of nursing practice, the role of the nurse in health care, and the value of nursing.

nursing standards Desired nursing behaviors established by the profession and used to evaluate nurses' performance.

obligations Demands made on individuals, professions, society, or government to fulfill and honor the rights of others. Obligations are often divided into two categories—moral and legal (welfare).

omission Failure to fulfill a duty or carry out a procedure recognized as a standard of care; often forms the basis for claims of malpractice.

oncology Area of health care that deals with the treatment of cancer.

open curriculum Educational system that allows a student to enter and leave the system freely; often uses past education and experiences.

open system System that can exchange energy, matter, and information with the environment and with other systems.

ordinance Local or municipal law.

outcome criteria Standards that measure changes or improvements in clients' conditions.

out-of-pocket expenses Amount the client is responsible for paying for a health-care service.

output Matter, energy, or information released from a system into the environment or transmitted to another system.

palliative Type of treatment directed toward minimizing the severity of a disease or illness rather than curing it; for example, for a client with terminal cancer, relief of pain is the main goal (palliative), rather than cure.

panel of approved providers A list of physicians, nurse practitioners, pharmacies and other health care providers that are approved by an insurance plan and to whom reimbursement will be made by the insurer.

patient Client; an individual seeking or receiving health-care services.

patient day Client day; the 24-hour period during which hospital services are provided that forms the basis for charging the patient, usually from midnight to midnight.

pediatrics Study and care of problems and diseases of children younger than the age of 18.

peer review Evaluation against professional standards of the performance of individuals with the same basic education and qualifications; formal process of review or evaluation by co-workers of an equal rank.

perceived role image The individual's own definition of the role, which is usually more realistic than the ideal role, involving rejection or modification of some of the norms and expectations of society.

percussion Physical examination involving the tapping of various parts of the body to determine density by eliciting different sounds.

performed role image The actual duties performed by the practitioner of a role. Often produces reality shock in new graduate nurses.

perjury Crime committed by giving false testimony while under oath.

permissive licensure Law that allows individuals to practice a profession as long as they do not use the title of the profession; no states now have permissive licensure.

phenomenology Philosophical approach that holds that consciousness determines reality in space and time.

plaintiff Individual who charges another individual in a court of law with a violation of the individual's rights; the party who files the complaint in a lawsuit.

point-of-service plans Insurance plans in which consumers can select providers outside of a prescribed provider panel if they are willing to pay an additional fee.

political action Activities on the part of individuals that influence the actions of government officials in establishing policy.

political involvement Group of activities that, individually or collectively, increase the voice of nursing in the political or health-care policy process.

politics Process of influencing the decisions of others and exerting control over situations or events, includes influencing the allocation of scarce resources.

practical nursing program Vocational nursing program; a program of study leading to a certificate in practical nursing, usually 12 to 18 months in length; these programs are located in a vocational or technical school or in a community or junior college; after passing the NCLEX-LPN CAT examination, students become licensed practical nurses (LPNs).

precedent Decision previously issued by a court that is used as the basis for a decision in another case with similar circumstances.

preceptor Educated or skilled practitioner who agrees to work with a less educated or trained individual to increase the individual's knowledge and skills; often staff nurses who work with student nurses during their senior year.

precertification Approval for reimbursement of services prior to their being rendered.

preferred provider organization (PPO) Method of payment for employee health-care benefits in which employers contract with a specific group of health-care providers for a lower cost for their employees' health-care services but require the employee to use the providers listed.

premium Amount paid on a periodic basis for health insurance or HMO membership.

prescriptive authority Legal right to write prescriptions for medications, granted to physicians, veterinarians, dentists, and advanced practice nurses.

preventive care Well care; nursing care provided for the purpose of maintaining health and preventing disease or injury, often through community health clinics, school nursing services, and storefront clinics.

primary care Type of health care for individuals and families in which maintenance of health is emphasized; first-line health care in hospitals, physicians offices, or community health clinics that deal with acute conditions.

primary care nurse Hospital staff RN assigned to a primary care unit to provide nursing care to a limited number of clients, who are followed by the same nurse from admission to discharge.

primary intervention Health promotion, illness prevention, early diagnosis, and treatment of common health problems.

private-duty nurse Nurse in private practice; nurse self-employed for providing direct client care services either in the home or the hospital setting.

privileged communication Information imparted by a client to a physician, lawyer, or clergyman that is protected from disclosure in a court of law. Communication between a client and a nurse is not legally protected, but nurses can participate in privileged communication when they overhear information imparted by the client to the physician.

profession Nursing; an occupation that meets the criteria for a profession, including education, altruism, code of ethics, public service, and dedication.

professional review organization Multilevel program to oversee the quality and cost of federally funded medical care programs.

professionalism Behaviors and attitudes exhibited by an individual that are recognized by others as the traits of a professional.

prospective payment system (PPS) System of reimbursement for health-care services that establishes the payment rates before hospitalization based on certain criteria, such as diagnostic-related groups (DRGs).

protocol Written plan of action based on previously identified situations; standing orders are a type of protocol often used in specialty units that have clients with similar problems.

provider Person or organization who delivers health care including health promotion and maintenance and illness prevention and treatment.

provider panel Health-care providers selected to render services to a group of consumers within a managed-care plan.

proximate cause Nearest cause; the element in a direct cause-and-effect relationship between what is done by the professional and what happens to the client. As, for instance, when a nurse fails to raise the side rails on the bed of a client who has received a narcotic medication, and the client falls out of bed and breaks a hip as a result.

public policy Decision made by a society or its elected representatives that has a material effect on citizens other than on the decision makers.

quality Level of excellence based on pre-established criteria.

quality assurance Activity conducted in health-care facilities that evaluates the quality of care provided to ensure that it meets pre-established quality standards.

quasi-intentional tort A violation of a person's reputation or personal privacy.

reality shock (transition shock) A sudden and sometimes traumatic realization on the part of the new graduate that the ideal or perceived roles do not match the actual performed role.

recertification Periodic renewal of certification by examination, continuing education, or other criteria established by the accrediting agency.

reciprocity Endorsement; a state's acceptance of a license issued by another state.

registration Listing of a license with a state for a fee.

registry Published list of those who are registered; the agency that publishes the list of individuals who are registered.

regulations Rules or orders issued by various regulatory agencies, such as a state board of nursing, which have the force of law.

rehabilitation Restoration to the highest possible level of performance or health of an individual who has suffered an injury or illness.

relative intensity measures (RIMs) Method for calculating nursing resources needed to provide nursing care for various types of clients; helps determine the number and type of staff required based on client acuity and needs.

respondent superior Legal doctrine that holds the employer or supervisor responsible for the actions of the employees or of those supervised; for example, under this doctrine, RNs are held responsible for the actions of unlicensed assistive personnel under their supervision.

responsibility Accountability; the concept that all individuals are accountable for their own actions and for the consequences of those actions.

restorative care Curative care; nursing care that has as its goal cure and recovery from disease.

resume Curriculum vitae; a summary of an individual's education, work experience, and qualifications.

retrospective payment system Payment system for health care in which reimbursement is based on the actual care rendered rather than on preset rates.

right Just claim or expectation that may or may not be protected by law; legal rights are protected by law, whereas moral rights are not.

risk management Evaluating the risk of clients and staff for injuries and for potential liabilities and implementing corrective and preventive measures.

secondary care Nursing care usually provided in short-term and long-term care facilities to clients with commonly occurring conditions.

secondary intervention Acute care designed to prevent complications or resolve health problems.

secured settings Any institutional setting imposing restriction of movement, confinement, and limitations to activity and access; jails, locked units or locked mental institutions, prisons.

service insurance Health insurance in which services are provided for a prescribed fee that is established between the providers and the insurance company.

sexual assault nurse examiner (SANE) A registered nurse specializing in care of victims of sexual assault, performing physical and psychosocial examination, collection of physical evidence, and therapeutic interventions to minimize trauma.

significant other Individual who is not a family member but is emotionally or symbolically important to an individual.

slander Oral defamation of character.

sliding-scale fees Fees for services that are based on the client's ability to pay.

slow-code order Physician's order that the efforts for resuscitation of a client who is terminally ill should be initiated and conducted at a leisurely pace; the goal of a slow-code order is to allow the client to die during an apparent resuscitation. Slow-code orders are not acceptable practice and do not meet standards of care.

staff nurse Nurse generalist who works as an employee of a hospital, nursing home, community health agency, or some other organization providing primary and direct nursing care to clients.

standards Norms; criteria for expected behaviors or conduct.

standard of best interest A type of decision made about an individual's health care when he or she is unable to make the informed decision for his or her own care, based on what the health-care providers and/or the family decide is best for that individual.

standards of care Written or established criteria for nursing care that all nurses are expected to meet.

standards of practice Written or established criteria for nursing practice that all professional nurses are expected to meet.

standing order Written order by physician for certain actions or medication administration to be initiated or given in certain expected circumstances; similar to protocols.

statute Law passed by a government's legislature and signed by its chief executive.

statute of limitations Specific time period in which a lawsuit must be filed or a crime must be prosecuted; most nursing or medical lawsuits have a 2-year statute of limitations from the time of discovery of the incident.

statutory law Law passed by a legislature.

stereotype Fixed or predetermined image of or attitude toward an individual or group.

stress Crisis situation that causes increased anxiety and initiation of the flight-or-fight mechanism.

stressor Internal or external force to which a person responds.

structure criteria Physical environmental framework for client care.

subpoena Court document that requires an individual to appear in court and provide testimony; individuals who do not honor the subpoena can be held in contempt of court and jailed or fined.

subsystem Smaller system within a large system.

summary judgment Decision by a judge in cases in which no facts are in dispute.

sunset law Law that automatically terminates a program after a pre-established period of time unless that program can justify its need for existence.

support system Environmental factors and individuals who can help an individual in a crisis cope with the situation.

systems theory Theory that stresses the interrelatedness of parts in any system in which a change in one part affects all other parts; often, the system is greater than the sum of its parts.

taxonomy Classification system.

team nursing Method of organizing nursing care in which each client is assigned a team consisting of RNs, LPNs, and nursing assistants to deliver nursing care.

technician Individual who carries out technical tasks.

technology Use of science and the application of scientific principles to any situation; often involves the use of complicated machines and computers.

teleology Utilitarianism; an ethical system that identifies the right action by determining what will provide the greatest good for the greatest number of persons. This system has no set, unchanging rules; rather, it varies as the situation changes.

tertiary care Nursing care usually provided in long-term care and rehabilitation facilities for chronic diseases or injuries requiring long recovery.

tertiary intervention The provision of advanced and long-term health care services to acutely ill clients, including the use of advanced technology, complicated surgical procedures, rehabilitation services and care of the terminally ill.

testimony Oral statement of a witness under oath.

theory Set of interrelated constructs (concepts, definitions, or propositions) that presents a systematic view of phenomena by specifying relations among variables with the purpose of explaining and predicting phenomena.

third-party payment Payment for health-care services by an insurance company or a government agency rather than directly by the client.

third-party reimburser An organization other than the client, such as an employer, insurance company or governmental agency that assumes responsibility for payment of health care charges for services rendered to the client.

throughput Matter, energy, or information as it passes through a system.

tort Violation of the civil law that violates a person's rights and causes injury or harm to the individual. Civil wrong independent of an action in contract that results from a breach of a legal duty; a tort can be classified as unintentional, intentional, or quasi-intentional.

tort-feasor Person who commits a tort.

total quality management (TQM) A method for monitoring and maintaining the quality of health care being delivered by a particular institution or health-care industry.

trial Legal proceedings during which all relevant facts are presented to a jury or judge for legal decision.

Tri-Council Nursing group composed of the American Nurses Association (ANA), National League for Nursing (NLN), American Association of Colleges of Nursing (AACN), and American Organization of Nurse Executives (AONE).

two plus two (2+2) program Nursing education program that starts with an associate (2-year) degree and then moves the individual to a baccalaureate degree with an additional 2 years of education.

Uniform Anatomical Gift Act Legislation providing for a legal document signed by an individual indicating the desire to donate specific body organs or the entire body after death.

unintentional tort A wrong occurring to a person or that person's property even though it was not intended. Negligence.

universal health-care coverage Health-care reimbursement benefits for all United States citizens and legal residents.

universal precautions Body substance isolation; guidelines established by the Centers for Disease Control and Prevention (CDC) and the Occupational Safety and Health Administration (OSHA) to protect health-care professionals and clients from diseases carried in the blood and body fluids, such as HIV and hepatitis B; involves the use of gloves whenever in contact with blood or body fluids and masks, gowns, and eye covers if a chance exists of contact with aerosol fluids.

upward mobility Movement toward increased status and power in an organization through promotion.

utilitarianism Teleology; an ethical system that identifies the right action by determining what will provide the greatest good for the greatest number of persons. This system has no set, unchanging rules; rather, it varies as the situation changes.

utilization guidelines Guidelines that stipulate the amount of services that can be delivered by a health-care provider.

value Judgment of worth, quality, or desirability based on attitude formed from need or experience; a strong belief held by individuals about something important to them.

values clarification Process by which individuals list and prioritize the values they hold most important.

veto Signed refusal by the President or a governor to enact a bill into law. If the President vetoes a bill, the veto may be overridden by a two-thirds vote of the membership of both the House and Senate.

veracity The principle of truthfulness. It requires the health-care provider to tell the truth and not intentionally deceive or mislead clients.

vicarious liability Imputation of blame on a person for the actions of the other.

victimization Experience of physical, emotional or psychological trauma in which the individual suffers injury, fear, self-blame and/or other dysfunction.

vocational nursing program Licensed practical nursing program in Texas and California; a program of study leading to a certificate in vocational nursing, usually 12 to 18 months in length; these programs are located in a vocational or technical school or a community or junior college; after passing the NCLEX-LPN CAT examination, students become licensed vocational nurses (LVNs).

APPENDIX A National Council of State Boards of Nursing, Inc.

Boards of Nursing

Alabama
Alabama Board of Nursing
P.O. BOX 303900
Montgomery, Alabama 36130-3900
Phone: (334) 242-4060
Fax: (334) 242-4360
Street Address:
RSA Plaza, Suite 250
770 Washington Avenue
Montgomery, Alabama 36130-3900

Alaska
Alaska Board of Nursing
Department of Commerce and Economic
 Development
Division of Occupational Licensing
3601 C Street, Suite 722
Anchorage, Alaska 99503
Phone: (907) 269-8161
Fax: (907) 562-5781
NCNET: NCZ026
Alaska Board of Nursing
P.O. Box 110806
Juneau, Alaska 99811-086
Phone: (907) 465-2544
Fax: (907) 465-2974
Linda Gohl, Licensing Examiner

American Samoa
American Samoa Health Service
Regulatory Board
LBJ Tropical Medical Center
Pago Pago, American Samoa 96799
Phone: (684) 633-1222, ext. 206
Fax: (684) 633-1027
Telex: #782-573-LBJ TMC

Arizona
Arizona State Board of Nursing
1651 E. Morten Avenue, Suite 150
Phoenix, Arizona 85020
Phone: (602) 255-5092
Fax: (602) 255-5130

Arkansas
Arkansas State Board of Nursing
University Tower Building, Suite 800
1123 South University
Little Rock, Arkansas 72204
Phone: (501) 686-2700
Fax: (501) 686-2714

California–RN
California Board of Registered Nursing
P.O. Box 944210
Sacramento, California 94244-2100
Phone: (916) 322-3350
Fax: (916) 327-4402
NCNET: C. Puri 132:NCZ030
Street Address:
400 R Street, Suite 4030
Sacramento, California 95814-6200

California–VN
California Board of Vocational Nurse and
 Psychiatric Technician Examiners
2535 Capitol Oaks Drive, Suite 205
Sacramento, California 95833
Phone: (916) 263-7800
Fax: (916) 263-7859

Colorado
Colorado Board of Nursing
1560 Broadway, Suite 670
Denver, Colorado 80202
Phone: (303) 894-2430
Fax: (303) 894-2821

Connecticut
Connecticut Board of Examiners for
    Nursing
410 Capitol Ave, MS 12 NUR
P.O. Box 340308
Hartford, Connecticut 06106
Phone: (860) 509-7264
Fax: (860) 509-7650
For Examination Information:
Examinations and Licensure Division of
    Medical Quality Assurance
Connecticut Department of Health Services
150 Washington Street
Hartford, Connecticut 06106
Phone: (203) 566-1032

Delaware
Delaware Board of Nursing
Cannon Building, Suite 203
P.O. Box 1401
Dover, Delaware 19903
Phone: (302) 739-4522
Fax: (302) 739-2711

District of Columbia
District of Columbia Board of Nursing
614 H Street, N.W.
Washington, District of Columbia 20001
Phone: (202) 727-7468
Fax: (202) 727-7662
For Examination Information:
Phone: (202) 727-7454

Florida
Florida Board of Nursing
4080 Woodcock Drive, East, Suite 202
Jacksonville, Florida 32207
Phone: (904) 858-6940
Fax: (904) 858-6964

For Examination Information:
Same as above

Georgia–PN
Georgia State Board of Licensed Practical
    Nurses
166 Pryor Street, S.W.
Atlanta, Georgia 30303
Phone: (404) 656-3921
Fax: (404) 651-9532
For Examination Information:
Exam Development & Testing Unit
Phone: (404) 656-3903

Georgia–RN
Georgia Board of Nursing
166 Pryor Street, S.W.
Atlanta, Georgia 30303
Phone: (404) 656-3943
Fax: (404) 651-7489

Guam
Guam Board of Nurse Examiners
P.O. Box 2816
Agana, Guam 96910
Phone: 011-(671) 475-0251
Fax: 011-(671) 477-4733

Hawaii
Hawaii Board of Nursing
P.O. Box 3469
Honolulu, Hawaii 96801
Phone: (808) 586-2695
Fax: (808) 586-2689

Idaho
Idaho Board of Nursing
P.O. Box 83720
Boise, Idaho 83720-0061
Phone: (208) 334-3110
Fax: (208) 334-3262
NCNET: ID NC2022

Illinois
Illinois Department of Professional
    Regulation

320 West Washington Street, 3rd Floor
Springfield, Illinois 62786
Phone: (217) 785-9465
(217) 785-0800
Fax: (217) 782-7645
For Examination Information:
Illinois Department of Professional
  Regulation
100 West Randolph, Suite 9-300
Chicago, Illinois 60601
Phone: (312) 814-2715
Fax: (312) 814-3154
Application Requests
Licensure Information
Assisting Nursing/Acting Coordinator
Phone: (217) 782-0458
(217) 782-8556
(217) 785-9465

Indiana
Indiana State Board of Nursing
Health Professions Bureau
402 West Washington Street, Room 041
Indianapolis, Indiana 46204
Phone: (317) 232-2960
Fax: (317) 233-4236

Iowa
Iowa Board of Nursing
State Capitol Complex
1223 East Court Avenue
Des Moines, Iowa 50319
Phone: (515) 281-3255
Fax: (515) 281-4825

Kansas
Kansas State Board of Nursing
Landon State Office Building
900 S.W. Jackson, Suite 551-S
Topeka, Kansas 66612-1230
Phone: (913) 296-4929
Fax: (913) 296-3929
Departments:
General Information
Continuing Education
Practice or Disciplinary

Phone: (913) 296-4929
(913) 296-3782
(913) 296-4325

Kentucky
Kentucky Board of Nursing
312 Wittington Parkway, Suite 300
Louisville, Kentucky 40222-5172
Phone: (502) 329-7000
Fax: (502) 329-7011

Louisiana–PN
Louisiana State Board of Practical Nurse
  Examiners
3421 N. Causeway Boulevard, Suite 203
Metairie, Louisiana 70002
Phone: (504) 838-5791
Fax: (504) 838-5279

Louisiana–RN
Louisiana State Board of Nursing
3510 N. Causeway Blvd., Suite 501
Metairie, Louisiana 70002
Phone: (504) 838-5332
Fax: (504) 838-5349
NCNET: NCZ018

Maine
Maine State Board of Nursing
24 Stone St.
State House Station #158
Augusta, Maine 04333-0158
Phone: (207) 287-1133
Fax: (207) 287-1149
NCNET: NCZ010

Maryland
Maryland Board of Nursing
4140 Patterson Avenue
Baltimore, Maryland 21215-2299
Phone: (410) 764-5124
Fax: (410) 358-3530

Massachusetts
Massachusetts Board of Registration in
  Nursing

Leverett Saltonstall Building
100 Cambridge Street, Room 1519
Boston, Massachusetts 02202
Phone: (617) 727-9961
Fax: (617) 727-2197

Michigan
Bureau of Occupational and Professional
  Regulation
Michigan Department of Commerce
Ottawa Towers North
611 West Ottawa
Lansing, Michigan 48933
Phone: (517) 373-9102
Fax: (517) 373-2179
For Examination Information:
Office of Testing Services
Michigan Department of Commerce
P.O. Box 30018
Lansing, Michigan 48909
Phone: (517) 373-3877
Fax: (517) 335-6696

Minnesota
Minnesota Board of Nursing
2700 University Avenue, West #108
St. Paul, Minnesota 55114
Phone: (612) 642-0567
Fax: (612) 642-0574

Mississippi
Mississippi Board of Nursing
239 N. Lamar Street, Suite 401
Jackson, Mississippi 39201
Phone: (601) 359-6170
Fax: (601) 359-6185

Missouri
Missouri State Board of Nursing
P.O. Box 656
Jefferson City, Missouri 65102
Phone: (573) 751-0681
Fax: (573) 751-0075
Street Address:
3605 Missouri Blvd.
Jefferson City, Missouri 65109

Montana
Montana State Board of Nursing
111 North Jackson
P.O. Box 200513
Helena, Montana 59620-0513
Phone: (406) 444-2071
Fax: (406) 444-7759
NCNET: NCZ032

Nebraska
Bureau of Examining Boards
Nebraska Department of Health
P.O. Box 94986
Lincoln, Nebraska 68509
Phone: (402) 471-4376
Fax: (402) 471-3577
Street Address:
301 Centennial Mall South
Lincoln, Nebraska 68508

Nevada
Nevada State Board of Nursing
P.O. Box 46886
Las Vegas, Nevada 89114
Phone: (702) 739-1575
Fax: (702) 739-0298
Street Address:
4335 S. Industrial Road, Suite 430
Las Vegas, Nevada 89103
Nevada State Board of Nursing
  (2nd Office)
1755 East Plumb Lane, Suite 260
Reno, Nevada 89502
Phone: (702) 786-2778
Fax: (702) 322-6993

New Hampshire
New Hampshire Board of Nursing
Health & Welfare Building
6 Hazen Drive
Concord, New Hampshire 03301-6527
Phone: (603) 271-2323
Fax: (603) 271-6605

New Jersey
New Jersey Board of Nursing
P.O. Box 45010

Newark, New Jersey 07101
Phone: (201) 504-6586
Fax: (201) 648-3481
Street Address:
124 Halsey Street, 6th Floor
Newark, New Jersey 07102

New Mexico
New Mexico Board of Nursing
4206 Louisiana Blvd., N.E., Suite A
Albuquerque, New Mexico 87109
Phone: (505) 841-8340
Fax: (505) 841-8347

New York
New York State Board of Nursing
State Education Department
Cultural Education Center, Room 3023
Albany, New York 12230
Phone: (518) 474-3843/3845
Fax: (518) 473-0578
For Examination Information:
Division of Professional Licensing Services
State Education Department
Cultural Education Center
Albany, New York 12230
Phone: (518) 474-6591

North Carolina
North Carolina Board of Nursing
P.O. Box 2129
Raleigh, North Carolina 27602
Phone: (919) 782-3211
Fax: (919) 781-9461
NCNET: NCZ014
Street Address:
3724 National Drive
Raleigh, North Carolina 27612

North Dakota
North Dakota Board of Nursing
919 South Seventh Street, Suite 504
Bismarck, North Dakota 58504-5881
Phone: (701) 328-9777
Fax: (701) 328-9785

Northern Mariana Islands
Commonwealth Board of Nurse Examiners
Public Health Center
P.O. Box 1458
Saipan, MP 96950
Phone: (011)-670-234-8950 through 8954
Fax: (011)-670-234-8930
Telex: 783-744
Answer back code: PNESPN744.
When calling, ask for Public Health Center
   (ext. 2018 or 2019)

Ohio
Ohio Board of Nursing
77 South High Street, 17th floor
Columbus, Ohio 43266-0316
Phone: (614) 466-3947
Fax: (614) 466-0388

Oklahoma
Oklahoma Board of Nursing
2915 North Classen Boulevard, Suite 524
Oklahoma City, Oklahoma 73106
Phone: (405) 525-2076
Fax: (405) 521-6089

Oregon
Oregon State Board of Nursing
800 N.E. Oregon Street, Box 25, Suite 465
Portland, Oregon 97232
Phone: (503) 731-4745
Fax: (503) 731-4755

Pennsylvania
Pennsylvania State Board of Nursing
P.O. Box 2649
Harrisburg, Pennsylvania 17105-2649
Phone: (717) 783-7142
Fax: (717) 787-0250
Street Address:
124 Pine Street
Harrisburg, PA 17101
For Examination Program/Contract
   Requirements:
Use same address as Pennsylvania State
   Board of Nursing

Puerto Rico
Commonwealth of Puerto Rico
Board of Nurse Examiners
Call Box 10200
Santurce, Puerto Rico 00908
Phone: (787) 725-8161
(787) 725-7904
Fax: (787) 725-7903

Rhode Island
Rhode Island Board of Nurse Registration
   & Nursing Education
Cannon Health Building
Three Capitol Hill, Room 104
Providence, Rhode Island 02908-5097
Phone: (401) 277-2827
Fax: (401) 277-1272

South Carolina
South Carolina State Board of Nursing
220 Executive Center Drive, Suite 220
Columbia, South Carolina 29210
Phone: (803) 731-1648
Fax: (803) 731-1647
NCNET: NCZ023
Departments:
Legal & Disciplinary Services
Education/Examination/Accounting/
   Computer Services
Phone: (803) 731-1667
Fax: (803) 731-1648

South Dakota
South Dakota Board of Nursing
3307 South Lincoln Avenue
Sioux Falls, South Dakota 57105-5224
Phone: (605) 367-5940
Fax: (605) 367-5945

Tennessee
Tennessee State Board of Nursing
426 Fifth Ave North
1st Floor, Cordell Hull Building
Nashville, Tennessee 37247-1010
Phone: (615) 532-5116
Fax: (615) 741-7899

Texas–RN
Texas Board of Nurse Examiners
P.O. Box 140466
Austin, Texas 78714
Phone: (512) 305-7400
Fax: (512) 305-7401
Street Address:
9101 Burnet Road
Austin, Texas 78758
Departments:
Practice & Compliance
Administration/Education/Examination
Phone: (512) 835-8686
Fax: (512) 835-8650

Texas–VN
Texas Board of Vocational Nurse
   Examiners
William P. Hobby Bldg, Tower 3
333 Guadalupe St, Suite 3-400
Austin, Texas 78758
Phone: (512) 305-8000
Fax: (512) 305-8101

Utah
Utah State Board of Nursing
Division of Occupational and Professional
   Licensing
P.O. Box 45805
Salt Lake City, Utah 84145-0805
Phone: (801) 530-6628
Fax: (801) 530-6511
Street Address:
Heber M. Wells Building, 4th Floor
160 East 300 South
Salt Lake City, Utah 84111

Vermont
Vermont State Board of Nursing
109 State Street
Montpelier, Vermont 05609-1106
Phone: (802) 828-2396
Fax: (802) 828-2484
For Mailing by UPS or FedEx:
81 River Street
Montpelier, Vermont 05602-1106

Virgin Islands
Virgin Islands Board of Nurse Licensure
P.O. Box 4247, Veterans Drive Station
St. Thomas, U.S. Virgin Islands 00803
Phone: (809) 776-7397
Fax: (809) 777-4003
Street Address:
Plot #3, Kongens Gade
St. Thomas, U.S. Virgin Islands 00803

Virginia
Virginia Board of Nursing
6606 West Broad Street, Fourth Floor
Richmond, Virginia 23230-1717
Phone: (804) 662-9909
Fax: (804) 662-9943

Washington
Washington State Nursing Care Quality
    Assurance Commission
Department of Health
P.O. Box 47864
Olympia, Washington 98504-7864
Phone: (360) 753-2686
Fax: (360) 586-5935

West Virginia–RN
West Virginia Board of Examiners for
    Registered Professional Nurses
101 Dee Drive
Charleston, West Virginia 25311-1620
Phone: (304) 558-3596
Fax: (304) 558-3666

West Virginia–PN
West Virginia State Board of Examiners for
    Practical Nurses
101 Dee Drive
Charleston, West Virginia 25311-1688
Phone: (304) 558-3572
Fax: (304) 558-3666
(Please indicate for PN Board)

Wisconsin
Wisconsin Department of Regulation &
    Licensing
1400 East Washington Avenue
P.O. Box 8935
Madison, Wisconsin 53708-3935
Phone: (608) 266-2112
Fax: (608) 267-0644
Tom Neumann, Administrative Officer
For Application Information:
Examinations:
Phone: (608) 266-0070
Endorsement:
Phone: (608) 266-8957

Wyoming
Wyoming State Board of Nursing
2020 Carey Ave, Suite 110
Cheyenne, Wyoming 82002
Phone: (307) 777-7601
Fax: (307) 777-6005

APPENDIX B Specialty Nursing Organizations

Academy of Medical-Surgical Nurses
(AMSN)
North Woodbury Road, Box 56
Pitman, New Jersey 08071
Phone: (609) 589-6677
Fax: (609) 589-7463

American Academy of Ambulatory Care
Nursing (AAACN)
North Woodbury Road, Box 56
Pitman, New Jersey 08071
Phone: (609) 582-9617
Fax: (609) 589-7463

American Association of Critical-Care
Nurses (AACN)
101 Columbia
Aliso Viejo, California 92656-1491
Phone: (800) 899-2226/(714) 362-2000
Fax: (714) 362-2020
http://www.aacn.org

American Association of Diabetes
Educators (AADE)
444 N. Michigan Avenue
Suite 1240
Chicago, Illinois 60611-3901
Phone: (312) 664-2233/(800) 644-2233
Fax: (312) 644-4411

American Association of Neuroscience
Nurses (AANN)
224 N. Des Plaines #601
Chicago, Illinois 60661
Phone: (312) 993-0043
http://www.aann.org

American Association of Nurse
Anesthetists (AANA)
222 South Prospect Avenue

Park Ridge, Illinois 60068-4001
Phone: (708) 692-7050
Fax: (708) 692-6968

American Association of Occupational
Health Nurses (AAOHN)
50 Lenox Pointe
Atlanta, Georgia 30324
Phone: (404) 262-1162
Fax: (404) 262-1165

American Association of Spinal Cord Injury
Nurses (AASCIN)
75-20 Astoria Boulevard
Jackson Heights, New York 11370-1177
Phone: (718) 803-3782
Fax: (718) 803-0414

American College of Nurse-Midwives
(ACNM)
1522 K Street, N.W., Suite 1000
Washington, DC 20005
Phone: (202) 289-0171
Fax: (202) 289-4395
http:www.acnm.org

American Nephrology Nurses Association
(ANNA)
North Woodbury Road, Box 56
Pitman, New Jersey 08071
Phone: (609) 589-2187
Fax: (609) 589-7463
http://www.inurse.com/anna

American Psychiatric Nurses' Association
(APNA)
6900 Grove Road
Thorofare, New Jersey 08086
Phone: (609) 848-7990
Fax: (609) 848-5274

American Society of Ophthalmic Registered
   Nurses, Inc. (ASORN)
655 Beach Street
PO Box 193030
San Francisco, California 94119
Phone: (415) 561-8513
Fax: (415) 561-8575

American Society of Plastic and Recon-
   structive Surgical Nurses, Inc. (ASPRSN)
North Woodbury Road, Box 56
Pitman, New Jersey 08071
Phone: (609) 589-6247
Fax: (609) 589-7463

American Society of Post Anesthesia
   Nurses (ASPAN)
11512 Allecingie Parkway
Richmond, Virginia 23235
Phone: (804) 379-5516
Fax: (804) 379-1386

American Urological Association Allied, Inc.
   (AUAA)
11512 Allecingie Parkway
Richmond, Virginia 23235
Phone: (804) 379-1306
Fax: (804) 379-1386

Association for Practitioners in Infection
   Control (APIC)
505 E. Hawley Street
Mundelein, Illinois 60060
Phone: (708) 949-6052
Fax: (708) 566-7282

Association of Operating Room Nurses, Inc.
   (AORN)
2170 S. Parker Road, #300
Denver, Colorado 80231-5711
Phone: (303) 755-6300
Fax: (303) 750-2927
http://www.aorn.org

Association of Pediatric Oncology Nurses
   (APON)

11512 Allecingie Parkway
Richmond, Virginia 23235
Phone: (804) 379-9150
Fax: (804) 379-1386

Association of Rehabilitation Nurses (ARN)
5700 Old Orchard Road, First Floor
Skokie, Illinois 60077-1057
Phone: (708) 966-3433
Fax: (708) 966-9418
http://www.rehabnurse.org

Association of Women's Health, Obstetric,
   and Neonatal Nurses (AWHONN)
700 14th Street, NW, Suite 600
Washington, District of Columbia 20005-
   2019
Phone: (202) 662-1600
Fax: (202) 737-0575

Dermatology Nurses' Association (DNA)
North Woodbury Road, Box 56
Pitman, New Jersey 08071
Phone: (609) 582-1915
Fax: (609) 589-7463

Emergency Nurses' Association (ENA)
216 Higgins Road
Park Ridge, Illinois 60068-5736
Phone: (708) 698-9400
Fax: (708) 698-9406
http://www.ena.org

International Society of Nurses in Genetics,
   Inc. (ISONG)
University of North Dakota
Department of Pediatrics/Genetics
501 Columbia Road
Grand Forks, North Dakota 58203
Phone: (701) 777-4243

Intravenous Nurses Society, Inc. (INS)
Two Brighton Street
Belmont, Massachusetts 02178
Phone: (617) 489-5205
Fax: (617) 484-6992

National Association of Nurse Massage
 Therapists (NANMT)
6851 Yumuri Street, #8
Coral Gables, Florida 33146
Phone: (305) 667-6821

National Association of Nurse Practitioners
 in Reproductive Health (NANPRH)
2401 Pennsylvania Avenue, NW #350
Washington, DC 20037-1718
Phone: (202) 466-4825
Fax: (202) 466-3826

National Association of Orthopaedic Nurses
 (NAON)
North Woodbury Road, Box 56
Pitman, New Jersey 08071
Phone: (609) 582-0111
Fax: (609) 589-7463

National Association of Pediatric Nurse
 Associates and Practitioners (NAPNAP)
1101 Kings Highway North, Suite 206
Cherry Hill, New Jersey 08034
Phone: (609) 667-1773
Fax: (609) 667-7187

National Association of School Nurses, Inc.
 (NASN)
PO Box 1300
Scarborough, Maine 04070-1300
Phone: (207) 883-2117
Fax: (207) 883-2683

National Flight Nurses Association (NFNA)
6900 Grove Road
Thorofare, New Jersey 08086-9447
Phone: (609) 384-6725
Fax: (609) 848-5274

National Nurses Society on Addictions
 (NNSA)
5700 Old Orchard Road, First Floor
Skokie, Illinois 60077-1057
Phone: (708) 966-5010
Fax: (708) 966-9418

Oncology Nursing Society (ONS)
501 Holiday Drive
Pittsburgh, Pennsylvania 15220-2749
Phone: (412) 921-7373
Fax: (412) 921-6565
http://www.ons.org

Society of Gastroenterology Nurses &
 Associates, Inc. (SGNA)
1070 Sibley Tower
Rochester, New York 14604
Phone: (716) 546-7241
Fax: (716) 546-5141

Society of Otorhinolaryngology and Head-
 Neck Nurses, Inc. (SOHN)
116 Canal Street, Suite A
New Smyrna Beach, Florida 32168-7004
Phone: (904) 428-1695
Fax: (904) 423-7566

Affiliate Members

American Association of Nurse Attorneys
 (TAANA)
720 Light Street
Baltimore, Maryland 21230
Phone: (410) 752-3318
Fax: (410) 752-8295

American Holistic Nurses Association
 (AHNA)
4101 Lake Boone Trail, Suite 201
Raleigh, North Carolina 27607
Phone: (919) 787-5181
Fax: (919) 787-4916
http://ahna.org

National Association of GCRC Nurse
 Managers (NAGCRCNM)
Clinical Research Center
The Center for Health Sciences
27-066 CHS 169747

10833 Le Conte Avenue
Los Angeles, California 90024-169747
Phone: (310) 825-5225
Fax: (310) 206-9440

National Association for Health Care
Recruitment (NAHCR)
PO Box 5769
Akron, Ohio 44372

Phone: (216) 867-3088
Fax: (216) 867-1630

National Student Nurses' Association, Inc.
(NSNA)
555 West 57th Street
New York, New York 10019
Phone: (212) 581-2211
Fax: (212) 581-2368

INDEX

Page numbers followed by b *indicate boxes; page numbers followed by* f *indicate figures; page numbers followed by* t *indicate tables.*

515